Internship Textbook for
General Nursing and Midwifery

Internship Textbook for
General Nursing and Midwifery

As per the INC Syllabus for GNM

THIRD EDITION

I CLEMENT

MSc (N) MSc (Psy) MA (Sociol) MA (Childcare and Edu) PhD (N) PGDHA

Professor and HOD Research and Development
RV College of Nursing, Bengaluru
Former Professor and Principal
Columbia College of Nursing, Bengaluru
VSS College of Nursing, Bengaluru, Karnataka, India

Professional Life Member
PhD Society of India, Chennai, Tamil Nadu
Nursing Research Society of India, New Delhi
Trained Nurses' Association of India, New Delhi
Christian Medical Association of India, New Delhi
Indian Society of Psychiatric Nurses, Bengaluru, Karnataka
Medical Surgical Nursing Society of India, Chennai
Indian Society of Neuroscience Nursing, New Delhi
Asian Association of Cardiac Nurses, Kolkata, West Bengal

Health Organization Member
Indian Red Cross Society
St John's Ambulance Association
General Secretary—Indian Society of Medical Surgical Nurses
Bengaluru, Karnataka, India

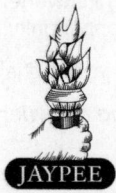

JAYPEE

JAYPEE BROTHERS MEDICAL PUBLISHERS
The Health Sciences Publisher
New Delhi | London

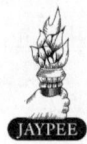

Jaypee Brothers Medical Publishers (P) Ltd

Headquarters

Jaypee Brothers Medical Publishers (P) Ltd
EMCA House, 23/23-B
Ansari Road, Daryaganj
New Delhi 110 002, India
Landline: +91-11-23272143, +91-11-23272703
+91-11-23282021, +91-11-23245672
Email: jaypee@jaypeebrothers.com

Corporate Office

Jaypee Brothers Medical Publishers (P) Ltd
4838/24, Ansari Road, Daryaganj
New Delhi 110 002, India
Phone: +91-11-43574357
Fax: +91-11-43574314
Email: jaypee@jaypeebrothers.com

Overseas Office

J.P. Medical Ltd
83 Victoria Street, London
SW1H 0HW (UK)
Phone: +44 20 3170 8910
Fax: +44 (0)20 3008 6180
Email: info@jpmedpub.com

Website: www.jaypeebrothers.com
Website: www.jaypeedigital.com

© 2022, Jaypee Brothers Medical Publishers

Inquiries for bulk sales may be solicited at: jaypee@jaypeebrothers.com

Internship Textbook for General Nursing and Midwifery

First Edition: 2003

Second Edition: 2018

Third Edition: **2022,** Reprint: 2024, 2025

ISBN: 978-93-5465-939-3

Printed in India at Sterling Graphics Pvt. Ltd.

Dedicated to

Smt KS Geetha
Founder and Chairman
JK College of Nursing and Paramedical
KSG Group of Institutions
Coimbatore, Tamil Nadu, India

Preface to the Third Edition

It gives me immense pleasure to revise the third edition of *Internship Textbook for General Nursing and Midwifery*. Nursing is a challenging profession where every nurse has to be competent enough to handle any crisis situation, after three year course of general nursing. This period fills the gap that is created during the 3 years, obviously there is slight lack of theoretical knowledge with lag in research, trends and issues, hospital administration and management including health economics care taught in internship which really help each general nursing student to withstand in growing technology and manage this work setup. This book is enriched with subjects as per INC standards and will definitely fulfill the need of internship students since all the subjects are filled up in one nutshell.

This text includes:
Section 1: Nursing Education.
Section 2: Nursing Research.
Section 3: Professional Trends and Adjustment.
Section 4: Nursing Administration and Ward Management.

Each chapter is drafted in simple easy English. Students can easily dig on and prepare themselves for their internal exams and score well. This internship period not only nourishes them with practical exposure, but also the theory added in this period really prepares them, moulds them in such a way that creates a knowledge skill which helps them to tackle problems faced as soon as they enter the job. Career opportunities in local and abroad are wide and they prefer general nurses fortified with this kind of knowledge so that they can be a good educator, researcher, administrator, manager, finally a highly qualified professional nurse with knowledge of health economics. I wish all the best to all the teachers, especially students who go through this book.

I Clement

Preface to the First Edition

Internship is a period of 26 weeks/6 months conducted after successfully completing the 3 years of general nursing course. This period fills the gap that is created during the 3 years, obviously there is slight lack of theoretical knowledge with lag in research, trends and issues, hospital administration and management including health economics care taught in internship which really help each general nursing student to withstand in growing technology and manage this work setup.

This book is enriched with subjects as per INC standards and will definitely fulfill the need of internship student since all the subjects are filled up in one nutshell.

This text includes:

Section 1: Educational Methods and Media for Teaching in Practice of Nursing (Chapters 1-3).

Section 2: Nursing Research (Chapters 4-11).

Section 3: Administration and Ward Management (Chapters 12-21).

Section 4: Professional Trends and Adjustments (Chapters 22-26)

Section 5: Health Economics (Chapters 27-35)

Annexure: Practical Guidelines for Clinical Practice.

Each chapter is drafted in simple, easy English. Students can easily dig on and prepare themselves for their internal exams and score well. This internship period not only nourishes them with practical exposure, but also the theory added in this period really prepares them, moulds them in such a way that creates a knowledge skill which helps them to tackle problems faced as soon they enter the job.

Career opportunities in local and abroad are wide and they prefer general nurses fortified with this kind of knowledge so that they can be a good educator, researcher, administrator, manager, finally a highly qualified professional nurse with knowledge of health economics.

I wish all the best for all the teachers, especially students who go through this book.

I Clement

Acknowledgments

I am thankful to the Lord Almighty who strengthens me with His abundant blessings through innumerable means, helping me in all my accomplishments.

My heartfelt thanks to Shri Sommana, Former Minister of Karnataka and Chairman of VSS Group of Institutions for his constant support and encouragement.

My sincere thanks to my guru Dr BT Basavanthappa, Principal, Rajarajeswari College of Nursing, Bengaluru, Karnataka, India, and a great philosopher and internationally renowned teacher of nursing, who helped me in discovering the world of knowledge Professor PV Ramachandran, Chairman, College of Nursing, Sri Ramachandra University, Chennai, Tamil Nadu, India. I am thankful to Ms Shylaja Sommana (Managing Director), Dr BS Naveen, Dr BS Arun and Ms Divya from VSS Group of Institutions, Bengaluru, Karnataka, India, for their support and encouragement.

I am also grateful to Dr BC Bhagavan, Syndicate Member of Rajiv Gandhi University of Health Sciences, Bengaluru, and Professor, Department of Surgery, Kempegowda Institute of Medical Sciences, Bengaluru, Karnataka, India, and Dr Aswathnarayanan MLA, Chairman, Padmashree Group of Institutions, Bengaluru, Karnataka, India.

Special thanks to Dr TV Ramakrishnan, Professor, Department of Anesthesiology and Head of Clinical Services, Department of Accident and Emergency Medicine, Sri Ramachandra University, Chennai, India. Dr Jeyaseelan Manickam Devadassan, Syndicate Member, The Tamil Nadu Dr MGR Medical University, Chennai and Dean, Annai JKK Sampoorani Ammal College of Nursing, Erode, Tamil Nadu, India. Dr Tamilmani, Principal and Mrs Jessie Sudarsanum, Head, Department of Medical Surgical Nursing of Annai JKK Sampoorani Ammal College of Nursing, Erode, Tamil Nadu, India, and all my teachers and students.

I convey my sincere thanks to my beloved parents, brothers and sisters and my wife Nisha Clement for her constant support and encouragement in each step of my life. I take this opportunity to thank my little ones, Cibin, Cynthia and Cavin. I extend thanks to my beloved friend and brother Mr Regi T Kurien.

I am very grateful to the whole team of M/s Jaypee Brothers Medical Publishers (P) Ltd, New Delhi, India, for all their support to work in this project and make it a success. Without their cooperation, I could not have completed this project: Shri Jitendar P Vij (Group Chairman), Mr Ankit Vij (Managing Director), Mr MS Mani (Group President), Dr Madhu Choudhary (Director–Educational Publishing), Ms Pooja Bhandari (Production Head), Ms Sunita Katla (Executive Assistant to Group Chairman and Publishing Manager), Ms Samina Khan (Executive Assistant to Director–Educational Publishing), Ms Jitika Royal (Development Editor), Mr Rajesh Sharma (Production Coordinator), Ms Seema Dogra (Cover Visualizer), Ms Geeta Srivastava (Proofreader), Mr Om Prakash Mishra (Typesetter), Mr Radhe Shyam Singh (Graphic Designer).

Contents

Section 3: Professional Trends and Adjustment

Section 4: Nursing Administration and Ward Management

Placement: Internship (3rd year Part II)　　　　　**Time: 120 Hours**

Nursing Education: 20 hours

Nursing Research: 30 hours

Professional Trends and Adjustment: 30 hours

Nursing Administration and Ward Management: 40 hours

NURSING EDUCATION

Course Description

This course is designed to introduce the students to the concept of teaching as an integral part of nursing practice.

General Objectives

Upon completion of this course, the student shall able to:

1. Explain the concept of teaching
2. Describe techniques used for teaching

Total Hours: 20

Unit	Learning Objectives	Contents	Hr	Teaching-Learning Activities	Method of Assessment
I	Describe the concept of education	**Introduction** a. Education 　－ Meaning, aims, scope and purposes	2	Lecture cum discussion	Short answers Objective type
II	Explain the process of teaching and learning	**Teaching-learning process** a. Basic principles b. Characteristics of teaching and learning c. Teaching responsibility of a nurse d. Preparation of teaching plan	4	Lecture cum discussion	Short answers Objective type Evaluation of teaching plan
III	Narrate the methods of teaching. Describe the clinical teaching methods	**Methods of teaching** a. Methods of teaching b. Clinical teaching methods 　－ Case method 　－ Bedside clinic 　－ Nursing rounds 　－ Nursing conference (individual and group) 　－ Process recording	14	Lecture cum discussion	Short answer Objective type Evaluation of planned as well as incidental health teaching

NURSING RESEARCH

Course Description

This course is designed to develop fundamental abilities and attitude in the student towards scientific methods of investigation and utilization of research finding so as to improve practice of nursing.

General Objectives

Upon completion of this course, the student shall able to:
1. Describe the use of research in the practice of nursing
2. Describe the scientific methods of investigation used in nursing
3. Participate in research activities in the health care settings.

Total Hours: 30

Unit	Learning Objectives	Contents	Hr	Teaching-Learning Activities	Assessment Methods
I	Discuss the importance of research in Nursing	**Introduction** a. Definition b. Terminology related to research c. Need and importance of nursing research d. Characteristics of good research	3	Lecture cum discussion	Short answers Objective type
II	Describe the research process	**Research process** a. Purposes and objectives b. Steps in research process	3	Lecture cum discussion	Short answer Essay type
III	Describe the various research approaches	**Research approaches and designs** a. Types b. Methods c. Advantages and disadvantages	5	Lecture cum discussion	Short answer Essay type
IV	Describe the various data collection methods	**Data collection process** a. Meaning b. Methods and instruments of data collection	5	Lecture cum discussion	Short answer Essay type
V	List the steps involved in data analysis	**Analysis of data** a. Compilation b. Tabulation c. Classification d. Summarization e. Presentation and interpretation of data using descriptive statistic	6	Lecture cum discussion Reading the research articles	Short answer Essay type
VI	Describe the importance of statistics in research	**Introduction to statistics** a. Definition b. Use of statistics c. Scales of measurement d. Frequency distribution e. Mean, median, mode and standard deviation	6	Lecture cum discussion	Short answer Essay type

Unit	Learning Objectives	Contents	Hr	Teaching-Learning Activities	Assessment Methods
VII	Describe the utilization of research in nursing practice	Utilization of research in nursing practice – Evidence-based practice	2	Lecture cum discussion	Short answer Essay type

PROFESSIONAL TRENDS AND ADJUSTMENT

Course Description

This course is designed to help students develop an understanding of the career opportunities available for professional development.

General Objectives

Upon completion of this course, the student shall able to:
1. Describe nursing as a profession
2. Identify various professional responsibilities of a nurse
3. Describe various professional organizations related to nursing
4. Identify the need for in-service and continuing education in nursing
5. Demonstration skills in application of knowledge of professional etiquettes in the practice of nursing in any healthcare setting.

Total Hours: 30

Unit	Learning Objectives	Contents	Hr	Teaching-Learning Activities	Assessment Methods
I	Describe nursing as a profession	**Nursing as a profession** a. Definition of profession b. Criteria of a profession and nursing profession c. Evolution of nursing profession in India d. Educational preparation of a professional nurse e. Qualities/Characteristics and role of a professional nurse	4	Lecture cum discussion	Short answer Objective type Essay type
II	Explain various aspects of professional ethics	**Professional ethics** a. Meaning and relationship of professional ethics and etiquettes b. Code of ethics for nurse by ICN c. Standards for nursing practice (INC) d. Etiquettes for employment: locating posting, applying and accepting a position, resignation from a position	6	lecture cum discussion Assignment: Application for job acceptance and job resignation	Short answer Essay type

Unit	Learning Objectives	Contents	Hr	Teaching-Learning Activities	Assessment Methods
III	Discuss the importance of continuing education in personal and professional development	**Personal and professional development** a. Continuing education – Meaning and importance – Scope – Identifying opportunities b. Career in nursing – Opportunities available in nursing in hospital, community teaching and other related special organization c. In-service education – Definition – Value – Need participation in committee procedures – Nursing in the future	10	Lecture cum discussion Draw a career ladder in nursing in reference to international influence and financial aid	Short answer Essay type
IV	Discuss the significance of legislation in nursing	**Legislation in nursing** a. Purpose and importance of laws in nursing b. Legal terms c. Common legal hazards in nursing d. Laws and regulations related to healthcare providers in India at different levels e. Service and institutional rules f. Regulation of nursing education g. Registration and reciprocities	5	Lecture cum discussion	Assignment
V	List the various organizations related to health and nursing profession and briefly describe their function	**Profession and related organizations** a. Regulatory bodies: Indian Nursing Council, State Nursing Council b. Professional organizations: – Trained Nurses Association of India – Students Nurses Association – Nurses league of the Christian Medical Association of India – International Council of Nurses (ICN) – International Confederation of Midwives, etc.	5	Lecture cum discussion Observational visits to State Nursing Council and Local TNAI office	Report of visit to the council Short answers Essay type

Unit	Learning Objectives	Contents	Hr	Teaching-Learning Activities	Assessment Methods
		c. Related organization and their contribution to nursing: World Health Organization, Red cross and St. john's Ambulance, Colombo plan, UNICEF, World Bank, etc.			

NURSING ADMINISTRATION AND WARD MANAGEMENT

Course Description
This course is designed to help the student to understand the basic principles of administration and its application to the management of ward and health care unit.

General Objectives
Upon completion of this course, the student shall able to:
1. Describe the meaning and principles of administration
2. Apply the principles of administration in practice of nursing
3. Plan the nursing service in the ward and community health settings
4. Describe the importance of good administration in the day to day nursing service in varied health care setting

Total Hours: 40

Unit	Learning Objectives	Contents	Hr	Teaching-Learning Activities	Assessment Methods
I	Describe the meaning, philosophy and principles of administration	**Introduction** a. Administration and management – Meaning – Philosophy – Elements and principles – Significance	4	Lecture cum discussion	Short answers Objective type Essay type
II	Describe the management process	**Management process** a. Planning – Importance – Purpose – Types of planning b. Organization – Principles of organization – Organization chart of hospital/ward/PHC/Sub center c. Staffing – Scheduling – Recruitment, selection, deployment, retaining, promotion, superannuation – Personnel management	15	Lecture cum discussion Companion of organization charts	Short answers Essay type Objective type Written test Evaluation of the organization chart prepared by students

Unit	Learning Objectives	Contents	Hr	Teaching-Learning Activities	Assessment Methods
		– Job description – Job specification – Staff development and staff welfare d. Directing e. Coordination and control – Quality management f. Budgeting g. Policies of hospital and various department of the hospital			
III	Explain the administration of different health care units	**Administration of hospital/ department/unit/ward** a. Health center/unit physical layout b. Safety measures for prevention of accidents and infections c. Legal responsibilities of a nurse d. Leadership styles e. Problem solving: process and approach, steps and methods of dealing with complaints of patients and other health team members f. Records and reports: meaning, types, importance	9	Lecture cum discussion Role play Group work on physical layout Reading notes	Short answers Objective type Essay type
IV	Discuss the importance of maintaining supplies and equipment for effective administration	**Management of equipment supplies** a. Maintenance of supplies and equipment (preventive maintenance) b. Handing over and taking over of inventory c. Indent and ordering of supplies and equipment d. Problem solving: process and approach, steps and methods of dealing with supplies and equipment	7	Lecture cum discussion Role play Group project on problem solving	Short answers Objectives type Essay type Evaluation of the report on Group project
V	Discuss the cost and financing of health services in India	**Cost and financing of health care** a. Cost of health care b. Health financing c. National health plans (annual and five year plans) and outlays, role of state and central government in allocation of funds d. Health insurance–types, issues etc	5	Lecture cum discussion	Short answer Test

1
SECTION

Nursing Education

TERMINOLOGY

Education: Education is the manifestation of divine perfection already existing in man.

Teaching: It is an active process in which one person shares information with others to provide them with the information to make behavioral changes.

Learning: It is the process of assimilating information with a resultant change in behavior.

Teaching-learning process: It is a planned interaction that promotes behavioral change that is not a result of maturation or coincidence.

Andragogy: It is the art and science of helping adults learn.

Idealism: Idealism idolizes mind and self. Idealism believes in universal mind. Idealism regards man as a spiritual being. The world of ideas and values are more important than the world of matter. Real knowledge is perceived in mind.

Naturalism: Naturalism believes that education should be according to the nature of the child. Naturalism advocates the creation of conditions in which the natural development of a child can take place in a natural way.

Pragmatism: The term pragmatism derives its origin from a Greek word meaning to do, to make, to accomplish. Experience is central here; everything is tested on the touchstone of experience.

Existentialism: According to existentialists, the primary aims of education is the making of a human person as one who lives and make decisions about what the learners will do and be.

It is an attitude and outlook that stress human existence that is the distinctive qualities of individual persons rather than man in abstract on nature and the world in general

Realism: Realism is concerned with the study of the world we live in realism believes that all knowledge is derived from experience. The realist believes that everything that exists in the universe is matter or energy or matter of motion.

Humanism: Humanism is a movement to gain for man a proper recognition in the universe. Man is a free agent.

Humanistic existentialism: Humanistic existentialism is the youngest philosophy. Existentialism may be described as a modern philosophy which is primarily build upon the work of the scholars of the twentieth century.

Experimentalism: Experimentalism is unreservedly a philosophy of change and of process. It teaches that everything is changing continually—man, morality, democracy and education; experience is the only reality.

Neorealism: Neorealism is a theory which excludes philosophy and theology as source of knowledge and truth; it looks to science as its primary source.

Eclectic tendency in education: It is a process of putting together the common view of different philosophies, into one comprehensive whole is eclectic tendency in education. It is the fusion or synthesis of different philosophies of education, is known as eclectic tendency in education.

Progressivism: The term progressivism in education is an American philosophy, which is a revolt against the formal, conventional and traditional system of education.

Reconstructionism: Reconstructionism has its origin in Plato; his republic is his vision of an ideal society. Reconstruction is of two forms; total change or desirable change.

Eclecticism: The dictionary meaning of the word eclectic means selecting or borrowing the best out of everything. According to eclectic tendency in education, modern education wants to synthesis the brief form of all the past movements into new structure.

Perennialism: Perennialism is a very constructive and inflexible philosophy of education. It is based on the view that reality comes from fundamental fixed truths, especially related to god.

Lecture: The lecture is a teaching procedure consisting of clarification or the explanation of facts, principles or relationships, which the teacher wishes the class to understand.

Demonstration: Demonstration is a method of teaching by exhibition and explanation combined to illustrate a procedure or experience. Demonstration can be divided into 3 phases namely the planning and preparation phase, performance phase and evaluation phase.

Group discussion: Group discussion is a cooperative; problem solving activity seeks a consensus regarding the solution of a problem. Discussion may formal or informal. Discussion method is commonly used for teaching selected topics and to enrich lectures, observation visits and case presentation.

Seminar: Seminar can be classified into four types namely: mini seminar, main seminar, national seminar and international seminar.

Symposium: Symposium is the most preferred method to discuss controversial issues such as professional status of nursing, impact of consumer protection act on nursing and like.

Panel discussion: The panel discussion method is a discussion in which a few persons carry on a conversation in front of an audience. This method is used when the group is too large to work effectively through the usual round-table procedure.

Role play: Role playing is a form of drama in which learners spontaneously act out roles in an interaction involving problems or challenges in human relations for subsequent discussion by the whole.

Project method: Project is a whole-hearted purposeful activity proceeding in a social environment. Also a project is a problematic act carried to completion in its natural setting. Project method gives an opportunity for self-expression; it gives an opportunity for relating the self to the community.

Field method: It is one of the natural methods of teaching, in which the student studies first hand objects and materials in their natural environment field trip correlate and blend school life with the outside world, providing direct touch with person and with community situations.

Workshop: The term workshop which is using in education, refers to a group of individuals who work together the solution of problems in a given subject matter field during a specific period of time.

Programmed instructions: The programmed instruction is a process of arranging material to be learned in a series of small steps designed to lead a learner through self-instruction from what he knows to the unknown of new and more complex knowledge and principles.

Computer assisted learning: Computer assisted instruction is a method of instruction in which there is a purposeful interaction between a learner and the computer device (having useful instructional material as software) for helping the individual learner achieve the desired instructional objectives with his own pace and abilities command.

Exhibition: Exhibitions are familiar items in our environment to day. When we go round an exhibition, our attention is often focused on a group of objects and materials that are displayed according to a deliberate plan.

Micro-teaching: Micro-teaching as a scaled down teaching encountered in class size and class time. The number of students is from 5-10 and the duration of period rangers from 5-20 minutes. A training procedure aimed at simplifying the complexities of regular teaching process.

Simulation: Simulation is a teaching technique used particularly in management education and training in which a real life situation and values are simulated be substitute displaying similar characteristics.

Case method: Nursing case study is one of the common and useful methods of teaching in clinical area. It is a form of qualitative and quantitative analysis involving a very careful and complete observation of a patient and his situation.

Nursing rounds: Nursing rounds are conducted by the head nurse/nursing teacher for the members of her staff/student. To be successful every nurse must be prepared to participate in the discussion of nursing care.

Bedside clinic: Bedside clinic is an organized clinical instruction in the presence of the patient. Based on the topic, it can be medical, nursing or combined. Bedside clinic is a method of clinical teaching. It always entails the presence of the patient.

Individual and group conference: Individual conference means, it is a clinical teaching method which focuses on the overall development of the individual student with special emphasis to the development of clinical skills.

Process recording: Process recording is a verbatim account of a visit for purposes of bringing out the interplay between nurses and the patient in relation to the objects of the visit.

1
CHAPTER

Introduction to Education

INTRODUCTION

The word education derived from the Latin word educare which means to lead out. The root meaning of education can be given as making manifest the inherent potentials in child. The idea of education is not merely to impart knowledge to the pupil in some subjects but to develop in him those habits and attitudes with which may successfully face the future. Education is the process of helping the child to adjust with this changing world. By means of education the child is subjected to certain experiences that are intended to modify his behavior in order to bring about proper adjustment with the changing environment. In fact, education is the basis of life. For leading a purposeful and ideal life is needed.

DEFINITION

The concepts of education as given by prominent Indian educationist are as follows:

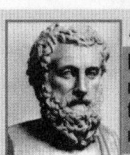

Aristotle

Education is the process of training man to fulfill his aim by exercising all the faculties to the fullest extent as a member of society

Fig. 1.1: Aristotle.

- *Rigveda:* 'Education is something which makes man self-reliant and selfless.
- *Upanishad:* 'Education is that whose end product is salvation.'
- *Bhagavad Gita:* 'Nothing is more purifying on earth than wisdom.'
- *Shankaracharya:* 'Education is the realization of self.'
- *Kautilya:* 'Education means training of the country and love of the nations.' 6. Panini: 'Human education means the training which one gets from nature.'
- *Gandhi ji:* 'By education, I mean all round drawing out the best in a child and man by body, mind and spirit.'
- *Swami Vivekananda:* 'Education is the manifestation of the device perfection, already existing in man.
- *Rabindranath Tagore:* 'Education is that which makes one's life in harmony with all existences.'

Concepts of 'Education' as Defined by Western Philosophers:

- *Socrates:* 'Education means the bringing out of the ideas of universal validity which are latent in the mind of every man.'
- *Plato:* 'Education is the capacity to feel pleasure and pain at the right moment. In develops in the body and in the soul of the

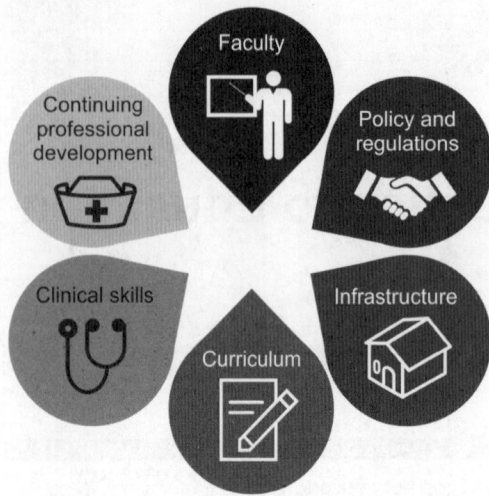

Fig. 1.2: Application of education in nursing.

integration, for delight, for leisure, for an obscure enjoyment, for ornament and for vocation. Education is for culture, for respecting human values, for refinement and sophisticate in characterization, for bringing up the posterity in a knowledgeable manner, for material prosperity, for employment, for building up a healthy society, for understanding human right, human duties and human dignity, for inculcating discipline, for quelling the savage and brutish qualities in the human being, for complete living so on and so forth are the main tenets of education, to name but a few. Education emancipates the human beings from oddities and infirmities. It is also a process of self-realization hind emancipation.

pupil all the beauty and all the perfection which he is capable of.'

- *Aristotle:* 'Education is the creation of a sound mind in a sound body.'
- *Rousseau:* 'Education of man comments at his birth; before he can speak, before he can understand he in already instructed.'
- *Herbert Spencer:* 'Education is complete living.
- *Pestalozzi:* 'Education is the natural, harmonious and progressive development of man's innate powers.'
- *Froebel:* 'Education is leading out of hidden power of man.'
- *UNESCO:* 'Education includes all the process that develops human ability and behavior.

CONCEPT OF EDUCATION

Education is for knowledge and know-how, for the development of esthetic and ethical skills, for artistic and intellectual creativity, for artistic and moral development, for self-discovery, for pursuit in search the truth, for intellectuality, for social equality and social efficiency, for ability, for emancipation and eternal happiness, for integrated growth and international understanding, for good citizenship, for democracy, for national

MEANING OF EDUCATION

- Education modifies the behavior. It brings such changes in the behavior of a child which is for his good. In the past, the education of a child meant the filling up of the child's mind with stuffed knowledge.
- The modern education aims at the harmonious development of the personality of the child. The schools and the teachers are to create such situation where the personality can be developed freely and fully.
- Education is a social process; its main concern is the modification of behavior. Thus educational psychology studies the human behavior as it is influenced by the social process of education.

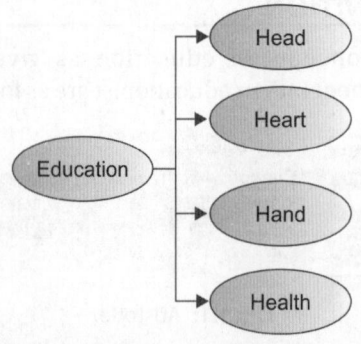

Fig. 1.3: Modern concept of education.

- It also studies and investigates those processes that lead to the understanding of the way in which behavior is modified through education.

PURPOSE OF EDUCATION

- Formation of healthy social and/or formal relationships among and between students, teachers and others.
- Capacity/ability to evaluate information and to predict future outcomes.
- Development of mental and physical skill: Motor, thinking, communication, social and Aesthetic
- Capacity/ability to earn a living: Career education
- Capacity/ability to be a good citizen.
- Cultural communication: Art, music and humanities.
- Acquisition/clarification of values related to the physical environment.
- self-realization/self-reflection: Awareness of one's abilities and goals.
- Capacity/ability to seek out alternative solution and evaluate them.
- Knowledge of moral practices and ethical standards acceptable by society/culture.
- Respect: Giving and receiving reorganization as human being.
- Capacity/ability to live a fulfilling life.
- Sense of well-being: Mental and physical health.
- Capacity/ability to think creativity.
- Understanding of human relations and motivations.
- Acquisition/clarification of personal values.
- Self-esteem/self-efficacy.

NATURE OF EDUCATION

- **Educational aims are not fixed for all times:** Education is not a single aim of activity. It has many aims. It is not limited to a particular stage of individual life. It is for different stages and for different levels. When educational aims are formulated, the educators should consider the unique

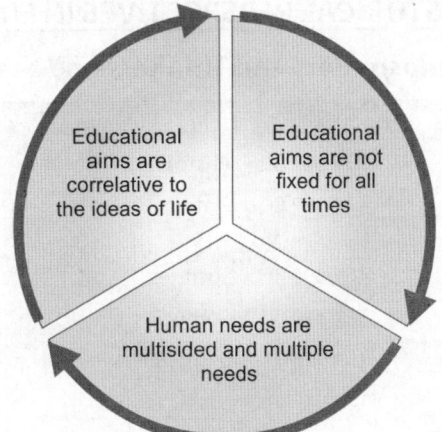

Fig. 1.4: Nature of education.

needs, characteristics and the level of mental development of individual child. For example, the aims of education for primary stage are not the same as that of the secondary or university stage.

- **Human needs are multi-sided and multiple needs:** Single aim of education cannot meet the requirements of the multilateral nature of man. For example, the teacher cannot attend to the body ignoring mind and spirit. Similarly we cannot afford to give training for a profession which ignores morality. He should follow an educational programme which can meet the multiple needs of the child.

- **Educational aims are correlative to the ideas of life:** The ideas of life change from time to time and country to country according to the changes in political, social, economic and physical conditions. So educational aims are also change according to the different schools of philosophies, religious, social, and scientific influences. It is clearly stated in the report of secondary education commission that, as political, social and economic conditions change and new problems arise. It becomes necessary to re-examine carefully and re-state clearly the objectives which education at each stage should keep in view.

HISTORICAL PERSPECTIVES IN EDUCATION

Philosophers and Thinkers and their Views

Sl. No.	Year	Philosopher	Views
1.	384-322 BC	Aristotle	Creation of a sound mind in a sound body
2.	427-347 BC	Plato	Developing the body and the soul of all the perfections which they are capable of
3.	469-399 BC	Socrates	Dispelling error and discovering truth
4.	551-478 BC	Confucius	Development of the whole man
5.	1592-1670	Comenius, John Amos	Development of the whole man
6.	1632-1704	Locke, John	Attainment of a sound mind in a sound body
7.	1672-1719	Joseph Addison	Believed, what Sculpture is to a block of marble, education is to a human being
8.	1746-1827	Pestalozzi JH	Natural, harmonious and progressive development of man's innate powers
9.	1776-1841	Herbart, Johann Friedrich	Developing morality
10.	1782-1852	Fröbel, Friedrich	Leading and guiding for peace and unity with god
11.	1872-1950	Aurobindo Sir	Building of human mind and spirit
12.	1824-1883	Dayananda Swami	Formation of character
13.	1859-1952	Dewey, John	Increasing social efficiency
14.	1803-1882	Emerson, Ralph Waldo	Controlling the mind
15.	1820-1903	Spencer, Herbert	Preparing for complete living
16.	1861- 1941	Tagore, Ravindranath	Making life in harmony with existence
17.	1863-1902	Vivekananda Swami	Manifestation of divine perfection already existing in man
18.	1869-1948	Gandhi MK	An all round drawing out of the best in the child and man-body, mind and spirit
19.	1870-1952	Montessori, Maria	Helping in the complete unfolding of the child's individuality
20.	1888-1975	Radha Krishnan, Sarvepalli	Training the intellect, refinement of the heart and discipline of the spirit

EDUCATION IN ANCIENT INDIA

Vedas, Aranyakas and the *Upanishads* give us the glimpses of the values and ideals of learning and educational system during the ancient period. When we go through these texts, one thing which comes to our mind, is the teacher who was worthy of highest reverence next only to one's parents. System was to lay great emphasis on acquisition of knowledge, discipline of the mind and body.

The father was considered as the first teacher and the home as the first school. Vidyarambha (starting of education) was an important ceremony to initiate the primary education.

Education was always started with keeping in mind the auspicious day in the

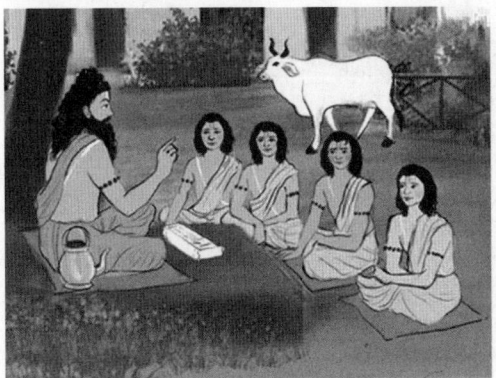

Fig. 1.5: Gurukul-Ancient Education System.

fifth year, i.e., akhsharamba. The next step was Upanayana a ceremony to mark the beginning of upper three classes. It was assumed as the second birth, i.e., dhviaja. A person achieves spiritual and cultural re-birth through a life of learning, austerity, discipline of body and mind through brahmacharya. According to thinkers in ancient India, Vidya or knowledge or learning or education was considered the third eye of man, which gives him an insight into all affaires and teaches him how to act; it leads us to our salvation: in the mundane sphere, it leads us to all round progress and prosperity. The concept of education is like a diamond which appears to be of different colors (nature) when seen from different angles-points of view or philosophy of life.

CHARACTERISTICS OF EDUCATION

General Characteristics

- It is a sociological process.
- It is a psychological process
- It is not only training of the intellect.
- It has to be compared both in formal and informal way.
- It is developing of knowledge, skill and attitude.
- It is a bipolar and in-polar process.
- It is a lifelong process.
- It is a child centered process.
- It is more than teaching and instruction.
- It is more than giving information.

Chief Characteristics of Education

- Education is a bipolar as well as tripolar process.
- Education is a child-centered process.
- Education is a psychological process.
- Education is not literacy.
- Education is a sociological process.
- Education is a life-long process.
- Education is more than instruction and teaching.
- Education is a deliberate as well as informal process.
- Education is more than giving information's.
- Education is developing knowledge, skills and attitudes.

GENESIS OF MODERN TEACHING AND ITS PIONEERS

Sl. No.	Year	Philosopher	Views
1.	1515-1568	Roger Ascham	An English Scholar and Author. He worked treatise an education. The school master in which he talked about the relation between teacher and pupil, the nature of children, the teaching of grammar, the development of morals and the selection of those who can become scholars
2.	1531-1611	Richard Mulcaster	An English scholar. He believed in the principle of individual differences and the principle of readiness. His revolutionary idea was regarding teacher's training
3.	1533-1592	Montaigne	French essayist and scholar. He set down his views in his two essays, on the education of children and on pedantry. He said this great world is true mirror wherein we must look in order to know ourselves as we should

Contd...

Contd...

Sl. No.	Year	Philosopher	Views
4.	1561-1626	Bacon, Francis	English philosopher, he would like the man to be the architect of his own success. He pleaded for the liberal education
5.	1592-1670	Comenius, John Amos	Czechoslovian educationist, textbook writer a pioneer of modern educational sciences. He believed in the process of natural growth of the child
6.	1596-1650	Descartes, Rene	French mathematician and philosopher. He penned his views in his Le Monde (The world). He advanced the revolutionary theory that the earth was in motion
7.	1632-1704)	Lock, John	English philosopher. In an essay concerning human understanding, he was concerned primarily with the question of how the mind acquires knowledge and he emphatically
8.	1712-1778	Rousseau, Jean-Jacques	Swiss educational reformer. True education, he said, is simply the development of the original nature of man. Therefore he stressed that child should be treated as a child a taught according to his nature
9.	1723-1790	Basedow, Johann Bernhard	Swiss educator. He was of the view that all education should be by means of play, pleasant and entertaining. Games were devised for teaching the languages and to develop motor control
10.	1746-1827	Pestalozzi, Johann Heinrich	Swiss educator. He named his direct method of acquiring knowledge as Anschauung which stands for direct knowledge acquired by the pupils own experience
11.	1776-1841	Herbart, Johann, Friedrich	German educator and philosopher. He is best known for his formal steps of lesson planning. He wrote several books-relation of school to life, encyclopedia of philosophy
12.	1782-1852	Fröbel, Friedrich, Wilhelm August	German educator and founder of the kinder garden method
13.	1803-1882	Emerson, Ralph Waldo	American educator, moralist. Essayist and poet. The drill and discipline, Emerson whished, should be made parts of a process which arouses the child to exercise his natural vigour
14.	1820-1903	Spencer, Herbart	English educator and philosopher. He recorded some important maxims of teaching- from simple to complex, from known to unknown from concrete to abstract, etc.
15.	1857-1911	Binet, Alfred	French experimental psychologist. He is noted for Binet-Simson scale. Regarding the proper foundation of pedagogy he said believe that the determination of aptitudes of children is the greatest business of instruction and education
16.	1859-1952	Dewey, John	American educators, philosopher and writer. He is best known for his pragmatic philosophy which has been variously termed as experimentalism, instrumentalism, and operationalism or functional

Contd...

Contd...

Sl. No.	Year	Philosopher	Views
17.	1861-1941	Tagore, Rabindranath	Indian poet and educational practitioner. The traditional school to him was more like a pigeon holed box than a human habitation. His publication a poet's school shows the place of nature in life and education. He established his famous school Santiniketan on the model of ancient ashrams in sylvan surroundings
18.	1861-1947	Whitehead, Alfred North	American educator. He wrote do not teach too many subjects. What you teach thoroughly
19.	1869-1948	Gandhi MK	Indian freedom fighter, patriot, philosopher, statesman, educator and originator of basic system of education which has dealt with separately
20.	1870-1948	Montessori, Maria	Italian educator known for her Montessori method which is discussed separately
21.	1871-1965	Kilpatrick, William Heard	American educator. He promoted the concept of the project method
22.	1880-1968	Keller, Helen Adams	A pioneer in the education of the deaf
23.	1872-1950	Aurobindo, Sir	Indian philosopher, sage and educator. He wrote every child is an inquirer, an investigator, and analyzer. The chief aim of teaching should be to help the growing soul to draw out
24.	1976-1925	Lane, Homer Tyrrel	British educator. He was a firm believer in self-government in educational institutions and for caring out his ideas into practice; he started the little commonwealth a reformatory school in 1912
25.	1887-1937	Parkhurst, Helen	Originator of the famos Dalton planner Contract plan, based on three principles of freedom, cooperation and budgeting the time
26.	1918-1970	Sukhomlinsky Vasily	Russian educator. He analyzed collective influences among their children. His most important publication is To Children I Give My Heart

Independent India

Sl. No.	Year	Philosopher	Views
1.	1948	Dr Radhakrishnan	University Education Commission of 1948, Dr Radhakrishnan was the chairman of this commission
2.	1952-53	Dr Mudaliar	Secondary Education Commission of 1952-53, Dr Mudaliar was the chairman
3.	1964-66	AS Kothari	Kothari education committee of 1964-1966, chairman was AS Kothari

TYPES OF EDUCATION

- **Formal:** It is pre-planned, direct, organized and given in specific educational institution such as schools and colleges. It is limited to a specific period and it has well-defined curriculum. It is given by qualified and trained teacher. Formal

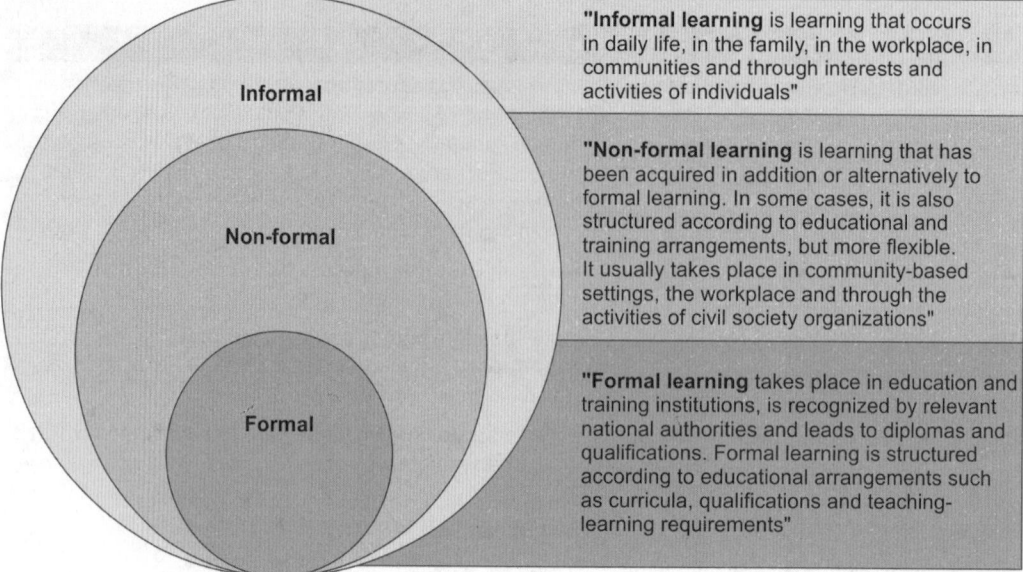

Fig. 1.6: Types of education.

education observes strict discipline; it also includes any types of vocational or general education imparted by teacher or the mother at home or by the teacher in or outside the school. While the church or temple tries to inculcate standards of values and modes of good behavior conscious by, the state makes laws to determine the conduct of its citizens.

- **Informal education:** It is not planned. It is the type of education which the child gets while moving and living in the community with other persons. He/She picks up the ways and habits of the adult member of his community and tries to adopt them. Informal education is indirect, incidental and spontaneous. There are no specific agencies or institutions like schools to impart this type of education. There is no prescribed time table or curriculum and no formal ends or goals or objective. Informal education does not need to have qualified or trained teachers and no examinations according of curriculum.
- **Nonformal education:** It falls within the formal and informal education. Nonformal education is intentional incidental and given outside the formal system, i.e.,

school. It is consciously deliberately planned, organized and systematically implemented.

AIMS AND OBJECTIVES OF EDUCATION

The aim of education as visualized by Rabindranath Tagore is "Enabling the mind to find out that ultimate truth which emancipates us from the bondage of dust and gives the wealth not of things but of inner light, not of power, but of love, making thus its own and giving expression to it. With the advent of modern civilization, there appears to be erosion in the moral values. With a view to surmount this irreparable loss, education should serve as a catalyst in bringing the equilibrium. It is at this juncture the assiduous efforts of the teacher for value based education is mostly a planned and purposeful activity it must have clear aims and objectives, in view. An aim is predetermined goal which inspires the individual to attain it through appropriate activities. Similarly without an end or objective no purposeful activity will have the real force which directs it, and makes it meaningful.

Sl. No.	Topics	Description
1.	Need for the aims	• Education is a purposeful and organized activity which deliberately endeavors to **modify the behavior** of educed. • Acting with an aim is all one with acting intelligently. The aim makes us act with a meaning. • The aims help us to measure our success and failures. • The aim of education, keep both the teacher and the taught on the right track.
2.	Factors determine	• **Philosophy:** Philosophy determines the aims of education. • **Elements of human nature** are always considered for the determination of educational aims. • **Religious factors:** Buddhism emphasized the inculcation of the ideals of that religion. • **Political ideologies:** The educational aims of a democratic political system can be quite different from that of an autocratic political setup. • **Socioeconomic factors** and problems of a country. • **Cultural factors:** Socio-cultural heritage of a country have a great influence on the aims of education. • **Exploration of knowledge:** Education today is science-oriented and technology based. It has to aim at exploring new information.
3.	Educational aims in relation to time and space	Educational aims cannot be fixed for all times all places. • Education is not a single-aim activity. • Human nature is multisided with multiple needs. • Educational aims are correlated to ideals of life. • The different types of education, such as general, technical, nursing, medical, commercial, etc., have separated aims for themselves.
4.	Individual aims of education	Education should aim at the training and development of the individual. The individual aim of education is stressed on the following grounds, i.e., biological, naturalists, psychological, spiritual and progressive. • **Biological:** Every child that comes to this world is a new and a unique product and a new experiment with life. The biologist believes that every individual is different from others. • **Naturalistic standpoint:** According to the naturalist, the central aim of education is the autonomous development of the individual. It is therefore, that education should be according to nature which would make an individual what he ought to be. • **Psychological standpoint:** The psychologists are of the opinion that education is an individual process. No two children are identical in intellectual capacity and emotional disposition. • **Spiritual or moral standpoint:** Since spiritual development of man is individual, the man function of education should be leaded the individual to self-realization and the realization of higher values in life. • **Progressive standpoint:** The progressivist is of the opinion that the progress and advancement of mankind is due to great individuals, born in different periods of history. They include great scientist, inventors, explorer, religious leaders, social reformers, philosophers and the like.
5.	Social aims of education	Individuality is of no value and personality a meaningless term apart from the social environment in which they are developed and made manifest. • **State socialism:** The state has the right to mould and shape the individual so as to suit its purposes and progress. It uses education as the most convenient means for preparing individuals to play different roles in society.

Contd...

Contd...

Sl. No.	Topics	Description
		• **Willing obedience to authority:** Social aims in their extreme form tell us that state is an idealized metaphysical entity over and above the individual citizen superior to him in every way, transcending him in all his desires and aspirations. • **Social aim of education:** Historical evidence: – Ancient Sparta where each man was born for himself but for his country, having not a wish but for country, affords a perfect example. – Modern Germany also before Second World War had a fanatical belief in the absolute value of the state and educational system there, like that of sparta, was merely material. – Roman Catholic doctrine also affords such an example. The slogan of extreme social aim has been everything of the state, for the state and by the state. • The social aim of education is interpreted as education for social service or education for citizenship. – Society is considered to be efficient only when it is physically strong, intellectually enlightened, economically self-sufficient and morally high. – It is only such individuals can contribute richly toward the welfare of that society. In democratic countries, therefore education aims at developing socially-efficient individuals who are ready to sacrifice their own desires if their satisfaction is harmful to others or if does not contribute to social progress. – John Dewey says, in the democratic and technological environment, the aim of education should be to enable the individual to control his environment and fulfill his possibilities.
6.	Specific aims of education	• **Vocational development:** – It makes one economically self-sufficient. – Vocational aim purpose to educational activity. – Vocational education is the only hope of children with lower intelligence. – Vocational education is essential for bridging the gap in society. • **Cultural aim:** Human race has a rich heritage in the form of traditions, manner and customs which is called culture. It is to be conserved and transmitted to the raising generalization through the agency of education, which is both a conservative and a dynamic force. • **Spiritual aim:** ancient Indian educators defined education as a means for salvation. The idealist proclaims that the only aim of education is to develop the spiritual side of an individual. • **Moral aim:** Mahatma Gandhi, the embodiment of morality says, education of heart, or moral education is the prime most function of education to provide. If it is to be worthy of its name.
7.	Aims of education in independent India	The Secondary Education Commission of 1952 (Mudaliar commission) suggested the following aims of education in free India. • Democratic citizenship-clear thinking, speech, writing for growth of nation. • Development of personality- all round development. • Development of leadership- should train the youth. • Vocational efficiency- creates a new attitude towards work. • Initiating students to the art of living- learn the art of harmonious living. The Kothari Education Commission of 1964-66 proposed some more aim of education in India. • Education for increased productivity-production of man power.

Contd...

Contd...

Sl. No.	Topics	Description
		• Social and national integration-inculcate the feeling of oneness and belongingness. • Education for modernization-update scientific and technological advancement. • Education for social, moral and spiritual values-the curriculum should include instruction in these subjects.
8.	Aims of nursing education in India	Nursing education has its aims in common with the aims of education in general as well as its specific aims. • Nursing manpower development-well qualified professions. • Knowledge aim-impart scientific and up-to-date knowledge. • Leadership aim-preparation of nurses as good leader. • Professional development aim- ethics and standards • Personality development aim- all round development. • Nursing research-scientific investigation is essential. • Democratic citizenship- responsible and contributing citizen of the country.

Importance of Aims of Education

- Education is purposeful, useful and planned activity.
- It is undertaken by the educator (teacher) and the educed (child) to achieve the clear cut aims of life.
- Without aims purposeful activity cannot be achieved. Absence of aims makes the activity haphazard, confused and chaotic.
- Without aims neither an individual nor an institution can realize the potentialities of education.

Advantages of Aims of Education

- An aim of education directs the child to accomplish the goals of life.
- It gives fore-sight to the education for effective planning.
- It stimulates both teacher and taught to know what the out-come will be before the completion of an activity.
- It makes the individual child to act with meaning and intelligence.
- It keeps both the teacher and taught on right path.

PRINCIPLES OF EDUCATION

As teaching and learning are the main part of education, these principles appropriately shall guide the students in future.

- Develop independent and interdependent lifelong learning strategies.
- Nurture the aspirations like confidence, curiosity, imagination, self-respect and responsibility for others.
- Explore and adapt new ideas in both work and leisure.
- Understand social change and individual development and take responsibility for sustaining both.
- Accept the constancy of change, cope, adapt and manage change effectively in all areas of one's life.
- Possess self-determination with a realistic assessment of one's aptitudes and inclinations.
- Recognize how the foundation of one's ideals and values emanate from one's particular background and experience.
- Participate in communities as both teacher and learner, connecting with others, sharing thoughts and creating knowledge while taking advantage of an open environment that values critical thinking and civil discourse.
- Enhance one's understanding of various forms of discrimination and oppression while embracing the principles of access to promote equitable opportunity for all in the teaching and learning experience.
- Explore, understand, and respect the tenacity and validity of diverse values and heritage.

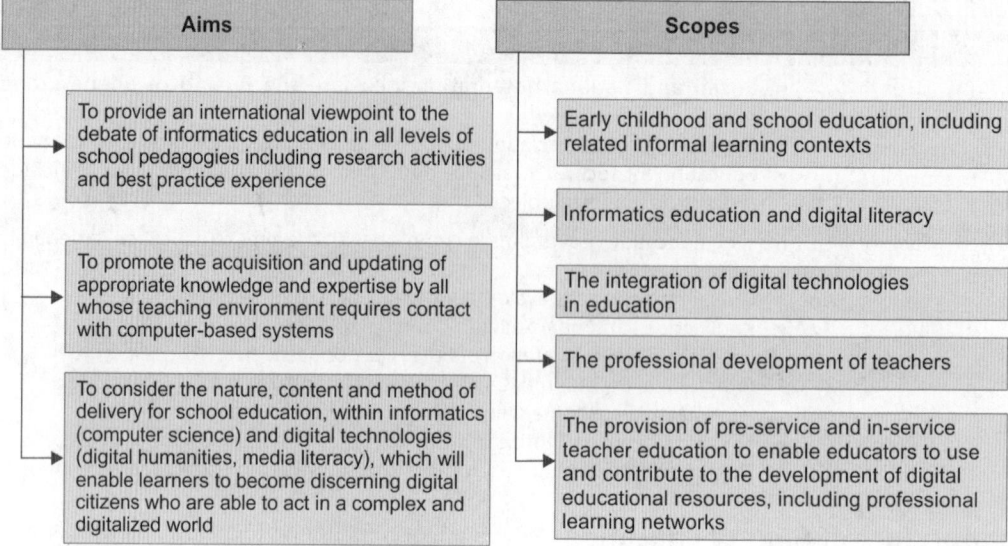

Aims	Scopes
To provide an international viewpoint to the debate of informatics education in all levels of school pedagogies including research activities and best practice experience	Early childhood and school education, including related informal learning contexts
	Informatics education and digital literacy
To promote the acquisition and updating of appropriate knowledge and expertise by all whose teaching environment requires contact with computer-based systems	The integration of digital technologies in education
	The professional development of teachers
To consider the nature, content and method of delivery for school education, within informatics (computer science) and digital technologies (digital humanities, media literacy), which will enable learners to become discerning digital citizens who are able to act in a complex and digitalized world	The provision of pre-service and in-service teacher education to enable educators to use and contribute to the development of digital educational resources, including professional learning networks

Fig. 1.7: Aims and scope of education.

- Appreciate the interconnection of global events and issues and one's place in the web of life.
- Develop an environment that encourage active learning and values the differing approaches of all community members.
- Enhance literacy in all areas—reading, listening, viewing, writing, speaking, creating, and movement.
- Reason quantitatively, using numerical data to meet personal and vocational needs and to respond to a world increasingly dependent on the understanding of a broad range of quantitative concepts and processes.
- Identify a need for information and know how and where to find it.
- Access, organize, interpret, evaluate, synthesize and apply information.
- Reflect on and assess information and knowledge from differing perspectives.
- Develop knowledge of one's feelings, values and biases and their relation to one's thinking and behavior.
- Integrate knowledge from multiple disciplines to make thoughtful and informed decisions.
- Base decisions on factual and affective evidence rather than on unexamined opinions.
- Determine the nature of a problem, analyze the problem and implement an appropriate solution, applying scholarly theories and methods where appropriate.
- Evaluate, integrate and adapt to technological change.

AGENCIES OF EDUCATION

Society depends upon education for the community development and progress of its physical and social life. Each generation has to hand over experiences, customs, thoughts and values of its own as well as those that it has inherited from the past generation to such succeeding generation.

Kinds of agency of education: Agencies of education may be said to be formal and informal on one hand, active and passive on the other.

- **Formal agencies:** The formal agencies which are developed with scientific and exclusively for imparting education are called formal agencies of education. They are deliberately, purposefully planned programme. The procedure and performance of their activity are fixed and well-defined. Such agencies include school, the church, the state organized recreational centers. etc.

- **Informal agencies:** Informal agencies are those which group up spontaneously. They do not observe formation of rules and regulations of rules. They directly exercise great educational influences on members. Such agencies are known as informal agencies. The family, the society, the play group, etc.
- **Active agencies:** The agencies which provide education through the interaction of persons are called active agencies. Education is two way process. Here, there is an inter action between the educator and educand, the individual and the group. They aim at controlling and guiding the social process. Family, church, school, sports, clubs, social welfare agencies are some agencies of this type.
- **Passive agencies:** Passive agencies are those which imply one way process. The influence on the individual but not influenced by him. However they are subjected to public control, public taste and state censorship. For example, e.g., cinema, radio, press, and television, etc.

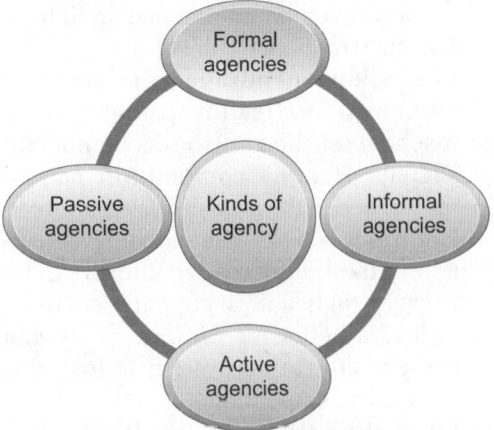

Fig. 1.8: Kinds of educational agency.

FUNCTIONS OF EDUCATION

Philosophers and educationists propose the following functions of education.

- **To complete the socialization process:** The main social objective of education is to complete the socialization process. With the emergence of nuclear families, the role of school and other institutions in the socialization process has increased considerably. The school trains the child to develop honesty, consideration for others and ability to distinguish between right and wrong. Socialization process also enables

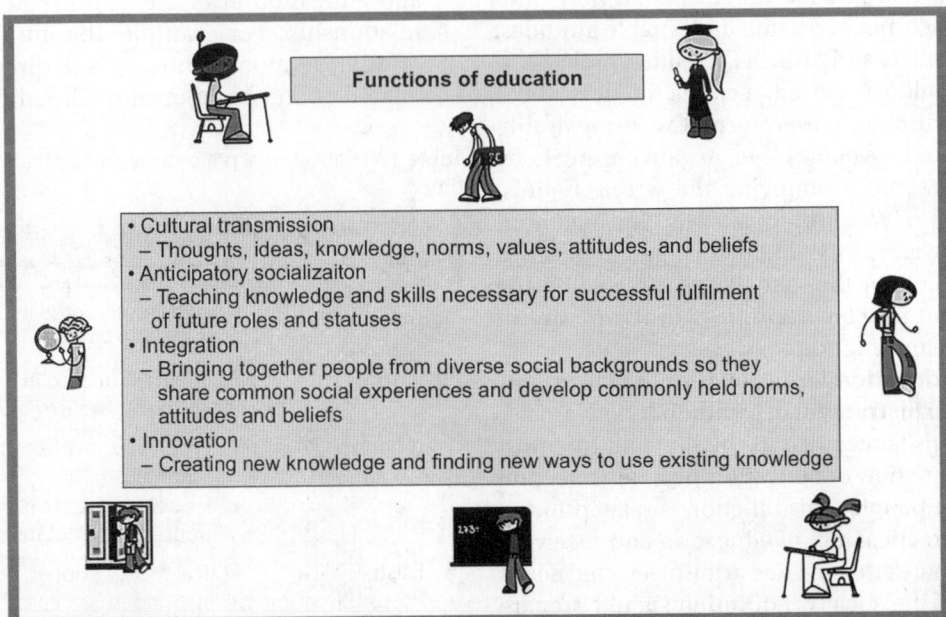

Fig. 1.9: Functions of education.

the child to cooperate with others and to grow as a good citizen by respecting the laws framed by the society. Socialization is achieved through textbooks and learning experiences intended to develop social skills.

- **To transmit the cultural heritage:** All societies are proud to uphold or highlight their cultural heritage and ascertain that the culture is preserved and transmitted through social organizations to future generations. All types of education and all agencies of education have to carry out the function of cultural transmission in an earnest way by teaching the elements of culture like literature, history, art, and philosophy, etc.
- **Formation of social personality:** Personality of individual members in a society shares some common features of the culture. Along with the process of transmitting culture, education also contributes to the formation of social personality. Formation of social perso-nality helps man to adjust with his environment and flourish himself in co-operation with others.
4. **Reformation of attitude:** In the developmental process, child may have incorporated some undesirable attitudes, beliefs and disbelief, loyalties, prejudices, jealousy, hatred, etc. It is the duty of the education to reform the undesirable attitudes and other negative aspects by means of removing the wrong beliefs, illogical prejudices and unreasoned loyalties from the child's mind. A collective effort by the school and home will bring out spectacular results in the matter of reforming attitudes.
- **Education for occupational placement-an instrument of livelihood:** Now-a-days, this is regarded as the first and foremost function of education by a large section of people. This function is related to the practical aim of education and receiving more attention due to the diversified needs of the society. Education should prepare students not only to foresee the future

occupational position but also enable them to attain it in an impressive way. The relevance of this function is evident from the importance we are giving to vocational training.

- **Conferring of status:** It is understood that an individual's status in the society is determined by the amount and type or kind of education he has received. In the current situation, the kind of knowledge one is gaining is important than the amount. For example, a graduate nurse or a diploma nurse can flourish anywhere in the world compared to a person holding PhD in a traditional subject.
- **Education encourages the spirit of competition:** Healthy competition is essential for the growth of a democratic society. Healthy competition can be manifested in the form of quality products and services. From the school level itself students should realize the need for engaging in healthy competition in order to lead a better life. Unfortunately, our present education system is fostering unhealthy competition
- **Education trains in skills that are required by the economy:** Economy and education always enjoy a bilateral relationship. For example, the number of well functioning hospitals is directly related to the number of qualified and

Table 1.1: Educational philosophy and educational theory.

Educational Philosophy	Educational Theory
Idealism	Perennialism (rooted in Idealism and Realism)
Realism	Essentialism (rooted in Idealism and Realism)
Pragmatism	• Progressivism (rooted in Pragmatism) • Reconstructionism (rooted in Pragmatism)
• Existentialism • Postmodernism	Critical theory (rooted in Postmodernism and Existentialism)

competent nurses passing out from the nursing institutes. More patients will be admitted to a hospital which is providing quality nursing care. This will lead to more money transactions and ultimately results in the economical development of the nearby areas of the hospital.

- **Fosters participant democracy:** In participant democracy, ordinary citizen is aware about his rights and duties and participates actively in the democratic process. Literacy is essential to nurture participant democracy and literacy is the product of education. Thus, education fosters participant democracy.
- **Education imparts values:** Education helps the students to realize the role of values in leading a good life as a social being. Through various activities education imparts values such as cooperation, team spirit, obedience, etc.
- **Education act as an integrative force:** Education act as an integrative force in society by communicating values that unite different sections of the society. By and large students learn social skills from the educational institutions. In India, through education we are teaching the concept of 'unity in diversity' as a part of developing this integrative force.
- **Values and orientation which are specific to certain:** Professions are also provided by education. This function deals mainly with the professional education. For example, in nursing institutes, nursing students are educated in a particular way to meet the health needs or the society.

SCOPE OF EDUCATION

The scope of education is meant to help people deal with various challenges that they come across in life. The scope of education can be explained by its various processes.

- **Education by accretion or storage:** According to this view, education is the process of gradually filling up the empty mind of the child with grains of knowledge. The teacher's mind and the books are the store houses of mental granary of the child. This is called the gow-sack theory. The theory is narrow and unsound.
- **Education as formation of mind:** Education as formation tries to form the mind by a proper presentation of materials. It is formation of mind by setting up certain association or connection of content by means of a subject-matter.
- **Education as preparation:** Education as preparation is a process of preparation or getting ready for the responsibilities and privileges of adult life. Preparation for complete living. This theory is the outcome of modern scientific tendency in education.
- **Education as mental discipline:** The theory of mental discipline is a traditional concept of education. According to this theory, the process of learning is more important than the thing learned. This theory is based upon the traditional 'Faculty Theory' of psychology according to which the mind is divided into a good number of separate faculties such as memory, attention, reasoning, imagination, perception, thinking, etc.
- **Education as growth and development:** It is a modern concept of education change is the law of nature. Man undergoes changes and transformations from cradle to grave. These changes may be of different types such as physical, mental, moral and emotional. Whenever there is change there is growth.
- **Education as direction:** Educate a child means directing the child in the proper direction. The young learners have innate powers, attitudes, interests and instincts. It is the essential function of education to direct those inborn instincts and power properly in socially acceptable and desirable channels.
- **Education as adjustment and self-activity:** Adjustment is essential to an individual for self-development. Education gives an individual the power of adjustment in an efficient manner

- **Education as social change and progress:** A society is composed of individuals and when the ideas of individuals change the society is bound to change. Change is the law of human life and society. The function of education is to maintain this progressive trend.

- **Education as a process of socialization:** After birth the child becomes a member of the society and the process of socialization begins then. Then the formal education of the child begins. Besides formal education the child continues to learn and gather experiences in informal or incidental way.

IMPORTANT PHILOSOPHIES IN EDUCATION

Sl. No.	Concept	Description
1.	Idealism	Idealism idolizes **mind and self**. Idealism believes in universal mind. Idealism regards man as a spiritual being. The world of ideas and values are more important than the world of matter. Real knowledge is perceived in mind.
2.	Naturalism	Naturalism believes that education should be according to the **nature** of the child. Naturalism advocates the creation of conditions in which the natural development of a child can take place in a natural way. The different forms of naturalism are physical naturalism, mechanical naturalism and biological naturalism.
3.	Pragmatism	The term pragmatism derives its origin from a Greek word meaning to do, to make, to accomplish. **Experience** is central here; everything is tested on the touchstone of experience. The basis of all teaching is the activity of the child.
4.	Existentialism	According to existentialism, the primary aim of education is the making of a **human** person as one who lives and makes decisions about what the learners will do and be.
5.	Realism	Realism is concerned with the study of the world we live in realism believes that all knowledge is derived from experience. The realist believes that everything that exists in the universe is matter or energy or matter of motion.
6.	Humanism	Humanism is a movement to gain for man a proper recognition in the universe. Man is a free agent.
7.	Humanistic existentialism	Humanistic existentialism is the youngest philosophy. Existentialism may be described as a modern philosophy which is primarily build upon the work of the scholars of the twentieth century.
8.	Experimentalism	Experimentalism is unreservedly a philosophy of change and of process. It teaches that everything is changing continually- man, morality, democracy and education; experience is the only reality.
9.	Neorealism	Neorealism is a theory which excludes philosophy and theology as source of knowledge and truth; it looks to science as its primary source.
10.	Eclectic tendency in education	It is a process of putting together the common view of different philosophies, into one comprehensive whole is eclectic tendency in education. It is the fusion or synthesis of different philosophies of education, is known as eclectic tendency in education. According to Munroe, the eclectic tendency is that which seeks the harmonization on principles, underlying various tendencies and rationalization of educational practices.
11.	Progressivism	The term progressivism in education is an American philosophy, which is a revolt against the formal, conventional and traditional system of education. The progressivism in education advocates that the education of the child should be for the present life it self and not for a future life.

Contd...

Contd...

Sl. No.	Concept	Description
12.	Reconstrutionism	Reconstrutionism has its origin in Plato; his republic is his vision of an ideal society. Reconstruction is of two forms; total change or desirable change. The present educational system does not represent Indian cultures and traditions. The primary aim of education is an all round development of personality.
13.	Eclecticism	The dictionary meaning of the word eclectic means selecting or borrowing the best out of everything. According to eclectic tendency in education, modern education wants to synthesis the brief form of all the past movements into new structure.
14.	Perennialism	Perennialism is a very constructive and inflexible philosophy of education. It is based on the view that reality comes from fundamental fixed truths, especially related to god. It believes that people find truth through reasoning and revelation and that goodness is found in rational thinking.
15.	Existentialism	Existentialism is an attitude and outlook that stress human existence that is the distinctive qualities of individual persons rather than man in abstract on nature and the world in general. It a type of philosophy which endeavors to analyze the basic structure of human existence in its essential freedom.

RELATION BETWEEN PHILOSOPHIES AND EDUCATION

Education is the deliberate and systematic influence extorted by the mature person upon the immature through instruction, discipline and the harmonious development of all the powers of the human being, physical, social, intellectual, esthetic, and spiritual, according to their essential hierarchy, by and for their individual and social use, and directed toward the union of the educand with his creator as the final end. Philosophy and education are so closely connected that one without the other is meaning. Many bonds unite education with philosophy. A brief discussion of some of these bonds will help to point out the close relationship between philosophy and education.

- **Natural bonds:** A natural bond signifies an association between two or more things or processes that is rooted in their very nature. There is a natural association between spiritual life and education, as well as the ideals and the cultural standards of the adult generation.
- **Logical bonds:** The core or heart of any given system of education is found in the ideals it sets out to attain. These ideals are determined through the philosophy. Once ideals have been established, it may be said to follow logically that a system of education must be set up in order to perpetuate them.
- **Social bonds:** Education aims at the perpetuation of social institutions which are based on a philosophy of the life and the process of society. History is the authentic method of recording, in the interests of posterity, human's activities and the progress of human society.

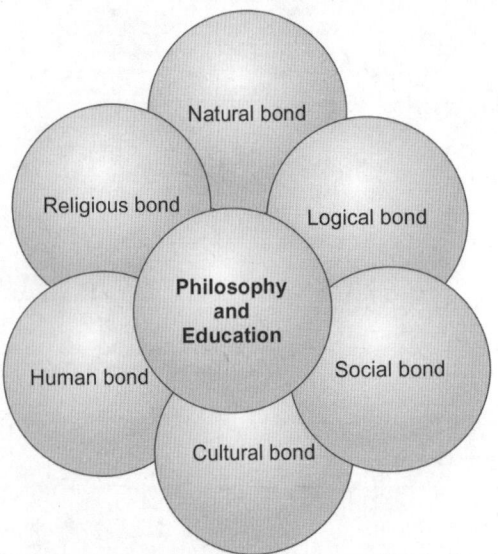

Fig. 1.10: Relation between philosophies and education.

- **Cultural bonds:** Culture embraces not only the sum total of people's accomplishments but the ideals and the virtues after which they strive. Therefore, there is a cultural bond between philosophy and education.
- **Human bonds:** Psychology, or the dealing in human relationship, is the basis for education. A recognized aim of education is to develop the personality of the student. This is done by knowing the individual student and the ideal that will best serve as a model for his education.
- **Religious bonds:** Philosophy and education are joined by religious bonds in addition to those bonds already mentioned, for education realizes its finest expression in religion. Man attains not merely an ordinary philosophy of life in religious education but a philosophy inspired from on high

CONCLUSION

Education is a complex process of controlling and modifying behavior. Education takes place in a variety of settings like institutions, families, museums, religious institutions, places of work, hospitals, community centers, etc. Education is conceived as a lifelong process. According to one definition, "Education is a deliberate, systematic influence exerted by a mature person upon an immature person, through instruction, discipline and harmonious relationship" in a wider sense, all experience is education. Education is life. That which broadens one's horizon deepens the insight, refines reactions, stimulates thought and feeling and develops the physical, intellectual, aesthetic, social and spiritual powers of man, is education

BIBLIOGRAPHY

1. Gabor D. First contact body language. How to start a conversation and make friends. Revised Edn. Rockefeller Center, New York: Fireside Publications, 2001:21.
2. Grant, Child development in India, 3rd edition, Ashish publishing house, New Delhi, 1992.
3. Santrock, J, W, Child Development, 7th edition, Brown and Bench Mark Publishers, Sydney, 1996.
4. Skinner E Charles. Educational Psychology. Fourth Edition, Prentice-hall of India Pvt. Ltd: New Delhi, 1996.
5. Taylor E Shelley. Health Psychology. Sixth edition, Tata McGraw-Hill Edition: New York, 2006.

2 CHAPTER

Teaching and Learning Process

INTRODUCTION

Teaching and learning is a process that includes many variables. These variables interact as learners work toward their goals and incorporate new knowledge, behaviors, and skills that add to their range of learning experiences. Over the past century, various perspectives on learning have emerged, among them-behaviorist (response to external stimuli); cognitive (learning as a mental operation); and constructivist (knowledge as a constructed element resulting from the learning process). Rather than considering these theories separately, it is best to think of them together as a range of possibilities that can be integrated into the learning experience. During the integration process, it is also important to consider a number of other factors—cognitive styles, learning style, the multiple natures of our intelligences, and learning as it relates to those who have special needs and are from diverse cultural backgrounds.

DEFINITION

- Teaching and learning involves the process of transferring knowledge from the one who is giving to the one who is receiving.
- Teaching is the process of attending to people's needs, experiences and feelings,

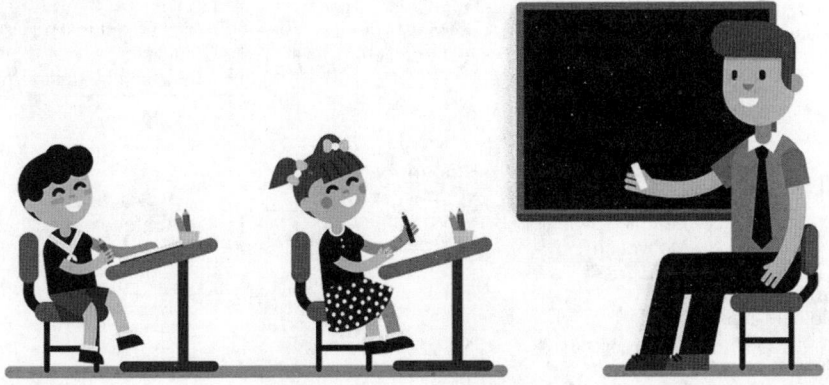

Fig. 2.1: Teaching and learning process.

and intervening so that they learn particular things, and go beyond the given. Teaching is one of the instruments of education and is a special function is to impart understanding and skill.

- It is deliberate intervention that involves the planning and implementation of instructional activities and teaching experiences to meet intended learner outcomes according to a teaching plan
- It can be defined as the relatively permanent change in an individual's behavior (knowledge, skill and learning attitude) that can occur at any time or place as a result of consciously

TEACHING-LEARNING PROCESS

Teaching-learning is a continuous process consisting of various steps. It is difficult to separate steps from one another. According to Wilson and Gallup the following are the steps in teaching-learning process (AIDCAS).

- Attention
- Interest
- Desire
- Conviction
- Action
- Satisfaction

Attention: The first task of the extension worker is to attract attention of the learners to the new and better ideas. Farmers are to be made aware of the improvement.

Interest: Once attention has been captured it becomes possible for the teacher to appeal to the basic needs or urges of the individual and arouse his interest in further consideration of the idea. Extension worker reveals how new practice will contribute to the farmer's welfare. The message should be presented attractively.

Desire: The desire is concerned with continuing farmer's interest in the idea or better practice until interest becomes a desire or motivating force. The extension worker explains the farmer that the information applies directly to the farmer's situation and doing of this would satisfy his needs.

Conviction: Action follows desire, conviction of the people, and prospects of satisfaction. In this step, the learner knows what action is necessary, and just how to take that action. He

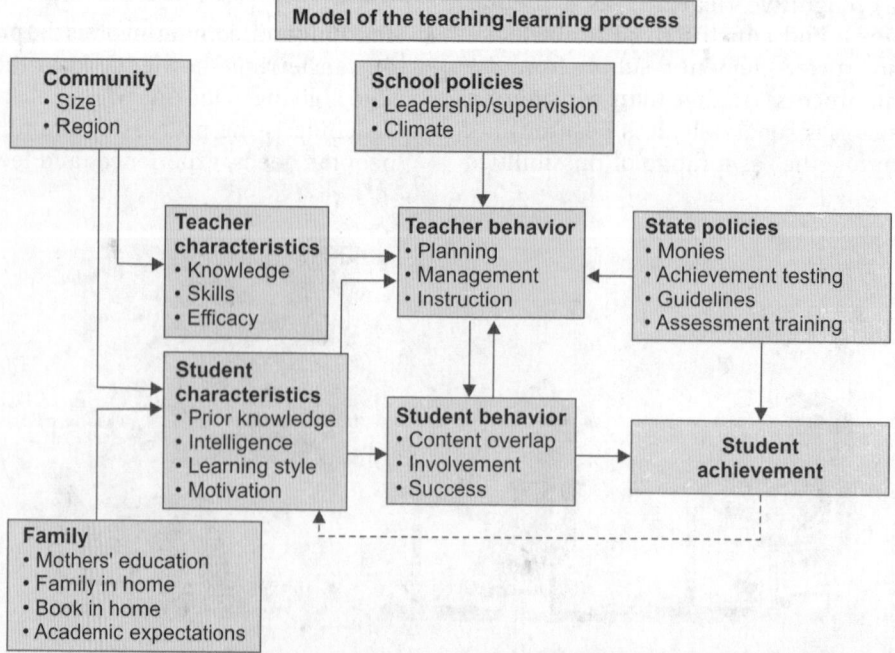

Fig. 2.2: Teaching-learning process model.

also makes sure that the learner visualizes the action in terms of his own peculiar situation and has acquired confidence in his own ability to do things.

Action: Unless conviction is converted into action the efforts are fruitless. It is the job of the extension worker to make it easy for the farmers to act. If new control measure is action oriented, the recommended chemical should be available within the farmers reach

Satisfaction: This is the end product of the process. Follow-up by the extension worker helps the farmers to learn to evaluate their progress and strengths. Satisfaction helps to continue his action with increased satisfaction. Satisfaction is the motivating force for further learning. "A satisfied customer is the best advertisement" will also apply to the extension worker.

> **Seven principles of effective teaching-learning process**
> « Encourages student-faculty contact
> « Encourages cooperation among students
> « Encourages active learning
> « Prompt feedback
> « Emphasizes time on task
> « Communicates high expectations
> « Respects diverse talents and ways of learning

ELEMENTS OF TEACHING AND LEARNING PROCESS

Teaching process cannot be performed if there is one element that is missing among the three of the teaching elements. There is what we called as elements of teaching and learning processes. These elements are necessary to be able to make teaching and learning possible. Without one of these elements, there could be no real teaching or learning process that will exist. It is so important that the presence of these elements is present in the process of teaching, considering that all of them play an important role in the system. The elements of teaching and learning process are the teacher, the leaner as well as the good learning environment. It is being considered that learning occur when there is established

relationship among these three elements. The teaching as well as the learning activity depends upon how these elements works together.

- **Teacher:** The teacher is considered as the element that has the main role in the teaching-learning process. He/she is considered as the so-called prime mover of the educational processes, thus he she directs the flow of the whole process. The teacher is the one that facilitates the whole process of leaning. He or she directs its flow and serve as main control of the teaching learning process.

- **Learner:** The learners are considered as the key participant in the teaching and learning process. They are considered as the primary subject or the main reason why the process is implemented. The knowledge that acquired by the learners will decide if the teaching and learning objectives are achieved. Learners vary from one another in the aspects of learning. There are those learners that learn fast while there are those learners that learn in average or slower.

- **Favorable environment:** The favorable environment, participates in the teaching-learning process by providing a place where there is a smooth flow of communication, avoiding some common barriers between the teacher and the learner. The presence of a good environment is so much important in the teaching and learning

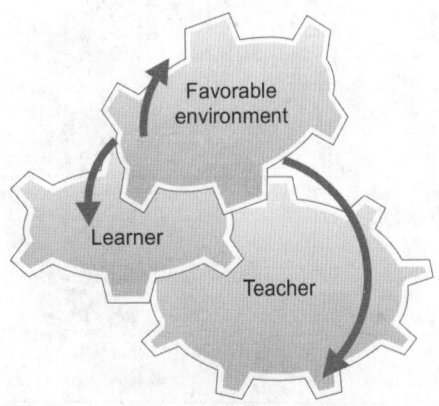

Fig. 2.3: Element of teaching and learning process.

process. The good environment provides a smooth flow of communication between the learners and the teachers, thus it facilitates a well executed teaching and learning process. A good environment is necessary for learning. The reason why we should make sure that we should have this kind of environment, as we teach or we learn.

TEACHING AND LEARNING STRATEGIES

The 6 E's and S (Engage, Explore, Explain, Elaborate, Evaluate, and Standards) lesson plan format was developed by teachers in consultation with faculty from schools of education and is based on a constructivist model of teaching. The lesson plans are based on constructivist instructional models with activities and sections of the plan designed to have the students continually add (or construct) new knowledge on top of existing knowledge.

Each of the 6 E's describes a phase of learning, and each phase begins with the letter 'E': Engage, Explore, Explain, Elaborate, Evaluate. The 6 E's allows students and teachers to experience common activities, to use and build on prior knowledge and experience, to construct meaning, and to

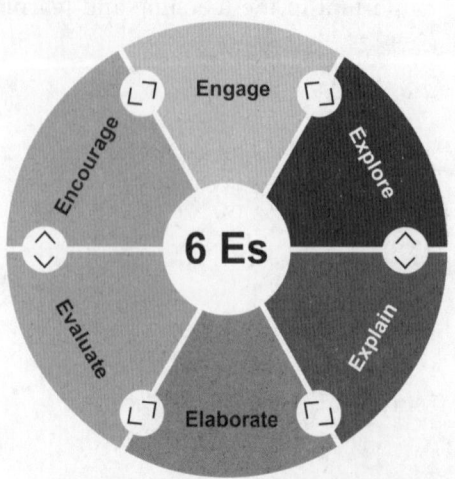

Fig. 2.4: 6 Es+S model of instruction.

continually assess their understanding of a concept.

Engage: An 'engage' activity should make connections between past and present learning experiences, anticipate activities and focus students' thinking on the learning outcomes of current activities. Students should become mentally engaged in the concept, process, or skill to be learned. Each lesson plan has an 'essential question' that is the basis for their inquiry. Normally, the section will include a few key questions to help direct some of the research in the Explore section.

Explore: Here the student investigates the topic more thoroughly. What is important is that the students are given the opportunity to 'free wheel' their way through the materials and not be over directed. They will need some direction and the teacher can circulate, asking important questions, listening to their interactions and ensuring that they remain on task.

Explain: This phase helps students explain the concepts they have been exploring. They have opportunities to verbalize their conceptual understanding or to demonstrate new skills or behaviors. This phase also provides opportunities for teachers to introduce formal terms, definitions, and explanations for concepts, processes, skills, or behaviors.

Elaborate: Here the students are expected to work directly on the given assignment. It is their opportunity to demonstrate their application of new information and to present their findings or conclusions to others. It is a good time for submitting materials for evaluation, doing presentations and completing the project or assignment.

Evaluate: While it is expected that evaluation will continue throughout the process, this is the section where the teacher evaluates the learning that has occurred. Students normally submit their work or assignments at this point. It is very important at this stage that the students be encouraged to engage in self-evaluation, group evaluation and develop their own tools to do so.

Table 2.1: 6 E's describes a phase of learning.

Engage	This lesson mentally engages students with an activity or question. It captures their interest, provides an opportunity for them to express what they know about the concept or skill being developed, and helps them to make connections between what they know and the new ideas.
Explore	Students carry out hands-on activities in which they can explore the concept or skill. They grapple with the problem or phenomenon and describe it in their own words. This phase allows students to acquire a common set of expreiences that they can use to help each other make sense of the new concept or skill.
Explain	Only after students have explored the concept or skill does the teacher provide the concepts and terms used by the students to develop explanations for the phenomenon they have experienced. The significant aspect of this phase is that explanation follows experiences.
Elaborate	This phase provides opportunities for students to apply what they have learned to new situations and so develop a deeper understanding of the concept or greater use of the skill. It is important for students to discuss and compare their ideas with each other during this phase.
Evaluate	The final phase provides an opportunity for students to review and reflect on their own learning and new understandings and skills. It is also when students provide evidence for changes to their understandings, beliefs and skills.
Encourage	Encouraging words and actions are often internalized by students and have the power to motivate them to succeed. Encouragement can even be the difference between students completing school and giving up on themselves.

Encourage: This section contains some suggestions for taking the students beyond the lesson. The purpose is to examine ways in which they can bring their findings to others or apply their understanding to new and unfamiliar circumstances. Normally, this type of activity will grow out of their excitement for what they have accomplished. This section is highly student driven, though teachers may want to gently suggest that the students enter their work in a competition or take their displays to other locations outside of their own school.

Standards: Standards are currently in the process of being integrated, lesson plan by lesson plan. In this section, the lessons are matched with state, provincial and/or national standards. It is primarily for the information of the teacher and should provide the information necessary to incorporate the lesson into the local board, district or school curriculum.

FACTORS AFFECTING TEACHING-LEARNING PROCESS

- **Intellectual factor:** The term refers to the individual mental level. Success in school is generally closely related to level of the intellect. Pupils with low intelligence often encounter serious difficulty in mastering schoolwork. Sometimes pupils do not learn because of special intellectual disabilities.

- **Learning factors:** Factors owing to lack of mastery of what has been taught, faulty methods of work or study, and narrowness of experimental background may affect the learning process of any pupil. If the school proceeds too rapidly and does not constantly check up on the extent to which the pupil is mastering what is being taught, the pupil accumulates a number of deficiencies that interfere with successful progress.

- **Physical factors:** Under this group are included such factors as health, physical development, nutrition, visual and physical defects, and glandular abnormality. It is generally recognized that ill health retards physical and motor development, and malnutrition interferes with learning and physical growth.

- **Mental factors:** Attitude falls under mental factors attitudes are made up of organic and kinesthetic elements. They are not to be confused with emotions that are characterized by internal visceral disturbances. Attitudes are more or less of definite sort. They play a large part in the mental organization and general behavior of the individual. Attitudes are also important in the development of personality. Among these attitudes and interest, cheerfulness, affection, prejudice,- open mindedness, and loyalty. Attitudes exercise a stimulating effect upon the rate of learning and teaching and upon the progress in school.

- **Emotional and social factors:** Personal factors, such as instincts and emotions, and social factors, such as cooperation and rivalry, are directly related to a complex psychology of motivation. It is a recognized fact that the various responses of the individual to various kinds of stimuli are determined by a wide variety of tendencies. Some of these innate tendencies are constructive and others are harmful. For some reason a pupil may have developed a dislike for some subject

because he may fail to see its value, or may lack foundation. This dislike results in a bad emotional state.

- **Teacher's personality:** The teacher as an individual personality is an important element in the learning environment or in the failures and success of the learner. The way in which his personality interacts with the personalities of the pupils being taught helps to determine the kind of behavior which emerges from the learning situation.

- **Environmental factor:** Physical conditions needed for learning is under environmental factor. One of the factors that affect the efficiency of learning is the condition in which learning takes place. This includes the classrooms, textbooks, equipment, school supplies, and other instructional materials.

- **Technology** has long been used as a support for learning, e.g., the use of radio, film, film strips, and overheads. During the past several decades, however, the advancement of technology has led to comprehensive meeting and teaching

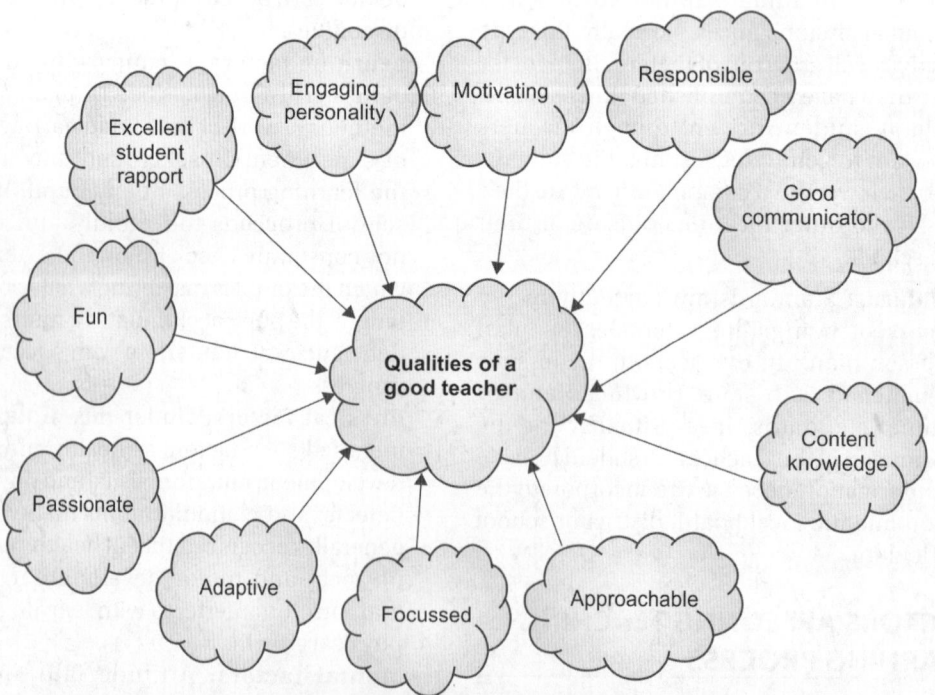

Fig. 2.5: Qualities of good teacher.

via more advanced technologies like audio-conferencing, video-conferencing, web conferencing and online learning management systems (LMS).

FUNCTIONS AND QUALITIES OF A GOOD TEACHER

As described in the words of Joseph Payne (1808-1876) "The teacher's part in the process of instruction is that of a guide, director or superintendent of the operation by which the pupil teaches himself." Swami Vivekananda (1863-1902) described the role of the teacher in teaching as, "The true teacher is someone who helps a person to get on the right path, who is there to lead them in making the best decisions for themselves." Both of the educationists have given importance to the pupils in fulfilling the role of a teacher which can service the basis for determining her functions and qualities. These are described as under:

Functions of a Teacher

- Creating and maintaining desirable learning environment.
- Motivating students to learn.
- Arranging for conditions which would provide opportunities to develop desired comprehension, competencies and attitudes.
- Utilizing the initiatives and natural urges of students to facilitate learning.
- Guiding and helping students to develop creative abilities.
- Guiding and helping students to develop inductive and deductive abilities.
- Diagnosing learning problems of students.
- Planning and implementing remedial measures.
- Evaluating records and reports
- Participating in planning and organizing of curriculum.

Qualities of a Good Teacher

A good teacher possesses the following qualities. A good teacher:
- Has mastery of the subject matter,

- Is skillful and artistic in teaching methods and in guiding learning,
- Treats each individual as unique and recognizes individual differences,
- Encourages self-learning,
- Keeps the students active and disciplined,
- Is kind and sympathetic,
- Plans her/his teaching carefully in advance but is not very rigid with the plan,
- Is approachable and seeks the co-operation of the leaner.

CHARACTERISTICS OF GOOD TEACHING

One set of characteristics of good teaching, extracted from research studies and summarized from the individual lecturer's point of view (Ramsden, 2003) includes:
- A desire to share your love of the subject with students
- An ability to make the material being taught stimulating and interesting
- A facility for engaging with students at their level of understanding
- A capacity to explain the material plainly
- A commitment to making it absolutely clear what has to be understood at what level and why

---

Box 2.1: Characteristics of good teaching.

1. It gives desirable information.
2. It creates self-motivation for learning.
3. Effective planning is essential for good teaching.
4. The students remain active in good teaching.
5. It focuses on selected information.
6. It is based on democratic ideals.
7. It is sympathetic and full of pity.
8. It is directional in nature.
9. It is based on the co-operation of teacher and students.
10. It is based on previous knowledge of teacher.
11. It is progressive.
12. It includes all sorts of teachers' performances and teaching methods.
13. It produces emotional stability.
14. It attempts to adjust the students with the environment.

- Showing concern and respect for students
- A commitment to encouraging independence.
- An ability to improvise and adapt to new demands
- Using teaching methods and academic tasks that require students to learn actively, responsibly and co-operatively
- Using valid assessment methods
- A focus on key concepts, and students misunderstandings of them, rather than covering the ground
- Giving the highest quality feedback on student work
- A desire to learn from students and other sources about the effects of teaching and how it can be improved.

NEED OF TEACHING AND LEARNING PROCESS

Involving themselves in the teaching-learning process requires the learner to pay attention, observe, memorize, understand, set goals and assume responsibilities which can be realized when they are build on their natural desire to explore. Understand things and master them. This can be realized by providing students with hands on activities. Encouraging their participation in the teaching-learning process and collaborative activities besides guiding them how to make decisions about what to learn and how and creating learning goals consistent with their interest and aspirations.

Social interaction is one of the main activities for effective learning. What children learn through interaction with their parents enables those becoming effective members of the society, internalizing the activities, habits, vocabularies and idea of the community in which they live. Children learn new things, collaborative and co-operative atmosphere in the school is very essential for effective learning. School collaboration influences academic accomplishment of the children, since it keeps them involved in academic endeavors. They take sincere efforts to improve

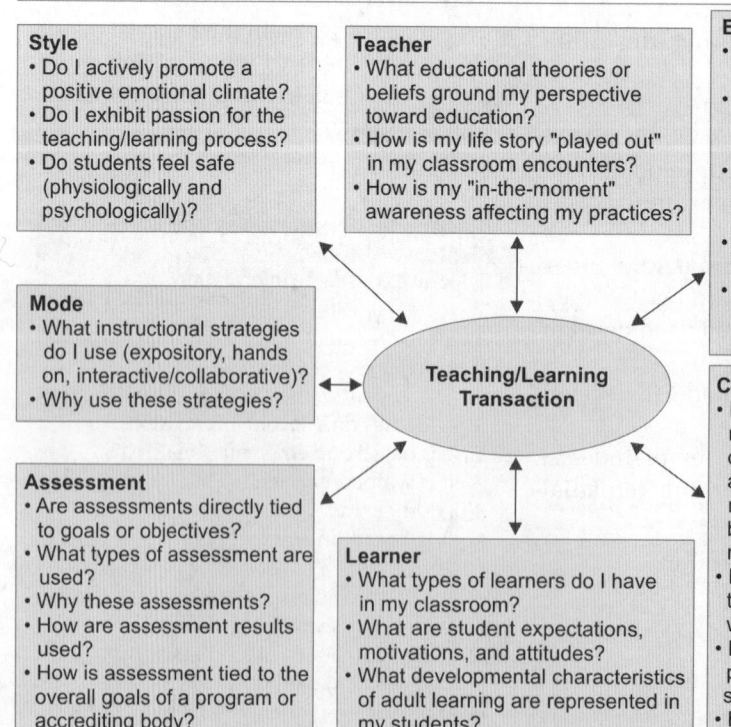

Fig. 2.6: Teaching/learning transaction model.

the quality of their academic achievement realizing that their knowledge is going to be shared with their fellow students in their classroom.

Social interaction among children can be improved if they assume leadership role by providing guiding and support to the group of their peers. Creating conductive environment in the classroom with adequate resources. Providing good models for how to co-operative with each other and linking the learning activities with the community at large teachers can enlarge the opportunity to the students for effective social interaction.

PSYCHOLOGICAL PRINCIPLES OF TEACHING

- **Principle of activity or learning by doing:** Children are active by nature and they process or method that is not based upon the student activity is not in accord with the progressive educational theories. Activity does not mean mere physical activity. If a pupil is to develop all sides of his personality, then it is necessary for him to be active in all.

Principles of Teaching

01	The goal of education is to improve learning for all learners, including teachers
02	Learning is enhanced when learning experiences are meaningful, engaging, and hands-on
03	Learning improves in an environment of positive social interaction and collaboration
04	Students learn best when they have a choice and adaptive options on learning and demonstrating their learning
05	Ongoing assessment designed to improve learning is the most helpful assessment for students
06	Engaging parents and families in student learning strengthen the learning experience

Fig. 2.7: Six teaching principles.

- **Principle of play way:** This principle is closely related to the principle of learning by doing. According to Froebel, play is the chief activity of childhood. It gives joy, freedom, contentment and inner and outer peace. It holds the source of all that is good. But without rational conscious guidance. Froebel says, childish activity degenerates into aimless play instead of preparing for those tasks of life for which it is designed. Play comes from within. It is a voluntary activity and is the manifested of creative urge.

- **Principle of motivation:** The teacher will do his best to motivate all children in the lesson. Motivation arouses the interest of children and once they become interested, they are willing to concentrate and work. Motivation is developed by following techniques: (a) utilizing the instinctive tendencies of the children in an effective manner, (b) satisfying the curiosity of children, (c) utilizing all the senses of children, (d) relating closely body and mind, (e) linking teaching-learning with life.

- **Principle of self-education:** Best teaching is enabling the child learn by his own efforts. Teacher must fire the imagination of their students. Children we are told, must be left free to express themselves for the best education is self education. Teachers, we are told, must stand aside. They must talk less, explain less and direct less.

- **Principle of individual differences:** No two children are alike. Teaching to be effective must cater to individual differences of children.

- **Principle of goal setting:** A definite goal must be set before each child according to the standard expected of him. Short-term or immediate goals should be set before small children and distant goals for older ones. It must be remembered that goals should be very clear and definite and the children must understand these goals.

- **Principle of stimulation:** Burton has said, teaching is the stimulation, guidance, direction and encouragement of learning. Ryburn emphasizes these aspects in these words; the guidance of the teacher is mainly a matter of giving the right kind of stimulus to help him to learn the right things in the right way.

- **Principle of association:** Thorndike points out those things we want to go together should be put together. Many different things or ideas which we want to go together should be associated with each other. They should form a part of one process. Then it becomes easier to make the student's understand their relationship.
- **Principle of readiness:** This principle is indicative of learner's state of mind to participate in the teaching-learning process. Readiness is preparation for action. A teacher must be alive to his principle.
- **Principle of effect:** This principle states a response is strengthened if it is followed by pleasure and weakened is followed by displeasure.
- **Principle of exercise or repetition:** According to it, the more a stimulates induced response is required, the longer it will be retained. Other things being equal, exercise strengthens the bond between situation and response. Conversely a bond is weakened through failure to exercise it. Thus the principle has two sub-parts, (a) Principle of use, and, (b) Principle of disuse.
- **Principle of change and rest:** Psychological experiments in learning have demonstrated that fatigue, lack of attention and monotony can be overcome by making appropriate provision for change, rest and recreation. While farming the time table it is kept in view that subjects and activities are provided in such a way that the students do not experience boredom and fatigue. Usually two consecutive periods of a subject are not provided in a class.
- **Principle of feed-back and reinforcement:** Learning theories point out that the immediate knowledge of the results and positive reinforces in the form of praise, grade, certificates, token money and other

incentives can contribute to make the task of learning joy able.

- **Principle of training senses:** Senses are said to be the gateways of knowledge. The power of observation, discrimination, identification, generalization and application can only be appropriately developed through the effective functioning of senses.
- **Principle of group dynamics:** Under the influences of group behavior, appropriate changes in the behavior of the members of the group can take place. Individuals composing the group think and feel as the group feels, do as the group does. A suitable climate for group dynamics is to be created in the classroom environment.
- **Principle of creativity:** Opportunities should be provided the student to explore things and events and find cause-effect relationships. The principle envisages that every student possesses some element of creativity which must be explored and developed to the maximum extent.
- **Principle of correlation:** Gandhi was of the firm view that correlation should be the basis of all work. He advocated that correlation of the learning task should be established with the craft, physical and social environment.

GENERAL PRINCIPLES OF TEACHING

Successful teaching necessitates that the teacher comes down to the level of the pupils and at the same time assists them in rising above it. To a great extent, the principles of teaching to be followed depend upon the age of the pupils, the subjects and topic of the lesson. However, there are certain general principles which should underline the teaching of all subjects. As already stated, there is no clear-cut dividing line between psychological and general principles of teaching.

- **Principle of definite goals or objectives:** Destination or goals of teaching-learning must be clear to the teachers and students. Goals and objectives keep the teacher and students on the track. Definiteness of goals helps in planning, executing and evaluating every step, phases or act of the teaching-learning process.

- **Principle of child centeredness:** The entire teaching endeavor is for the child. Therefore, it is essential that teaching strategies should cater to the aptitude, interest and abilities of the students. In the drama of education, child should be assigned the role of hero.

- **Principle of linking with life:** Teaching can never be performed in vacuum. It is always in a social context. In the teaching of all the school subjects, examples from everyday life should be given their due place.

- **Principle of correlation:** Knowledge is one whole. Various ideas and events are interrelated. There exist links among various subjects. Correlation of the present events can be made with the past similarly future can be visualized on the basis of the present happenings or state of affairs. Gandhi propounded his system of basic education with correlation as its cornerstone-correlation with the craft, correlation with the physical environment and correlation with social environment.

- **Principle of active involvement and participation of students:** Teaching and learning is a two-way traffic. Traditional teaching was almost teacher-centered. There was very little scope for the involvement of the students. The teacher taught and the students listened to him passively. The new teaching emphasizes that the students must actively participate in all the stages and steps of teaching-learning.

- **Principle of co-operation:** Classroom environment becomes lively when the teacher and taught work in unison, helping each other in carrying out the task of teaching and learning. All the participants have the same common interest. Naturally, they must cooperate with teacher.

- **Principle of remedial teaching:** All students do not learn with the same speed and accomplishment. Some lag behind and need extra coaching. The teacher has to find out where the fault lies and think for positive measures. He may have to arrange for remedial or compensatory or extra teaching for any particular group of students for removing their specific difficulties.

- **Principle of creating conductive environment:** Physical as well as social

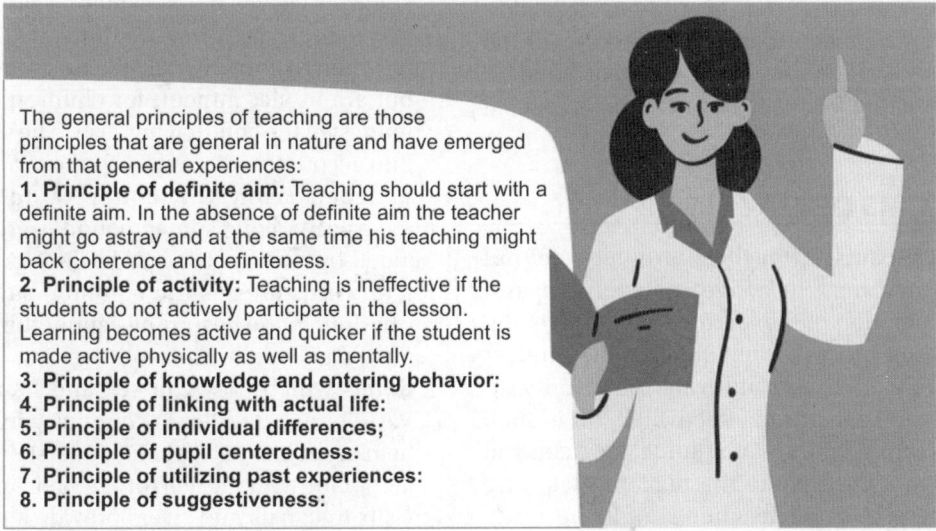

The general principles of teaching are those principles that are general in nature and have emerged from that general experiences:

1. Principle of definite aim: Teaching should start with a definite aim. In the absence of definite aim the teacher might go astray and at the same time his teaching might back coherence and definiteness.

2. Principle of activity: Teaching is ineffective if the students do not actively participate in the lesson. Learning becomes active and quicker if the student is made active physically as well as mentally.

3. Principle of knowledge and entering behavior:

4. Principle of linking with actual life:

5. Principle of individual differences;

6. Principle of pupil centeredness:

7. Principle of utilizing past experiences:

8. Principle of suggestiveness:

Fig. 2.8: General principles of teaching.

environment of the classroom plays a vital role in motivating the learners. Arrangement of light and furniture, etc., should be properly attended to. There should be proper discipline and order. The teacher should be sympathetic but firm.

- **Principle of planning:** Planning determines the quality or success of any task. Planning in teaching involves the preparation of the lesson notes.
- **Principle of effective strategies:** Teaching process to be effective must adopt proper means, strategies and tact's. A teaching strategy is a generalized plan for a lesson which includes structure, desired learning behavior in terms of goals of instruction and outline of planned tactics necessary to implement the strategy.
- **Principle of flexibility:** Strategies should serve as guides for effective teaching. Strategies may have to be changed if the classroom situations or warrant. Teaching is a complex task and a live phenomenon. The possibilities of alternation in planned strategies cannot be ruled out at the execution stage. A teacher must be quite imaginative and resourceful for adopting himself and his teaching to be requirements of the teaching-learning environment.
- **Principle of variety:** A variety of teaching aids and strategies should be adopted to motivate and sustain the interests of the students. Variety serves as great tonic for creating fresh environment and checking boredom and lethargy.

MAXIMS OF TEACHING

The maxims of teaching are very helpful in obtaining the active involvement and participation of the learners in the teaching learning process. They quicken the interest of the learner and motivate them to learn. They make learning effective, inspirational, interesting and meaningful. They keep the students attentive to the teaching-learning process. A good teacher should be quite familiar with them. Now we proceed to discuss them.

- **Proceed from the known to the unknown:** The most natural and simple way of teaching a lesson is to be proceed from something that the students already know to those facts which they do not know. What is already known to the students is great use to the students. This means that the teacher should arouse the interest in a lesson by putting questions on the subject matter already known to the pupils. The teacher is to proceed step by step to connect the new matter to the old one. New knowledge cannot be grasped in a vacuum.
- **Proceed from simple to complex:** The simple task or topic must be taught first and the complex one can follow later on. The word simple and complex are to be seen from the point of view of the child and not that of an adult. We would be curbing the interest and initiative of the children by presenting them complex problems before the simpler ones are presented.
- **Proceed from easy to difficult:** We must graduate our lessons in order of ease of undertaking them. Student's standards must be kept in view. This will help in sustaining the interest of the students. In determining what is easy and what is difficult we have to take into account the psychological make-up of the child. Logically viewed one skill may be easy but psychologically it may be difficult. There are many things which look easy to us but are in fact difficult for children. The interest of the children has also to be taken into account.
- **Proceed from the concrete to the abstract:** A child's imagination is greatly aided by a concrete material. Things first and words after is the common saying. Children in the beginning cannot think in abstracts. Small children learn first from things which they can see and handle. Very young pupils learn counting with the help of pebbles, etc., a child understands is aeroplane with the help of a model. Actual visits to canals and rivers provide a clear idea of them. A lesson in geography can be made interesting with the help of models,

Box 2.2: Maxims of teaching.

- Simple to Complex
- Known to Unknown
- Concrete to Abstract
- Analysis to Synthesis
- Induction to Deduction
- Near to Far
- Whole to Part
- Psychological to Logical
- Particular to General
- Empirical to Rational
- Actual to Representative

pictures and illustrations of bridges, rivers and mountains, etc. Care must be taken exercised to ensure that the students do not remain at the concrete stage all the times. This is only the initial step for children with a view to reach the higher stage of abstraction as they advance in age.

- **Proceed from particular to general:** Before giving principles and rules, particular examples should be presented. As a matter of fact a study of particular facts should lead the children themselves to frame general rules. The rules of arithmetic, of grammar, of physical geography and almost of all sciences are based on the principle of proceeding from particular instances to general rules.

- **Proceed from indefinite to definite:** Ideas of children in the initial stages are indefinite, incoherent and very vague. These ideas are to be made definite, clear, precise and systematic. Effective teaching necessitates that every word and idea presented should stand out clearly in the child's mind as a picture. For classifying ideas, adequate use of actual objectives, diagrams and pictures. Every possible effort should be make the children interested in the lesson.

- **Proceed from empirical to rational:** Observation and experience are the basis of empirical knowledge. Rational knowledge implies a bit of abstraction and arguments approach. The general feeling is that the child first of all experiences knowledge in his day to day life and after that he feels the rational basis. For instance, plane

geometry makes better sense when taught in the context of everyday life instead of it in the format of a highly abstract theory. It is always better to begin with what the children see, feel and experience than arguing and generalizing.

- **Proceed from psychological to logical:** Logical approach is concerned with the arrangement of the subject matter. Psychological approach looks at the child's interests, needs, mental makeup and reactions. When we treat a subject logically, we are usually thinking of it from our own point of view and not from the point of view of the child. In psychological approach, we proceed from the concrete to the abstract, from the simple to the complex and from known to unknown. We start reading by teaching the child to read a whole sentence as it is for the adult.

- **Proceed from whole to parts:** Whole is more meaningful to the child than the parts of the whole. The learner sees a relationship between the central ideas of the material to be learner. The whole unit or passage for slow learner should be smaller than the whole for the fast learners.

- **From near to far:** A child learns well in the surroundings in which the resides. So he should be first acquainted with his immediate environment. Gradually he may be taught about things which are away from his immediate environment. In a geography lesson we start from the local geography and then take up tehsil, district, state, the country and the world gradually.

- **From analysis to synthesis:** Analysis means breaking a problem into convenient parts and synthesis means grouping of these separated parts into one complete whole. Complex problems can be made simple and easy by dividing it into units.

- **From actual to representative:** When actual objectives are shown to children, they learn easily and retain them in their minds for a longer time. This is especially suitable for younger children. Representative objectives in the form of pictures, models, etc., should be used for the grownups.

- **Proceed inductively:** This maxim include almost all the maxims stated above. In the inductive approach, we start from particular examples an establish general rules through the active participation of the learners. In the deductive approach, we assume a definition, a general rule or formula and apply it to particular examples. An example will make this distinction very clear. The farmers in India are very poor's is a general statement in the deductive type of reasoning.

TEACHING RESPONSIBILITIES OF A NURSE

Nurse educators are registered nurses with advanced education who are also teachers. Most work as nurses for a period of time before dedicating their careers (part-time or full-time) to educating future nurses. Nurse educators serve as faculty members in nursing schools and teaching hospitals, sharing their knowledge and skills to prepare the next generation of nurses for effective practice. They develop lesson plans, teach courses, evaluate educational programs, oversee students' clinical practice and serve as role models for their students.

They may teach general courses or focus on areas of specialization, such as geriatric nursing, pediatric nursing or nursing informatics. Most nurse educators have extensive clinical experience, and many continue caring for patients after becoming educators. Even if they no longer practice, nurse educators must stay current with new nursing methods and technologies, which keep them on the leading edge of clinical practice. With experience, nurse educators may advance to administrative roles, such as managing nurse education programs, writing or reviewing textbooks and developing continuing education programs for working nurses.

Box. 2.3: Educational activities of a nurse.

- Providing direct clinical care
- Clinical teaching
- Competency assessment
- Curriculum development
- Education program planning and co-ordination
- Classroom teaching
- Relief of other nursing roles

Responsibilities: Nurse educators typically work in academic settings at nursing schools, community colleges and technical schools. Some also work in health care settings as staff development officers or clinical supervisors. They may work a nine-month academic calendar or all year long. Nurse educators typically do not have to work 12-hour shifts or overnight hours, as clinical nurses often do. Much of a nurse educator's day is spent in an office or a classroom, preparing for classes, giving lectures, advising students, grading papers, attending faculty meetings, handling administrative work and keeping up with current nursing knowledge. Educators who oversee students in clinical settings may divide their time between campus and a nearby hospital or other health care facility. Many faculty members are also actively engaged in research efforts, which add to the scientific base for nursing practice.

Academic life is demanding and can be filled with unexpected pressures, including multiple, competing demands on the educator's time. There are often research and publishing requirements to be met. Nurse educators are often expected to participate in professional organizations and attend or speak at conferences. They may serve on peer review and other academic committees or be asked to write grant proposals to bring new funding to the school. Still, most nurse educators are highly satisfied with their work. They find interaction with students rewarding, and they take pride in the role they play in preparing nurses to care for patients.

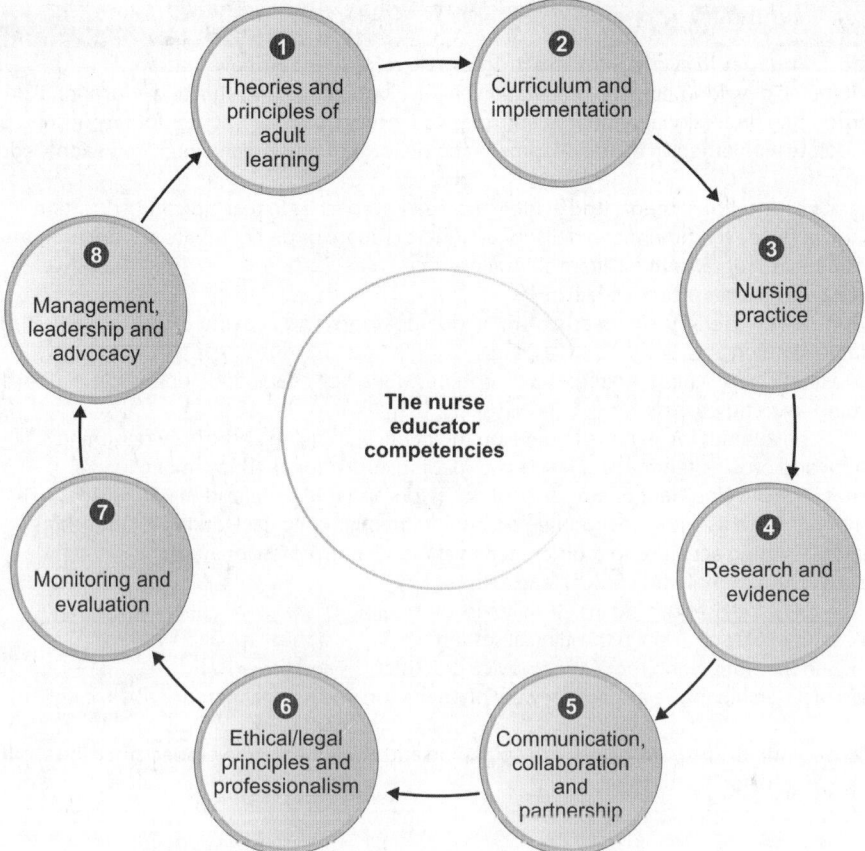

Fig. 2.9: Competencies of nurse educator.

DUTIES OF NURSE EDUCATOR

Nurse educators teach and mentor the next generation of nurses. They are the role models for nursing students, guiding students through the challenges of learning what it means to be a nurse. Prepared at the master's or doctoral level, they are the faculty at colleges, universities, vocational/technical schools and hospital-based diploma programs.

- **Academic programs:** Nurse educators ensure that students who pass through their hands are prepared for a constantly changing health care environment. They design the academic programs at their institutions in accordance with the state regulations regarding nursing instruction. In addition to teaching the courses, nurse educators evaluate the effectiveness of the programs and revise them as necessary. Nurse educators teach in formal academic programs as well as in continuing education programs for graduate nurses.

- **Supervision:** Nurse educators lecture in the classroom and work in clinical settings such as hospitals, clinics and nursing homes. Most institutions maintain clinical labs where students learn to perform basic nursing tasks such as medication administration, dressing changes or other hands-on skills under the direct supervision of the nurse educator. Once students have mastered these skills, they move into real life clinical settings, where they perform nursing tasks while the nurse educator supervises their practice and continues to teach them as they work with patients.

- **Coaching and mentoring:** A nurse educator tailors the learning experience to the student. She may carefully coach an

---

Box 2. 4: Duties of nurse educator.

Subscale 1. Engages in curriculum and program development and evaluation
- Facilitate the development, implementation and evaluation of curriculum and educational programs incorporating professional standards, attitudes and values that reflect contemporary nursing practice
- Collaborate with others in the development and delivery of nursing and interprofessional education programs
- Integrates educational theory and evidence based approaches in teaching and education
- Engage in the development and delivery of undergraduate or postgraduate tertiary programs
- Participate in programs to facilitate clinical practice

Subscale 2. Facilitates effective learning
- Recognize and identify the needs of individual learners and provide resources and support to facilitate learning
- Use a variety of teaching strategies appropriate to learner needs and contexts in supporting the teaching-learning process
- Foster opportunities for learners to develop their critical thinking and critical reasoning skills
- Monitor and provide feedback to learners regarding educational achievement
- Facilitate the development of professional behaviors and role socialization
- Promote positive learning environments through effective collegial working relationships
- Facilitate learning activities to promote teamwork and interprofessional practice

Subscale 3. Educational and clinical leadership
- Act as a role model, engaging in self-reflection, modeling critical and reflective thinking
- Work as an expert clinician in the clinical setting
- Engage in mentoring and motivating novice practitioners and other staff
- Provide leadership in the ongoing review of education and clinical practice at a facility or regional level
- Undertake primary responsibility for the planning and implementation of specialist clinical education in your hospital or health service

anxious student through her first catheter insertion or provide a more experienced and confident student with a challenge that will help her learn new skills. The educator's goal is to choose learning opportunities that help her students build on their strengths and overcome personal or scholastic limitations. Nurse educators provide regular feedback and advice to their students to help them improve their practice.

- **Other Responsibilities:** Nurse educators often have other responsibilities, especially in academic settings. They may perform research and present the results of their work at nursing conferences. Most participate in professional organizations or have leadership roles in the academic community. They may perform peer review- a form of quality management—or write grant proposals in addition to their teaching duties. Nurse educators must also maintain their clinical skills and may work part-time in direct patient care to do so.

- **Administration:** Some nurse educators move into administrative work and become deans of nursing programs. Their responsibilities include developing nursing programs in collaboration with instructors, assuring funding for programs, developing budgets, and hiring and supervising staff. The dean of a nursing program assures the content of the nursing instruction will meet the changing health care environment and collaborates with the health care facilities in her community that provide clinical experiences for the nursing students to assure relevant and meaningful educational experiences.

LESSON PLANNING

Lesson plan is a plan prepared by a teacher to teach a lesson in an organized manner. It is a plan of action and calls for an understanding on the teacher's part, about the students, knowledge and experience about the topic being taught and her/his ability to use effective methods.

Definition

- Lesson plan is a plan prepared by teacher to teach a lesson in organized manner.
- Lesson plan is a plan of action calls for an understanding on teacher's part about the student's knowledge and expertise about the topic being thought and the ability to use effective method.

Purpose of Lesson Plan

- It helps the teacher to be systematic orderly in teaching a subject matter.
- It provides confident and self-reliance to the teacher.
- She sets the objective that she is developed in students through certain activities.
- It encourages continuity in teaching process and avoids repetition.
- The interest of the students can be maintained throughout lesson plan.
- It ensures a definite objective the day's work and a clear visualization of that objective.
- It helps to clarify the ideas.
- It helps the teacher to delimit the teaching field, keeps boundaries within which the teacher has to work and thereby saves the time and labor.
- It is a best technique to judge the outcome of instruction.
- Provides guidelines for the teacher in teaching-learning process.
- Provides awareness of structure, content with which the teacher is involved in the direction to achieve the objectives.
- Develops the reasoning, imagination and decision making ability of the teacher.
- Facilitates micro-teaching.
- It is essential for effective teaching.

Characteristics of Good Lesson Plan

- It should be written
- It should have a clear aims.

- It should be linked with previous knowledge.
- It should show the techniques of teaching.
- It should cover the exact scope.
- It should show illustrative ideas.
- It should contain suitable subject manner.
- It should be divided into units.
- It should provide for activity.
- It should provide the continuity in the teaching process.
- It should provide for individual difference.
- It should be flexible.
- It should include the summary.
- It should refer to reference material.
- It should include assignments for students.
- It should provide for self-evaluation.

Advantages of Planning a Lesson

- It helps the teacher to be systematic, orderly in the treatment of the subject matter.
- It provides confidence and self-reliance to the teacher. She set fourth some definite aims that she is to develop in students through certain activities or some other means.
- It encourages the continuity in the teaching process and unnecessary repetition is avoided.
- The interest of the students can be maintained throughout the lesson when it is well planned.

Steps Involved in Planning a Lesson

There are few steps which should be followed while making a lesson plan. These are,

- **Preparation/introduction:** This in fact, is a means of exploration of the student's knowledge which helps to lead them onto the lesson. The teacher needs to prepare the students to receive new knowledge. She can introduce the lesson by testing the pervious knowledge of the student by asking questions. This in turn may reveal their, ignorance; arouse interest and curiosity to learn new matter. Charts, maps, diagrams, pictures also can be used.
- **Presentation:** The aim of lesson plan should clearly state before the presentation

of the subject matter, which helps both the teacher and the student to have a common pursuit.

- During presentation in this stage both the teacher and the student must actively participate in the teaching learning process. The students must get some new ideas and knowledge.
- Questioning, discussion, appropriate examples from real life situations should feature in presentation to make the presentation interesting and to motivate the students to learn.
- *Teaching aids:* Teaching aids should be used to make the lessons meaningful, clear, explanatory and comprehensive.
- Black board summary can be developed side by side.

- **Comparison or association:** This step is important where the students are given examples and they are asked to observe carefully and compare them with other set of examples and facts. These will enable the student to deduce definition and arrive at generalizations on their own.
- **Generalization:** This step involves reflective thinking. The knowledge presented through the lesson should be thought provoking, innovating and stimulating to assist the students to generalize and untested formula, etc.,
- **Application:** The students make use of the knowledge acquire in familiar and unfamiliar situations and at the same time it tests the validity of the generalizations arrived at by the students. The students of nursing especially need to develop the skill of learning to apply the knowledge and skills gained in the classroom in their day to day nursing practice in the wards, clinic and home situations. This makes learning more permanent and worthwhile.
- **Recapitulation:** This being the last step in the planning of a lesson, understanding and comprehension of the subject matter taught by the teacher can be tested by asking suitable, stimulating and provotal questions to be students on the topic.

This also gives a feedback to the teacher regarding the efficacy of the methods of teaching adopted by her. It tells whether further explanation, clarifications, etc., are needed or not, as well.

Suggested performa for a lesson plan: There are various performa which can be used as an outline for lesson plan. Whatever format is used the essential elements which should feature in a lesson plan are

- Statement of central and contributory objectives.
- Relationship of the present lesson with the previous lesson.
- Inclusion of learning objectives (refer to student activities).
- Inclusion of learning activities (refer to teacher activities).
- Methods of teaching to be used.
- Audio-visual aids to be used.
- Summary of the lesson being taught.
- Evaluative questions.
- Assignments for students.
- References on the topic of the lesson.

COURSE PLAN

Course content and learning experiences need to be organized so that they serve the educational objectives. The concept of student centered learning, problem solving, nursing process and a variety of modes of learning may have to be considered for vitalizing the teaching and learning activities for the students. The key to successful teaching is good planning. It serves as a guideline for the teacher as well as for the student in creating the atmosphere.

Definition: A course may be defined as complete serious of studies leading to graduation or a degree in case of BSc (N) course requiring completion of several short courses.

Purposes of Course Planning

- To ensure autonomy.
- It gives stability.
- It helps to solve the problem.
- It supports the curriculum process.

- It secures future progress.
- It brings about improvements.
- It promotes utilization of resources.
- It contributes to general planning.

Principles of Course Planning

- **State the objectives** in behavioral terms which are to be achieved.
- **Establish sequence:** Arrange the content, according to the learning experiences from simple to complex, known to unknown, whole to part. Should be based on prerequisites of learning, arranged in time sequence. Place the content materials into some sort of order of succession, e.g., in teaching bed making, plan teaching of simple open bed first, admission beds next and then to more complex bed making like post-operative beds and fracture beds, renal beds, etc.
- **Ensure logical and psychological continuity:**
  - Organize the course focusing around students rather than the subject matter.
  - It should be adapted to the level of the students.
  - It should allow variation from students (individual differences).
  - It should encourage logical memory and problem solving.
  - Combining logical and psychological requirements help the teacher to
    - Organize content into fewer units.
    - Helps the student to develop easy understanding of important concepts.
    - To avoid automized learning and repetitions.

  For example, teaching different types of diets be arranged from teaching about balanced diet, fluid diet to different therapeutic diets prepared in various diseased conditions. The students may learn to prepare some of these diets.
- **Provide cumulative learning:** Provide reinforcement by continuing the use of these concepts and activities which have been acquired either through practice or through use in a new context, such as reinforcement on communication skills, problem solving approach, community orientation, and patient centered teaching, personalized care, approach decision making. For example, student nurses learn to give bed bath in first year the same experience in reinforced in various other clinical situations where patient with different condition/disease need to be given a bed bath using different techniques according to availability of recourses, condition of patient, etc., the concepts which need constant and continuing reinforcement are included in core curriculum content.
- **Plan for integration:** Integration or transfer of learning is not necessarily spontaneous, pointing out application of learning acquire in one situation into another situation/field results in likely transfer of learning. Integration happens within an individual but teacher have plan related courses horizontally so that knowledge of one area can be transferred to another area. For example, teaching of baby in hospital under midwifery nursing and baby bath at home in community health nursing, simultaneously. Again application of learning that anxiety causes stress and stress is detrimental towards patient's response to recovery in actual nursing care of patients is transfer of learning. Through knowledge helps us to remember but the best way to retain what is learnt its to use it, otherwise learning gets rested too.
- **Unity curriculum:** Combine closely related subjects so as reduce unmanageable bulk of specialized subjects and bring some unity into atomized specialization, e.g., gynecological nursing and maternity nursing can be effectively combination in order to reduce bulk. Focusing center determines the ideas that will stand out the ideas to be put together. It also reduces the unit to manageable size and serves as a center of organization. We have combined psychology, educational psychology,

sociology and economics in group title behavioral sciences.

- **Select an approach** that is acceptable to all teachers, e.g., problem solving.
- **Provide variety in modes of learning:** Include innovative ideas in modes of learning. Group discussion, independent study modules, and problem solving approaches facilitate better learning. The assignments planned should be thought provoking and not just copying from books. Encourages library utilization reading of nursing journals of India by the teachers as well as by the students.

Content for a course plan: For organized and systematic preparation of course plan there are a few essential contents which should feature in the plan.

- Mention the objectives or outcomes to be achieved through the given course, e.g., pediatric nursing, community health nursing, midwifery, etc.
- Specify the level of learner (1st year, 2nd year, 3rd year).
- For a course in nutrition—this would give a brief course description (the general purpose for the course), e.g., this course is designed of total health care programme.
- Mention the placement of the course within the curriculum, e.g., in GNM Programme the courses an anatomy and physiology, physics, chemistry, fundamentals of nursing are placed in the 1st year.
- Organize the organization, content topic wise, unit wise or lesson plan wise.
- Describe the resources materials and methods of teaching, i.e., classroom, clinical teaching, laboratory teaching including simulation and learner centered methods of teaching.
- Give the plan of learning activities for students (e.g., assignment).
- Does the procedure for ongoing and terminal evaluation.
- Give references for teachers as well as for students.
- Schedule, place length of experience, experience record, observations, procures,

plan for rotation and clinical teaching in cases of the courses associated with field experiences, supervised and guided practice.

Process of organization learning experience: Certain steps involved in the organization, which are:

- Agreeing upon the general scheme of organization, the staff concerned for teaching the course must discuss and agree on the general scheme of organization of the course for its smooth implementation.
- There should be an agreement regarding the general principles of organization, i.e., community, sequence and integration.
- The basic units should be included.
- Flexible plans should be developed which can be bundled each teacher.
- The plan should be used for particular activities for a particular course.

Elements of course planning: A course planning would contain

- Objectives.
- Specification for the level of learners.
- Placement in the curriculum.
- Resource materials needed for the course.
- Unit plans.
- Evaluation measures.
- Bibliography.

Characteristics of course planning: According to Elliot and Mosier,

- Plan must be a continuous process.
- Plan must find a definite place in educational organization.
- Plan should take into consideration resources and establish conditions of work.
- It must be realistic and practical.
- It must involve active and continuing participation of all interested individual/ groups.
- The content and scope of plan should be determined by the needs of the individuals and groups to be served.
- It should utilize the services of specialties without allowing them to dominate.
- It should provide opportunity for all persons and groups to understand and appreciate the plan.

- Course plan should provide continuous evaluation.
- It should have opportunity for modification for future action.
- Efficient and effective planning saves time, effort and money.
- Planning needs redefinition of educational objectives.
- It has to decide priorities.
- It has to equalize the educational opportunities.

The teacher roles in course planning:
- Teacher plan units of work.
- She should select materials and learning activities according to the level of students.
- She should plan carefully.
- She should avoid gaps and non-projective repetition in subject matter content.
- She should provide for inforcement you previous learning.
- She has to setup working groups.
- She has to arrange the teaching learning environments and seek to move student's forward goals that often are not at all explicit.
- She should formulate the objectives prior to the planning.
- She should possess knowledge adequately.
- She should have skills related to the area that they are teaching.
- The teacher's plan should focuses on general objectives of the course, the unit and class plan.
- She should be efficient in preparing course plan.
- The teacher plans carefully by bringing into synthesis those conditions that are known to her.
- She should be accountable every step of planning.
- She should plan equally to all the students.

UNIT PLAN

A unit may be small covering only four hours of activity, or it may be large covering several weeks or even months of activities. For example, the unit on normal labor may take 2-3 weeks because it consists of learning about stages of labor, physiological changes, management of labor including practical experiences. A number of lessons may be required to complete the unit. Each lesson is a part of the whole unit and leads to the development to subsequent lesson in the unit.

Definition: Planning the unit is known as 'unit planning'. A unit consists of a comprehensive series of related and meaningful activities to achieve the purpose, educational objectives by providing significant educational experience that would result in appropriate behavioral changes in the learners.

Characteristics of Unit Plan

- Takes place in terms of whole rather than fractions.
- Provides for verbal and horizontal organization of learning experiences.
- Take place effectively with understanding and acceptance of goals.
- Provide a sound basis for evaluation.

Criteria of Good Unit Plan

- The needs, capabilities and interests of the students should be kept in view.
- A variety of experiences like field trips, experiments, demonstrations, projects etc.,
- A previous experience and background of the students should be taken into account.
- It should provide to new experiences which students have not gained before.
- Familiar and related topics should be included in the unit.
- It should be related to the social and physical environment of the students.

Essential Activities in Planning a Unit

There are certain activities which are involved while planning and developing all teaching-learning units.

- **Selection and statements of objectives:** Educational objectives are the statements of the outcome in terms of desirable changes in behavior which are manifested as a result of specific teaching learning activities.

- **Selection of content:** The knowledge or the content components of the unit plan refers to all the knowledge in the form of facts, concepts, and principles, etc., which are required to attain the objectives of the unit. The content and learning experience for a unit vary according to the type of unit, objectives, and the field of study.
- Distribution of time and the allotment of time
- Organization of content of the unit.
- Selection of teaching and learning activities.
- Teachers experience.
- Selection of methods of evaluation.
- Selection of references.

Advantages of Unit Plan of Instruction

- Unit plan idea adds more meaning to the learning activities in the institution because of the purposefulness of the unit activities and their interrelatedness.
- As unit serves as an organizing principle for the materials and the procedure of learning, the unit plan organizes the classroom work/activities.
- Unit plan shows direction to learning by centering specific aims, objectives and goals.

- Schörling states, it is easier to provide for individual differences, directed study, socialization and remedial teaching in the unit plan of instruction; it is also possible to have a sensible balance between individual or independent work and co-operative or group activities.
- The unit plan vitalizes learning. The teacher can plan activities which can change the classroom, from an isolated social situation into a vital laboratory of life by basing selection and organization of a material on human needs and the persistent problems of life.

COMPARISON BETWEEN EDUCATION PROCESS AND NURSING PROCESS

Differences comparison between process elements: Nursing education process education process and nursing process.

- Assessment appraise physical and ascertain (determine) learning needs psychological needs. Readiness (willing) to learn and learning styles.
- Planning develop care plan based develop teaching plan based on mutually goal setting mutually predetermined behavioral to meet individual needs. Outcomes to meet individual needs.

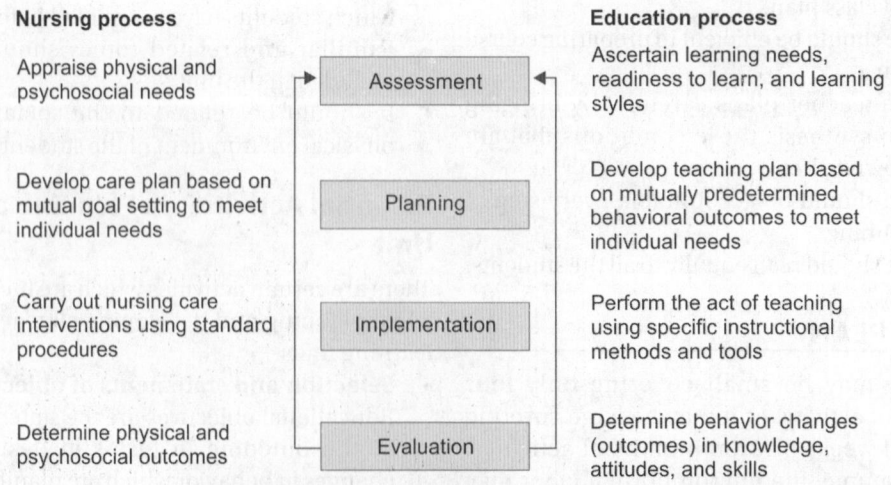

Nursing process		Education process
Appraise physical and psychosocial needs	Assessment	Ascertain learning needs, readiness to learn, and learning styles
Develop care plan based on mutual goal setting to meet individual needs	Planning	Develop teaching plan based on mutually predetermined behavioral outcomes to meet individual needs
Carry out nursing care interventions using standard procedures	Implementation	Perform the act of teaching using specific instructional methods and tools
Determine physical and psychosocial outcomes	Evaluation	Determine behavior changes (outcomes) in knowledge, attitudes, and skills

Fig. 2.10: Education process parallels nursing process.

- Implementation carryout nursing care perform the act of teaching using interventions using specific instructional methods.
- Evaluation: Determine physical and determine behavioral changes psychological outcomes (Outcomes) in knowledge, attitude and practical skills.

Similarities

- They are consisting of the four basic elements of (assessment, planning, implementation and evaluation).
- They are logical, scientifically-based frame works for nursing.
- They provide a rationale basis for nursing practice rather than an intuitive (spontaneous) one.
- They are methods for monitoring and judging the overall quality of educational process and nursing interventions based on objective, data and scientific criteria.
- If the outcomes in either process are not achieved, as determined by evaluation, the nursing process or the education process can and should begin again through reassessment, re-planning and re-implementation.

CONCLUSION

Teaching and learning is a process that includes many variables. These variables interact as learners work toward their goals and incorporate new knowledge, behaviors, and skills that add to their range of learning experiences. It is a combined process where a teacher assesses understanding needs, establishes particular learning objectives, formulates teaching and memorizing strategies, enforces a plan of work, and assesses the outcomes of the instruction.

BIBLIOGRAPHY

1. Brown H, Ciuffetelli DC (Eds). Foundational methods: Understanding teaching and learning. Toronto: Pearson Education 2009.
2. Cooper, James M. Classroom teaching skills. Boston, New York: Houghton Mifflin Company.
3. Mayer R. Thinking, Problem Solving, Cognition. WH Freeman and Company, New York 1983.
4. Mason D. Promoting health literacy: Patient teaching is a vital nursing function. American Journal of Nursing, 2001;101(2): 7.
5. Rankin SH, Stallings KD. Patient Education: Principles and Practices. 4th ed. Philadelphia: Lippincott 2001.

3

CHAPTER

Teaching Methods in Education

INTRODUCTION

Education must begin with the child and must be adapted to the needs and requirements of the child as he grows. Only in this manner, an individual will be made socially efficient. Progressive methods of teaching provide suitable opportunities for 'learning by doing', for 'experimentation' and for 'co-operation'. Every teacher must devise his own method, good method can result only from the following up of broad principles, e.g., orderly arranging of procedure in teaching, arrangement of subject matter which will avoid waste of time and energy. A method must link up the teacher and her pupils into an organic relationship with constant mutual interaction.

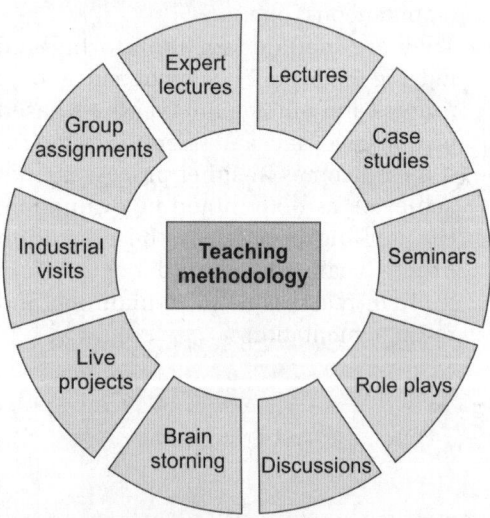

Fig. 3.1: Types of teaching methods.

DEFINITIONS

- The method of teaching in which approaches most likely to the method of investigation. **—Burke**
- A device implies the external modem or form which teaching may take from time-to-time.
- A teaching method comprises the principles and methods used by teachers to enable student learning. These strategies are determined partly on subject matter to be taught and partly by the nature of the learner.

MEANING OF METHODS OF TEACHING

The procedural dimension in the educative process refers to the methods and techniques, which may he used by the teacher or the learner to achieve the desired educational objectives. The dimensions like substantive, the environmental, the human relations and the procedural dimensions are interrelated. Knowledge environment and human relations all affect the procedural aspect of education. Teaching in nursing encompasses both cognitive, and artistic aspects. Teaching skill and technical competency in teaching have effect on student's learning. Art in teaching is necessary and can be developed. Systematic attention to methods and materials of teaching and learning as well as mastery of the subject matter are essential for the development of artistic teaching.

OBJECTIVES OF METHODS OF TEACHING

- Aim at developing, 'love for work'.
- Inculcates the desire to do work with the maximum efficiency which one is capable of.
- Develops the capacity for clear thinking.
- Provides adequate opportunities for participation in freely accepted projects and activities in which cooperation and discipline are constantly in demand.
- Expands students' interest.
- Provides opportunities to pupils to apply practically the knowledge and skill acquired by them.
- They should adapt to the 3A's—Age, Ability, and Aptitude of the student.
- Eagerness of the inspectorate: Officers in education department are personally eager to see experimentation within reasonable limits.
- General support of the profession.
- Teamwork and a sense of security.
- Mastery of the subject-matter.
- Provision for a good library and teaching-learning material.
- Role of teachers' training institutes.
- Cooperation of the parents.

PRINCIPLES FOR SELECTION OF TEACHING METHODS

- Methods should be suited to the objectives and the content of the course.
- Methods should be adapted to the capacity of the student.
- Methods should be in accord with sound psychological principles.
- Methods should suit the Teacher personally and capitalize on her special assets.
- Methods should be used creatively.

CLASSIFICATIONS OF METHODS OF TEACHING

- **Inspirational methods:** Based on high activity on the part of the teacher, e.g. simulation and micro-teaching.
- **Expository methods:** Cognitive emphasis is high, while student activity and emphasis on experience is low, e.g. lecture method.
- **Natural learning method:** Learning takes place in a natural way, e.g. field trips.
- **Individualized methods:** Main emphasis is for each learner to learn at his own pace, e.g. programmed instruction, self-study, case method, and computer oriented instruction.
- **Encounter methods:** Providing experience through confrontation or through encounter effective for change in basic behavioral patterns and developing new ways of looking at things, e.g. role play, simulation.
- **Discovery methods:** These methods are high on all dimensions like learner activity, experience, experimentation by the learner and cognitive understanding, e.g. problem-solving technique.
- **Group methods,** e.g. project method, socialized classroom method.

CHARACTERISTICS OF METHODS OF TEACHING

- Imparting knowledge in an efficient manner.
- Inculcates desirable values and proper attitudes and habits of work in the students.
- Create a genuine attachment to work and a desire to do it as efficiently, honestly, and thoroughly as possible.
- The principle of 'verbalism and memorization' activity and, project method' should be assimilated in school practice.
- Provides opportunities for students to learn actively and to apply practically the knowledge that they have acquired in the classroom.
- Clear thinking and clear expression both in speech and writing has to take place.

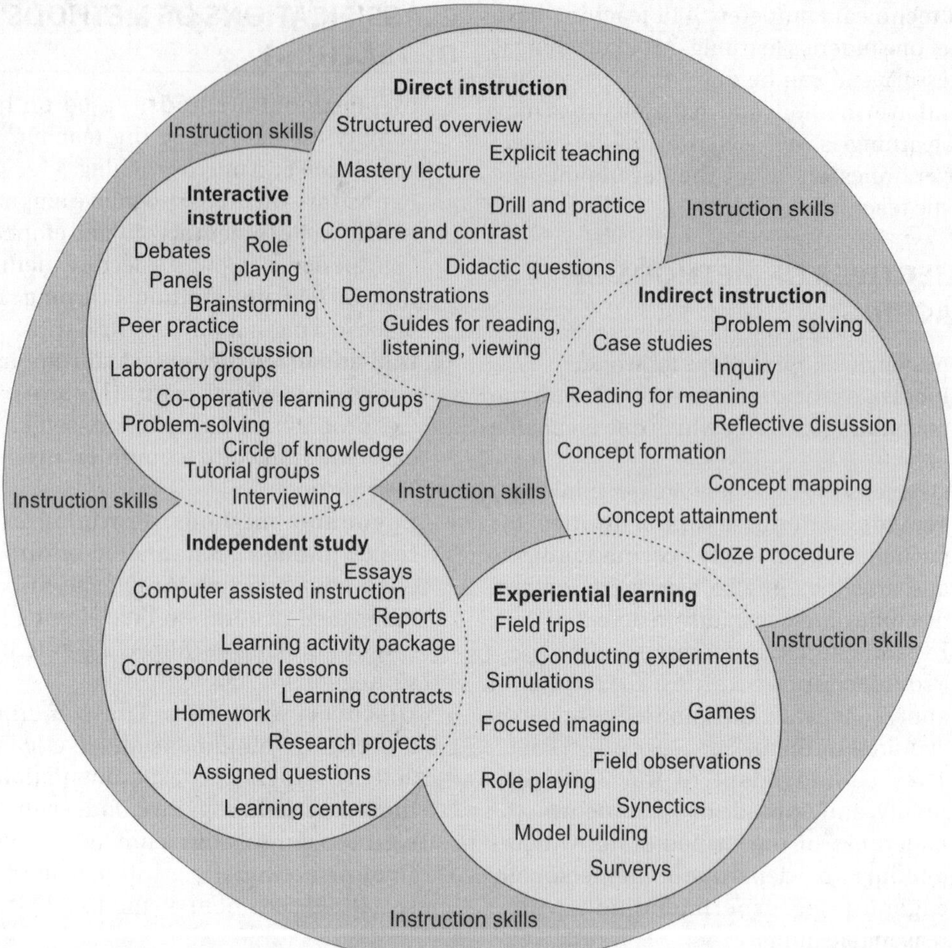

Direct instruction
Structured overview
Instruction skills
Explicit teaching
Mastery lecture
Interactive instruction
Drill and practice
Instruction skills
Compare and contrast
Debates Role playing
Panels
Didactic questions
Brainstorming
Demonstrations **Indirect instruction**
Peer practice
Guides for reading, Problem solving
Discussion listening, viewing Case studies
Laboratory groups Inquiry
Co-operative learning groups Reading for meaning
Problem-solving Reflective disussion
Circle of knowledge Concept formation
Tutorial groups Concept mapping
Instruction skills Interviewing Instruction skills Concept attainment
Independent study Cloze procedure
Essays
Computer assisted instruction **Experiential learning**
Reports Field trips
Learning activity package Conducting experiments Instruction skills
Correspondence lessons Simulations
Learning contracts Games
Homework Focused imaging
Research projects Field observations
Assigned questions Role playing
Learning centers Synectics
Model building
Surverys
Instruction skills

Fig. 3.2: Instructional skills.

Flowchart 3.1: Approaches/methods of teaching.

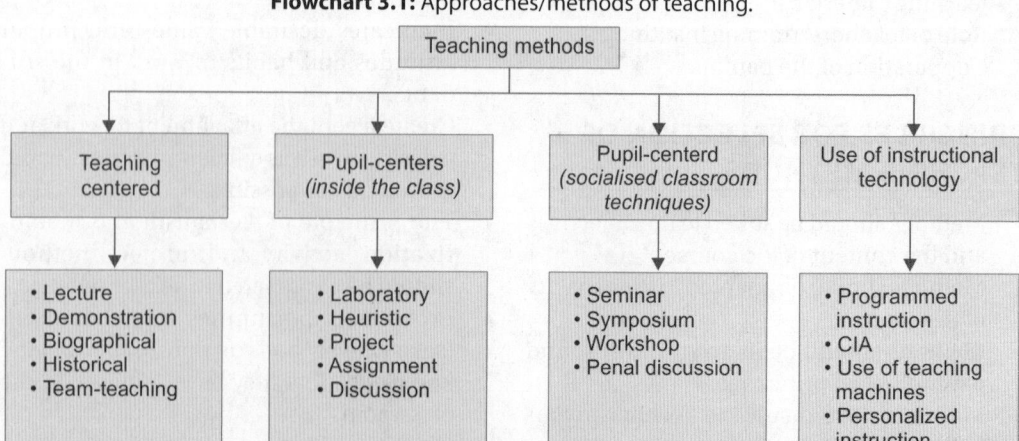

Teaching centered	Pupil-centers (inside the class)	Pupil-centerd (socialised classroom techniques)	Use of instructional technology
• Lecture • Demonstration • Biographical • Historical • Team-teaching	• Laboratory • Heuristic • Project • Assignment • Discussion	• Seminar • Symposium • Workshop • Penal discussion	• Programmed instruction • CIA • Use of teaching machines • Personalized instruction

- Trains the learners in the techniques of study, methods of acquiring knowledge through personal effort and initiative.
- A well-thought-out attempt should be made to adopt methods of instruction in order to benefit all categories of students.
- Opportunity for the students should be provided to work in groups and to carry out group projects and activities to develop in them the qualities necessary for group life and for cooperative work.

LECTURE METHOD

The lecture method has been the earliest known method of instruction. At present, the method is used to a greater extent in colleges only. Many peoples, young people cannot stand sustained narration since their span. The lecture method is a one-way communication system and in a classroom, only the teacher remains active and the students passive.

Definitions of Lecture Method

- Lecture method is talk giving specified information to the class or long serious speech.   **—Oxford Dictionary**
- The lecture is an excellent method for presenting information to a large number of persons in a short period of time.
          — A Adivi Reddy

Purposes of Lecture Method

- Lecture method is only appropriate method for making available to a large class.
- It draws the attention of the student in its vital elements and bring students abstract of development in the forefront of research.
- It helps to promote the students with factual basis from which to build concepts by concrete examples.
- Students can feasible involving in arriving at the general information like formulation of laws.

Principles of Lecture Method

- **Principle of aim:** Lecture is based on aim, nobody likes aimless lecture. Even the best teacher will fail if his lecture is not based on some objectives.
- **Principles of activity:** If you want to learn a thing you have to actively participate.
- **Principle of correlation:** The lecture is not effective lecture is scientific planning. The subject matter of the topic which is sort to be taught should be well planned.
- **Principles of looking ahead:** Good lecture is always prognostic on the basis of the past experiences of a teacher; certain predictors are made about the future of the child.

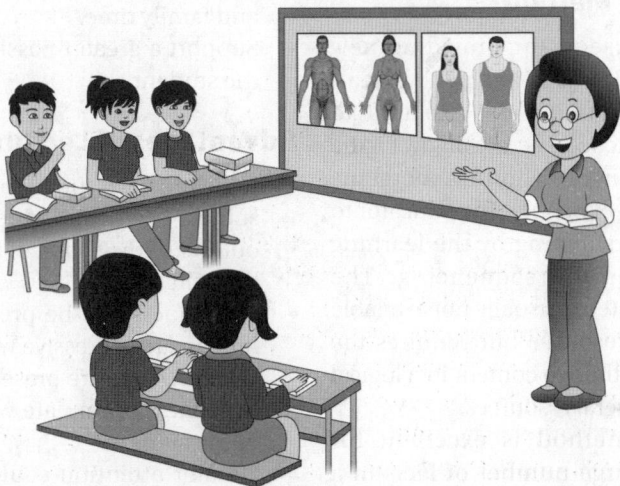

Fig. 3.3: Lecture method of teaching.

Table 3.1: Uses, advantages and disadvantages of lecture method.

Lecture Method		
Uses	**Advantages**	**Disadvantages**
• To orient students. • To introduce a subject. • To give directions on procedures. • To present basic material. • To introduce a demonstration, discussion, or performance. • To illustrate application of rules, principles, or concepts. • To review, clarify, emphasize, or summaries.	• Saves time. • Permits flexibility. • Requires less rigid space requirement. • Permits adaptability. • Permits versatility. • Permits better center over contact and sequence.	• Involves one-way communication. • Poses problems in skill teaching. • Encourages student passiveness. • Poses difficulty in gauging student reaction. • Require highly skilled instructors.

- **Good lecture needs effective preparation:** The lecture has to be prepared physically, socially, emotionally, and spiritually to enable him to take the lecture.

The chief characteristics of the lecture methods are as follows:

- Usually, it is an organized presentation.
- It can be used to cover thoroughly the subject matter.
- It is adaptable to large groups.
- It conserves time.
- Results are easy to cheek.
- Listeners sometimes absorb information without thinking.

Uses of Lecture Method

- Lectures are useful for providing new information, such as a new policy, treatment, protocol or concept related to professional practice. Lectures allow for the transmission of information in a short time to a large group of people. The educator to promote understanding by the learning group controls the sequencing. The material presented is usually not available from a single resource bur requires the educator to synthesize content in a logical format from several resources.
- The lecture method is excellent for presenting a large number of facts in a short period.

- It is useful in introducing new subjects in summarizing the literature in a field in reviewing, integrating different ideas and concepts into an orderly system of thought. It is often useful for advanced students.
- It is difficult to meet individual needs by the lecture method, as there is little personal relationship between teacher and students.
- A lecture should be well-organized with ideas developed in sequence. Local experience should be used to illustrate statements.
- A lecture should relate past, present, and future materials on the subject.
- Most economical interns of use of space and family time.
- Support a greater passivity on the part of the student.

Advantages of Lecture Method

- A proper perspective and orientation subject can be presented and the general outline of the scope of the subject can be brought out.
- Many facts can be presented in a short time in an impressive way.
- When lecture are presented in series, it is possible to stimulate very goods interest in the subject.
- Greater attention could be secured and maintained as interest leads to attention.

- The language may be made suitable to all members of audience.
- The spoken word has a greater weight than the mute appeal by books.
- Lectures can be advantageously made use of for presenting a number of facts belonging to the different subjects and the impressions thus created would be of a longstanding value.
- Lectures facilitate inter-disciplinary approach to topics.

Criticism of the Lecture Method

- **The lecture is time-consuming:** It is all too true that the lecture offers no advantage and takes up much valuable time when it covers self-explanatory information that can be found easily in the textbook.
- **The lecture provides little student activity:** While this may appear to be a basic fault, it actually is not. It is true that the teacher prepares, organizes, and presents the lecture and it is equally true that the student sits, listens and takes notes.
- **The lecture requires special skill:** This fault is in itself, proof of the fact that the lecture, not the method is weak. There must be mastery of subject matter before a lecture can be successful, but that is not a fault of the lecture.
- **The lecture is not readily analyzed and summarized by the student:** When this is the case, it is generally the fault not of the method but of the teacher. For if the teacher plans her lecture carefully, organizing it under sub-heading and then delivering it slowly, stating the major points with emphasis, the student will be able to take good notes.
- **The lecture is sometimes poorly adapted to the perceptive ability of the students:** It seems impossible that a teacher can spend a whole term lecturing on a subject without creating understanding in the students, yet this sometimes happens.
- **The lecture is likely to become a sustained dictation exercise:** This obvious not a weakness but an abuse of the lecture method and a frequent one in the school of nursing.

Hints for Successful Lecturing

- Present an outline of the lecture (use the black board, overhead transparency or handout) and refer to it as you move from point to point.
- Repeat point in several different ways.
- Use short sentences.
- Stress important points (through your tone or explicit comments).
- Pause to give listeners time to think and write.
- Use lecture to compliment, not simply repeat the text.
- Avoid racing through the last part of the lecture. This is a common error made by the instructor wishing to give too much information into the allotted time.
- Schedule time for discussion in the same or separate class periods as the lecture.
- Preparation reduced stress, frustration, insecurity and consequent and ineffective.

Disadvantages of Lecture Method

- It is a waste of time to repeat the matter already presented in books. Independent reading will be disturbed as a result if this.
- The teacher to make the lecture impressive may care more for the manner and style and very little for the content matter.
- If the lecture is very fast in lecturing, the pupils cannot easily take notes and will not have any written record of the salient points made out by them.

| The lecture is time consuming |
| The lecture provides little student activity |
| The lecture requires special skill |
| The lecture is not readily analyzed and summarized |
| The lecture is sometimes poorly adapted |
| The lecture is likely to become a sustained dictation exercise |

Fig. 3.4: Criticism of lecture method.

- Lectures are said to kill the imitative of pupils and their problem-solving attitude disappears.
- Lectures create mental inertia in class rooms, i.e., non-analysis of the lecture will result in non-co-operation between the minds of the pupils and teacher.
- The lecture may lose sight of the subject matter.
- Dictation would become prominent in the course of lectures.

Guidelines for a Teacher for Lecturing

- Maintain good eye contact. Make the learners feel what you have to say is directed to each one personally. Your eyes as well as your voice communicate to them; and their eyes, facial expressions, and reactions communicate to you. Watch for indications of doubt, misunderstanding, a desire to participate, fatigue, or a lack of interest.
- Maintain a high degree of enthusiasm.
- Speak in a natural, conversational voice. Enunciate your words clearly. Make certain the learners can hear every spoken word.
- Emphasize important points by the use of gestures, repetition, and variation in voice inflection.
- Check learners' comprehension carefully throughout the presentation by watching the faces of the learners and by questioning. Observing facial expressions as an indication of doubt or misunderstanding is not a sure way of checking on learner's comprehension. The best time to clear away mental fog is when the fog develops. Mental fog tends to create a mental block that prevents the learners from concentrating on the subject matter being presented.
- Instruct on the class level. Use words, explanations, questions, and the like, directed to the needs of the average learner in the class. Identify and prepare instructional aids to illustrate the points.

- Stimulate learners to think. Think, as used here, refers to creative thinking rather than to a mere recall of facts previously learned. Use a number of instructional devices for stimulating learners thinking. Among those devices are thought—provoking questions, class discussions.
- Provide examples to link the subject matter to the lives of the learners.
- Sequence the content logically, systematically, and sequentially building upon previous content areas.
- Avoid being prescriptive and try to be provocative.
- Maintain time stipulations.
- A diverse range of instructional materials can be used to support the content, such as slides, charts, posters, flannel and so on.

DISCUSSION METHOD

A discussion is a conversation with a focal point, such as a specific topic, question, concept, or problem, in which there is a sincere desire to arrive at a decision. It is basically a co-operative, problem-solving activity which seeks a consensus regarding the solution of a problem rather than decision by majority of vote. That is, it is the working together in the search for the solutions of a problem of common concern rather than just talking about a topic.

General Principles of Discussion

The general principles relating to the organization of discussion are given below:
- There should be a clearly defined objective which is understood by all the participants.
- There should be a leader to guide and co-ordinate the proceedings.
- The main points in the discussion should be recorded as it is going on either on the blackboard or by a 'recorder' elected by the group.
- Every person should feel free to participate.
- Timid persons should be encouraged to contribute.
- All points of view should be fairly considered.

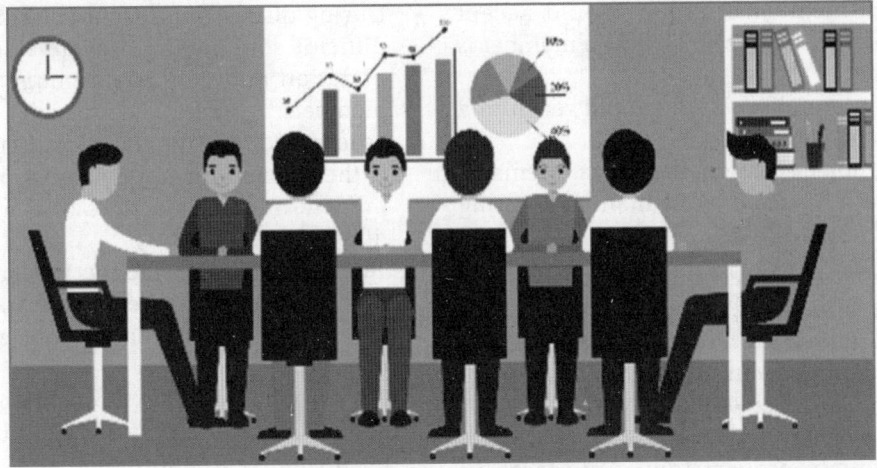

Fig. 3.5: Discussion method.

Table 3.2: Uses, advantages and disadvantages of discussion method.

Discussion Method		
Uses	**Advantages**	**Disadvantages**
• To develop imaginative solutions to problems. • To stimulate thinking and interest and to secure student participation. • To emphasis, main teaching points. • To supplement lectures, reading, or laboratory exercises. • To determine how well student understands concepts and principles. • To prepare students for application of theory of procedure. • To summaries clarify points or review.	• Increase students interest. • Increase student's acceptance and commitments. • Utilise student knowledge and experience. • Results in more permanent learning because high degree of student participation.	• Require highly skilled instructor. • Requires preparation by student. • Limits content. • Consumes time. • Restricts size of groups.

- Discussions should keep to the point.
- The discussion should be properly closed with a report, decision, recommendation, or summing up of the matters discussed.
- The members of the group should come to the discussion with a basic knowledge of the topic to be discussed.

Discussion Technique

A well conducted group discussion with adequate resources is very effective in reaching decisions based on the ideas of all students. It is effective in changing the attitude and behavior of students.

Rules to be followed for group discussion:
- Ideas or views expressed by the group members should be clear and concise.
- The members have to listen to each other what is discussed among them.
- There should not be any interruption when the member of the group is discussing or speaking.

- Each member of group should accept the criticism gracefully, if by a member is done.
- The group discussion should reach to a conclusion.
- In group discussion, the relevant remarks should be made by its members during discussion.

Group discussion technique involves:

- Proper planning of topic with objectives and guidelines. Proper planning of the environment in which discussion is arranged, i.e. environment should be non-threatening.
- Adequate preparation of students in relation to topic to be discussed is required for the success of group discussion.
- Role of each member of group, leader of group and role of teacher need to be clarified.
- Teacher opens the discussion session with brief introduction of topic to be discussed with objectives and guidelines.
- Students are invited to express their ideas or view points.
- During discussion, teacher assumes the role of facilitator.
- One of the students among group records the proceedings.
- Teacher controls the group discussion by discouraging over talkative students and involving the passive students in discussion.

- During discussion, teacher clarifies the difficult statements to avoid misinterpretation and confusion among group members.
- Teacher redirects the course of discussion, if the discussion is deviated from the predetermined objectives or if wasting time.
- Teacher guides the students in relation to pros and cons of the view points and after analyzing the view points, a consensus is reached.
- After group discussion, a concluding note in the form of summary of the discussion, performance of students and a few words of appreciation to encourage the students to participate in forthcoming discussions.

Advantages of Discussion Method

- Group discussion method involved active participation of students and promote learning abilities of students.
- Students self-esteem is enhanced as their view points or suggestions are accepted.
- Help the students to develop problem solving technique.
- Develops self-confidence among members of group.
- Provides an opportunity to students to express views or skills.
- Develops social skills and a feeling of team activity.

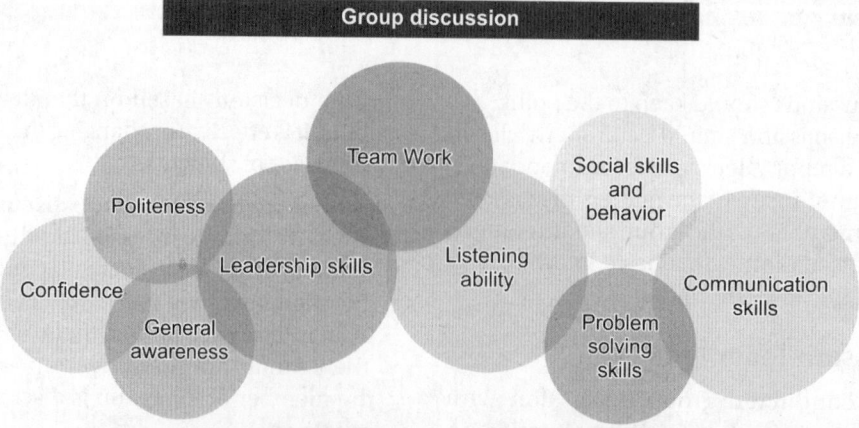

Fig. 3.6: Group discussion techniques.

- Develops ability among students to compare and contrast the knowledge on particular topic.

Disadvantages of Discussion Method

- Group discussion method is time-consuming as it is difficult to complete the discussion within time.
- Without adequate preparation of students, group discussion method is not so useful as meaningful exchanges of views will not occur among students.
- Sometimes, over talkative students overcome others and make other members passive.
- Group discussion method is not effective for a larger group i.e. more than twenty members.

Forms of Discussion

- **Class discussion:** Sometimes, the teacher may select the discussion method for teaching a particular topic, with the whole class participating as one group. This can be managed quite efficiently if the class is not too large. The teacher, acting, as leader, will present the topic, guide and direct the discussion, note the main points on the blackboard and assist the group in summing up. This is a useful method when the students have a prior knowledge of the subject; it can also serve as a learning experience for students on how to conduct discussions.
- **Group discussion (6-20 members):** When a class is large or when it is desirable to discuss several aspects of a topic, it is useful to divide the class into groups. The teacher may act as a Chairman, introducing the topic for discussion, helping the students to organize themselves into group being available to assist the group as required, receiving the reports at the end of the allotted time, leading general discussion, clarifying points and summarizing up. Each group should appoint its own leader and recorder.

The following rules are followed during discussion:
- Express the ideas clearly and concisely.
- Listen to what others say.
- Do not interrupt when others are speaking.
- Make only relevant remarks.
- Accept criticism gracefully.
- Help to reach conclusions.

- **Panel discussion:** In a panel discussion, a small group of 4–8 persons qualified to talk carry on group conversation in front of large audience. When audience is large and total participation is not feasible, the panel retains the advantages of discussion group. It is more formal than a discussion and less formal than a lecture. A panel consists of a few members who come prepared to exchange ideas and views on a particular subject under the leadership of a chairman. When used as a method of teaching, the panel may be a group of experts on the subject. They prepared the subject in advance. The chairman opens the discussion by introducing the member/speakers and presenting the topic and invites the first person to speak. This discussion is carried on in conversational way, with the chairman making sure that all keep to the point. When necessary, the chairman may clarify any issue or misunderstanding or may introduce another thought so that subject will be fully covered. The discussion may

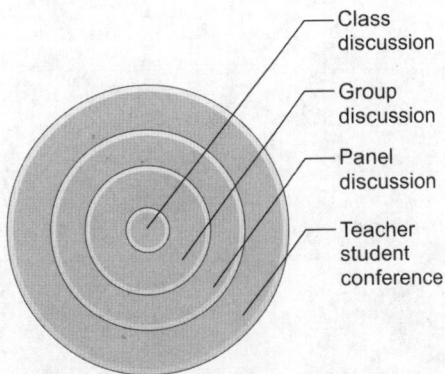

Class discussion

Group discussion

Panel discussion

Teacher student conference

Fig. 3.7: Forms of discussion.

or may not be thrown open to the floor. It is the chairman who should continue as a leader and at the end should draw together that than points and sum up the discussion.

- **Teacher student conference:** It is a personal exchange of ideas and information to help the student function in his or her professional environment. It may be used to plan more effective approach to the acquisition of subject content, or to seek information related to problems of a personal nature, which influence the student's professional success. As a method of teaching, a conference is a meeting of the teacher with a small number of, students as a group for discussion of problem, or a selected situation or before or after and observation visit.

DEMONSTRATION METHOD

Demonstration method is very important in teaching of nursing then in any other fields. It is very instructional method that is chosen depends on the learning needs of the student's time available to teach. The setting the resources and the teacher own comfort. An experienced and skilled teacher uses a variety of a techniques depends on the subject on the topic.

Objectives of Demonstration

- To give a vivid picture of the related nursing care.
- To make specific observation by the student.
- To provide a deal situation to learn the particular procedure thoroughly.
- To get a realistic idea about the procedure.
- To stimulate and encourage for the development of initiation among the students.
- To obtain active participation among the students.

Meaning of Demonstration

- Demonstration means to show procedure.
- Demonstration means performing an action to demonstrate the correct way to be done.
- Demonstration means activity that describes.
- Demonstration means program or intervention that is being tested.

Definitions of Demonstration

- Demonstration is an activity that describes or illustrates by experiment or practical application during which one displays, operates, and explains.
- Demonstration is a technique, which is often used by all the teachers to teach various subjects.
- Demonstration method is itself learning through observation and uses the several senses.
- Demonstration gives a visual representation of ideas, facts, or process.

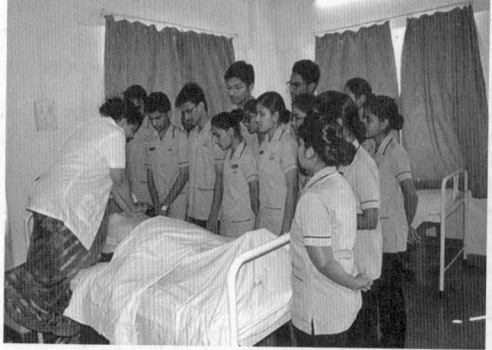
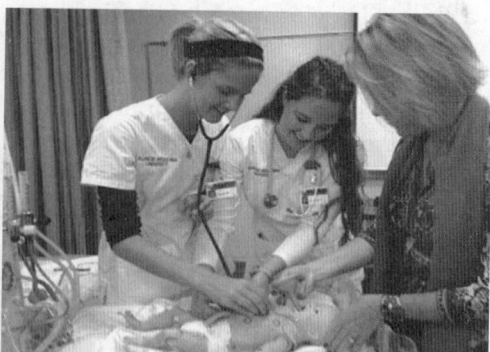

Fig. 3.8: Demonstration method of teaching.

- Demonstration means to show are performing and action to demonstrate the correct way as to be done.

Purposes of Demonstration

- To show a demonstrate method.
- To teach psychomotor skill.
- To orient a new equipment/procedure.
- To render tender loving care.
- To educate the patients.
- To promote learning by doing/imitation.
- To utilize the sense of sight and touch.
- To present the procedure with skills.

Types of Demonstration

- Individual demonstration, e.g., TPR.
- Group demonstration, e.g., lifting and transporting.
- Lecture cum demonstration, e.g., CPR, television teaching, rehabilitation procedures.
- Demonstration cum practice, e.g., TPR in ward or demonstration room.

Characteristics of Demonstration

- Demonstrator should encourage the audience and see that people understand and learn to do what is being demonstrated.
- Before starting actual working, he should tell the audience: what is being demonstrated.
- The audience, especially the interested points, the importance of the practice being demonstrated.

- The audience to go through the steps of demonstration so that they can repeat the process themselves without further helps.
- Invite questions and create an atmosphere that the audience may clarify its doubts.
- A demonstrator should be well prepared in the subject himself, and should take the help of his colleagues and teachers, whenever necessary.

Important Steps in Good Demonstration

- Preliminary assessment.
- Preparation of the patient unit and articles.
- Procedure.
- After the procedure care of the patient and articles.
- Recording and reporting.
- Know the students well; whom do you wish to teach. What is the level of the knowledge and literacy and their sphere of influence.
- Keep ready the resources.

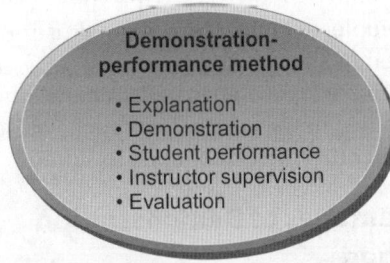

Fig. 3.9: Phases of effective demonstration.

Table 3.3: Uses, advantages and disadvantages of demonstration method.

Demonstration Method		
Uses	**Advantages**	**Disadvantages**
• To teach manipulative operations or procedures • To teach troubleshooting • To illustrate principles • To teach operation or functioning of equipment • To teach teamwork • To set standards of workmanship • To teach safety procedures	• Minimize damage and waste • Saves time • Can be presented to large groups	• Require careful preparation and rehearsal • Requires special classroom arrangements

- Remember that changing people's practices is a more delicate than surgery.
- Check whether there is sufficient staff equipment, transport, inputs, etc., before carrying over the demonstration.
- Ask oneself can freely provide knowledge inputs when needed.
- Don't try to show too much one or two variables are usually can be demonstrate at one time.
- Keep watch and demonstrate their interaction of the variable.
- Maintain proper cheeks to illustrate efficiency of the practice.
- Plan and inform campaign to ensure contact with the target students.
- Choose your co-operator carefully; be sure the co-operator cooperates with you.
- Get them involved and keep them informed.
- Consider location and accessibility both for the lay formers and VIPs.
- Involve the agencies, individuals and others in all the operations. This lens creditability to the demonstration.
- Organize field day trips and visits of people, who may be potential user of the demonstration and its results.
- Keep records prepare talks, charts, photos, slides, news, stories, technical bulletins and other aids, frequently use them.

Advantages of Demonstration Method

- It activates several senses. Teaches by exhibition any explanation. This increases learning because the more senses used, the opportunities for learning.
- It trains student in the art of careful observation a quality which is so essential to good nurse. It is method in itself learning through observation and it uses several of the senses.
- It provides opportunity for observational learning. The student not only hears the explanation, but also can see the procedure or process. It projects a mental image in the student mind, which fortifies verbal knowledge.

- It clarifies the underlying principle by demonstrating the 'why' of the procedure.
- It commands interest by use of concrete illustrations.
- It correlates theory with practice.
- It gives the teacher an opportunity to evaluate the student's knowledge of procedure and to determining reteaching is necessary.
- It points out that students must have knowledge and must be able to apply it immediately serves as strong motivation.
- Return demonstration by the student under supervision of the teacher provides an opportunity for well-directed practice before the student must use the procedure on the ward.

Uses of Demonstration Method

- To demonstrate experiments and the use of experimental equipment in the science laboratory, medical, nursing, etc.
- To demonstrate procedure in the classroom and the ward to review or revise procedure to meet a special situation or to introduce a new procedure.
- To teach the patient/client a procedure to treatment which he must carry out in the home.
- To demonstrate a procedure at the bedside or in the ward conference room, demonstration of a procedure in natural setting has more meaning.
- To demonstrate different approaches in establishing support with client, the more effective nurse-patient relationship may be established.

Steps to Demonstrating a Psychomotor Skill

I. Before demonstration:
- Formulate behavioral objectives.
- Perform a skills analysis and determine the sequence.
- Assess entry behaviors of learners, and determine pre-requisites.
- Formulate the lesson plan, with particular reference to:

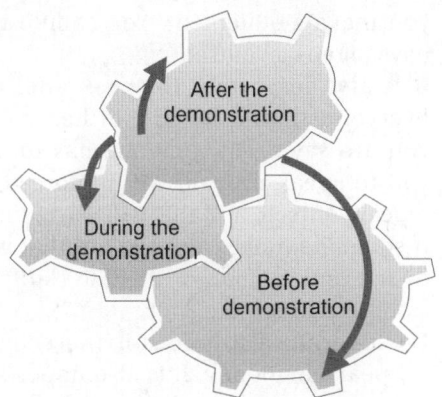

Fig. 3.10: Steps to demonstrating psychomotor skill.

a. Ensuring optimum visibility
b. Preparation for all materials

II. During the demonstration:
- State the objectives to the learner.
- Motivate them by explaining why the skill is important.
- Demonstrate the total skill at normal speed.
- Write the sequence of part skills on the chalkboard, as a checklist for the step-by-step demonstration.
- Demonstrate each part skill slowly, in the correct sequence.
- Obtain feedback by questioning and observation of non-verbal behavior.
- Avoid the use of negative examples and variations in technique.

III. After the demonstration:
- Provide immediate supervised practice, with adequate time allowance.
- Provide verbal, rather than physical guidance.
- Make the environment psychologically safe by providing a friendly atmosphere and constructive criticism.
- Remember that initial interest may wane so provide motivation and encouragement.
- Remember that learners will acquire that skill at different rates, so individualize the planning to cater for the fast and slow learner.
- Replace the both.
- Discuss.

Disadvantages of Demonstration
- Demands energy, time, and skill.
- Poor demonstration yields poor learning.
- Demands the same condition where the skill is to be performed.
- Demands interest, motivation, and knowledge.
- Does not cover all aspects of cognitive learning.

GROUP DISCUSSION

In its simple meaning, the term group discussion stands for the discussion held within a group. In this sense, group discussion as teaching strategy may be defined as some sort of discussion, i.e. interchange of ideas between students and the teacher or among a group of students, resulting into active learning for the realization of the predetermined teaching-learning objectives. This group discussion, in no way, occurs occasionally or incidentally but is planned and organized with deliberate efforts on the part of the teacher and students for achieving the set goals.

Organizational Procedure

In this strategy, students of a class may form a group along with the subject teacher. The teacher is the leader of this group on account of his status, functions, and responsibilities fulfilled by him in the organization of group discussion. Usually, the following three stages and steps are involved in the employment of group discussion at a teaching strategy:
- Planning and setting the proper stage for discussion.

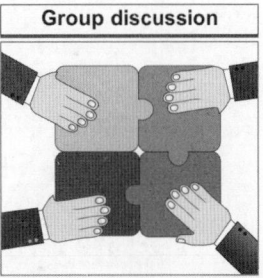
Group discussion

Fig. 3.11: Group discussion method of teaching.

- Ensuring active, democratic, and useful participation of the group members.
- Evaluating the outcomes of the discussion in the light of the realization of objectives.

At the first stage, the teacher induces the need of holding group discussion and sets the stage to make necessary assignment for facilitating the application of group discussion as a teaching strategy.

At the second stage, an environment for the proper implementation of the strategy is ensured. The teacher, at this stage, ensures that every member of the group plays active role in the group discussion. The discussions are held in a perfectly democratic style providing full and free exchange of ideas within the group. The teacher, as a group leader controls and monitors the progress of the discussion in a perfectly democratic way with his least involvement in the discussion. The aim remains to make the members engaged in useful discussion for achieving the desired teaching-learning objectives.

As happens with all the methods and strategies, the group discussion strategy also carries strengths and weaknesses as pointed out in the following way:

General Instruction

- **It is important to make sure you speak clearly.** It is also important to be concise. Speak in a manner that will allow the other members to understand exactly what you are saying. This should occur the first time you make a statement. You should not have to repeat yourself.
- **It is also important to speak audibly.** Everyone should be able to hear what you are saying. If someone has to ask you to speak up, you will be forced to repeat yourself, and this will waste time. If someone makes a statement that you do not understand, ask them to clarify in a polite manner.
- **During group discussions,** it is not enough to speak eloquently. It is also important to make sure you speak in a proper tone. While speaking harshly, it can send across the wrong message to others who are participating in the discussion. This could lead to conflicts, and it is important to avoid this. The tone of your voice and the way you speak will say a lot about how you feel about a certain topic, and it will also show how well you can speak.
- **If you do not speak in an intelligent manner,** the other members may assume that you are unintelligent, even if that is not the case. If you need to interrupt someone who is speaking, it is always important to interject their conversation in a pleasing way. Some groups may require you to raise your hand and be called upon before you can comment on a statement or idea.
- **If a statement has to be disagreed,** do it in a manner that is tactful. Always talk in a manner that is courteous to others. If you are the head of the discussion group, it is

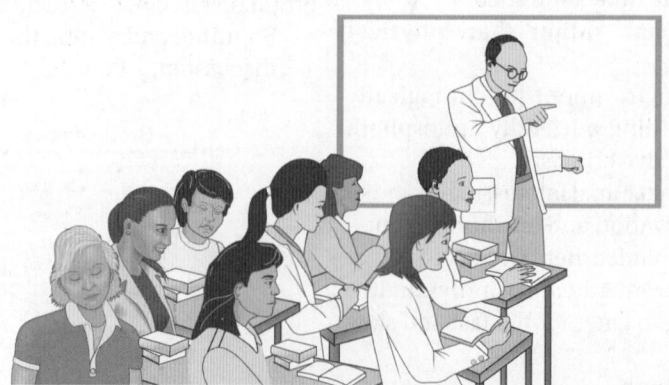

Fig. 3.12: General instruction in group discussion.

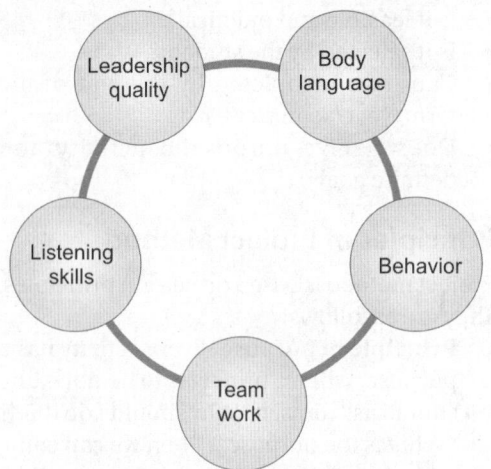

Fig. 3.13: Skills needed in group discussion.

as well as an effective leader. When a group member speaks others listen to it with patience and try to show respect for his opinion, but at the same time, they may also put up their own views in a quite democratic way.

- It teaches the students not to accept any idea blindly but to weigh it with all its pros and cons and consequences before practicing.
- It provides good training for verbal communication, expression of ideas and creative and constructive thinking.
- A free and democratic discussion provides proper check over the wrong information, ideas and ways of problem-solving.

very crucial for you to speak properly. Even though the group should be responsible for making the final decision, the members will look to you to lead them. If you cannot speak in a proper manner, your leadership abilities may be questioned. If you have to repeat yourself to the group, this will delay the amount of time it takes for the group to achieve important goals.

- **While it is important to speak eloquently,** avoid using technical terms that are not understood by the group. Being able to explain complicated concepts in a simple manner will allow the group to quickly grasp what you are trying to tell them.
- **The cultural background of an individual** will also play a role in how they speak.

Advantages of Group Discussion

Group discussion strategy has the following advantages:

- It ensures the active participation of the students in the process of teaching-learning.
- It trains the students for carrying out group activities and cooperative tasks. The qualities linked to proper social development and democratic living is also developed with the adoption of this strategy.
- It provides opportunities to the students for imbibing the qualities of a good listener

Disadvantages of Group Discussion

Group discussion, as a strategy, may suffer from the following drawbacks and limitations:

- The teacher, as a group leader, may take all initiative in his hand by unnecessarily interfering in the thought process of the members or talking too much.
- The group discussion may go out of track by paying little considerations to the set objectives.
- It requires facilitation and if facilitation is poor then the process is vitiated.
- It requires more space than for lecture.
- It is time-consuming.
- It is difficult to monitor the progress of many small groups.
- When dominant members are not controlled it can affect the participation of other members in the group.

PROJECT METHOD

Projects and the project method have been applied to almost every kind of teaching, new or old, and to almost impossible to derive a meaning for the term that can be said to be truly its own. The word project in education was its application to an objective type of training that was developed by boys' and girls' agricultural clubs and in the vocational courses established in high schools. The essential elements of the project as used here

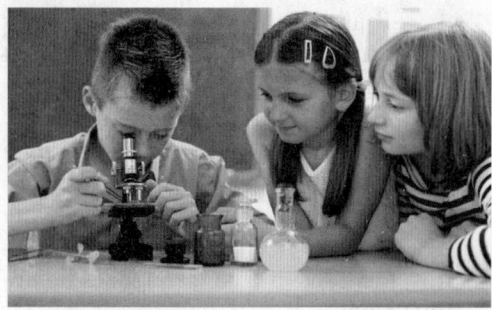

Fig. 3.14: Project method.

was the activity of the individual and the production of tangible results.

Definitions of Project

- According to Stevenson (1922), "A project is a problematic act carried to completion in its most natural setting."
- According to Kilpatrik (1921), "A project is a whole-hearted purposeful activity proceeding in a social environment."
- Ballard, H (1936) says, "A project is a bit of real life that has been imported into school."

Essentials for a Project: Learning activity should be:

- Problematic in nature.
- Aimed at a definite, attainable.
- Purposeful, natural and life like in its procedure to attain the goal.
- Directed and planned by the student.
- Practical in nature with emphasis on a single, complete unit of purposeful activity, resulting in concrete achievement.

Criteria for Selection of Projects

Every potential project should be carefully studied with the following questions in mind:

- Does it have definite educational values? Is it worthwhile?
- Is it challenging and does it require a reasonable amount of effort?
- Is it adapted to the needs and ability of the student?
- Are the cost and availability of material, as well as the time required for execution, commensurate with the educational values to be derived?

- Is it feasible and practical?
- Is it selected by the student?
- Can it be completed by the end of the term/year/semester?
- Does it give purposeful activity and definite goals?

Principles of Project Method

Project method is based on certain principles. They are as follows:

- **Principle of purpose:** Every activity has a purpose, when a project is to be done one should ask himself "Why should I do this"? "What is the purpose"? Then we can come out with the purpose of doing a project which leads to learning.
- **Principle of activity:** "Learning by doing an activity" gives a long lasting learning. Child becomes an active participant of both physical and mental activities. As far as possible activity should be done under the guidance of a teacher.
- **Principle of experience:** Project method provides an opportunity to learn through experience, group activities, if organized, help in developing social skills, such as communication, team spirit, good habits in the students. By doing a project, the child gains experiences which also help in self-learning.
- **Principle of reality:** Project method provides a real life situation to-work with. It is

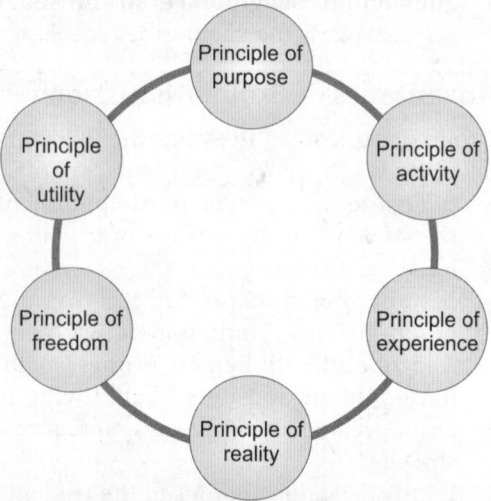

Fig. 3.15: Principles of project method.

a kind of transfer of classroom learning to real situation.

- **Principle of freedom:** Project method provides opportunities with freedom to the children to be creative according to their interests, abilities, aptitudes, etc. Children can choose the projects of their own choice.
- **Principle of utility:** Project method makes use of the principles of utility, letting children work on various projects which can be useful in their lives.

Characteristics of Project Method

The following are the special characteristic of this project method:

- **The project method is the embodiment of a new way of looking** at the pupil and of a new way of teaching him to live. The method aims at teaching the child to get the best out of life, not in the future, not when he is grown up, but here and now, "to the traditionalist, education is preparation for life to Dewey education is part of living and not a preparation for future living."
- **The project method is an attempt to use experience** because it is the trust and best master and one too whose lessons we never target.
- **The project method aims at bringing out what is in the child** and at allowing him to develop himself. It gives an opportunity for self-expression; it gives an opportunity for relating the self to the community. It tries to make the school the best place the child knows.
- **The experiments of the project method want to reset** the whole curriculum where the activity that is chosen becomes the

Principles of project method
• Principle of definite **purp**   • Principle of **freedom**   • Principle of **utility**   • Principle of **experience**   • Principle of **activity**   • Principle of **reality**   • Principle of **social experience**

Fig. 3.16: Principles of project method.

core and all knowledge that is acquired becomes incidental.

- **The project method purposes not merely the abstract solving** of a problem but the whole sequence of activities involved in a complete undertaking. It is just a problem. Situation which has not only to be solved but the activity involved is actually carried to completion. The idea underlying the method was that children should develop their knowledge through trying out theories in the practical solution of problems in the course of which they would come to appreciate the principles involved. Fresh knowledge is to be acquired only as a result of the felt needs of the pupils.
- **The project, in other words, the activity purposeful act** may be of any character annual or motor or both. It may take form of preparing and presenting a play. It may be running of a school hospital. We cannot restrict the project method to experience of the "doing" type, as it will be contrary to good pedagogy and sound psychology.
- **The activities when made the sole means of education** will inevitably cut across the time table organization to which we are accustomed as well as across the ordinary classroom organization. For example, in preparing to present a play, the pupils will have their own particular jobs to do, the actors to learn and rehearse their parts the young electricians and some painters to prepare the effects, the dressmakers to make and fit the clothing, etc.
- **A project is a play activity and children engaged in the carryout** of a project are undoubtedly children at play, though they may be getting through a lot of apparently hard and monotonous error. There is a marked contrast between the boy making bricks for the room has building and the labourer doing exactly the same thing as his daily. One is playing, the other is working.
- **The project method is a complete surrender to a child's point of view**. It seeks to offer the pupil complete freedom

Types of project method
Dr. W.H. Kilpatrick, in his paper on "The project method" (1918), has classified projects on the basis of tasks involved. • Problem type: A project that involves investigation and solution of practical problems (e.g., doing a project on the problem of low literacy level in a nearby village, investigating pollution problems, investigating community health problems, etc.) • Product type: A project that involves construction of a useful material object or article to embody some idea or plan in external form. (e.g.,) making a model of the wooden cantilever bridge over the Phochu river in Punakha) • Consumer type: A project that provides opportunities for experience on a particular area/field and writing an account of it. (e.g., attending a festival in a village and writing an account on its aesthetic value) • Drill type: A project that provides opportunities for mastery of skill or knowledge on a particular area/field. (e.g., writing a critical analysis "on the system of government during the rule of first and second Desis")

Fig. 3.17: Types of project method.

of choice of problem to be solved as well as the means to be employed in solving it. The fundamental principle is the educative use of occupations that are suitably doctored to meet the requirements of the ordinary school. The result is that in place of externally imposed tasks of the traditional kind, the pupil's activities are centered round a number of spontaneous projects.

- **In the project method, the procedure of the school** is liable to be determined by the technique of workshop, because it is believed that the child learns much better from his own activity than from constant instruction.
- **An attempt is made to establish a positive relation** with life. For Kilpatrick, a project may be said to represent a whole-hearted purposeful actively carries on is a social milieu.

Types of Project

Project are classified as:
- **Individual project:** Project which is planned for each student.
- **Group project:** Project for the class as a unit.
- **Model:** These are projects for production of some physical material.
- **Learning purpose project:** Projects such as waking a fracdude tured bed or CPR

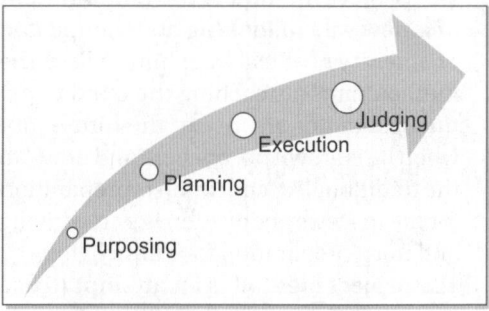

Fig. 3.18: Steps in developing project.

where the main aim is acquisition of some ability.
- **Project showing solution of patient's problem:** These types of projects are for intellectual development and emphasis is on student's creative thinking.

Steps in Developing a Project

For developing a project, there are four steps as discussed below:
- **Purposing:** The project should be based on the purpose of learning. The students should be able to acquire knowledge as well as skill from preparation of project. So the purpose of preparing the project should be clear.
- **Planning:** Once the purpose of the project is clear, start planning the project in terms

of money, material, manpower, and time. Plan about the material required, from where to get material, cost of project and about the time in which it can be completed by the utilization of how much manpower.

- **Execution** the project planned should be started to prepare so that students can learn and acquire knowledge.
- **Judging:** It is the best way to know about the project, whether it has met the criteria for which purpose it was prepared or not. By this, further improvements, if required can be made in the project.

Steps in Doing a Project

There are six steps involved in project method of teaching. In school age small projects can be taken up, projects selected at professional colleges may vary with vast depth in knowledge. Projects selected at undergraduate programme in nursing may include projects related to community, clinical area, and education or administration areas.

The steps involved in project method of teaching are given below:

- **Providing a situation:** In a school, there can be a number of situations that can be used as a project. Invite suggestions from the students on the possible projects which they would like to take up. A general brainstorming session can be organized where teachers may also give some ideas, (but never force the students to take up any project of teacher's choice). It should be left to the students to decide an area they would like to work on.
- **Choosing the topic and framing the objectives:** From broad area of work specific topic should be chosen. Once a specific topic is chosen, the objectives of the project should be spelt out in detail. Objectives should be very specific.
- **Planning:** The teacher has to motivate the student to plan the specific details of the project in relation to duration, budget, procuring and maintenance of items,

etc. Neglect of any detail in the plan may lead to the project's failure. Plan must be discussed by the teacher and students. A good plan with all the necessary details is extremely essential for success of a project.

- **Implementation:** Execution of a project demands teamwork in which each participating student is assigned specific responsibilities, if it is a group project. Activities should be divided among the team members according to their capacities, abilities, and interests. If student finds any problem in carrying on the project the teacher must deal with it and help the student to sort out.
- **Evaluation:** Evaluation of a project should be done taking into account its objectives as well as its planning. Evaluate whether the implementation could be carried on according to the plan, record any failures occurred, and how they could be overcome. Experience sharing among the students is very helpful.
- **Recording:** Students must keep a record of all the activities associated with the project. Project report should be prepared for future references detailing the topic, objectives, plan, execution, evaluation, results and learning experience.

Advantages of Project Method

- Stimulate and arouse interest among students.
- Keep the students on freedom of thoughts and action while working.
- Provides creative and constructive thinking.
- Helps the students to think logically and scientifically before starting the project.
- Teaches the students to evaluate complete work.
- Develops team spirit and co-operation among students.

Disadvantages of Project Method

- It is time-consuming.
- Sometime students have misconception about the term project.

- Cost of the project comes to high due to cost of material and sometimes the material for preparation of project is not available.

ROLE PLAY

Role playing is a method by which learners participate in an unrehearsed dramatization. They are asked to play assigned parts of character as they think the character would act in reality. This method is a technique to arouse feelings and elicit emotional responses in the learners. It is used primarily to achieve behavioral objectives in the affective domain. Role playing is the spontaneous acting out of a clearly defined situation by two or more persons for subsequent discussion by the whole class. It is a method of teaching usually stimulating interest among students and permits the teacher to evaluate their understanding and concepts.

Definitions of Role Play

- Role play is the spontaneous acting out of a clearly defined situation, usually done in front of a group with time allotted at conclusion for discussion and used to practice real life situations.

- Role playing is the technique where the teacher puts student in situation about which they want to teach to the students.
- Role playing is based on a particular theme, performed before the audience to spread the message to the people.
- Role playing is a dramatization along with verbalization.
- Role playing is relatively new educational techniques in which people spontaneously act out problems of human relations and analyze the enactment with the help of other role players and observes.

Purposes of Role Play

- To develop communication skills for successful interpretation.
- To involve everybody to work co-operatively for a common goal.
- To try new behaviors in the presence of co-learner.
- To experience the situation emotionally and to develop insight into the problem.
- To develop new skills for dealing with problems.
- To encourage thinking and creativity.
- It helps the participants to get inside the character and enact the meaning of the character.

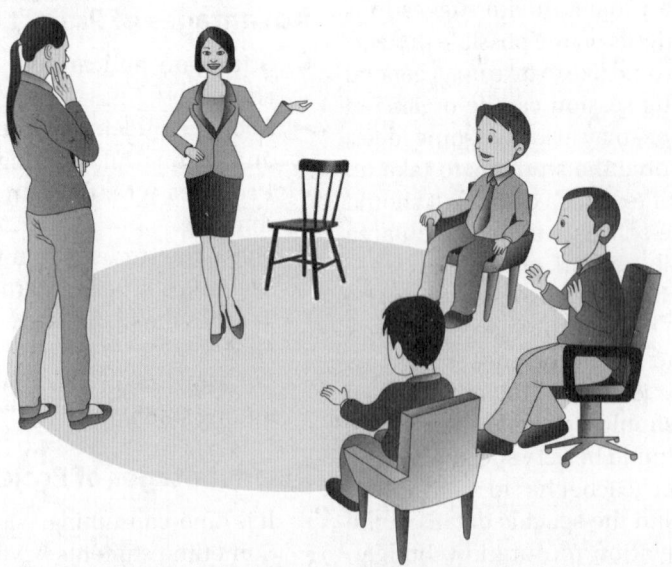

Fig. 3.19: Role play method of teaching.

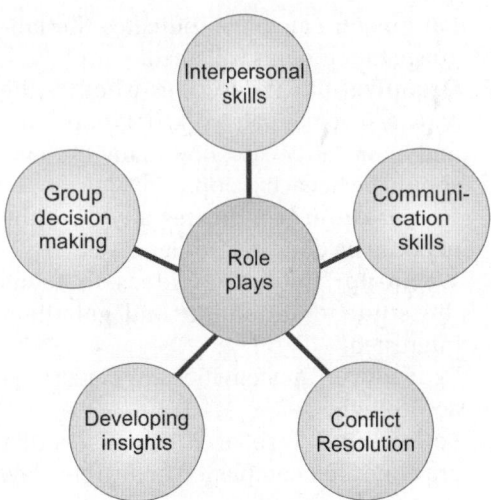

Fig. 3.20: Skills need for role play.

- To create the motivation and involvement necessary for learning to occur.

Characteristics of Role Play

- The role play should have clear objectives.
- It should analyze the needs in a stimulated real life situation.
- It should encourage independent thinking.
- The actors are not allowed to project their own life in the role.
- It should make the audience to participate actively.

Steps of Role Play

According to Richards (1985), the following are the steps of role play:

- **Preliminary activity:** Role play starts with a problem. This may be recognized by the learner or the teacher. Role playing centers around the needs and concerns of the group. The group is involved in some way in developing the background situation. The situation should increases the group's insight and deepen the ability to see the situation. So, the preliminary activity includes selection of a situation, and selection of the participants. It is best to ask for volunteers, unless there is a special reason for assigning certain roles. After actors are chosen, they are briefed as to their roles and the group has a warming up session. This prepares them for critical observation and analysis of the situation.

- **Model dialogue:** The model dialogue is presented depending upon the level of the participants. It should be simple and clear so that the audience can able to understand the concepts in the role play. The dialogues are also in such a way that it does not harm anyone in the audience.

- **Learning to perform the role play:** After the roles have been decided, the participants are given written descriptions about their roles and setting. The scenes are described and discussed with them briefly. The actor should understand who he is and he should be given sometime to think, so that he can add some of his views.

- **Performing the role play:** The role play is performed under a director. The director introduces the scene and also the roles of the participants. In introducing role playing to a group it is best to keep the problem and the situation as simple as possible, involving a familiar and non-threatening situation. All members of the group should be helped to understand what is happening and actively involved. The group members will enact their roles

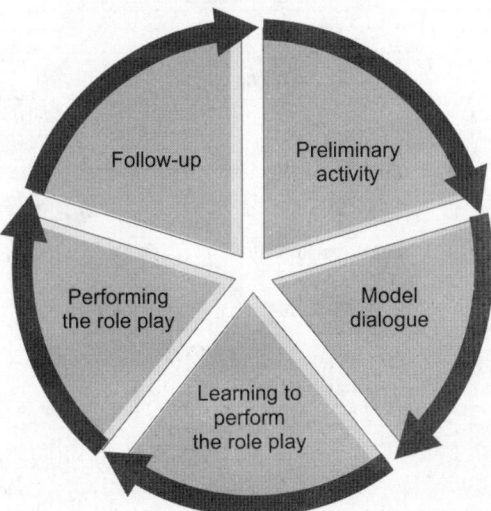

Fig. 3.21: Steps of role play.

and the audience is actively concerned with the drama. They are supposed to pay attention to what is going on. The scene should be succinct. Elaborate dialogue and irrelevant material is avoided. The scene is cut when it has served its purpose.

- **Follow-up:** After the roleplay action has ended, both the participants and audience can discuss the action. This gives them the opportunity to explore their feeling and negates possibility of feeling threatened when the group makes their observation. Following discussion, an attempt is made to summarize and evaluate the insights derived and make plans to provide an opportunity to put into effect, the behavior implied.

Factors Influencing Role Play

- **Level:** It indicates the minimal level at which the activity can be carried out.
- **Time:** Time depends on whether the students need to read articles, reports, etc.
- **Aim:** Aim indicates the broader objectives of each activity.

- **Language:** Language indicates the language the students will need.
- **Organization:** It describes whether the activity involves pair work, or group work, and in the latter ease, how many students should be in each group.
- **Preparation:** It indicates anything the needs to be done before class.
- **Warm-up:** It involves ideas to focus the student's attention and get them interested.
- **Procedure:** The activities are performed accordingly.
- **Follow-up:** It involves the activities that are done after completion of the role play.

Uses of Role Play in Nursing

- It helps in developing leadership skills and social interaction.
- It helps in problem-solving.
- It develops to identify to observe and analyze situation.
- To practice selected behavior in real life situation.
- It helps to identify critical issues.

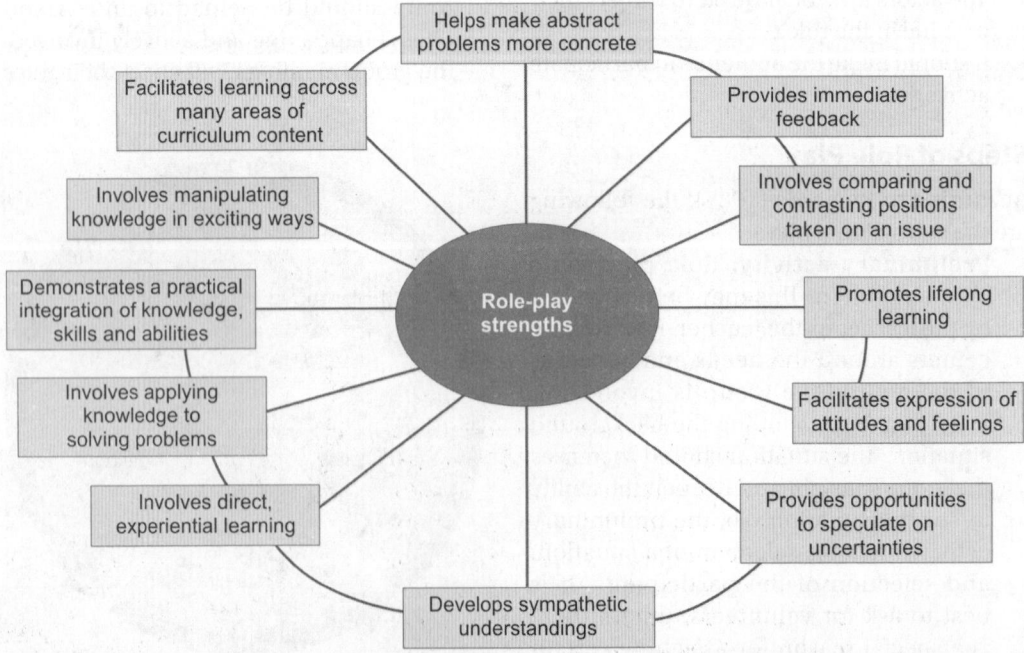

Fig. 3.22: Strengths of role play.

- It encourages independent thinking and action.
- It helps the nurse to observe and understanding patient's problems and solves them.

Guidelines for an Effective Role Play

- Faculty should plan meticulously for the role play; they also are required to be prepared to monitor and modify student actions and reactions, if needed.
- Good scenario can be created by incorporating situations that involve conflicting emotions.
- Three stages of role play are as follows:
  a. **Briefing:** Setting the stage and explaining the objectives, which is usually the shortest stage.
  b. **Running:** Acting out the role play, which may take 5–20 minutes.
  c. **Debriefing:** Discussion, analysis, and evaluation of role playing experience. Which may last 30-40 minutes or more.
- Debriefing stage is more important where students are provided the platform to clarify, take decisions and alternative decisions can be understood; enhance observational skills and other interpersonal reactions.
- Video or audio taping of role play may be supplementing in debriefing stage.
- This method works best with small groups of students where all students involved in the role play can become active observers.
- Students should be encouraged to respond naturally to the role play and avoid phoney acting.

- Criticism should be focused on the behaviors exhibited in the role play and not directed towards specific students.

Values of Role Play for a Teacher

Role play helps the teacher in the teaching learning situation. It helps to:
- Note individual student needs in a simulated real life situation.
- Assist the student in meeting her own needs by giving her spot suggestions. She can encourage the peer group to give their suggestions.
- Encourage impendent thinking and action by keeping herself back stage and allowing the student to perform.

Advantages of Role Play

- It provides an opportunity to practice new skills.
- It helps in group problem-solving.
- It helps to develop sensitivity and feeling by having the opportunity to put oneself.
- It encourages the students in independent thinking.
- It makes a situation in an effective manner, where it cannot be expressed in words.
- It promotes activity and interest in the students.
- It instills confidence in the students.
- It is good for developing initiative and creative.

Disadvantages of Role Play

- It is time-consuming.
- Requires careful planning, preparation and rehearsal.

Table 3.4: Uses, advantages and disadvantages of role plays.

Role Plays		
Uses	*Advantages*	*Disadvantages*
• Exploring and improving interviewing techniques and examining complexities and potential conflicts of groups. • To consolidate different lessons in one setting.	• Good energizers. • Promotes empathy of trainees for other situation. • Encourages creativity in learning.	• Participants might be reluctant. • May not work with trainees who do not know each other well.

- Learners may have difficulty in acting their roles.
- The group members may be too shy in participating.
- Role playing should not be used when pressure of time is present.

PANEL DISCUSSION

Panel discussion is discussion in which 4 to 8 qualified personnel sit and discuss the topic in front of large group or audience. Panel discussion has a chairperson (moderator) and 4 to 8 speakers. The success of the panel discussion depends upon the chairperson. He is the one who has to keep the discussion going and develop train of thought.

Concepts of Panel Discussion

- A panel consists of a few members who come prepared to exchange ideas and views on a particular subject under the leadership of a chairman. When used as a method of teaching, the panel may be a group of 'experts' on the subject or may be selected students who have requested and have prepared the object in advance.
- The chairman opens the discussion by introducing the members and the topic is announced and if it is broad in scope, limits of discussion are stated. The chairman remains seated after inviting the first person to speak.

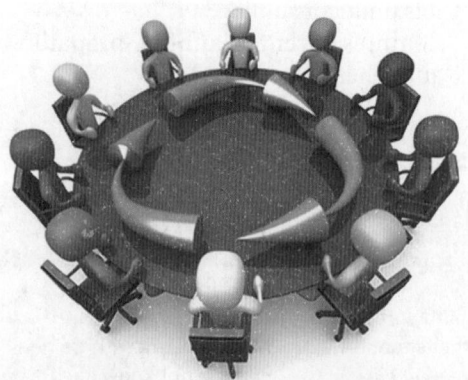

Fig. 3.23: Panel discussion method of teaching.

- The discussion is executed in a conversational way, with chairman making sure that all keep to the point. When necessary the chairman may clarify any issue or misunderstanding or may introduce another thought so that the subject will be fully covered.
- The panel discussion should provide a natural setting in which the audience will have the opportunity to ask questions, evaluate replies and make constructive contributions.
- The discussion may or may not be thrown open to the floor. If it is, the chairman should continue as leader and at the end, should draw together the main points and sum up the discussion.

Panel Discussion Techniques

- One chairperson and 4-8 speakers sit in front of large audience.
- Chairperson opens the meeting, welcomes the group and introduces panel speakers.
- Topic is introduced briefly by chairperson and then invites the panel speakers to present their view.
- In panel discussion, there is no specific agenda, no order of speaking and no set of speeches. The chairperson can interact in the form of question or simple statement related to topic to any of the speaker without any order form.
- At end, after exploration of main aspects of subject by speaker, the chairperson opens the discussion for audience by inviting them to participate in discussion.

Advantages of Panel Discussion

- It is an extremely effective method of education, if it is properly planned.
- Information reaches to a large number of audiences.
- Spontaneity of the panel discussion arouses interest among audience to participate in discussion, at end of panel discussion.
- It allows experts to present different opinions.
- It provokes better discussion.

- Frequent change of speaker keeps attention from lagging.
- Can provoke better discussion than a one person discussion

Disadvantages of Panel Discussion

- Experts may not be good speakers.
- Personalities may overshadow content.
- Subject may not be in logical order.

SYMPOSIUM

Symposium is a type of socialized technique whereas each of participants is expected to present a well-reasoned argument or point at view with respect to the problem being discussed. The point of view may be presented through speakers or paper reading. Fact and feeling of each presentation vary with the speakers and with the situation. This makes symposium constant in form but flexible in method.

Meaning of Symposium

Symposium is a Greek term for drinking party symposia were very frequent at Athens. Their enjoyment was heightened by agreeable conversation, by introduction of music and dancing, sometimes philosophical subjects were discussed at them.

Derivation of word: Syn- together, Posis- a drinking.

- A drinking parting at which there was intellectual conversation.
- Any meeting or social gathering at which ideas are freely exchanged.
- Conference or meeting to discuss a particular academic subjects.
- A collection of opinion especially a published group of essay on a subject given.

Definition of Symposium

Symposium is a method of group discussion in which two or more persons under the direction of chairman present separate speeches which gives several aspects of one question.

Aims and Objectives of Symposium

- To clarify thought in debatable questions.
- To investigate a problem from several points of view.
- To acquire increased knowledge, intellectual abilities, and skills.
- To increase interest towards the subject.
- To change attitudes and values towards common goal.
- For better personnel and social adjustments.
- To get good co-operation.

Principles of Symposium

- Chairman has to introduce the topic and has to lead the meeting.
- Discussion among symposium members is not allowed.
- Chairman takes charge over the topics distributed to the speakers and allots them sufficient time for presentation of particular topic.
- Speakers present the topics through speech or paper reading.
- Chairman should start symposium with short introduction of the topic and speakers.
- To the conclusion chairman is responsible for summarizing the topic.
- Doubts clarified at the end of discussion.

Members involved in symposium: 1. Chairman, 2. Speaker, and 3. Audience.

Role of Chairman

- Selection of topic
- Distribution of topic.
- Guide the speaker towards goal.
- Control over the group.
- Summarizing and giving conclusions.

Qualities of a Chairman

- Responsible for planning and coordinating the program.
- Good counselor.
- A researcher.

- A resource person.
- A representative to professional nursing organization.

Role of a Speaker

- Preparation of the topics.
- Presentation of the topic.

Role of Audience

- Listens over the program.
- Arising questions and clarifying the doubts during the end.

Uses of Symposium

Used in:
- Political meeting,
- Professional conventions,
- Association meetings,
- Co-acting group, and
- Conference.

Techniques of Symposium

- Success depends largely on personnel involved and degree of preparation.
- Experts in various field experiences can yield more informations.
- Good planning and organizations.

- All the members should know the objectives.
- Teachers should have a conference with student speaker regarding topic presentation prior to prevent overlapping.

Merits of Symposium

- Symposium method generally presents wider basis for discussion then lecture method.
- It has greater organization than other discussion.
- Greater advantage in political meeting professional organization.
- Persons involved have different roles to play which avoids conflicts and misunderstanding among them.
- Audience can get wide sets of knowledge from different exposure.
- It acts or a disciplined way of both teaching and learning.

Demerits of Symposium

- No discussion among symposia members.
- Topics should be given by chairperson.
- Inadequate opportunity for all the students to participate actively.

Symposium
Principles
• The speeches may be persuasive, argumentative and informative.
• Original presentation is objective and accurate.
• The method always includes a summary at conclusion.
• Each speed proceeds without interruption.
• The chairman of the symposium introduces the topic, suggests its importance and sometimes indicate the general approaches.
• All members of the symposium performing group can sit in a straight line behind the table; or in adjoining chairs with the chairman in the middle or to one side of the speakers.
• The symposium presents two conflicting points of view, the reading arrangement can separate the speakers on the platform to indicate differences in opinion or to preserve peace.

Fig. 3.24: Principles of symposium.

Symposium
Advantages

- Symposium can be used to address a large group or class.
- This method can be frequently used to present broad topics for discussion at conventions and organization of meetings.
- In symposium, the principle of organization is high as the speeches are prepared beforehand.
- It gives a deeper insight into a topic.
- It directs the students to continuous independent study.
- This method can be used in political meetings.

Fig. 3.25: Advantages of symposium.

- Speakers are limited to 15 to 20 minutes and therefore each one is seriously hampered in development of her topics.
- Absence of rehearsal of the program.

SEMINAR

The word seminar is derived from the Latin word seminarium, meaning 'seed plot'. This method of instruction is based on the teaching method of Socrates and the Greek work "paideia" which means the general knowledge or learning of values needed by all humans. Seminar is, generally, a form of academic instruction, either at a university or offered by a commercial or professional organization. It has the function of bringing together small groups for recurring meetings, focusing each time on some particular subject, in which everyone present is requested to actively participate. This is often accomplished through an ongoing socratic dialogue with a seminar leader or instructor, or through a more formal presentation of research.

Definitions of Seminar

- Seminar is a group of members come together to exchange views of current problems of to share with others their own experiences, experiments, discoveries, etc.
- Seminar is a small discussion group that provides an opportunity for knowledge. Integration at high level.
- Seminar is an advanced type of socialized techniques; each individual in the seminar group either takes part in carrying out of separate individual investigation or assumes a share of a large project.

Objectives of Seminar

- To give students the opportunity to participate in methods of scientific analysis and research procedures.
- To promote deeper understanding about attitudes, interests and develop desirable interpersonal relationships- desirable group process.
- To help the students to develop skills in reading and comprehension of scientific writing of verbal presentations.

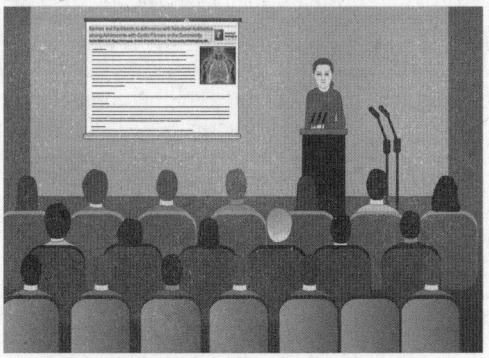

Fig. 3.26: Seminar method of teaching.

- In enables that students to gain experience in self-evaluation end in evaluation of others.
- In enables the students to gain additional information, insights and other approaches to problem-solving.

Purposes of Seminar

- It helps the student to study the subject matters.
- It requires a background of knowledge skills in library work.
- It helps in problem-solving skills.
- It helps the students to participate in methods of scientific analysis and research procedures.
- It helps in students to increase their responsibilities.
- It helps the students to change their attitudes and values.

Areas Involved in Seminar

Seminar format is useful in:
- Teaching professional development
- Administrative abilities, and
- Ethical and legal issues.

Goals of Seminar

Students will:
- Increase their understanding of ideas as presented by the work at hand.
- Talk to one another, not just to the teacher alone.

- Be actively involved in their own learning.
- Think more deeply about issues in a clear and concise way.
- Speak more articulately.
- Question each others opinions.
- Listen better.
- Read more thoroughly.
- Learn to justify/qualify opinions.
- Be exposed to extensive literature related to the topic.

Elements of Seminar

- The group should be heterogeneous.
- Critical physical arrangement.
- The environment should be safe for open discussion.
- Should be enveloped with deep questioning.
- Discussion of profound works of human endeavor.
- Leader not active in discussion; does not offer his/her own opinions.
- Higher level of questions; more analysis, synthesis, evaluation; fewer right/wrong answers.
- Discussion constantly tied to work under discussion.
- Motivation level of student is improved.
- Sparse use as instructional tool.
- Process/evaluation of seminar by participants.
- Profound learning experience for everyone involved.

Table 3.5: Uses, advantages and disadvantages of seminar method.

Seminar Method		
Uses	*Advantages*	*Disadvantages*
• To provide general guidance for a group working on an advanced study or research project. • To exchange information on techniques and approaches being explored by members of a study or research group. • To develop new and imaginative solutions to problems under study by the group.	• Provides motivation and report. • Stimulates active participation. • Permits adaptive instruction.	• Requires highly competent instructor. • Poses evaluation problems. • Is more costly than instruction, most other methods.

Steps in Implementing a Seminar

- Establish a safe environment.
- Coach students on expectations.
- Choose a selection carefully; assign it to the class.
- Read and study selection carefully, making notes where necessary.
- Prepare the opening, core, and closing questions.
- Prepare the room physically by arranging chairs/desks in circle.
- Begin the seminar.
- Process and evaluate the seminar with the class afterwards.
- Reflect personally on the experience, fine-tuning for future use.

Guidelines of Seminar Presentation

- A seminar presentation is a short informal talk giving the about the topic proposed with extensive search of literature. Share the ideas and discoveries in a way that gives seminar participants an opportunity for discussion. These presentations form a normal part of the teaching and learning process.
- Do not think of the presentation as a test. The act of investigating sources, digesting information, and summarizing other people's work will help to clarify these matters in your mind.
- Develop confidence in handling information, making useful notes, and presenting an argument.
- Topics can be chosen according to own particular interests or with the assistance of tutor. They might are:
  - Reading of a set text from the course, applying one critical theory.
  - An account of one critical theory and how it can be applied to a couple of set texts.
  - A response to one of the tutorial topics from the course materials.
  - An account of the publishing history or the critical reception of one of the set texts.
- A seminar presentation should not try to imitate an essay. It is better to offer a

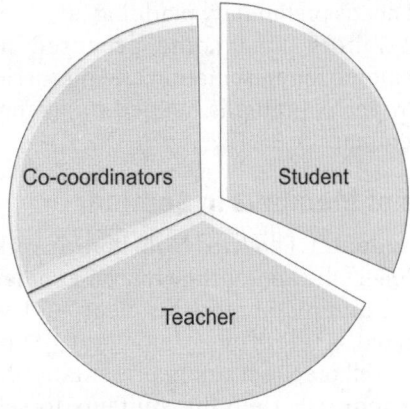

Fig. 3.27: Role of members in seminar.

presentation on something smaller and more specific, rather than the type of general question posed in a coursework essay.

- Do not write down the presentation verbatim. Make outline notes and then speak to these notes using the set text, any critical theory, and own extended notes as backup material.
- If you have the resources, it is a nice courtesy to provide other members of the group with a copy of your outline notes.
- Overhead projection facilities will often be available. Otherwise, photocopies of any illustrative material will be perfectly acceptable.

Advantages of Seminar

- Seminar helps the student to increase their responsibilities.
- It gives opportunity to participate in methods of scientific analysis and research procedure.
- It helps to do thorough study on subject.
- It helps to improve leadership qualities.
- It is an effective method of problem-solving.
- It will help to improve curriculum there by the profession.

Disadvantages of Seminar

- It is useful only upper division students as it needs high skills for performing library work.

- It needs preliminary planning.
- Members must come prepared with material for presentation and discussion.
- Proper planning is needed to arrange a seminar.

Role of Members in Seminar

I. **Student:** 1. Expected to do library work, 2. Collect the appropriate relevant contents, 3. Contents should be clear and well stated, 4. Utilize the AV aids, and 5. Should be well prepared before presentation.
II. **Teacher:** 1. Help the students to select appropriate topic, 2. Guide the students to select the contents, and 3. Suggest available sources of information.
III. **Co-coordinators:** 1. Select problem is solved analyzed and critically evaluate and concluded by coordinator, and 2. The coordinator has to organize the seminars.

FIELD TRIP

The teacher is a person responsible to provide conductive environment to students so that they engage themselves in useful and constructive activities through own experiences and it is possible through field trip. A teacher cannot do an effective teaching in a classroom alone but it is possible if the teacher does not ignore the outside world experience and its influence of pupil apart from classroom teaching.

Definitions of Field Trip

- Field trip is defined as an educational procedure by which the student studies first hand objectives and materials in the natural environment. **—Heidgerken**
- Field trip is defined as most concrete and the real best visual techniques which bring the pupil into direct contact with real life situation. **—Bhatia**
- Field trip forms a concrete learning experience in a real situation which has been undertaken with a specific purpose. **—Nanda**
- Field trip can be defined as the fact it links works of both theory and practical experience.
- Field trip is essentially a visit to demonstration, plots, frames of progressive farmers, poultry, dairy, orchard model houses. **—Dahama**

Objectives of Field Trip

- To apply theory into practice.
- To evaluate the result of new practice.
- To enrich the classroom instructions.
- To develop observational skills.
- To improve social interaction among the students.
- To evaluate students according to domains, such as cognitive, psychomotor, and affective.
- To refresh students knowledge.
- To obtain a baseline data.
- To develop creativity skill among students.
- To obtain primary observation.
- To see the practice demonstrated.
- To see the students level of accomplishment.

Purposes of Field Trip

- It helps to furnish first hand information to supplement and enrich the classroom teaching.
- It helps to co-relate and blend school life without side world by providing a direct touch with community situation.
- It helps to distinguishes, differentiate and develop better understanding of housing, sanitation, economic condition, etiology factors of disease.
- It helps to develop keenness and observational skills.

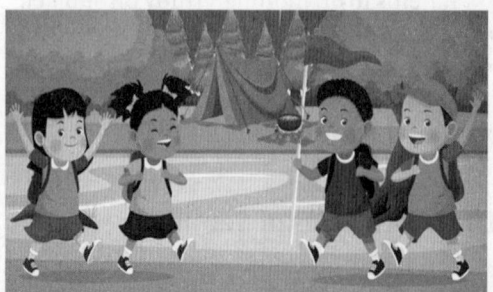

Fig. 3.28: Field trip method of teaching.

- Field trips provide opportunity to apply what is taught and verify what is learned.
- Field trip provides actual source material for study.
- Field trip provides vitalized instruction which help to arouse interest and motivation.
- Field trip affords an opportunity to solve problems arising from individual and group in a natural situation.
- Field trip serves in an effective means of co-relating the subjects of curriculum.
- Field trip helps to develop leadership qualities.
- Field trip helps to develop aesthetic sense in students.

Types of Field Trips

- *Local school trips:* This type forms half a day visit to section of school building and grounds to see procedures, equipments and materials, e.g. measuring distance, studying about trees, shrubs and flowers, practicing health and safety procedures. They are done during regular schedule period.
- *Community trip:* This is type of trip forms a whole day visit to nearby place like zoo, museum, hospital etc.
- *Tour (or) journey:* This type of trip forms for several days or a week, for example, distant projects arrange by block program

as Bharatyatra, visit to NIMHANS Bangalore, CMCH Vellore, etc.

- *Imaginary tour:* Details of real tours are investigated, studied and planned, materials collected, decisions taken on trip destinations regarding routes, cost, etc. but the destinations are seen by means of motion pictures, slides, photographs, objects, reports and recording, etc.
- *Inter school visits or inter college visit:* Medical students visiting the arts college for exchange of ideas, referring books to attain knowledge. A group of school students of music or science meeting corresponding organization of other school to gain knowledge in relation to mutual interest.
- *Individual trip:* This type of trip helps the student to take the responsibility to do the assignment in connection with curricular activity. This trip, for example, is famous for collecting biological specimens and fossils for the study of natural science and anthropology.

Organization of Field Trip

The success of the field trip depends upon efficient planning.

- Determine the specific aims of the field trips the students and teacher should be clear with objectives and purpose of trip.

Align with curriculum	Before the trip
• Stimulation for a unit	• Communicate goals and expectations
• Mode of learning content	• Stimulate interest in the trip
• Culmination or extension for a unit	• Establish questions to answer/ hypotheses to test
During the trip	**After the trip**
• Facilitate learning onsite	• Debrief by returning to questions/ hypotheses
• Structure observation, interaction and gathering of evidence	• Have students apply learning
• Use materials by museum educators	• Reflect on whole process
• Leverage museum guides/resources	

Fig. 3.29: Planning field trip.

- Determine of suitable place to visit and collect information regarding the place to be visited from various sources.
- Necessary permission for the trip to be secured from concerned authorities.
- Affordable cost of expenditure should be secured.
- Organization committee students should be formed to organize the trip.
- Teacher should work as a guide and should correlate the knowledge gained in the school and with field trip.
- Evaluation of field trip to be done on return from the journey.

Sequence in organizing the field trip it involves:

- **Knowledge:** Make a survey and obtain accurate information regarding the place to be visited which offer potential education experiences for nursing students and analyze the educational value of the field trip.
- **Rapport:** Establish and maintain cordial relationship with authorities in charge of institution (or) place to be visited, inform the concerned authority beforehand obtain a permission letter to avoid wastage of time, energy, and material.
- **Objectives:** Both student and teacher should be aware of objectives of the field trip, and it is responsibility of the teacher to make the student understand goal of field trip of facilitate the learning activity.
- **Time and transportation:** Make a needed arrangement for the time, place of meeting, duration of the visit, transport and its expenditure.
- **Preparation of the students:** The trip assignment is in the form of the unit assignment and must be based on good principles, establish the objectives and stimulate the student to think about its terms of importance, purpose, practice and personnel, student should be aware of objectives of the trip and direct the student to take down special points.
- **Supervision:** Careful supervision in needed to protect the student, safety rules are to be followed during field trips.

- Do not get on or off a moving vehicle weight it comes to complete stop.
- Do not put hands or head out of the moving vehicle.
- Cross streets on pedestrian crossing with green walking sign.
- Be alert for possible danger whenever traveling.
- Always stay with group don't go alone, inform the group leader when going out in a free time.
- Students should take their own responsibility of their health and safety during field trips.
- **Evaluation:** After the field trip, there should be a open discussion, students are asked to give the reports, questions asked by students are clarified by the teacher, experience of the students and information obtained through field trip is clearly co-relate and integrate with class subjects, activities of field trip documented for future references. Any modifications needed for future field trips are discussed through evaluation. Evaluation regarding the field trip can be alone through group discussion, quiz programme conducted by the teacher. Knowledge obtained through field trip can be elicited by flow diagrams, sketches and photographs in institution magazine for future references. After evaluation the teacher come to conclusion that students had gained accurate knowledge of things observed through a meaningful field trip.

Responsibilities of Teacher in a Field Trip

- Check the presence of all students and see that no student is missing.
- Adequate information should be given to the students regarding vehicle no time, where to get down from vehicle.
- Check the account of the group members and submit account.
- Guide and supervise the students during the trip.
- Safety rules to be followed strictly through-out the trip.

- Teacher should encourage unity, discipline among the group.
- First aid box should be taken and kept in the vehicle for the trip.
- Accuracy, clarity, brevity regarding the learning experiences in field trip should be fulfilled by the teacher.

Responsibility of Student in a Field Trip

- Each student is personally responsible to know place of visit, vehicle used for trip, time, and place of getting on and off the vehicle.
- Student should be punctual and obey the commands or instructions of the teacher.
- Student should wear suitable dress based on place of visit.
- Students should not misbehave and be considerate to others, professionally mature behavior is expected from each student.
- Questions should framed and kept ready, when given opportunity questions asked by the students relevantly.
- All luggages of the student should be labeled and should be ready on time for departure.
- Each student should keep account of his/her own expenditure and record fare for the vehicle used for the trip.
- Each student should take notes whenever they are instructed to take.

Advantages of Field Trips

- Observation of active participation with reality.
- Opportunity for co-operative group work and sharing responsibilities.
- It enable the students to develop self-confidence.
- It permits comparison between reality and theory.
- It develop qualities of observation and decision making.
- It ensure close contacts with reality.
- It increases the variability.
- It permits evaluation of degree to which educational objectives are attained.

- It is a good method for individual motivation.
- It is the most concrete and most real visual technique which help students to gain actual meaning to compact tendency of abstractness and simulate correct thinking.
- It gives relief from monotonous life of classroom.

Limitations of Field Trips

- Costly in time and transport.
- Field trip possible for limited audience only.
- Requires careful planning for its effectiveness.
- Distracters cannot be controlled.
- Advance knowledge regarding the place should be known to teachers; otherwise they will not be able to answer student's questions.
- A group discussion should follow field trip if not a complete learning will not be possible.
- Finding appropriate site may be difficult.
- Schedules are difficult to maintain.

Field Trip and Nursing Education

- Field trip plays an important role in molding and shaping the nursing students in promoting, enriching, vitalizing, and implementing content areas in nursing education.
- As a field trip in nursing education student attend clinics, visit various therapy departments.
- Nursing students gain firsthand knowledge of community agencies, health camps, first aid activities, and other function in relationship to hospital in helping those patients.
- It helps the nursing students to observe real thing and it helps them in active learning.

Following examples of field trip where nursing students can observe various situations:
- Rehabilitation centers,
- Water purification centers,

- Old age home,
- School for handicapped children, e.g. deaf and blind,
- Occupational nursing areas,
- Sheltered workshop.
- Commercial company, e.g., dairy centers,
- Specialized centers, such as hospitals, and
- Physical therapy in outpatient program.

WORKSHOP

A workshop is a meeting with group of individuals during which various experts and consultants find solutions to problems that have cropped up in the course of their work during the specific period of time. An essential feature of workshop is complete active involvement by each participant the whole point of attendance is to work and to learn from practical experience. One of the commonest methods used in the workshop is group discussion of selected problems, the size of the group being small enough to encourage full participation by each member and large enough for each member to gain from the experience of the others.

Definitions of Workshop

- Workshop is a large number of people belonging to a particular of discipline or allied disciplines collect together together to take up specific issues and problem for making recommendations for future action.
- Workshop is a making of people to work together is small groups upon problem which are of concern to them and relevant to them in their own spheres of activity and a find suitable solutions.
- Workshop is the name given to a noble experiment in education. It consists of series of meeting usually four or more with emphasis on individual work, within the group, with the help of consultants and resource personal.
- Workshop is a meeting during which experienced people in responsible positions come together with experts and consultants to fine solution to problem that have cropped up in the course of their work and they have had difficulty in dealing with on their own.
- Workshop is complete active involvement each participant; the cobble point of attendance is to work and to learn from the practical experience.
- Workshop is a meeting at which a group engages in intensive discussion and activity on a particular subject or project.

Purposes of Workshop

- It helps to improve the knowledge.
- It improves an opportunity for learning.
- These techniques will be employed to engage participation.
- It helps people with previous experience on subject especially departments, institutions and community.
- It helps in evolving policies, programs, and methodologies.
- It provides more interactions and discussion from the participants.
- It helps participants to express freely and exchange ideas.
- It is collective thinking process to solve the problems.
- It is introducing participant to a systematic approach to educational problems.
- It is stimulating a given proposition of participants to wish to reach at least those objectives set out in the educational aspects.

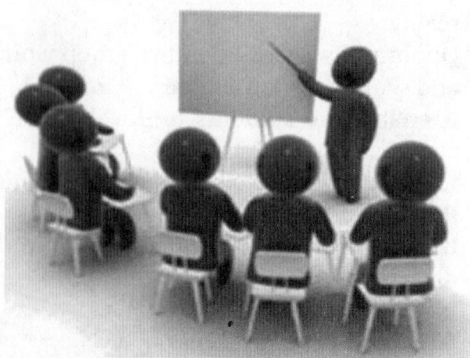

Fig. 3.30: Workshop method of teaching.

Principles of Workshop

Workshop method proposed it uses the systematic approach, it also relives on such educational principles as,

- Workshop allowing participants to prepare and select objectives to be reached will increase his motivation.
- Workshop gives the participants active role, it make teaching more effective.
- Proving the participants with regular opportunities to see the progress, it increases learning speed and improves the quality of the knowledge and skills he requires.

Working Methods of Workshop

- Free choice of personal objectives: in order to ensure that the workshop fully meets educational needs, invited to select the objectives you wish to reach before the end of the workshop.
- Preliminary reading assignments (oriented towards practical exercises).
- Clarifying sessions.
- Practical exercises.
- Group presentation.
- Next working day preview.
- Individual consultations.
- Formative evaluation (pre-test evaluation, day evaluation, evaluation questionnaire and long-term evaluation).

Advantages of Workshop

- Training program helps to reach the aim of educational point.
- It improves learning activities.

Disadvantages of Workshop

- It is time-consuming.
- It needs constant supervision.
- It needs manpower and enough material.
- It is mostly learning activity.

Evaluation and Workshop

As with any workshop, the progress of evaluation is of vital importance. Not only an assessment to make of how will the objectives have been met, but also there are decisions to be made about whether or not there might be merit in repeating various aspects, with or without modification. In the workshop that been described participants were asked for their reaction at the conclusion of the final sessions.

EXHIBITION

Exhibitions are familiar items in our environment today. When we go round an exhibition, our attention is often focused on a group of objects and materials that are displayed according to a deliberate plan. Exhibitions that are arranged in schools are

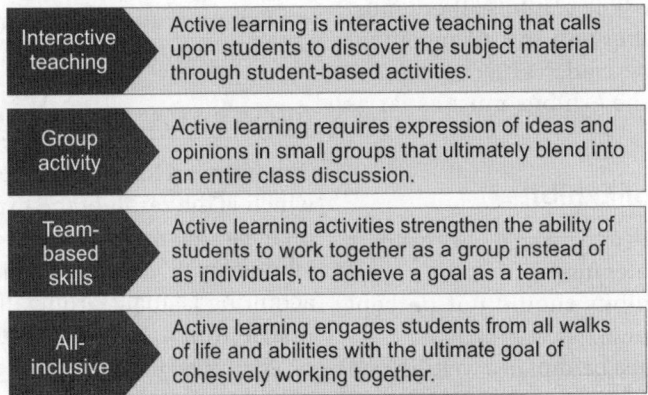

Fig. 3.31: Skills needed in workshop.

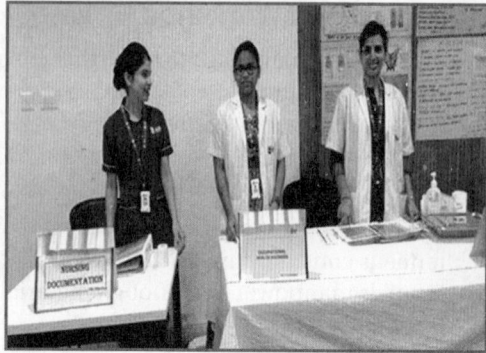 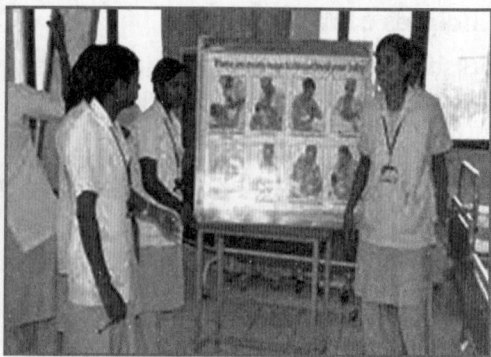

Fig. 3.32: Exhibition methods of teaching.

usually communicating something valuable to students, public, and parents.

The values of exhibitions are as follows:

- It is one of the effective modes of mass communication and instruction on a large scale.
- Self activity is fostered on the part of those who take part in the exhibition.
- The outcomes of different activities and processes are very well understood by pupils.
- Team spirit is encouraged as conduct of an exhibition is a co-operative effort.
- Parents and visitors can have an idea of the work done by the pupils and as such it fosters parent - school contacts.

Exhibitions must be an annual affair. The idea of holding an exhibition must be promoted even at the beginning of the year. Teachers must guide and lead the pupils in the preparation of possible exhibits. There must be effective labeling and the arrangement of the item may be made subject-wise. The explanations for the exhibits must as far as possible be brief.

Arrangement of Exhibits

- Popular, difficult and easier type of exhibits must be kept inter mixed.
- Too many exhibits should not be kept crowded in a room.
- The exhibits must be kept in a well-lighted place.
- Dynamic and static exhibits must be kept mixed so that overcrowding can be avoided.

- It is better to put one single idea in an exhibit.
- Colorful and moving exhibits will attract the attention of the people.
- Entire campus should be clean and should present a festive appearance.
- Student committees could be formed for different activities.
- There must be enough space for the visitors to move and the volunteers to stand and explain.

Planning the Exhibits

While planning the exhibits following points to be remembered:

- Put only one central idea in your exhibit.
- Place your exhibit where it is certain to be seen.
- An exhibit, is seen not read.
- Make your labels short and simple.
- Labels should be uniform and legible.
- Motion attracts attention.

PROGRAMMED INSTRUCTION

Programmed instruction is a new innovation which is the result of the experimental study of learning process in the psychological laboratory. It is a self-teaching technique for acquiring factual learning. It is an integrated instructional system which may employ programmed books, teaching machines, films in various forms of audio-visual devices.

- Programmed instruction is a self-instruction whereby learner proceeds through instructional materials in short steps at his own pace receiving immediate knowledge of the correctness of his answers.

- Programmed instruction is planned to control the students responses and to provide a feedback to the student in a pattern designed to accomplish maximum transfer of learning.

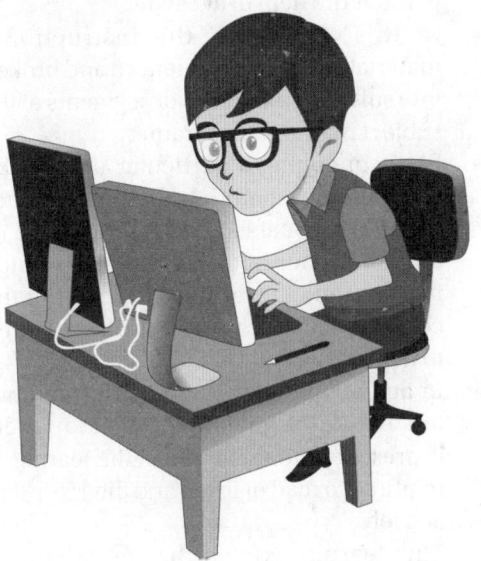

Fig. 3.33: Programme instruction teaching.

- Attempts were made since Socrates period; there were the attempts toward a systematic involvement of self-activity on the part of the learner in the learning process.
- But, today, the teaching machine focusing so much attention clearly and specifically on the value of student self-activity and on the importance of reinforcement in the learning process.
- Programmed instruction is self-sufficient. It is so very well planned and organized that when once it is programmed, it takes care of itself and leads the learner to successful learning without the intervention of the teacher.
- Programmed instruction is an instructional technique designed to suit the changing learning situations.

Definitions of Programmed Instruction

- **According to Kochhar, SK (1992),** It is a kind of learning in which a 'program' takes the place of a tutor for the student, and leads him through a set of frames of specified behaviors designed and

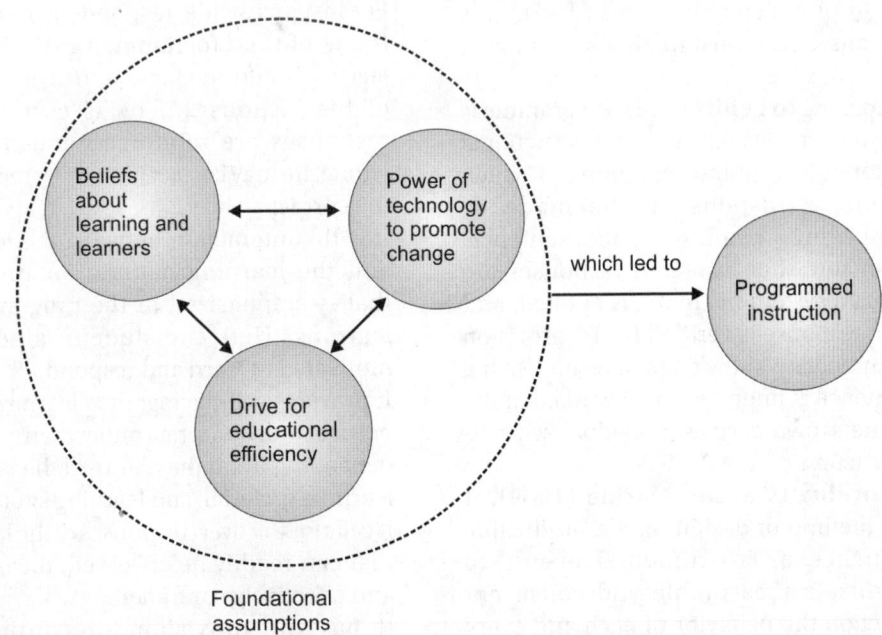

Fig. 3.34: Programme instruction strategy.

sequenced to make it more probable that he will behave in a given desired way.

- **According to American Writers,** "The programmed instruction is a process of arranging material to be learned in a series of small steps designed to lead a learner through self-instruction from what he knows to the unknown of new and more complex knowledge and principles".

- **According to Smith and Moore (1962),** Programmed instruction is the process of arranging the material to be learned into a series of sequential steps, usually it moves the students from a familiar background into a complex and new set of concepts, principles and understanding.

- **According to Jacobs and others (1966),** Self-instructional programmes are educational materials from which the students learn. These programmes can be used with many types of students and subject matter, either by themselves, hence the name "self-instruction" or in combination with other instructional techniques.

- **According to Espich and Williams (1967),** Programmed instruction is a planned sequence of experiences, leading to proficiency in terms of stimulus responses relationship, that have proven to be effective.

- **According to Leith (1966),** Programme is a sequence of small steps of instructional material (called frames), most of which require a response to be made by completing a blank space in a sentence. To ensure that expected responses are given, a system of cueing is applied, and each response is verified by the provision of immediate knowledge of result. Such a sequence is intended to be worked at the learners' own pace as individualized self-instruction.

- **According to Susan Markle (1969),** It is a method of designing a reproducible sequence of instrumental events to produce a measurable and consistent effect on the behavior of each and every acceptable student.

Characteristics of Programmed Instructions

- Programmed learning is a method or technique of giving or receiving individualized instruction from a variety of sources, such as programmed textbook, teaching machine, and computers with or without the help of a teacher.

- In this technique, the instructional material is logically sequenced and broken into suitable small steps or segments of the subject matter, called frames.

- For sequencing a particular unit of the instructional material, the programmer has to pay consideration for the initial or entry behavior of the learner with which it begins and the terminal behavior or the competence which the student is required to achieve.

- In actual operation, a frame (a small but meaningful segment of subject matter) is presented to the learner. The learner is required to read or listen and then respond actively.

- This learning system has an adequate provision for immediate feedback that is based on the theory of reinforcement. For instance, while responding to the first frame of the programmed material, the learner is informed about the correctness of his response. If he is correct, his responses are reinforced and if he is wrong, he may correct himself by receiving the correct answer.

- It is the interaction between the learner and the learning material or program that is emphasized in the programmed learning. Here the student is actively motivated to learn and respond.

- It provides self-pacing; thus learning may occur at individual rate rather than general, depending upon the nature of the learner, learning material, and learning situations.

- It calls for the overt responses of the learner that can readily be observed, measured, and effectively controlled.

- It has the provision for continuous evaluation that may help in improving the student's performance and the quality of programmed material.

Principles of Programmed Instruction

- **Principle of small steps:** This principle is based on the basic assumption that a person learns better if the content matter is presented to him in suitable small steps. Therefore, a programmer while preparing a program should try to arrange the subject matter into a properly sequenced and meaningful segment of information, called frames. These segments should be presented one at a time before the learner for responding.
- **Principle of active responding:** This principle rests on the assumption that a learner learns better by being active. In programmed learning, the learner may remain active if he responds actively to every frame presented to him. Therefore, a

good program should actively involve the learner in the learning process. It should be so formed that the learner may not feel much difficulty in moving from one frame to another and to remain meaningfully, busy and active by responding to the frames thus, acquiring the knowledge step-by-step.

- **Principle of immediate reinforcement:** The psychological phenomenon of reinforcement is the basis of this principle. One person learns better when he is motivated to learn by receiving infor- mation of the result just immediately after responding. Therefore, in a good program, appropriate consideration is always made for the provision of immediate reinforcement by informing him about the correctness of his response.
- **Principle of self-pacing:** Programmed learning is a technique of individualized instruction. It is based on the basic assumption that learning can take place better if an individual is allowed to learn at his own pace. So, a good program should always take care of the principle of self-pacing. The programming of the material should be done in view of the principle of individual difference and the learner should be able to respond and move from one frame to another according to his own speed of learning.

| Principle of small steps |
| Principle of active responding |
| Principle of immediate reinforcement |
| Principle of self-pacing |
| Principle of student-testing |

Fig. 3.35: Principles of programmed instruction.

Table 3.6: Uses, advantages and disadvantages of programme instruction.

Uses	Advantages	Disadvantages
• To provide remedial instruction. • To provide make-up instruction for late arrivals, absentees, or transients. • To maintain previously earned skills which are not performed frequently enough. • To provide retraining on equipment and procedures which have become obsolete. • To upgrade production. • To accelerate capable students. • To provide enough common background among student • To provide the review and practice. Of knowledge and skills.	• Reduce failure rate. • Improves end-of-course proficiency • Saves time. • Provides for self-instruction.	• Requires local or commercial preparation. • Requires lengthy programmer training. • Increases expenses. • Requires considerable lead.

- **Principle of student-testing:** For better learning, it is always good to seek continuous evaluation of the learning process. The principle of student testing meets this requirement. In the programmed learning, the learner has to leave the record of his response because he is required to write a response for each frame on a response sheet. This detailed record helps in revising the program. It may also prove a good source for studying and improving the complex phenomenon of human learning.

Advantages of Programmed Instruction

- Student is kept active and alert.
- The teacher gets relieved of doing ordinary jobs and she can play the important role of a guide, counselor, motivator, organizer.
- Social and emotional problems can be eliminated.
- The problems of discipline have been automatically solved by the use of self-instructional material.
- Programmed instruction makes learning interesting.
- Every student can work at his own place.
- Programmed instructions is useful in situations where the human instructions are not available.
- Intellectual and some motor skills will be taught more efficiently.
- More complex of the concepts can be known.

Types

There are two types in programmed instruction as given below:

Linear programming: Linear programming is based strictly upon a learning theory of conditioning. The primary objective is to bring the behavior of the learner under the control of a variety of stimuli through the use of easy steps, one at a time. Each step requires the student to participate actively by making a response.

Branching programming: Branching programming is not committed to any theory of learning. It is considered to be a technique for preparing written materials that will accommodate a wide range of educational purposes. It is primarily for diagnostic purposes, so that the student can be provided with specific remedial material needed as she selects responses.

Techniques of Programmed Instruction

- In programmed instruction, the student is presented with the necessary information broken down into very small steps.
- After understanding each step the student must take a response, answer a question, work out a problem or make a choice, usually by writing in a space provided.
- The student response is immediately checked with the right answer, than he goes on to the next step which, if the answer was correct, will follow on from the previous bit of information.

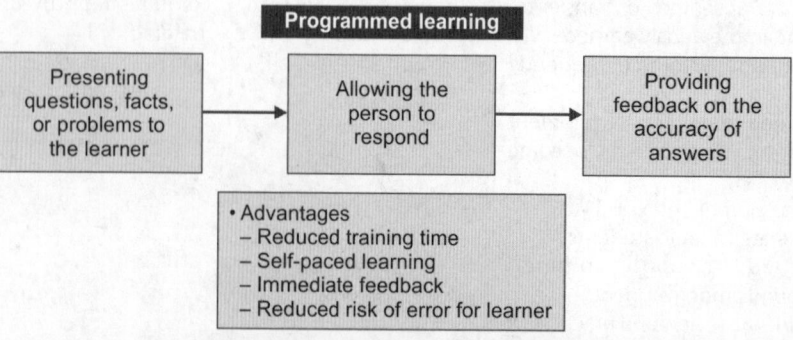

Fig. 3.36: Programmed learning steps.

- If the answer was incorrect, the student is now presented with the material specifically written to correct the error and then return to the original question for a second try, before going on to the next step.
- Programmed instruction is an attempt to provide effective instruction without requiring the physical presence of human teacher.
- The material presented to the learner and the activities in which he is engaged are selected, ordered, and arranged on the basis of empirical tests of effectiveness of the procedure adopted.
- This method of teaching that the reward of being right, encourages the students to learn.
- The programmed instruction is a new strategy of teaching. It is highly individualized instructional strategy for the modification of behavior.
- It is used for instructional purpose, but it can also be employed as a mechanism of feedback device for improving teaching efficiency.
- The theoretical knowledge of programmed instruction is essential to use it as feedback device for the modification of teacher behavior in nursing education programs.

Assumptions of Programmed Instruction

The programmed instruction has the following basic assumptions:
- A student learns better by being active.
- A student learns better if he is motivated to learn by confirming his responses.
- A student learns better if the content matter is presented in small steps.
- A student learns better if he commits minimum errors in his learning.
- A student learns better if the sequence of content is psychologically valid.
- The learning may be effective if the prerequisites are specified on the part of the learner.

Characteristics of Programmed Instruction

The following are the main features of programmed instruction strategy:
- It is not an audio-visual device. It is a part of education technology, i.e. instructional technology.
- It is not a test. It is a new strategy for teaching and learning.
- It is not the solution of educational problems. It is a new instructional problem. It is a new instructional strategy for the modification of behaviors of the learners.
- It cannot replace the teacher from the field of teaching but the effective teacher can prepare a good program.
- It requires more creativity and imaginative efforts to develop highly individualized instruction.

Steps for Development of Programmed Instruction

The development of programmed instruction is a very challenging job for a teacher. The mastery of the topic; knowledge and practice of programmed instruction are essential for it. The following steps are important in preparing programmed instruction material:
- Selection of the topic to be programmed.
- Identifying the objectives.
- Content analysis for developing the instructional procedure.
- Writing objectives (Emerging and Terminal) in behavioral terms.
- Construction of criterion test.
- Deciding appropriate paradigm and strategy of program.
- Writing program frames and individual try out.
- Group try out, revising, and editing the program and preparing final dealt.
- Master validation or evaluation of programmed in terms of internal and external criteria.
- Preparation of a manual of the program.

These steps are followed to prepare an effective program instruction material.

The procedure is very time-consuming and laborious. The programmed text is different from conventional text, because the workability of the material is determined on the basis of student's responses.

Disadvantages of Programmed Instruction

- It requires experts on programmed instruction.
- Preparation is difficult and time- consuming.
- Material is not available.
- It necessitates special educational competence.
- It costs high additional investment cost in teacher's time and money.
- There will be no group dynamics.

COMPUTER-ASSISTED LEARNING

Computer-assisted instruction (CAI), as the name suggests, stands for the type of instruction aided or carried out with the help of a computer as a machine. It is just one step ahead of the use of teaching machine and, probably, two of the use of programmed textbook in making the instructional process as self-directed and individualized as possible. Computer influence every sphere of human activity and bring many changes in education, health care scientific research, social sciences etc. usage of computers in health care system will save the time, economizes energy and help the nurses to provide quality nursing care.

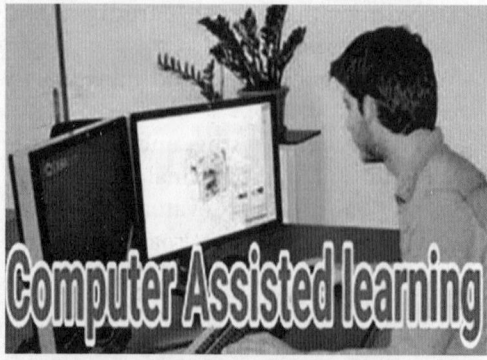

Fig. 3.37: Computer assisted learning.

Definitions of Computer-assisted Instruction

- **According to Hilgard and Bower (1977),** "Computer-assisted instruction has now taken as so many dimensions that it can no longer be considered as a simple derivative of the teaching machine or the kind of programmed learning that Skinner introduced".
- **According to Bhatt and Sharma (1992),** "CAI is an interaction between a students, a computer controlled display and a response entry device for the purpose of achieving educational outcomes."

This definition brings into limelight the following things:

- In CAI, there is an interaction between an individual student and the computer just as happens in the tutorial system between the teacher and an individual student.
- The computer is able to display the instructional material to the individual student.
- The individual student takes benefit of the displayed material and responds to it. These responses are attended by the computer for deciding the future course of instruction displayed to the learner.
- The interaction between the individual learner and the computer device helps in the realization of the set instruction objectives.

Importance of Computer in Education

The following are the areas in which computers are helping the educations:

- Computers take over the most of the drudgery of schooling like classifying children according to abilities, preparing time table, etc.
- Computers allocate learning resources to individuals and groups.
- Computers maintain progress cards and preserve them confidentially.
- They provide easy access to files of information for reference and guidance.
- They engage the students in tutorial interaction and dialogue.

Types of Computer-assisted Instruction Programs

- **Logo:** This system developed by Feurzeing and Papart provides instruction which can be used to produce pictures on an oscilloscope or make a little mechanical robot. Often students suggest their own tasks and then write appropriate programs.
- **Simulation and gaming:** This system enables the student mount an experiment in symbolic form.
- **Controlled learning:** Controlled learning involves the use of interesting adaptive strategies. It includes both drill and practice. Drill and practice programs are supplementary to the regular curriculum followed by the classroom teacher.

Basic Assumptions

The computer-assisted instruction, meant for auto-individualized instructions, rests on the following basic assumptions:

- **Instruction for a number of learners at a time:** CAI can serve at a time thousands of learners in an individualized way. What an individual needs according to his ability and interest in a particular subject or topic, and accordingly he can get the instructional material and help from the computer. Moreover, it is the best programmed instruction available to him in such a nice individualized way. Hence, the first assumption of CAI lies in its capacity of providing quality and quantity auto-instruction to a sufficiently larger number of the individual learners at a time.
- **Automatic recording of the learners' performance:** How does an individual learner react to the presented instructional material? What are his quarries and difficulties? What is his performance in terms of learning outcomes? All such things can be successfully and accurately recorded by the computer device. It helps much in further planning the needed instruction to the individual learner for this proper advancement.

  This timely and proper auto-recording is the second assumption underlying CAI.
- **Variety in the use of methods and techniques:** CAI assumes that every learner cannot be benefited through a single method and all the subjects or topics in a subject cannot be handled through a common method or strategies. It believes that there should be a wide variety of methods and approaches for imparting instruction in a particular subject or topic so that all the individual learners may be able to choose a particular method or approach

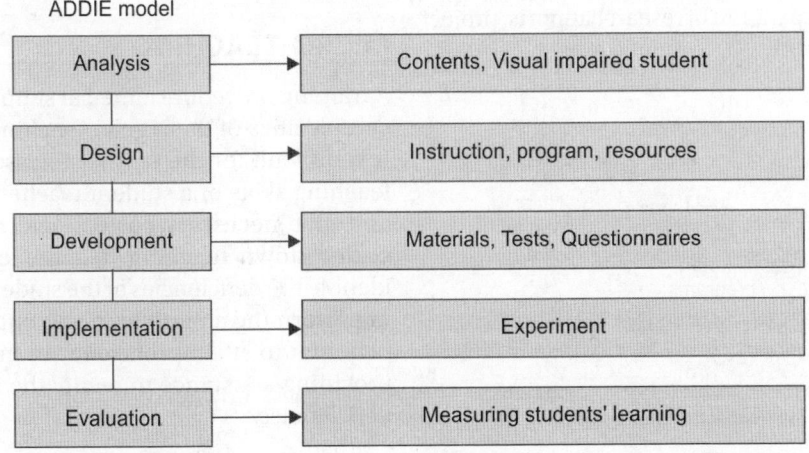

Fig. 3.38: ADDIE model.

according to their own interest, ability and nature of the instructional material.

Instructional Uses of Computer

Computer-assisted instruction programs are very useful in self-paced learning. The following are some of the areas where the computers prove to be effective in the instructional process.

I. **Drill and practice:** 1. Most common and least complex method, 2. A learner is presented with a series of questions or problems about materials, e.g. drug dosage calculation, I.V drip rate calculation, 3. Writing up of textbooks; collection of education materials, and 4. Library maintenance.

II. **Tutorial programs:** 1. Display new material, 2. Tutorial information, and 3. Feedback.

III. **Simulations:** 1. The real life situations will be presented to assist learners in problem solving and decision-making skills in a safe environment.
2. Interactive video instruction can provide learners with true to life simulation.
3. Video picture, graphics can be incorporated in the design of software.

IV. **Nursing Research:** Research works life
1. Review literature or search for related articles, e.g., Internet, search line.
2. Tool for data collection.
3. Dissemination of findings and results.
4. Tabulations.
5. Preparation of research reports, project report.

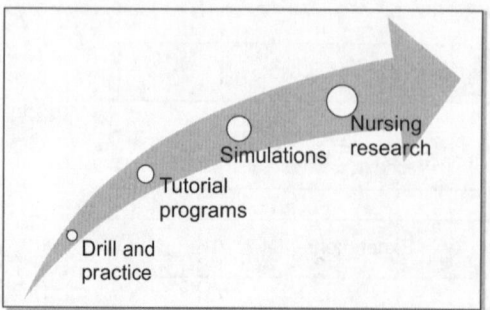

Fig. 3.39: Instructional uses of computer.

Advantages of Computer-assisted Learning

- It saves time in learning.
- It performs miracles in processing the performance data.
- It helps to determine subsequent activities in the learning situation.
- The large amount of information stored in the computer is made available to the learner more rapidly.
- The dynamic interaction between the student and instructional programme is possible.

Disadvantages of CAL

- Inadequate training of teachers and inadequacy of instructional material.
- It is prohibitively expensive.
- Computers inject a non-human quality into educational programs.
- The computer fails to appreciate the emotions of the students.
- The emotional warmth climate which is created by the teachers in the classroom interaction with the students are lacked in CAL.
- The peripheral equipment puts constraint in the ways on which a student can interact with the computer.
- CAT fails to develop essential features of language competency CAT is mechanical approach to education.

MICRO-TEACHING

A training procedure aimed at simplifying the complexities of the regular teaching process. It is difficult for the teacher to assess all the teaching skills of a student teacher at a time and give necessary corrections. By way of scaled down teaching, teacher can easily identify the deficiencies of the student teacher in performing a particular teaching skill and help him to attain proficiency in that skill by providing assistance to rectify the identified deficiencies.

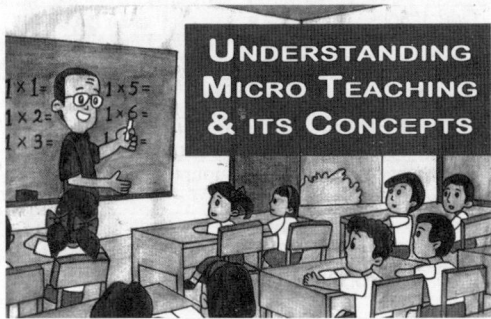

Fig. 3.40: Micro-teaching method.

Definitions of Micro-teaching

- **According to Allen,** "Micro-teaching as a scaled down teaching encounter in class size and class time". The number of students is from 5-10 and the duration of period ranges from 5-20 minutes.
- **According to DW Allen (1966),** Micro-teaching is a scaled down teaching encounter in class size and time.
- **According to Allen and Eve (1968),** Micro-teaching is defined as a system of controlled practice that makes it possible to concentrate on specific teaching behavior and to practice teaching under controlled conditions.
- **According to RN Bush (1968):** Micro-teaching is a teacher education technique which allows teachers to apply clearly defined teaching skills in carefully prepared lessons in a planned series of five to ten minute encounters with a small group of real students, often with an opportunity to observe the result on video tape.
- **According to McAleese and Unwin (1970),** The term micro-teaching is most often applied to the use of closed circuit television to give immediate feedback of a trainee teacher's performance in a simplified environment.
- **According to Clift and other (1976),** Micro-teaching is a teaching training procedure which reduces the teaching situation to a simple and more controlled encounter achieved by limiting the practice teaching to a specific skill and reducing teaching time and class size.
- **According to BK Passi and MS Lalita (1976),** Micro-teaching is a training technique which requires student teacher to teach a single concept using specified teaching skill to a small number of pupils in a short duration of time.

Characteristics of Micro-teaching

- It is relatively a new experience or innovation in the field of teacher education, more specifically in student teaching.
- It is a training technique and not a teaching technique. In other words, it is a technique or design used for the training of teachers (or makes them learn the art of teaching). It is not a method of classroom instruction or teaching like inductive-deductive, demonstration or question-answer method.
- It is micro- or miniaturized teaching in the sense that it scales down the complexities of real teaching with the provisions such as:
  a. Practicing one skill at a time.
  b. Reducing the class size to 5-10 pupils.
  c. Reducing duration of the lesson to 5-10 minutes.
  d. Limiting the content to a single concept.
- There is provision of adequate feedback in micro-teaching as it provides trainees due information about their performances immediately after the completion of their lesson.

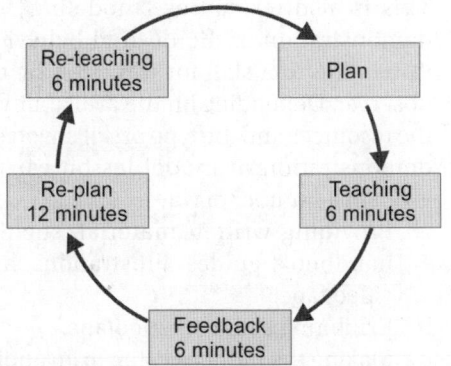

Fig. 3.41: Micro-teaching cycle.

- Teaching is said to be composed of very specific skills. These skills cannot be mastered through the traditional approach to teacher training. Micro-teaching provides opportunity to select one skill at a time and practice it through its scaled down encounter and then take other in a similar way.
- Micro-teaching is a highly individualized training device permitting the imposition of a high degree of control in practicing a particular skill.

  Looking at the above characteristics and features, the term micro-teaching may be defined appropriately as a technique or device of imparting training to the inexperienced or experienced teachers for learning the art of teaching by practicing specific skills through a "scaled down teaching encounter", i.e. reducing the complexities of real normal teaching in terms of size of the class, time and content.

Phases of Micro-teaching

- **Orientation:** In the beginning, the student teacher should be given necessary theoretical background about micro-teaching by having a free and fair discussion of the following aspects:
  a. Concept,
  b. Significance or rationale of using micro-teaching,
  c. Procedure, and
  d. Requirements and setting for adopting micro-teaching technique.
- **Discussion of teaching skills:** Under this step, the knowledge and understanding about the following aspects is to be developed:
  a. Analysis of teaching into component teaching skills.
  b. Discussion of the rationale and role of teaching skills in teaching.
  c. Discussion about the component teaching behavior comprising various teaching skills.
- **Selection of a particular teaching skill:** The teaching skills are to be practiced by taking them one at a time. Therefore, the student teachers are persuaded to select a

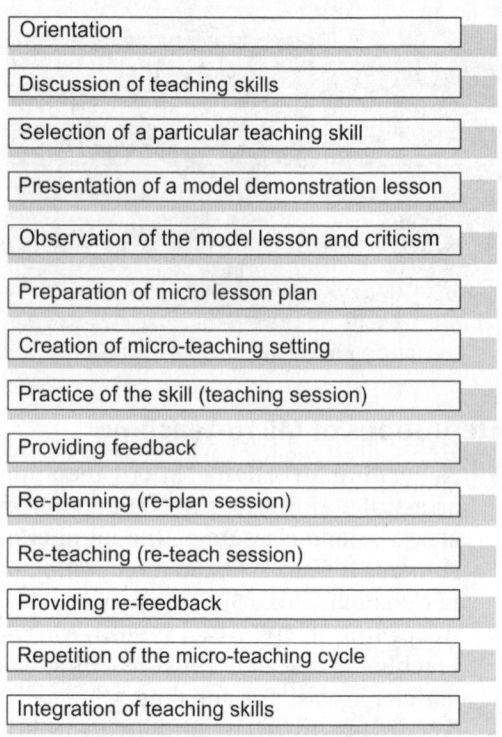

Orientation

Discussion of teaching skills

Selection of a particular teaching skill

Presentation of a model demonstration lesson

Observation of the model lesson and criticism

Preparation of micro lesson plan

Creation of micro-teaching setting

Practice of the skill (teaching session)

Providing feedback

Re-planning (re-plan session)

Re-teaching (re-teach session)

Providing re-feedback

Repetition of the micro-teaching cycle

Integration of teaching skills

Fig. 3.42: Phases of micro-teaching.

particular skill for practice. They are also provided with necessary orientation and processing material for the practice. Most of such material may be found in the literature available with NCERT. The student teacher may be given a necessary background for the observation of a model or demonstration lesson on the selected teaching skill.

- **Presentation of a model demonstration lesson:** Here, a demonstration or model lesson for the use of the selected teaching skill is presented before the trainees. This is also termed as "modeling", i.e. demonstration of the desired behaviors in relation to a skill for imitation by the observer. Depending on the availability of the resources and the type of skill involved, demonstration or model lesson can be given in a number of ways:
  a. Providing written material, such as handbook, guides, illustrations, and video tape.
  b. Exhibiting a film or videotape.
  c. Making the trainees listen to an audio-tape.

d. Arranging a demonstration from a live model, i.e. a teacher educator or an expert demonstrating the use of the skill.

- **Observation of the model lesson and criticism:** What is read, viewed, listened, and observed through a modeling source here is carefully analyzed by the trainee. In a demonstration given by an expert or teacher educator, the student teachers are expected to note down their observations. An observation schedule especially designed for the observation of the specific skill is distributed among the trainees and they are also trained in its use beforehand. Such an observation of the model lesson and its relevant criticism provide desired feedback to the person giving the model lesson.

- **Preparation of micro lesson plan:** Under this step, the student teachers are required to prepare micro lesson plans by selecting proper concept for the practice of demonstrated skill. For their preparation, help may be taken from the teacher educators and the sample lessons available in NCERT.

- **Creation of micro-teaching setting:** The following is the standard setting for a micro-class:
  a. Number of pupils: 5-10.
  b. Types of pupils: Real pupils or preferably peers.
  c. Types of supervisor: Teacher educators and peers.
  d. Time duration of a micro lesson: 6 minutes.

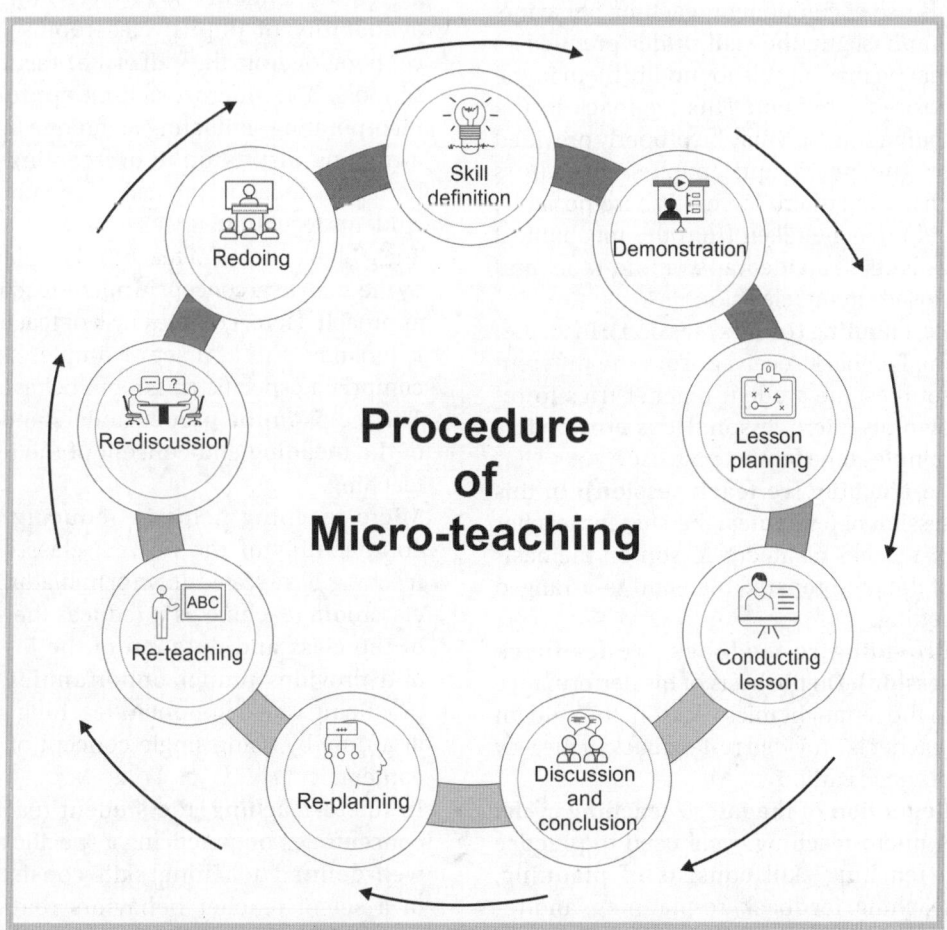

Fig. 3.43: Micro-teaching procedure steps.

e. Time duration of a micro-teaching cycle: 36 minutes.

- **Practice of the skill (teaching session):** Here, the student teacher teaches his prepared micro lesson for 6 minutes (prescribed time schedule for teach-session) a micro-class consisting of 5-10 real pupils or peers (Student teachers). It is supervised by the teacher educator and peers both with the help of appropriate observation schedule. Where possible, the student teacher may also have his lesson taped on a video or audio tape.

- **Providing feedback:** The greatest advantage of micro-teaching lies in providing immediate feedback to the student teacher on his teaching performance demonstrated in his micro-lesson. The feedback is provided in terms of his use of component teaching behaviors emphasizing the skill under practice so that he may be able to modify them in the desired direction. This feedback in the Indian situation may be properly provided by the peers and teacher educators observing micro lesson. Where possible, help may be taken from the mechanical gadgets like videotape, audio tape, and closed circuit television.

- **Re-planning (re-plan session):** In view of the feedback received from the different sources, the student teacher tries to re-plan his micro-lesson. He is provided 12 minutes time for this purpose.

- **Re-teaching (re-teach session):** In this session of 6 minutes, the student teacher re-teaches his micro-lesson on the basis of the pre-prepared plan and re-arranged setting.

- **Providing re-feedback (re-feedback session):** On the basis of his performance in the re-taught micro-lesson, the student teacher is provided re-feedback in the way outlined earlier.

- **Repetition of the micro-teaching cycle:** A micro-teaching cycle used to practice a teaching skill consists of planning, teaching, feedback, re-planning, and re-feedback operations

- The micro-teaching cycle is repeated and the student teacher is required to re-plan and re-teach his lesson till he attains mastery over the skill under practice.

- **Integration of teaching skills:** The last step is concerned with the task of integrating various teaching skills individually mastered by a student teacher. This helps in bridging a gap between training in isolated teaching skills and the real teaching situation faced by a student teacher.

Advantages of Micro-teaching

In the Indian context, micro-teaching has the following advantages over the traditional methods of learning the art of teaching:

- In our traditional mode of teacher training, a great dependence is observed on the availability of pupils, classrooms and cooperation from the staff of the practicing schools. The micro-teaching approach incorporating simulating technique helps a training institution in overcoming the hardships faced in the task of organizing students teaching.

- The global concept of teaching is replaced by the analytical concept in micro-teaching approach. Here, complex task of teaching is looked upon as a set of simpler skills comprising specific classroom behaviors. This helps in the proper understanding of the meaning and concept of the term teaching.

- Micro-teaching helps in reducing the complexities of the normal classroom teaching. It is a scaled down or miniaturized classroom teaching as it reduces the size of the class and duration of the lesson and provides proper opportunities for practicing one component teaching skill at a time by using single concept of the content.

- In micro-teaching, the student teacher concentrates on practicing a specific and well-defined teaching skill consisting of a set of teacher behaviors that are observable, controllable, and practicable.

Consequently, it provides a more appropriate technique of learning the art of teaching (although mastering one teaching skill at a time) than the traditional program.

- Micro-teaching helps in the systematic and objective observation by providing a specific observation schedule.
- Micro-teaching works as a laboratory exercise to focus training on the acquisition of teaching skills and instructional techniques. Here, a trainee can experiment with several alternatives in a limited time and resources. It is just like learning the art of operating human body parts in a medical laboratory by a student doctor before actually operating a patient.
- Micro-teaching provides economy in mastering the teaching skills. It saves the time and energy of the student teacher as well as of the pupils. It is not only easy for a student teacher to handle a micro-group (5-10 pupils) but it is also safe because they will have less problems of classroom discipline and subsequent mental tension as faced commonly in the traditional practice teaching program. It also saves the pupils from being unnecessarily used as guinea pigs for training student teachers.

BIBLIOGRAPHY

1. Ann JZ. Professional Adjustments and Ethics for Nurses in India. Bangalore: B.I. Publications, 6th edition.
2. Cunningham WF. Pivotal problems of education. Macmillian. New York 1940.
3. G Sripriya. Quality in nursing education, nursing journal of India.
4. Loretta EH. Teaching and Learning in Schools of Nursing, 3rd edition, 1996.
5. Macaden L. et al. Indian Nursing Journal of Continuing nursing educational, Nursing Education: Current scenario and future goals. Vol. I, No (1), July- December 2001.
6. Moore TV. The driving forces of human nature and the adjustments. Grune and Statton. New York 1948.
7. Nanda SK. Educational theory principles and methods, Jullundar, 1982.
8. Potter and Perry, Fundamentals of Nursing, London, Mosby Publishers, 4th edition.
9. Shields TE. Philosophy of education. Catholic university press. Washington 1921.
10. Zerwekh J. Nursing today, London: W.B.Saunders Company, 3rd edition.

4

Clinical Teaching Methods

INTRODUCTION

The clinical teaching is a type of group conference in which a patient or patients is (are) observed and studied, discussed, demonstrated, and directed towards the improvement and further improvement of nursing care. In nursing clinical teaching may be given by the doctor in order to discuss the medical aspects of a patient's condition more vividly than can be done in the classroom. Such a class will usually follow, or be followed by, a further consideration of the range of conditions to which the disease seen in the patient belongs.

The current movement is toward the development of theoretical research designs for the study of the processes of teaching and learning and their ultimate effects on self-appropriated learning. Teachers must rely on currently available information and their own resourcefulness in the selection, adaptation, and evaluation of effective teaching-learning methods and devices.

Educators continue to seek ways of having personal and close contact with master teachers who inspire through their ability to communicate their knowledge of the subject field and their understanding of the student as an individual.

COMMONLY USED CLINICAL TEACHING METHODS

In nursing commonly used clinical teaching methods include:

- Nursing clinics/bedside clinic.
- Nursing rounds.
- Nursing assignments.
- Nursing care conferences.
- Morning and afternoon reports.
- Team nursing conferences.
- Health team conferences.
- Individual conferences.
- Field visits.
- Process recording, etc.

PURPOSES OF CLINICAL TEACHING

- To provide individualized care in a systematic, holistic approach.

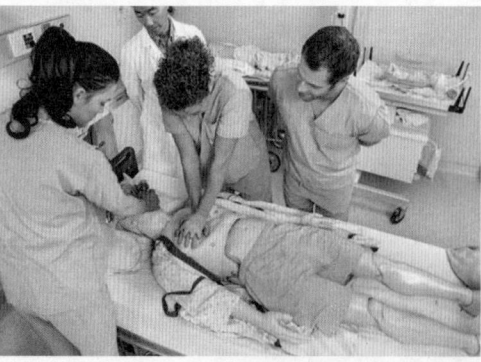

Fig. 4.1: Clinical teaching.

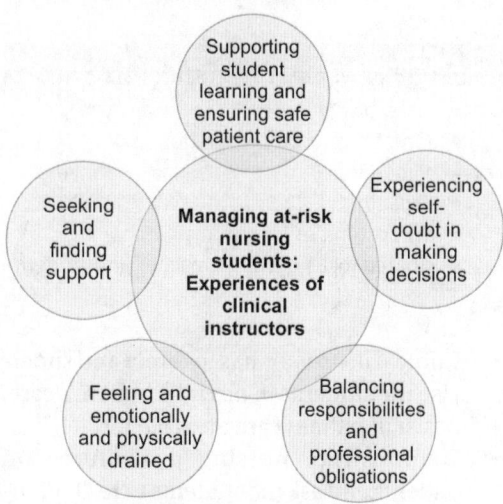

Fig. 4.2: Role of clinical instructor.

- To develop high technical competent skills.
- To practice various procedures.
- To collect and analyze the data.
- To conduct research.
- To maintain high standard of nursing practice.
- To become independent enough to practice nursing.
- To develop cognitive, affective and psychomotor skills.
- The students will develop the techniques, e.g., observation.

- To meet the needs of client.
- To improve standards of nursing practice.
- To develop various methods in delivering care.
- To identify the problems of clients.
- To learn various diagnostic procedures.
- To learn various skills in giving health education techniques to the clients and significant others.
- To help in integration of theoretical knowledge into practice.
- To develop communication skills and to maintain interpersonal relationships.
- To maintain inter-institutional relationship.
- To develop proficiency and efficiency in carrying out various nursing procedures.
- To assist physician in assisting procedures.
- To learn managerial skills.
- To become professionally active member.
- To encounter reality in the practice of nursing, synthesis learning, practice activities described in the course objectives.

ESSENTIALS OF GOOD CLINICAL INSTRUCTION

The clinical instructor or head nurse has to select a clinical area, where the clients require

Learner explanation
The learner explains their thinking process
The tutor observes the learner's reasoning ability
The tutor observes the process the learner takes to form a conclusion

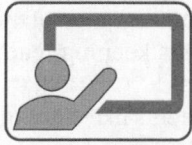

Role modelling
The tutor role models their thinking process
The tutor explains their process and how they came to form a conclusion

Questioning
The tutor should question the learner
"What if?" questions can promote reasoning

Fig. 4.3: Essentials of good clinical instruction.

Table 4.1: Challenges and advantages of clinical teaching.

Challenges	Advantages
• No formal teaching training • Learners of diverse backgrounds and motivation • Stressful healthcare environment—every case is a teaching case • Juggling stresses of personal role	• Case-based • One-on-one: preceptorship • Experiential • Meaningful • Opportunities for critique • Shared focus between teacher and student

good nursing care and also it should provide chance for the students to practice high standards of nursing care practice.

The clinical instructor and the head nurse should consider the needs of students to develop the individuals at a higher level of functioning.

They select the area where opportunities are available for the instructor to teach and the students to learn according to the requirements set by the institution.

Identify the nursing personnel (head nurse and staff nurse) who are interested in attending and sharing the discussion in nursing care conferences, nursing rounds and other sessions where clinical conditions were discussed.

Competent teacher should be available. The head nurse and instructor should cooperate with one another to plan and to provide improved nursing care practice.

FUNCTIONS OF THE CLINICAL INSTRUCTOR

- Set the objectives, standards for practice.
- Develop evaluation tools.
- Should take permission of the institute.
- Prepare master rotation plan.
- Set up the clinical area in an ideal manner.
- Keeps ready equipment in working condition to provide nursing care.
- Clinical instructor has the chief responsibility in planning, direction of instructional program within one clinical area of student's experience.
- Clinical instructor has to maintain the standards of nursing care practice.

- Clinical instructor has to direct and supervise the students in providing client's care.
- Assist in patient care and role model.
- Demonstrate nursing procedures on patients and ask the students to re-demonstrate procedures to develop skill and confidence.
- Develop an understanding of research for better patient care.
- Analyze the difficulties and guiding the students accordingly.
- Maintain high standards of patient care.
- Encourage, motivate and inspire students.
- Supervise and evaluate the performance of students.
- Maintain strict discipline.
- Maintain students' records, e.g., duty rosters, individual assignments, evaluation tools, clinical teachings and performance of students.
- Conduct individual conferences with the students to solve any problems arose and to meet their professional and personal needs.
- To attend the lectures (of doctors) which were arranged for students and make arrangements for presentation of the topic, e.g., bringing clients keeping ready overhead? Projectors, etc.
- Supervise assignments like ward teaching class, case study, health talks.
- Has to participate in faculty conferences.
- Focus attention of the students upon the medical and nursing problems of the clients to whom they are assigned.
- To help the students to develop ability to adjust general plans of care to the needs of individual patients.

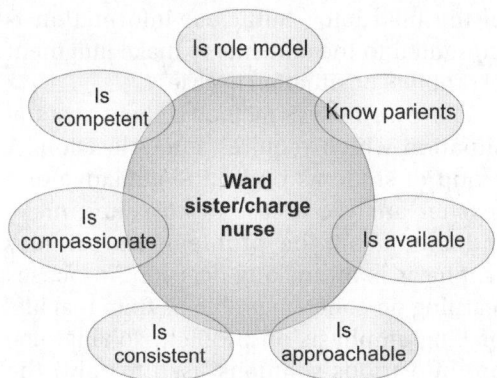

Fig. 4.4: Skills of ward sister.

- Assist the students in preparing teaching plans.
- To demonstrate skillfully the nursing procedures of special importance on the particular area.
- To guide the students in acquisition of new skills.
- To direct the students in their use of library resources for writing and preparing clinical assignments of students.
- To guide the students in conducting nursing research activities.
- To develop potentialities of each student.

QUALITIES OF A CLINICAL INSTRUCTOR

- She should enjoy bedside nursing.
- She should be an expert in bedside nursing.
- She should have good communication skills and develops good rapport among the nursing personnel.
- She must know methods of delivering the care.
- Confidence has to be maintained since success in clinical nursing rests upon her ability to win the cooperation of doctors, head nurse, staff nurse, other professional colleagues, technicians, the auxiliary staff, ability to work well with other persons.
- Should possess adequate theoretical background.
- Should possess advanced knowledge in educational psychology and other advanced areas, e.g., specialties.

- Should enjoy in teaching the students in hospital situation.
- She should be appointed on the basis of outstanding skills.
- Ability to implement the knowledge into practice.
- Ability to communicate the knowledge to others.
- Should have good teaching skills.
- Physically active.
- Very wholesome, healthy, smiling and pleasing personality.
- Neat, nicely dressed (good poise)
- Good conduct
- Empathetic, sympathetic in nature.
- Should understand total nursing program
- Should have detailed knowledge about area, in which she was placed.
- Should have positive philosophy of life.
- She must know teaching and evaluating methods.
- She has to maintain good working relations
- She should be responsible for all arrangements of experiences in her clinical area.
- She has to participate in professional activities.
- She has to maintain good conducive, democratic environment.
- She has to maintain freedom of speech.

CASE METHOD

Used in three forms: (1) Case study, (2) Case analysis, (3) Case.

Case Study/Case Presentation

The student will be given the opportunity to provide nursing care for specific client, after 4 or 5 days of careful study, the student nurse will prepare case study by comparing with the text, the student presents the case before the batch of companions, general discussion about the client will be dealt.

Definition

Case method is a method of clinical teaching in which a student/teacher presents a case. It is an oral report of a clinical case as compared with the literature.

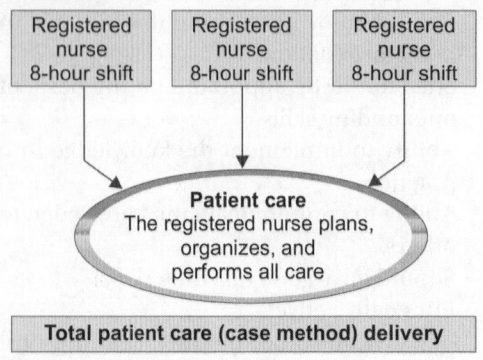

Fig. 4.5: Nursing care delivery by case method.

of the instructor. Sufficient information is presented to the students to make judgment of problem or situation in case.

The case analysis method is about a central situation which requires some decision. A group of students under the guidance of a teacher analyze a case discuss, and make judgments on the problem. Its primary emphasis is on making decision. It focuses learning on concrete problems from real life, placing emphasis on problem-solving, i.e., on the various solutions used to solve the problem.

Purpose

- To give first-hand information about the disease, investigation, treatment and nursing management.
- To learn about a particular patient thoroughly as a whole related to the disease and compare with the literature.
- To observe and interpret signs, symptoms reaction of the patient and assess prognosis.
- To compare and contrast case with a particular diagnosis with another care of similar diagnosis.

The case study method of teaching and learning originated many centuries ago.

Case Analysis

A concrete case for analysis and discussion by a group of students under the leadership

Objectives of Case Analysis Method

- Develop a mind that has the power to transfer from familiar types of problems to new ones and to be able to explain wisely the basis for a decision.
- Develop the ability to master a tangle of circumstantial evidence, selecting important factors from a whole set of facts and weighing their importance in the context of the base.
- Enlarge the ability to utilize ideas, to test them against the facts of the problem, to examine ideas and facts and to discuss ways which make them appropriate for the solution of the problem.
- Extend the ability to utilize data from experience as a test of validity of the ideas already obtained with flexibility to revise goals and procedures when the need arises.

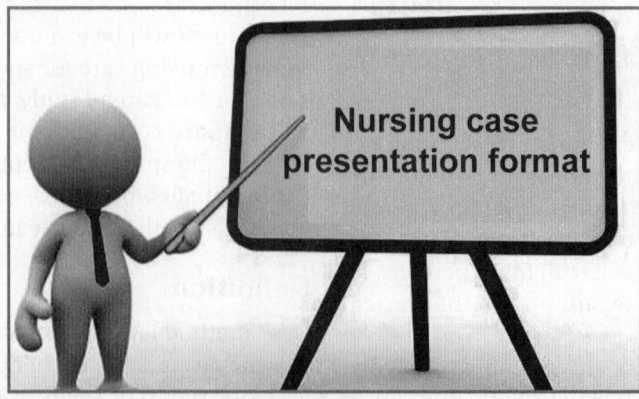

Fig. 4.6: Case method teaching.

- Expand the ability the communicate thoughts to others in a way which stimulates further thought.
- Develop the ability to use ideas in theoretical form, to create a framework of general propositions from problem-solving experiences.

Case Incident Technique

A critical incident technique which requires immediate decision and action is taken from a case and presented to the students for their analysis and decision. No background information is given to them regarding details of the incident at the time, it is presented. The instructor will have facts about the case, can be given as requested by the students. The case incident method of teaching is a modification of case analysis method which focuses on critical incident in a case which requires immediate decision and action. There is no background information. It just pinpoints the incident which requires solution. It was originated by Paul and Faith Pigors.

The Phases of Case Incident

Phase 1: The incidents: After discussing the various factors which influence the behavior of adult patients in the hospital, the class is presented with an incident taken from a life situation.

Phase 2: Getting the facts: The students are ask what information they need before they can make an effective decision. The leader has the facts of the case and given them as request by the group. The group members summarize it.

Phase 3: Determining the source of the problem and the consequences. The group determines which area of the problem needs immediate decision and consequences can occur if decision is not made.

Phase 4: Stating decision and reasons for decisions by individual students. Each student would be asked to write down what she would have done and give the reasons for her decision.

Phase 5: Identifying major decision and issues raised by the individual students through group discussion. Identifying and discuss major decisions raised by individuals and classify them into categories. The process of systematic thinking about the incident then should be reviewed and summarized.

Advantages of Case Method

- It is useful to get firsthand knowledge from a real situation.
- It recognizes problem, discuss solutions, develop insight.
- Sense of achievement develops when the student presents the case of others.
- Student gets an opportunity for family education.
- It improves self-confidence in the students.
- Student can compare the patient's condition with the literature, so better understanding is possible.
- Develops skills of presentation.

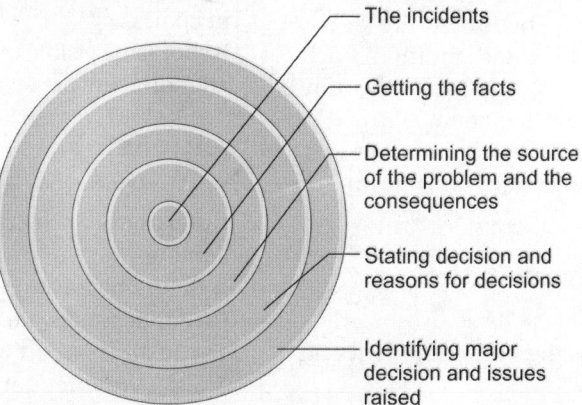

Fig. 4.7: Phases of case incident.

Limitations

- The patient may feel uncomfortable and may not like losing her privacy.
- Case method, if presented in unorganized manner may lose its effect.
- The group needs to be smaller as large groups may cause distraction.

CASE PRESENTATION

Case presentation is a method of teaching learning in which a case is presented by a student/teacher.

Meaning

- In-depth oral report of the clinical case for the purpose of learning is known as case presentation.
- It is a form of teaching-learning activity done by the teacher/student about the patient's condition as a whole which will be compared with the book picture.

Purpose

- To provide an ideal situation to learn about the disease, investigation, treatment and nursing management.
- To get a firsthand knowledge from a real situation.
- To learn about a particular patient thoroughly as a whole related to the disease and compare with the book picture.
- To get a realistic idea about the patients present condition and the nursing care to be implemented.
- To stimulate and encourage the deve_lopment of intuitive and ability in each member of the group and thereby obtaining active participation.
- To observe and interpret signs, symptoms, reaction of the patient and result of therapy.

Phases in Case Presentation

Teacher presentation:
- Be aware of objectives of the student and their level.
- Know the availability of cases.

- Choose appropriate case.
- Acquaint yourself with theoretical aspects of the disease.
- Learn the case yourself first.
- Give prior information to the students about the case.
- Select suitable case (patient) based on the level of nursing students and their specific objectives of learning that is knowledge, attitude and practice.
- The disease condition must be evident in the patient.
- The case should have received adequate medications, nursing care suitable for teaching.
- Informed consent of the patient is obtained for case presentation and encourage cooperation of the patient.
- Inform staff of particular ward.
- Develop adequate rapport with the patient.
- Prepare a plan in such a way that what to see question to be asked and points to be discussed.
- The teacher must establish a permissive, non-authoritarian atmosphere, so that students will feel free to discuss about a case.
- Treat the student with respect and tolerance.

Preparation of Audiovisual Aids

- It should be relevant to the content and patient condition.
- It should be in a attractive manner.
- It can be either in the form of flash card or charts.
- It should be visible to all (those who are all attending the presentation)

Physical Setup

- The presentation can be done near to the patient. So it should have adequate lighting.
- It should be free from noise.
- Cleanliness must be maintained.
- Ensure the comfort of the patient.
- Make sure adequate space is available near the bedside.

Table 4.2: Method of case presentation.

Case information to include	Examples in text
Patient demographics (age, gender, nationality, etc.)	"A 35-year-old man"; "a 1-month-old infant"; "a 12-year-old Somali girl," etc.
Presenting symptoms	"Demonstrated typical signs and symptoms of Huntington's disease"; "presented to the hospital with severe chest pain"; "experienced a burning sensation due to swollen leg muscles"
History of problems/symptoms	"Reported a long history of asthma"; "had a family history of colon cancer on the maternal side"; "reported that inflammation had begun one year prior"
Diagnoses	"Based on the characteristic appearance of the cutaneous lesions, a diagnosis of granuloma annulare was made"; "a clinical diagnosis of chronic respiratory disease was made"; "intestinal legions were consistent with severe Crohn's disease"
Treatment	"The patient was immediately intubated and antitubercular therapy was initiated"; "treatment was initiated with low-dose corticosteroids, anticoagulants, and vasodilators"
Procedures	"Following kidney biopsy, renal cysts were excised laparoscopically"; "the patient underwent three skin grafts"; "an emergency arteriogram showed smooth segmental narrowing and bilateral vasospasm"
Complications/challenges	"Additional history revealed that he had been ingesting ergotamine preparations for a number of years to relieve chronic muscle pain"; "laparoscopic access to the duodenum was inhibited by intra-abdominal fat"
Outcomes	"Patient was asymptomatic on subsequent visits"; "although scapular swelling subsided, she continued to report severe back pain for the following month"; "...resulting in significant improvement within 4 hours and resolution of symptoms within 48 hours"

- Around 6-8 students can effectively learn from case presentation in the ward setup.

Procedure of Presentation

- It should be suitable to the learning objective, students level and patient condition.
- Correlation and integration must be done between the patient condition and the book picture.
- There must be unity, continuity and sequence in presentation.
- It should be flexible, allowing students to reflect, question, etc.
- Be audible.
- Mutually introduce the patient and the student group to each others.
- Follow the sequence given in the format.
- Converse with the patient and make relevant observations.
- Help students observe any relevant signs and symptoms and clarify significant history.
- Make known what medical and nursing care had been done along with their rationales.
- Relate the findings and care with the literature.
- Discuss the nursing care of the case comprising with the idealistic care.
- Encourage objective evaluation of nursing care.
- The presentation should attract the student and make them to participate actively.
- Use appropriate visual aids illustrations which is relevant to the patient condition.
- Duration of case presentation can be 30–40 minutes.
- Involve patient in the process of case presentation.

- The instructor will minimize her own contribution to the discussion but at the same time will be prepared at any time to summarize the condition.
- Make conclusion with future plan for nursing action and care.
- Ensure the comfort of the patient and thank the patient for his participation.

Format for Case Presentation

History of the patient:
- Identification data
- Socioeconomic status.
- Family history.
- Family medical history.
- Personal history.
- Menstrual history (female patients).
- Marital history.
- Obstetrical history.
- Past medical history.
- Present medical history.
- Present surgical history.

Along with this information, content about the disease must be written in the form of:
- Definition of case
- Review of anatomy and physiology.
- Types (if any) (book picture/patient picture).
- Incidence (book picture/patient picture).
- Risk factors (book picture/patient picture)
- Etiology picture (book picture/patient picture).
- Pathophysiology (book picture/patient picture).
- Clinical manifestations (book picture/patient picture).
- Diagnostic evaluation (book picture/patient picture).
- Complication (book picture/patient picture)
- Management (book picture/patient picture).
- Dietary management.
- Drug management
- Surgical management.
- Nursing management.
- Health education.
- Summary
- Bibliography.

Advantages

- It is useful to get firsthand knowledge from a real situation.
- It recognize problem, discuss solutions, develop insight and see relationships.
- The student feels the thrill of achievement in presenting the case to others.
- It helps the student to receive and care a patient in future without fear.
- It helps in family education and rehabilitation.
- It helps in developing a good interpersonal relationship.
- It develops personal skill, knowledge and personality.
- It improves good speaking and organizing ability.
- It improves self-confidence.
- Gives an opportunity for teacher to check knowledge level of the student.
- It is helpful to correlate and integrate the patient picture and book picture. So that the student can understand well and the doubts will be clarified on the spot.
- Students can learn from each others.
- Student can take responsibility for their own learning.

Disadvantages

- An unorganized content can frustrate the listener.
- The patient may overhear the discussion.
- The patient may feel uncomfortable.
- If the group is so large, student cannot talk or discuss so loudly and also attention may be lost and cause distraction.
- If schedule in the morning, the case presentation will not be effective, it will be uncomfortable to both family and also hospital staff who will be busily doing procedures.

CASE STUDY

Nursing case study is one of the common and useful methods of teaching in clinical area. It is a form of quantitative and qualitative analysis involving a very careful and complete observation of a patient, and his situation.

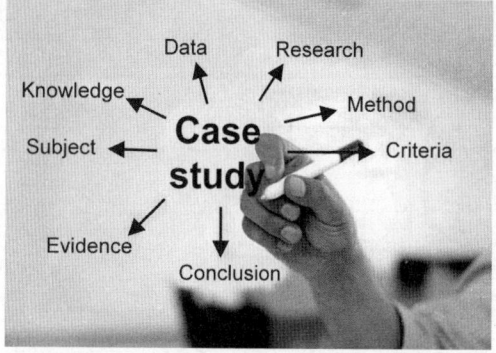

Fig. 4.8: Components of case study.

Meaning

- Case study is the intensive study of a phenomenon, including subjective information and objective information.
- Case study is an analysis of the nursing problems of an individual patient, which grow out of his diagnosis, his physical and mental condition, treatment, which are influenced by personality and socioeconomic development.
- Case study is a close, deep, cumulative and clinical study of a patient.
- Case study is a fairly exhaustive study of a person or group.

Criteria for a Good Case Study

- Continuity.
- Completeness of data.
- Validity of data.
- Confidential recording.
- Analysis and scientific synthesis.

Sources of Case Data

- Personal documental diaries, history of previous illness.
- Health team members.
- Related persons.
- Official records.
- Subject itself.

Principles

- It should include supportive and therapeutic care given to the patient.
- Emphasis should be on the individual needs of patients and how those are met.

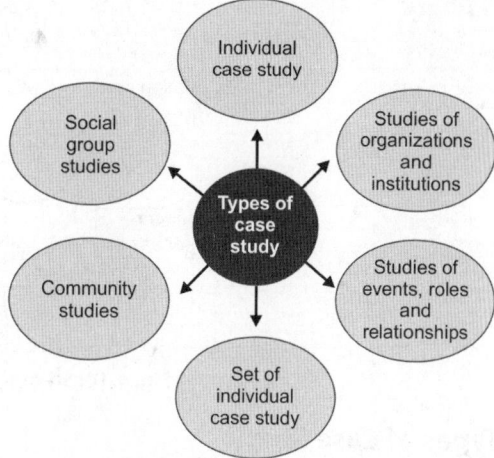

Fig. 4.9: Types of case study.

Steps in Nursing Case Study

1. **Selection of the case:** The level of knowledge of the students is taken into considerations while assigning patients. Selection of cases should be based on the level of care needed, e.g., wholly independent patient is not assigned for case study.
2. **Collection of data:** Collection of data is divided into two aspects:
   a. Subjective data: All the information, the patient himself gives.
   b. Objective data: Data which are documents through observation, investigation or intervention.
3. **Examination:** Examination of patient includes anthropometric measures, biological measures, clinical examination and dietary examination. History relevant to present and past conditions is collected using the relevant formats.
4. **Diagnosis and identification of casual factors:** Through laboratory investigations and invasive procedures, the casual factors are identified.
5. **Nursing process:** The nursing process includes assessment of the patient, forming nursing diagnosis on the basis of assessment, planning the care and implementation.
6. **Evaluation and follow-up:** The effectiveness of care rendered is identified here.

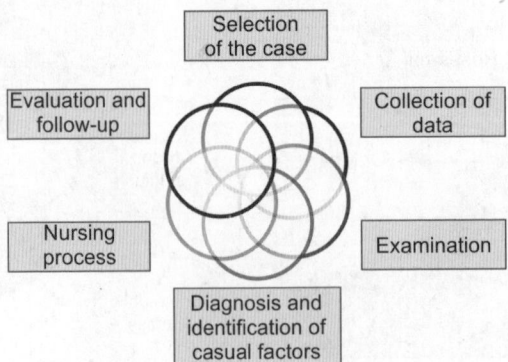

Fig. 4.10: Steps in nursing case study.

Types of Case Study

1. Oral case study.
2. Written case study.

Form and Presentation

- The case study which is in written form is generally considered best, to record in narrative form.
- Some form of outline should be used to guide the beginners. The older students may use an outline as a guide, but should be permitted to use her own initiative and creative ability in writing her study.
- Oral case study is one which is presented by one or more students in a form of verbal report to the clinical instructor.

Advantages of Nursing Case Study

- Case study is useful to the student's in planning and providing comprehensive nursing care to the patients.
- It permits the students to provide care and follow up the services for 3–5 days continuously.
- It is also useful in developing the self-expression in writing, regarding nursing care of patients.
- It helps the student to develop clinical knowledge by comparing the ideal book picture with realistic patient condition.
- Better nursing care results because of the concentrated effort on the part of the student in defining and solving the problem.
- Student gain a greater understanding and appreciation of human personality and the factors that influence.

- Collection and organization of information increases students understanding of nursing problems associated with disorder.
- It helps the students to learn and apply the problem-solving approach in nursing.
- It provides for individual differences of the study.
- It provides an opportunity for self-expression in writing.
- It provides a source of material for future references.

Disadvantages

- It is more time consuming and a costly method.
- It leaves no opportunity, once the study is completed, to branch out and incorporate new ideas.
- It requires a great deal of time to rewrite in to an acceptable form.

CARE PLAN

Planning process leads to success in achievement of goals and objectives, gives meaning to work life and provides direction for operational activities of the organization. Further planning may results in efficient and effective use of resources and assist in the formulation of visionary activities and the future direction of the agency. Thus, nursing of the highest quality can only be achieved when patient's needs are individualized through a proper and systematic nursing care plan.

Meaning

Nursing is the diagnosis and treatment of human response to actual or potential health problems. The nursing care plan serves as the organizational framework for the practice of nursing. The nursing care plan is a systematic method by which nurses plan and provide care for patients. This involves a problem-solving approach that enables the nurse to identify patient's problems and potential at risk needs (problems) and to plan, deliver, and evaluate nursing care in an orderly, scientific manner.

Definition

- The nursing care plan is the method by which nursing is practiced systematically and provides the means by which nurses demonstrates accountability and responsibility to clients and families.
- The nursing care plan is a blueprint for supporting patient's adaptive responses to illness (NANDA).
- A nursing care plan is a document that reflects collaborative exchange and patient's informed consent.

Principles for Constructing Care Plan

- In making the plan to be used by nurses in caring for patient it is necessary to take into account diagnosis, physical and mental condition, and the plan for medical care.
- Care plan should embody both patients and nurses concepts of health and values of health.
- They should address patient's primary concerns.
- Care plan should be drawn from patient's resources and capabilities.
- Care plan should be the outcome of a shared decision making process that empowers patients and communities' nurses respect for patient's individuality.
- Care plan should reflect patient's informed consent.
- Care plan should enhance patient's motivation to carry out the plan.
- Care plan should consider patient's individual characteristics his nationality, age, relationships and any handicaps he may have.
- It should be in brief compact statements.

Resources of Care Plan

- **Patients:** Active patient participation is necessary for developing effective care plans. Patients are the best source of information about their needs, and change that occur as their health status change. Likewise, patient values and beliefs cannot be overlooked when planning care. Patient needs, values, and beliefs strongly influence the problems addressed in a collaborative patient care plan.
- **Professional knowledge:** Nurses share with patients their professional recommendations about the patient problems they believe are important to address. They discuss the level of wellness that they believe the patient can achieve. They share ideas for nursing implementation and patient action to achieve this level of wellness.

Developing Patient Care Plans

In this phase of care plan development, nurses and patients examine the nursing diagnosis and research an agreement about the general nature of outcomes, implementations and evaluation criteria to include in the plan. While formulating a nursing care plan five dynamic and interrelated phases are to be considered—assessment, diagnosis, planning, implementation and evaluation.

Assessment

This is the first nursing care plan, where the nurse systematically gathers, verifies, and communicates data about a client to establish a data base about the client's level of wellness, health practices, past illness and related experiences and expectations.

Assessment phase is subdivided into:
- Data collection.
- Data validation.
- Data clustering.
- Data documentation.

Table 4.3: Application of nursing process steps in case study.

Cues	Inference	Nursing Diagnosis	Panning	Interventions	Rationale	Evaluation
S: • "Sumasakit ang aking tiyan" as verbalized by the client • Pain scale: 5/10 as 0 is the lowest and 10 is the highest • With the pain characteristics of moderate pain O: • With facial grimace • Verbal report of acute pain • Guarding behavior on the left lower extremity	External and internal factor aggravates the nerve endings in the lower extremity causing production of prostaglandin, bradykinin, histamine and progesterone to react on the specific region causing pain sensation felt by the client	Acute pain related to post-surgical as manifested by facial grimace, guarding behavior and verbal report of pain felt in the lower abdominal region	After series of nursing interventions the client should manifest a decrease in the pain scale of 5/10 to a manageable level of 0/10	• Assess the clients pain scale and perception • Encourage verbal report during and after the nursing interventions • Monitor V/S and pain scale • Teach client diversional activities • Advise breathing exercise • Administer etoricoxib 120 mg/tablet as prescribed by the physician	• To identify the intensity, onset, duration, quality, and quality of the pain • Pain is highly subjective and to identify the effectiveness of the interventions • Obtain baseline V/S, V/S changes during onset of pain, for future comparison after interventions • To divert clients attention from pain • To allow proper O_2 supply in the body, clients tend to stop breathing during pain • Relieve the client of pain using pharmacologic intervention	After series of nursing interventions goals are met as evident of the clients decrease in pain scale from 5/10 to 0/10 or with no pain and discomfort and positive verbal report of the client during the evaluation

Data can be of two types:
1. **Subjective data:** Subjective data are collected through interview and health history.
2. **Objective data:** Objective data are collected through:
   a. Physical examination.
   b. Observation of behavior.
   c. Diagnostic and laboratory data.
   d. Medical records.
   e. Other healthcare team members.

Nursing Diagnosis

This step enables the nurse to individualize care for the client. During diagnostic phase, the nurse analyzes and interprets data collected about the client using scientific and professional knowledge. The nurse then identifies the client's healthcare problems and writes nursing diagnosis, which form the basis for the care plan.

Steps of nursing diagnosis are:
- Identifying client problems.
- Formulating nursing diagnosis.
- Documenting diagnosis.

Planning

Planning is a category of nursing behavior in which client centered goals are established and strategies are designed to achieve the goals. Planning requires the nurse to use deliberate decision making and problem-solving skills to design nursing care for each client. During planning, priorities are set, goals are determined, expected outcomes are developed, and a nursing care plan is formulated.

Steps of planning:
- Identifying client goals.
- Establishing expected outcomes.
- Consulting.
- Writing nursing care plans.
- Establishing priorities.
- Selecting nursing actions.
- Delectating actions.

Implementations

Implementations are to carry out the nursing care plan developed in the previous component of the nursing process. Implementation is a category of nursing behavior in which the actions necessary for achieving the expected outcomes of nursing care are initiated and completed. Implementation includes performing, assisting or directing the performance of activities of daily living. Counseling and teaching the client of family, giving direct care to achieve client centered goal, supervising and evaluating the work of staff members and recording and exchanging information relevant to the client's continued health.

Types of nursing implementation include:
- Performing nursing action.
- Reassessing client.
- Reviewing and modifying existing care plan.

Evaluation

Evaluation measures the client's response to nursing interventions and the client's progress toward achieving goals. Evaluation determines if a client improves, remain stable or deteriorates. Another aspect of evaluation involves measurement of the quality of nursing care provided in health care settings. To objectively evaluate the degree of achieving a goal, the nurse should use following:
- Examine the goal statement to identify the exact desired client behavior or response.
- Assess the client for the presence of that behavior or response.
- Compare the established outcome criteria with the behavior or response.
- Judge the degree of agreement between outcome criteria and behavior or response.

Steps of evaluation:
- Comparing client response to expected outcomes.
- Analyzing reactions for results and conclusions.
- Modifying care plan.

Advantages of Nursing Care Plan

- It is a summative structure where at a glance all the information of the patient is received.
- It portraits about the patient as a person, a little about his home background, his interests, his known worries and fears.

- In addition to the description of the patient, the portraits gives suggestions for personal approach and tells the outstanding symptoms which the patient shows, so that, the new nurse will have enough information to give him with care and prevent a break in its continuity.
- It involves a collaborative team work—head nurse, shift nurses, patient and his family members.
- Enables students to plan the care according to priority.
- Students can practically experience the patient's disease condition and the associated signs and symptoms, so that they can make an effective plan.
- Students can correlate all the steps of nursing process read in theory and directly apply it practically.
- Students can prioritize the nursing care plans based on scientific principles.
- Writing patient care plans not only assist students to assimilate information, but also provides a vehicle for communicating student's knowledge to faculty.

Common Student's Problem

- **Incomplete database:** Gathering insufficient data leads to many errors in writing a care plan.
- **Stating outcomes as nursing behaviors rather than patient behaviors:** Stating nursing, rather than patient behavior is an error that occurs most often when students view nursing as a task oriented rather than problem-solving endeavor.
- **Selecting patient behaviors that are not observable and measurable:**
  - To consider patient resources and desires.
  - Writing nursing implementation statements insufficient in number of specialist.

Disadvantages of Care Plan

- It is time consuming.
- It cannot be formulated during emergency conditions, e.g., cardiac arrest.
- All plans cannot to implement because of the unavailability of resources.

NURSING ROUNDS AND REPORTS

There are several methods that can be used effectively in clinical teaching. Nursing rounds are conducted by the head nurse/nurse teacher for the members of her staff/students. To be successful every nurse must be prepared to participate in the discussion of nursing care.

Definition

Nursing rounds are conducted by the head nurse/nurse teacher for the members of her staff/students for a clear understanding of the disease process and the effect of nursing care for each patient.

Types of Ward Rounds

- Rounds with the doctors.
- Rounds to discuss psychological problem of patients.
- Social service rounds.
- Medical rounds for nurses.
- Rounds with the physical therapists.
- Nursing rounds.

Meaning of Nursing Rounds

To acquaint nurse with all patients in the ward in order that better understanding and more purposeful care may be achieved for each patient.

Purposes of Nursing Rounds

The purpose for ward rounds includes:
- To observe the physical and the mental condition of the patients and the progress made day to day.
- To observe the work of staff.

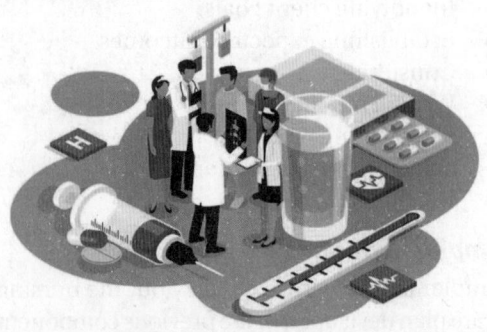

Fig. 4.11: Nursing rounds.

- To make specific observation of the patient and to give report to doctor, e.g., wound, drainage, bleeding, etc.
- To introduce the patients to the personnel and vice versa.
- To carry out the plan made for the care of the patients.
- To evaluate the results of treatment and the satisfaction of the patient with his care.
- To ensure the safety measures employed for the patient and personnel.
- To orient the nurse/student in handing over/taking over regarding patient's treatment, care done, care yet to be completed and condition of the patient.
- To teach the nursing students and the hospital aids regarding specific conditions.
- To check any preventable conditions present in the patient such as bedsore, foot drop, etc.
- To cheek the emergency equipment kept near the patient and to cheek their safety and working order.
- To compare the clinical manifestation of the patients having some disease so that the student understand in a better manner and gain better insight.

- To prescribe any modification in nursing action.

Nursing Rounds

- In nursing rounds the patient's history and the medical aspects of his care are included only as a background for the understanding of the nursing care.
- The nurse/teacher who have been caring for the patient during the week may present the background information and tell the points in nursing care which she considers to be most essential.
- She is then responsible for answering the questions of the class including these of the head nurse.
- In another method of conducting rounds, the head nurse/teacher may involve any nurse in the group to tell what she knows about the patient and his nursing care; other students make addition and suggestions and help to answer the questions.
- This method is a means of testing the student's knowledge and acquaintance with all the patients on the floor.
- Students prepare by studying indications and actions of drug.

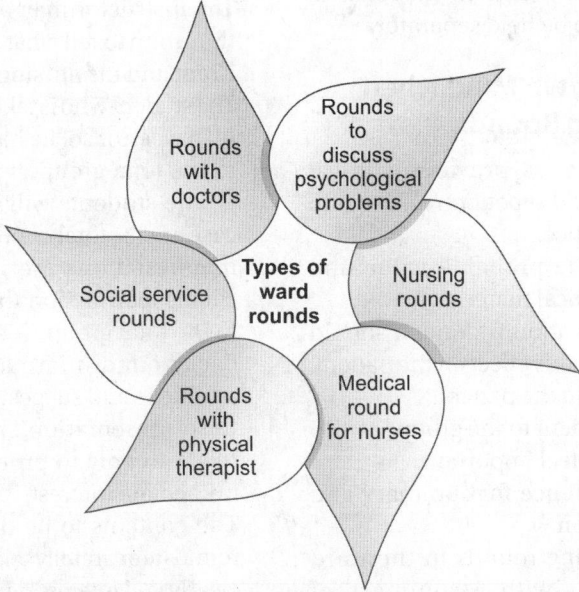

Fig. 4.12: Types of ward rounds.

- Students are told prior to rounds so that they may prepare themselves.

Preparation by the Head Nurse/Nurse Teacher

- In preparing for rounds the nurse selects the patients who are to be discussed in relation to the time which has been set aside for the purpose.
- Rounds should properly not last longer than 20 minutes.
- The head nurse needs to read the patient's progress and prognosis, their nursing care and its effectiveness.
- She should post the time for rounds at least a week in advance and indicates the type of preparation the nurse is to make, i.e., whether she is to know thoroughly the history, care and progress of her own patients or briefly that of all patients in the ward.
- Patient with similar diagnosis but with differing history, treatment, and prognosis may be selected or varied conditions existing in the same ward also can selected for teaching purpose.
- Rounds for staff nurses should be held separately from those for students since the background of the 2 groups vary widely.
- Rounds for students in their first clinical term may need to be held separately.

Factors to be Kept in Mind when Planning Nursing Rounds

- To consult student's previous clinical experience to avoid repetition and to add to earlier experience.
- Keep in mind the probable value and availability of clinical material.
- If some demonstration is done, it should not have a deleterious effect on the patient.
- Explain the plan to the patient.
- Introduce the patient to the group.
- Make the patient feel important.
- Have post-conference for summary and further explanation.
- Record the nursing rounds in the ward teaching records with a summary of nursing points stressed.

Ways of Conducting Rounds

- When true ward rounds are conducted, the teacher with the group of nurses goes to the patient's room.
- Outside the door, out of his hearing they discuss the objectives after which they go into see the patient and talk for a few moments with him.
- They then move on to the next patient.
- The discussion must have necessarily be brief including only the outstanding points. If the purpose is to visit all the patients in the ward.
- Nursing rounds is done in reporting style regarding patient's condition, nursing care, medical care and prognosis.

Procedure for Conducting Nursing Rounds

- Students have to be given information about ward rounds, so that, it will help them, to prepare themselves for the learning experience.
- Students will be following nursing rounds, the clinical instructor or ward supervisor will stop briefly at the bedside of each patient for a short discussion of the most significant nursing problem.
- The instructor may instruct any nurse in the group to tell what she knows about the client and his nursing care.
- The student who is taking care of the patient for a week or so, he has to present the case to the total group of the students so that all the students will be aware about the case and its total condition. If any cardinal manifestations are identified, with the clients' permission they can demonstrate to the total group. The presentation of the background information is followed by additions and suggestions from the group.
- Case presentation should be short and relate to only to problem or situation of immediate interest.
- The contents to be discussed in nursing rounds are carefully selected, well organized, clearly and interestingly presented, for each client only 3-4 minutes have to be spent.

Advantages of Nursing Rounds

- This method is a means of testing the student's knowledge and acquaintance with the entire patient's on the floor.
- The students, who are informed prior to rounds, benefit the maximum in real life teaching method.
- No other type of rounds is a substitute for nursing rounds.
- It is always be very valuable for the head nurse to go on regular nursing rounds with clinical instructor.
- An intelligent nurse with creative abilities may find many other ways of successfully assisting student nurses to develop nursing skills.
- Helps in orienting a new nurse/student to the patients.
- An interesting strategy involving the student, teacher and the patient.
- It offers a real life learning situation.
- Evaluation of nursing activity, hurdles faced by nurses in implementing or success nursing care can be appraised.

Disadvantages of Nursing Rounds

- The confidentiality of the patient is hampered.
- The patient may over hear the discussion and he may not like the thought that he is being talked about if he cannot hear.
- If the group is large the teacher may not able to speak loudly enough to be heard, in which case the attention of individuals who are on the fringes is lost.
- Distractions are present in ward.
- An unprepared nursing round has little teaching-learning value.
- Quality of nursing rounds on the quality and presentation of the nurse teacher/head nurse.

BEDSIDE CLINIC

The group visits the client or the client may be brought to the conference room during the discussion. This method is of helpful, when some members of the group are unfamiliar with the client or when there are special

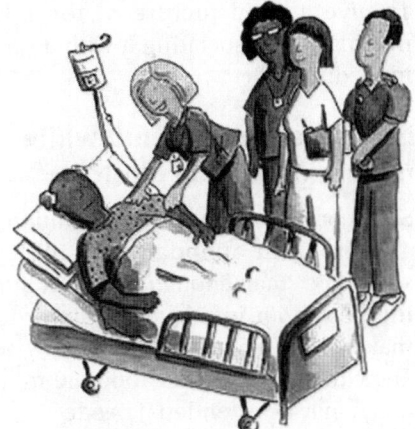

Fig. 4.13: Bedside clinic.

observations, which need to be made, to give the discussion in a more meaningful.

In this conference, when the client is to be visited is predetermined. The group knows the purpose of the visit and what to be observed.

Frequently the client is engaged in purposeful conversation, the teacher will use this opportunity to demonstrate and to help the client to identify his needs and the assistance can be given to him in handling his problems.

Client should feel ease; embarrassment of client should be avoided.

Client should know the group and what is expected from him, comfortable environment should be maintained, and minimum group members should be allowed.

Meaning

Bedside clinic is a method of clinical teaching. It always entails the presence of the patient. Either the group visits bedside or the patients is brought to the conference room. Nursing clinics are conducted by the head nurse or clinical instructor. In a nursing clinic the patient's medical history, medical and nursing managements are discussed briefly.

Purposes

- To portray the nursing problems typically associated with a particular disease or disorder.

- To give a vivid picture of the related nursing care associating it with a specific individual.

Points to be Kept in Mind while Conducting Bedside Clinic

- Select patients with typical conditions.
- The group in attendance at the clinic should be small enough to gather around the bed in an informal way in order to make the patient to feel at ease.
- The clinic usually lasts about 30 minutes and it may be extended if needed.
- Before starting the bedside clinic the instructor must fully be aware of the details of the patient like, personal characteristics, medical history and medical conditions.
- Instruct the group about necessary observations of the patient.

Preparation for Bedside Clinic

- The unit must be prepared.
- Prior permission must be taken from the patient and significant others.
- Any due care/drugs to be given during the period of discussion must be completed before discussion.
- All the reports of the patient may be kept ready.

- The group selected should be small in size.
- The time period should be around 30 minutes.
- Patient selection should be appropriate to the student's knowledge.
- Consent should be obtained from the patient and his family.
- The clinical instructor should be well versed with the patient's problems and its management.
- The environment should be conducive for teaching.
- Proper time should be selected for teaching, so as to prevent unnecessary interference with the patient's routine and student's work.

Steps

1. Students should gather around the patient. All the students should be able to view the patient and procedures like physical examination, if performed.
2. The clinical instructor will introduce the group to the patient and the patient to the group.
3. She explains the bio-data, medical history, treatment modalities being carried on and the response of the patient to the treatment.

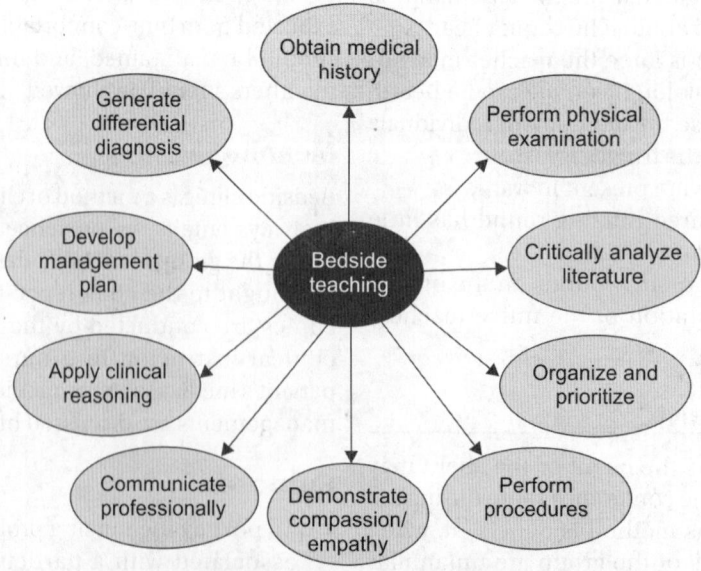

Fig. 4.14: Bedside teaching techniques.

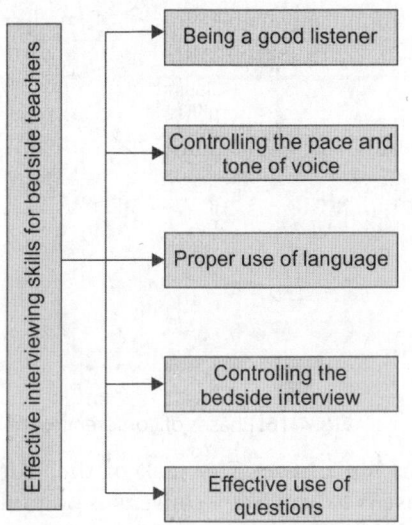

Fig. 4.15: Skills needed for bedside interview.

4. In between the patient may be involved and asked about his feelings towards the treatment and nursing care.
5. This is followed by discussion.

Method

Steps involved:
1. Students are made to stand in an informal way near the bedside.
2. Necessary observations of the patient are instructed to the student.
3. The clinical instructor first tells about the history, the physical and mental condition of the patient.
4. The nursing problems of the patient are presented to the students.
5. The management of such nursing problems is presented.
6. Lastly the patient's problems and its management are summarized.
7. The instructor calls on for discussion.

Advantages

- Helps in arousing interest and imitativeness in the students.
- Encourages discussion among the students about the patient's problems and its management.
- Gives an opportunity for the teacher to evaluate or assess the knowledge and skills in nursing care of the students in his/her ward.
- Each students gets chance to know the patient in general.

Disadvantages

- Patient may feel uncomfortable if large group of health team members are included.
- The patient may over hear the discussion and feel bad about his disease condition.
- Proper organized explanation is needed otherwise it loses the essence of such gathering.

CONFERENCE (INDIVIDUAL AND GROUP)

Nursing care conference is a method of teaching, which provides an opportunity for an informal discussion of a problem and free exchange of knowledge and experience about the common interest and it consists of a group discussion using problem-solving techniques or nursing process. Nursing care conferences are so "old hat" and so identified with basic nursing education that their potential value in staff development and continuing education is often unrecognized. Within the institution, particularly at the unit level, a nursing care conference can provide a good learning experience for all the staff who shares a common nursing problem in providing care to a specific patient.

Definitions

- A nursing care conference is designed around a consultation visit of a clinical nurse specialist. But more frequently they are designed for the staff of a specific nursing unit, and are planned around some aspect of nursing care or focus on a scientific nursing problem presented by a patient in that unit.
- A nursing care conference is a "course of action discussion, the focus is on assessing the nursing problem arriving at possible solutions, helping staff to examine a patient's problems from his point of view."

Planning and Preparation

- The organizers should prepare well in advance regarding particular conference.
- Before presenting, the student will have to collect all the data regarding the patient. She will have to work with that patient and collected information about the signs and symptoms since how long the patient is sick. What are the laboratory findings? What about his family backgrounds, socioeconomic conditions, etc.?
- The conference should be planned in relation to the objective of the conference and it should be spontaneous in nature.
- The student should be given ample opportunity to work in the ward for quite a good amount of time before she is assigned to present in the conference.

Technique

- The nursing care conference is used as a consultation tool to help in problem-solving.
- The teacher must be flexible and she will help the students during discussion.
- The conference should involve all the students in discussion. The teacher involves all the students by putting questions, giving guidance, if necessary.
- Teacher has to draw out the potentials of the students to the maximum in discussion. She will provide ample time for the students to think.

Phases

The nursing care conference is used as a consultation tool to help in problem-solving. It has got three phases. They are: (1) initial phase, (2) Working phase, and (3) Closing phase.

Initial phase: The opening phase can be defined as the first two minutes of the conference. The task here is to make a commitment to work on a problem relating to a particular patient. What happens during these few minutes often sets the tone for the entire session.

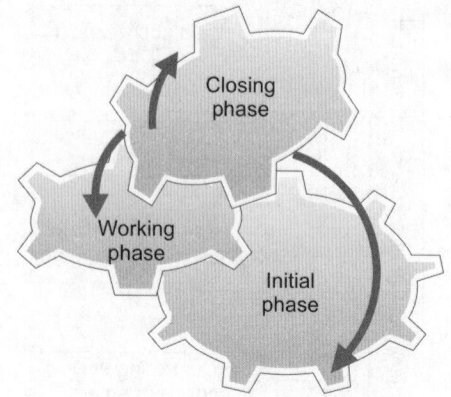

Fig. 4.16: Phases of conference.

Working phase: The task of the working phase is to arrive at a consensus on problem identification and solution. Once the patient is selected we have found that a great deal of time during this phase is spent in delineating the problem clearly. In some conferences there is a difference of opinion among the nurses, often the data are inconsistent or incomplete. It is helpful the group focus their discussion by asking direct questions, rephrasing what the group has said and summarizer. Sometimes, when data on the patient are incomplete the group will try to fill in. If the consultant and group view the absent data as critical to the solution, time is better spent in getting the facts than in speculation. Conference time can be used to identify just what information is needed. The problems are identified and the group can often reach its own solutions. Offering concrete solutions to problem, behavior allows the staff to feel they are getting something from the group and the consultant who offers alternatives and support to a frustrated staff establishes credibility and does them a great service and she should be careful to ask the group's opinion on the validity of her suggestions. The nurses can ventilate their anxiety by expressing their feeling.

Closing phase: Once the group has worked through problem-solving and has decided on solutions, the next phase is closure. The task here is to delegate responsibility to one or more of the staff to act on the problems.

Advantages

- It helps the students to collect the information in creative way, i.e., the students will be able to validate the data pertaining to the situation and appropriateness.
- It provides real practical learning environment to the students.
- It fortifies the thinking of students, thereby the creativity and judgment capacity will be increased.
- It provides free opportunity to think.
- Each member will be actively participating in the conference.

Disadvantages

- It will be of little use if the students do not accustom to such situation.
- There are chances of using these conference hours for classroom teaching.

Conference is an important method of clinical teaching. The nursing care conference is formed in formal or informal way. It uses problem-solving technique in discussion and the students will have to identify the problems and solutions for these problems. It provides students ample opportunity to think. The learning objectives could be best achieved, when it is used in a well-planned way. These will be much adding to the knowledge of students as many students give their contributions.

GROUP CONFERENCE

The group/team idea as applied in the field of nursing is of fairly recent origins, but groups of individuals in a loose knit pattern of organization with undefined relationship have existed in our hospital wards almost ever since inception. As nursing has advanced techniques aiming towards physical and psychological care of patients have multiplied infinitely and ultimately it has required a situation in which it has become impossible for the professional nurse to carry out all the tasks of nursing for her patient by herself.

Meaning of Conference

A conference is the act of consulting together. The conference is the nucleus of the in-service nursing program. At the conference there spring up spontaneously many teaching opportunities which are invaluable in terms of the application to specific patient problems. Techniques of group process and principles of interpersonal relationship are an integral part of the procedure. Observation made during nursing team conference offer unique opportunity for guidance of nursing service personnel.

Advantages of the Nursing Team Conference

- It is used to plan for the daily continuity of nursing care that best meets the patient's need.
- As a teaching tool, nursing team conference offers valuable opportunities for learning.
- It gives an ability to observe, report, and analyze significant findings input to its

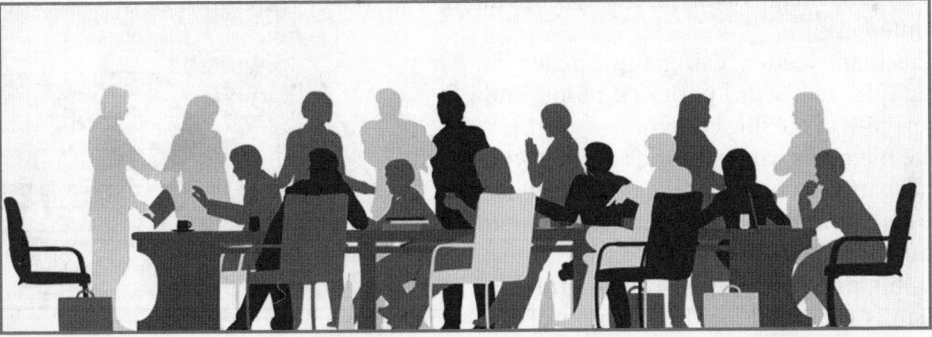

Fig. 4.17: Group conference.

greatest test as students are confronted with their daily responsibility.

Objectives of the Nursing Team Conference

Nursing Team Conference

- Identifies the patient nursing problem.
- Recognizes, ability and limitation of various team members.
- Help to communicate the ideas, information on related nursing care.
- Utilizes scientific information to influence the cause of nursing care
- Makes generalization from specific information that is factual.
- Helps to report, interpret, channelize and carry out hospital or healthcare problems.
- Teaches what is required to help team members fulfill their roles.
- Helps to plan nursing care cooperatively with other team members.
- Brings also maximum creative potential of the team.

Conference Procedure

- A time is planned each day for the members of the nursing team to meet as a group. During this period, patient's problems are identified and explored, and an approach is developed by the team.
- The nursing care plans are revised or further developed, according to changing needs of patients.
- Each member of the nursing team has recorded during the course of the day and the response of the patient to her care, questions and comments of the patient and individual notes are used as guides in conference.
- The team leader, using the Kardex as a guide, reads the patient's name and objective of nursing care.
- The members who have the contract with that particular patient discuss his response to his care and any additional information from the patient or his family.
- Problems are identified by the group; a plan is projected for the solution of the problems.

- The Kardex is revised and the objective is altered by the leader. The head nurse functions as a resource person and assist the team leader and the team members in identifying nursing problems and developing nursing care plans.
- The nursing team conference is the planning stage for the team and assignment of nursing personnel for the following day is developed during and immediately after the conference.

The Major Types of Conferences

- **Team leader direction conferences** are held at the beginning of a work shift and an hour prior to the ending of the shift. The purpose is to give and receive pertinent, accurate information concerning the care of the patients, and to create an environment that encourages collective and cooperative participation.
- **Patient-centered conferences** are planned meetings to identify problems and evaluate nursing care. These conferences provide a means for all the team who are directly contributing care to a group of patients, have benefit from the experiences of others. The members as a group aim to formulate nursing intervention for one or two patients analyze the nursing care given. The clinical nurse coordinator and the supervisor are important members of the patient-centered conferences.
- **Nursing service management conferences** should be part of the planned

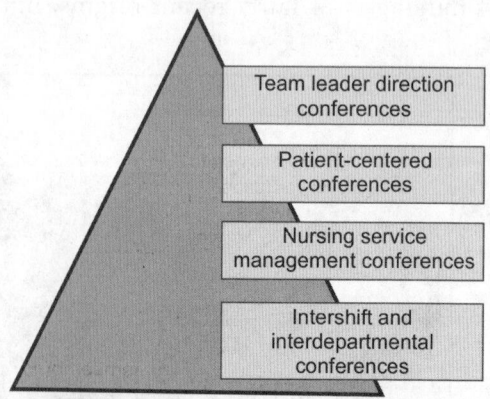

Fig. 4.18: Major types of conference.

scheduled meetings for each unit or section. The supervisor assisted by the clinical coordinator is the leader here. The topics presented are discussed may include standards of patient care and policies, procedures, safety measures, infection control, nursing audit evaluation, unit staffing measures and clarifications of new personnel policies.

- **Intershift and interdepartmental conferences** are necessary to pass on pertinent information from one individual or group to another.

Demands on the Professional Nurse

Demands were identified by Chao and Wilk's students of nursing educations of Columbia University. They are:

- **To identify the patient's nursing problem:** The team leader is first of all a listener, so that the leader can be able to assist the group to develop a whole plan out of varied contributions.

  The leader provides the team members with an opportunity to explore and evaluate the nursing care they have provided the patients.
- **To recognize ability and limitations of various team members:** The team leader must exercise professional judgment in evaluating the observations, contributions, and suggestions made by other members for the development of evaluation of nursing care. The leader must also help the team members to recognize their capabilities and limitations in the areas of skill, knowledge and judgment.
- **To communicate:** The professional nurse must continually be concerned not only with her own ability to communicate but with the ability of team members as well. It takes two people communicate—the speaker and the listener. Successful communication in the team depends upon how much understanding the professional nurse may have of the ability and limitation of other team members. The leader must

be prepared to employ approaches which will facilitate communication.

- **To use scientific information to influence the course of nursing care:** This is the expression of the professional status of nursing. It is this ability which makes it possible to plan for comprehensive or individualized nursing care. Professional knowledge and judgment are reflected in direct protection to the ability of the professional nurse to recognize any valuable clue in the work, attitude or thinking of non-professional member, and to identify and apply those scientific principles which would be helpful in making use of the worker's contribution.
- **To generalize from specific:** The leader, in evaluating the contribution of the team members, arranges and presents this information in such a way that it will be useful to the team members at a future date, should a similar situation arise. To report, interpret, channel and carry out hospital policies: Policies are necessary guides and as such are subject to interpretation. In team conferences, questions or problems relating to hospital policies are discussed as they apply to particular patients. One policy which frequently comes up for discussion is visiting hours.
- **To bring out "maximum creativity":** The team leader is responsible for creating a working environment which is conducive to the full participation of the members of the nursing team. She must be aware of the needs of the members of the group and must assist them to meet these needs. Through this process the team leader assists the other members to identify and solve problem, and to become more competent within the range of their ability.
- **To teach in conference what is required to help team members fulfill their roles:** One of the characteristics of a professional person of a broad scientific background which may be used in a variety of situations. The non-professional person is

dependent upon routines or techniques. It is important that the professional nurse recognizes which teaching is indicated and whether the teaching will be effective. Detailed teaching is not the responsibility of the team leader in conference.

- **To plan nursing care cooperatively with other team members:** This is the primary overall purpose of the nursing team conference. The team leader encourages all team members to participate in the planning, and guides the development of the plan on the basis of scientific principles.

PROCESS RECORDING TEACHING

The art of effective communication is a dynamic process. It comes naturally to some persons, but to others, it is acquired only by hard labor. Many times the student nurses communicate with patient's very superficially and stereotyped way rather than being of meaningful therapeutic nature. Thus the nursing student needs to develop more perceptiveness so that they can effect constructive intervention through verbal exchange.

Definition

- Walker defines process recording as "A verbatim between nurse and the patient".
- Hudson defines process recording as "An exact written report of the conversation between the nurse and the patient during the time they were together".
- Conen defines process recording as "A teaching—learning tool". Others used the words such as "interpersonal-relations recording". "Patient-nurse interaction interviews, etc., in place of process record. Though this process recording is used in arty field of nurse-patient relationship it is widely practiced in the field of psychiatric nursing. Regardless of the area in which the nurse functions she must be aware of the dynamics of human behavior and skill in using her own behavior and communication.

Uses of the Process Record

There are mainly three uses:
- As a teaching-learning tool.
- As an evaluation tool.
- As a therapeutic tool.

Different Phases in Process Recording

- Preparing the student for process recording.
- Recording nurse-patient interaction.
- Evaluating the interactions by nurse-teacher and the student.

Guidelines to Students

How to go about process recording (always use initials in referring patient's name):
- Your goals for working with assigned patients should be written down before starting the process recording.
- Note important factors in patient's personality development (get it from patient's history).
- Mention about the therapies which patient is getting—both past and present.
- Date of process recording should be mentioned.
- Amount of time you spent with patient should be recorded.
- A brief description should be written about the setting and situation before your conversation.
- Identify the patient's needs (as represented by patient behavior).
- Identify mental mechanisms that you think the patient are using and give examples.
- After completion of process record, give your comment on how well you were able to meet the goals which you set before starting your work.
- Evaluate the process record as a learning experience for you at the end of the assignment.

Statement of Goals or Objectives

Since a therapeutic interaction should be purposeful, the purpose should be specifically stated in terms of outcome so that the process can be evaluated effectively. Some of the examples of objectives are:

- To know the anxiety level of patient.
- To help the patient express his feelings towards hospitalization.
- To assess his feelings and thoughts related to a particular incident that happened.

Record of Interaction between Nurse and the Patient

Truthful recording of what the nurse said and did what the patient said and did, including any nonverbal behavior of the patient, such as changing the position, looking at various things, eye contact, biting the nails, pacing, etc.

Therapeutic Relationship

- A therapeutic interpersonal relationship is one where two or more people relate to each other with a purpose of change in behavior, reduction of anxiety, support, encouragement, caring and teaching. In a therapeutic relationship a helper and a person who needs help are involved.
- The major skill involved in therapeutic interpersonal relationship is observation and understanding of behavior and communication are of great importance.
- The aim is change towards growth of the client even though in this process the therapist may gain more understanding about himself and his interaction pattern, etc.
- A therapeutic relationship should help the client to meet his day-to-day needs, to learn to approach problem situations, to find out new ways of coping, and to move in the direction of fuller growth within himself.
- Therapeutic relationship may be more tasking on the nurse than any other part

of nursing, because there the nurse has to give a part of herself and not some medication or treatments.

- In order to be able to give a part of oneself, one has to be mature, has to have a fair understanding of self, and has to have certain abilities and attitudes.

Phases of Process-Recording

There are three main phases of process recording.

I. Preparing the student for process recording
II. Recording nurse-patient interactions.
III. Evaluating the nurse-patient interactions.

I. **Preparing the student:** The teacher must help the student to define objectives to be accomplished during nurse-patient interactions. The teacher should discuss the process record as a teaching learning tool. Teacher should help the student to learn how to go about writing a process record.

II. **Recording nurse-patient interactions**: There are four important parts in process recording of the nurse-patient interaction. There is the recording of:

1. The exact verbatim report of nurse-patient conversation.
2. The student's conscious feelings and her interpretation of the patient's feeling.
3. Analysis for meanings and clues to patient's needs.

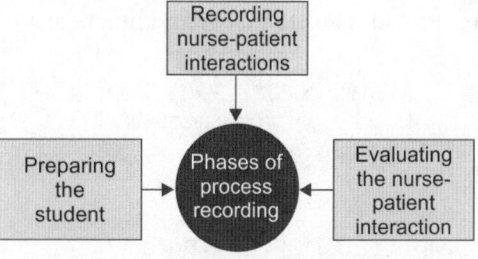

Fig. 4.19: Phases of process recording.

4. The instructor's and the student's evaluation of the total process recording experience.

Requirements for process recording:
- A minimum of 2 people.
- Reassurance of the patient regarding confidentiality of the interview.
- Recording of all verbal interaction.
- Notation of thoughts, feeling, and action's of student nurse.
- Notation of nonverbal communication of the patient.
- Notation of the interaction done as soon as possible after the interaction occurs (note the time lapse between interaction and actual recording).

III. **Evaluating the nurse-patient interaction:** After the interacting data have been collected by the student, the teacher and the students should analyze the data during which the objectives should be kept in focus.

The teacher should correct the recording and help the student to advance to the stage of self evaluation.

Merits

- Improves the skill of communication and technique of interaction.
- It improves the more specific therapeutic conversations.
- Improves the ability to face stressful situation.
- Helps understand the psychopathology of various illnesses.
- Understands the use of mental mechanism.
- Patients learn to listen to others.
- Provides link to theory and practice.

Demerits

- It is time consuming.
- Chances of changing the therapeutic relationship to social relationship.
- Needs strict confidentiality.

CONCLUSION

Teaching method is the stimulation, guidance, direction and encouragement for learning. Effective transfer of knowledge can be achieved by employing various student friendly teaching-learning methods. Progressive method of teaching provides uitable opportunities for effective teaching learning process. A teaching learning method will help the teacher to conduct teaching in an agreeable, student friendly and successful manner by maintaining link between the subject matter and the student.

BIBLIOGRAPHY

1. Billings D, Halstead J. Teaching in nursing: a guide for faculty, 3rd edition. St. Louis Mo: Saunders/Elsevier; 2009.
2. Craddock E. Developing the facilitator role in the clinical area. Nurse Education Today. 1993;13:217-24.
3. Davis D, Stullenbarger E, Dearman C, Kelley JE. Proposed nurse educator competencies: Development and validation of a model. Nursing Outlook. 2005;53(4):206-11.
4. Kalb KA. Core competencies of nurse educators: Inspiring excellence in nurse educator practice. Nursing Education Perspectives. 2008;29(4):217-9.
5. McGregor A. Academic success, clinical failure: struggling practices of a failing student. Journal of Nursing Education. 2007;46(11):504-13.

5

CHAPTER

Educational Media

LEARNING OBJECTIVES
- Meaning and objectives of Audiovisual (AV) aids
- Important values of AV aids
- Characteristics of good teaching aids
- Principles of AV aids
- Types or classifications of AV aids

INTRODUCTION

Audiovisual aids or devices or technological media or learning devices are added devices that help the teacher to clarify, establish, correlate accurate concepts, interpretations and appreciations and enable him to make learning more concrete, effective, interesting, inspirational, meaningful, and vivid. They help in completing the triangular process of learning viz, motivation-clarification-stimulation. The aim of teaching with technological media is clearing the channel between the learning and the things that are worth learning.

The basic assumption underlying audiovisual aids is that learning-clear understanding-stems from sense experience. The teacher must show as well as tell. Audiovisual aids provide significant gains in informational learning, retention and recall, thinking and reasoning, activity, interest, imagination, better assimilation and personal growth and development. The aids are the stimuli for learning why, how, when, and where. The

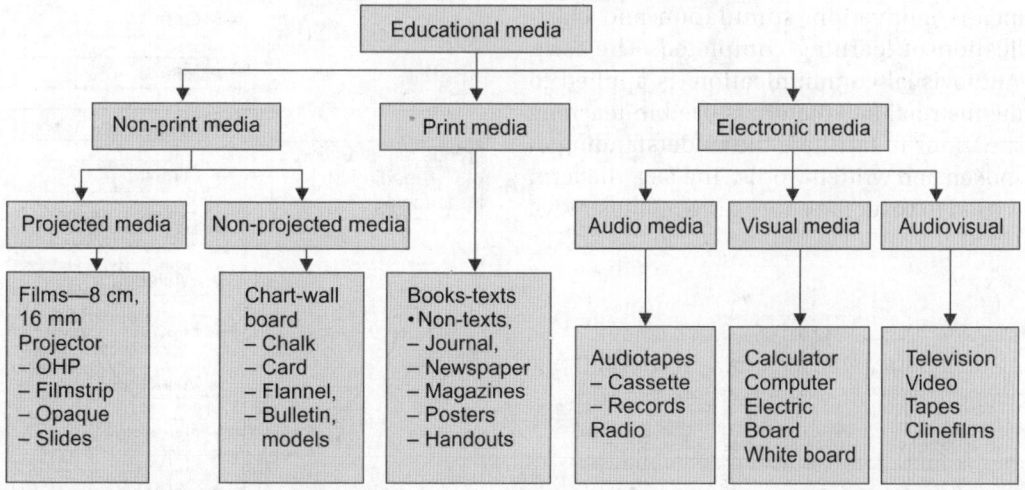

Flowchart 5.1: Educational media classification.

Educational media		
Non-print media	Print media	Electronic media

Projected media	Non-projected media		Audio media	Visual media	Audiovisual
Films—8 cm, 16 mm Projector – OHP – Filmstrip – Opaque – Slides	Chart-wall board – Chalk – Card – Flannel, – Bulletin, models	Books-texts • Non-texts, – Journal, – Newspaper – Magazines – Posters – Handouts	Audiotapes – Cassette – Records Radio	Calculator Computer Electric Board White board	Television Video Tapes Clinefilms

hard to understand principles are usually made clear by the intelligent use of skillfully designed instructional aids.

DEFINITIONS

- Audiovisual aids are those sensory objects or images which initiate or stimulate and reinforce learning. **—(Burton)**
- Audiovisual aids are those aids which help in completing the triangular process of learning, i.e., motivation, classification and stimulation. **—(Carter V. Good)**
- Audiovisual are those devices by the use of which communication of ideas between persons and groups in various teaching and training situations is helped. These are also termed as multisensory materials. **(Edger Dale)**
- Audiovisual aids are supplementary devices by which the teacher, through the utilization of more than one sensory channel is able to clarify, establish and correlate concepts, interpretations and appreciations. **—(Mckown and Robert)**
- Audiovisual aids are anything by means of which learning process may be encouraged or carried on through the sense of hearing or sense of sight. **(Kinder S James)**

MEANING OF AUDIOVISUAL AIDS

Audiovisual aids are those aids which help in completing the process of learning. It means motivation, stimulation and clarification of learning completed. The term 'Audiovisual communication' is applied to the instructional materials used in teaching situations to facilitate the understanding of spoken and written words. The fact, the term is used to cover the entire range of illustrative instructional materials like visual material—auditory materials and the combination of the two.

Audiovisual communication learning program; and the content of course, information, ideas, thought, etc., prepared for use in such program are called software, while the audiovisual aids and equipment are called hardwares. Audiovisual communication appeals to the senses of hearing and seeing. Audiovisual aids are generally used as learning aids complementary to the books and formal classroom instruction. Comenius was the first educator who prepared and used a book illustrated by pictures to give it a sensory appeal. He found that corrected learning to their experiences. There is more effective in focusing student's attention and make learning enjoyable.

OBJECTIVES OF USING AUDIOVISUAL AIDS

- To hold the attention of learner.
- To increase the effectiveness of teaching.
- To make the learning experience last longer.
- To save time

Flowchart 5.2: Types of instructional media.

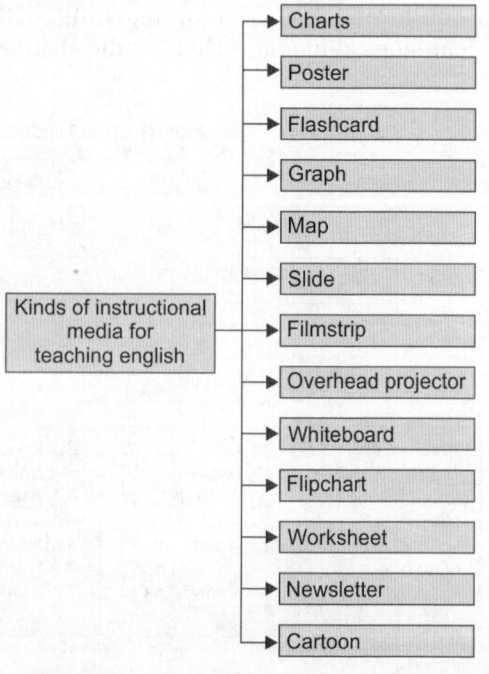

Fig. 5.1: Process of learning.

IMPORTANT VALUES OF AUDIOVISUAL AIDS

- **Antidote to the disease of verbal instruction:** They help reduce verbalism. They help in giving clear concept and thus help to bring accuracy in learning.
- **Best motivators:** They are the best motivators. The students work with more interest and zeal. They are more attentive.
- **Clear images:** Clear images are found when we see, hear, touch, taste and smell as our experiences are direct, concrete and more or less permanent. Learning through the sense becomes the most natural and consequently the earliest.
- **Vicarious experiences:** It is beyond doubt that the first hand experience is the best type of educative experiences. But it is neither practicable nor desirable to provide such experiences to pupils.
- **Variety:** Mere chalk and talk do not help. Audiovisual aids give variety and provide different tools in the hands of the teacher.
- **Freedom:** When audiovisual aids are employed, there is great scope for children to move about, talk, laugh and comment upon. Under such an atmosphere, the students work because they want to work and not because the teacher wants them to work.
- **Opportunities to handle and manipulate:** Many visual aids offer opportunities to students to handle and manipulate things.
- **Retentivity:** Audiovisual aids contribute to increase retentively as they stimulate response of the whole organism to the situation in which learning takes place.
- **Based on maxims of teaching:** The use of audiovisual aids enables the teacher to follow the maxims of teaching, such as concrete to abstract, known to unknown and learning by doing.
- **Helpful in attracting attention:** Attention is the true factor in any process of teaching and learning. Audiovisual aids help the teacher in providing proper environment for capering as well as sustaining the attention and interest of the students in the classroom work.
- **Helpful in fixing up new learning:** What is gained in terms of learning needs to be fixed up in the minds of students? Audiovisual aids help in achieving this objective by providing several activities, experiences and stimuli to the learners.
- **Saving of energy and time:** A good deal of energy and time of both the teachers and students can be served on account of the use of audiovisual aids as most of the concepts and phenomena may be easily clarified, understood and assimilated through their use.
- **Realism:** The use of audiovisual aids provides a touch of reality to the learning situation. By seeing a film show exhibiting the life of the people of the tundra region, students learn it more effectively in about 2 hours than by spending weeks by reading.
- **Vividness:** Audiovisual aids gives vividness to the learning situation. A film on Buddha provides a vivid picture of his life and teaching.
- **Meeting individual differences:** There are wide individual differences among learners. Some are ear-oriented; some can be helped through visual demonstrations, while others learn better by doing. The use of a variety of audiovisual aids help in meeting the needs of different types of students.
- **Encouragement to health classroom interaction:** Audiovisual aids, through their wide variety of stimuli, provision of active participation of the students, and vicarious experiences encourage healthy classroom interaction for the effective realization of teaching learning objectives.
- **Spread of education on a mass scale:** Audiovisual aids, such as radio and television help in providing opportunities for education to people living in remote areas. They also help in promoting adult education.
- **Promotion of scientific temper:** In place of listening to facts, students observe demonstrations and phenomena and thus cultivate scientific temper.
- **Development of higher faculties:** Verbalism promotes memorization. Use of

audiovisual aids stirs the imagination, thinking process and reasoning power of the students, and calls for creativity, and inventiveness and other higher mental activities on the parts of students and thus helps the development of higher faculties among the students.

- **Reinforcement to learners:** Audiovisual aids prove effective reinforces by increasing the probability of re-occurrence of the response associated with them and thus render valuable help in the teaching-learning process.
- **Positive transfer of learning and training:** Use of audiovisual aids helps in the learning of other concepts, principles and solving the real problems of life by making possible the appropriate positive transfer of learning and training received in the classroom.
- **Positive environment for creative disciples:** A balanced rational and scientific use of audiovisual aids develops motivation, attracts the attention and interests of the students and provides a variety of creative outlets for the utilization of their tremendous energy and thus keeps them busy in the classroom work. In this way, the overall classroom environment becomes conducive to creative discipline.

CHARACTERISTICS OF GOOD TEACHING AIDS

- They should be meaningful and purposeful.
- They should be accurate in every respect.
- They should be simple.
- They should be cheap.
- As far as possible, they should be improvised.
- They should be large enough to be properly seen by the students for whom they are meant.
- They should be up to date.
- They should be easily portable.
- They should be according to the mental level of the students.
- They should motivate the learner.

PRINCIPLES IN THE USE OF TEACHING AIDS

1. **Principle of selection:** Teaching aids prove effective only when they suit the teaching objectives and unique characteristics of the special group of learner. Following points may be kept in this regard.
   - They should suit the age-level, grade-level and other characteristics of the learner.
   - They should have specific educational valve besides being interesting and motivating.
   - They should be the true representatives of the real things.
   - They should help in the realization of desired learning objectives.
2. **Principle of preparation:** This principle requires that following points should be attended to
   - As far as possible, locally available material should be used in the preparation of an aid.
   - The teacher should receive some training in the preparation of aids.
   - The teacher themselves should prepare some of the aids.
   - Students may be associated in the preparation of aids.

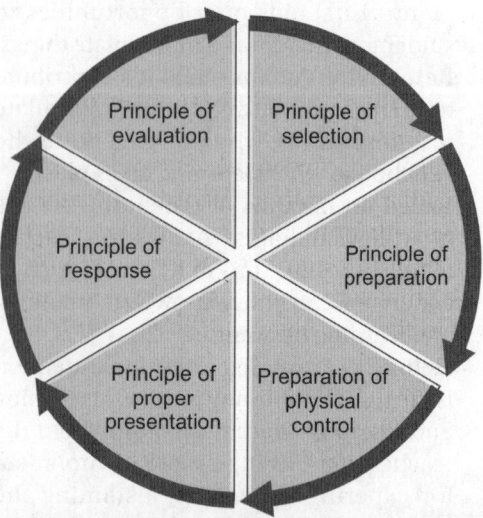

Fig. 5.2: Principles in the use of teaching aids.

3. **Preparation of physical control:** This principle relates to the arrangement of keeping aids safely and also to facilitate their learning to the teacher for use.

4. **Principle of proper presentation:** This principle implies the following points.
   - The teacher should carefully visualize the use of teaching aids before their actual presentation.
   - They should fully acquaint themselves with the use and manipulation of the aids to be shown in the classroom.
   - Adequate care should be taken to handle an aid in such a way as no damage is done to it.
   - The aid should be displayed properly so that all the students are able to see it, observe it and derive maximum benefit out of it.
   - As far as possible, distraction of all kinds should be eliminated so that full attention may be paid to the aid.

5. **Principle of response:** This principle demands that the teachers guide the students to respond actively to the audiovisual stimuli so that they drive the maximum benefit in learning.

6. **Principle of evaluation:** This principle stipulates that there should be continuous evaluation of both the audiovisual material and accompanying techniques in the light of realization of the desired objectives.

PROBLEMS IN THE USE OF TEACHING AIDS

While all these aids are becoming more and more popular day by day, there is still some problem to be faced and solved. These are:

- **Apathy of the teacher:** Teacher in general is yet to be convinced that teaching with words alone is very tedious, wasteful and ineffective.
- **Indifference of students:** The judicious use of aids arouses interest but when used without a definite purpose they lose their significance and importance.
- **Ineffectiveness of the aid:** Due to the absence of proper planning and the

Apathy of the teacher

Indifference of students

Ineffectiveness of the aid

Financial hurdles

Absence of electricity

Lack of facilities for training

Coordination between center and states

Language difficulty

Not catering to local needs

Improper selection of films

Fig. 5.3: Problems in the use of AV aids.

lethargy of the teacher and without proper preparation, correct presentation, appropriate application and discussion and the essential follow-up work, the aids do not prove their full usefulness. A film like a good lessons this various steps-preparation, presentation, application, and discussion.

- **Financial hurdles:** The central state and state government have set up boards of audiovisual education and have chalked out interesting Program for the popularization of teaching aids but the lack of finances is not enabling them to do their best.
- **Absence of electricity:** Most of the projectors, radio, and television cannot work without the electric current which is not available in a large number of schools.
- **Lack of facilities for training:** Training colleges or specialized agencies should make special provision to train teachers and workers in the use of these aids.
- **Coordination between center and states:** Good film libraries, museums of audiovisual education, fixed and mobile exhibition and educational melas should be organized both central and states.
- **Language difficulty:** Most educational films are in English. We should have these in Hindi and other important Indian languages.

- **Not catering to local needs:** Little attention is paid in the production of audiovisual aids to the local sociological, psychological and pedagogical factors.

- **Improper selection of films:** Films are not selected according to the classroom needs.

CLASSIFICATIONS OF TEACHING AIDS

Classification number-1: Projected and non-projected aids

Projected aids	Graphic aids	Display boards	3-D-aids	Audio-aids	Activity aids
Films	Cartoons	Blackboard	Diagrams	Radio	Computer-assisted instruction
Films strips	Charts	Bulletin	Models	Recording	Demonstration
Opaque projectors	Comics	Flannel board	Mock-ups	Television	Dramatics
Overhead projectors	Diagrams	Magnetic board	Objectives		Experimentation
Slides	Flashcards	Peg board	Puppets		Field trips
	Graphs		Specimens		Programmed instruction
	Maps				Teaching machines
	Photographs				
	Pictures				
	Postures				

Classification number-2: Audiovisual material, visual materials and audiovisual materials.

Audio material	Visual material	Audiovisual materials
Language laboratories	Bulletin boards	Demonstration
Radio	Chalkboards	Films
Sound distribution system sets	Charts	Printed materials with recorded sound
Tape and disco recording	Drawings, etc.	Sound filmstrips
	Exhibits	Study trips
	Film strips	Television
	Flash carts	Video tapes
	Flannel boards	
	Flip books	
	Illustrated books	
	Magnetic boards	
	Maps	
	Models	
	Pictures	
	Postures	
	Photographs	
	Self-instructional	
	Silent films	
	Slides	

Classification number-3: Big medias and little medias—

Big medias include computer, VCR, and TV.

Little media include radio, film strips, graphic, audio cassettes and various visuals.

Classification number-4: Three-dimensional aids—

- Models
- Mock-ups
- Specimens

Three-dimensional aids are the replicas or substitutes of real objective.

CONE OF EXPERIENCE

Edgar Dale, the chief exponent of audiovisual aids in teaching is the originator of the Cone of experience. All the learning experience which be utilized for classroom teaching are shown by Edgar Dale in a pictorial device-pinnacle form-which he called the cone of experience. In a simple language, it may be stated that the cone classifies the audiovisual aids according to their effectiveness in communication-aid at the base of the cone as most effective-relative effect gradually decreases.

At the pinnacle of the cone, the direct, purposeful experiences are represented. At the pinnacle of the cone, the verbal symbols are represented.

The experiences included in the cone are as indicated below:

- **Direct, purposeful experience:** The experiences gained through the senses are direct and purposeful. If has been amply observed, an ounce of experience is better than a tonne of theory, simply because it is only as an experience that any theory has vital and verifiable significance. This, direct experience is gained through the aids mentioned at the base of the cone.

- **Contrived experience:** When the real thing cannot be perceived directly, its simplification because necessary.

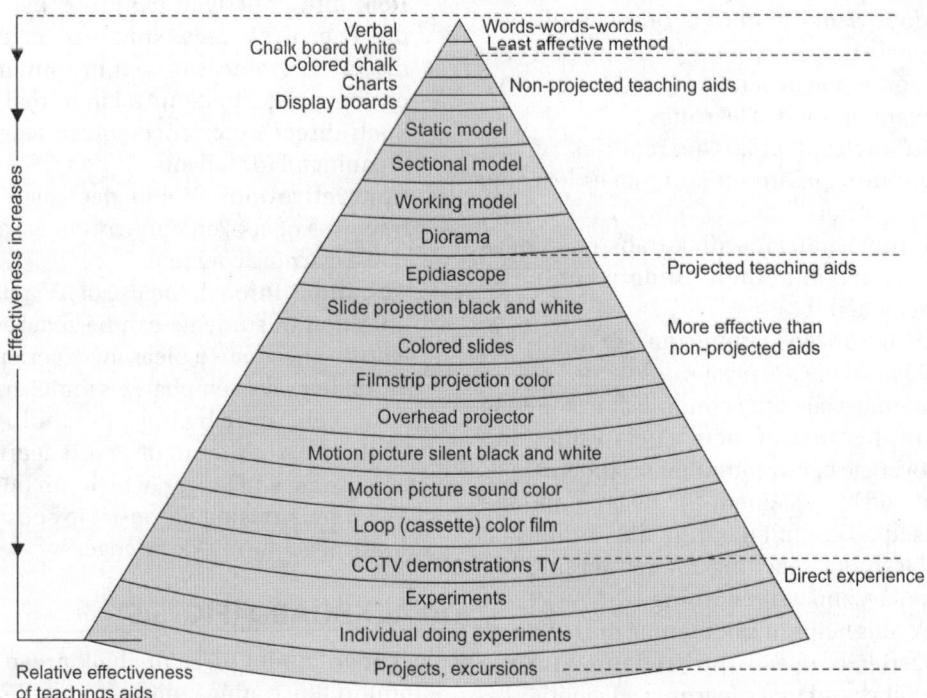

Fig. 5.4: Cone of experience.

Contrived experience is like a working model which is an editing of reality and differs from the original either in size or in complexity. The real object may be too small or to big, may be confused or concealed. In such a situation, imitation is preferred for better and easier understanding.

- **Dramatic participation:** In dramatics, certain real events are presented through the play, the pageant (kind of drama, usually based on local history), pantomime (actors do not speak, make movement), table an (picture line scene in which the characteristics stand still, silently), and the puppets.

SIGNIFICANTS OF AUDIOVISUAL AIDS IN CLASSROOM COMMUNICATION

- Audiovisual aids and equipments appeal to our senses and open better avenues to learning. It has been rightly observed that the senses gateways to all knowledge.
- Audiovisual materials because of their sensory appeal enable us to perceive information in better way and increase the retention span of learning.
- Audiovisual aids the realities of our world to classroom and makes learning purposeful.
- Audiovisual aids make abstract ideas contract and their understanding is facilitated.
- AV aids make learning quicker in this age of knowledge-explosion.
- AV materials are economical in the long turn because of their repeat values and coverage of large number of students
- AV aids supplement the teacher and are used as complementary aids to normal classroom teaching for reinforcing the spoken and written words.
- AV aids helps in overcoming the language barrier between the students and the teacher and make learning efficient.
- AV aids provide a variety of instructional methods and motivate children to learn independents of the teacher at times.

- AV aids reduces verbalism in the classroom & thus bourdon of students.

PSYCHOLOGICAL BASES OF AUDIOVISUAL AIDS

Psychological studies on learning and retention reveal that 80% of information and its retention are through auditory and visual senses. Because of the sensory appeal of audiovisual aids, the retention span of learning increases is attached to audiovisual aids.

- **Motivation:** The sensory appeal of audiovisual aids motivates and stimulates students to learn easily in a related atmosphere.
- **Curiosity:** The curiosity of students is aroused due to the novelty and variety in teaching aids when used for classroom teaching.
- **Interest:** Many AV aids give students the opportunity of manipulative their learning environment and their interest in learning sustained.
- **Real and contrived experiences:** With the use of AV aids, students have the direct experiences of real life situations or contrived situations a kin to real one. Such direct experiences make learning meaningful to students.
- **Concretization:** AV aids decreases abstractness of spoken and written words to make learning concrete.
- **Attention:** Through the use of AV aids the attention of students can be secured, as learning becomes a pleasant experience.

Psychology also emphasizes multisensory experiences in learning. Psychologists advocates the maximum of' 'more learning, faster learning and longer', which can only be achieved by arousing all possible senses or gateways of acquiring knowledge.

BLACKBOARD (FIG. 5.5)

Blackboard and a piece of chalk prove very helpful in illustrating concepts and ideas to the students. These can be used for drawing diagrams and sketches, etc. Blackboards are a simple and unique device which, in spite of

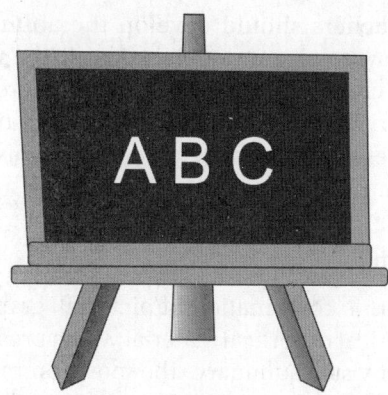

Fig. 5.5: Blackboard.

new devices and techniques in teaching, is irreplaceable as well indispensable. It is the oldest and best friend of a teacher.

It is the mirror through which students visualize all about the teacher's mind regarding as a while. It is the cheapest teaching device and continues to be the sine quo none of our educational system. It is most universally used aid. Writing on clay and sand was the ancient from of blackboard writing. It helps crystallizing the main points, summarizing and reviewing.

Main uses of the Blackboard

- The teacher can illustrate the main points of the lesson on the blackboard.
- Abstract statements can be clarified in the exposition stage and summer containing the salient features can be given at the recapitulate stage.
- Questions and problems can be listed on the blackboard.
- Pupil's interest in class work can be stimulated by blackboard writing and drawings.
- A teacher can use the blackboard for graphs, graphics, sketches, maps and statistics, etc.
- A blackboard provides a lot of scope for creative and decorative work.
- The teacher can erase writing and drawing and start afresh.
- It helps the teacher to focus the attention of his students on the lesson. It takes heed of varying capacities and rates of grasp of the students.

- A teacher can review the whole lesson for the benefit of the class with the help of the Blackboards.

Types of Blackboards

- **Fixed blackboards:** Fixed in the wall facing the class and normally made of wood or concrete cement.
- **Blackboard on easel:** A portable and adjustable blackboard put on a wooden easel can be taken out of the classroom while taking classes in the open.
- **Roller blackboard:** Made of thick canvas wrapped on a roller mostly used for teaching higher classes.
- **Graphic boards:** It has graphic lines and is used for teaching mathematics, science and statistics.
- **Magna board:** A board which enables teacher to make three dimensional demonstrations with objects on a vertical surface. Small magnets are used to hold suitable objects fixed whether they are put on this vertical surface.

Chalkboards of Different Types of Surfaces

- Paint-coated pressed wood
- Dull finished plastic surface
- Vitreous-coated steel surface
- Ground glass boards

Chalkboard of Different Colors and Color Chalks

Sl. No.	Color of the blackboard	Color of the chalk
1.	Green chalkboard	White or yellow chalk
2.	Gray board	Yellow
3.	Red chalkboard	Green, yellow
4.	Orange chalkboard	Blue or light green
5.	Yellow chalkboard	Blue
6.	Rose chalkboard	Purple, dark blue
7.	Black chalkboard	Any color

Effective use of Blackboard

Following points may be kept in view while using the blackboard:

- Blackboard should be kept clean so that writing on it could be easily read by the student from all parts of the room.
- Writing on the blackboard should be legible.
- Letters and drawing should be large enough to be seen from all parts of the room.
- Writing should be started from the top left corner.
- Writing should be in straight rows.
- Extreme lower corners of the blackboard should not be made use of as writing on it cannot be seen easily.
- Material on the blackboard should be covered by standing in front of it.
- Only salient points of the subject matter should be written on the blackboard.
- Diagrammatic visual presentation involves many processes should be prepared before the beginning of the lesson.
- It should be ensured that blackboard is well lighted by natural or artificial means.
- Everything needed for the blackboard should be got together before the class begins, i.e., collection of chalk, rules, T square, compass, projector, etc.
- While writing on the blackboard, the teacher should ensure that the class is attentive.
- Duster and not hand or handkerchief should be used in cleaning the blackboard.
- Occasionally, students may be asked to write or draw diagram on the blackboard.

- Teachers should develop the ability to draw freely on the blackboard. The map or chart or diagram that grows before the very eyes of the students in much more useful and valuable than a well finished map, chart or diagram.

CHART

A chart is combination of pictorial, graphic, numerical or vertical material which presents a clear visual summary. The most commonly used types of charts include outline charts, tabular charts, flowcharts and organization charts. Other types of charts are technical diagrams and process diagrams. Flip charts and flowcharts are also being used. Readymade charts are available for use in teaching in almost all areas in all subjects. But charts prepared by a teacher himself in co-operating his own ideas and lines of approach of the specific topic are more useful.

Purposes of Charts

- For showing relationship by means of facts, figures and statistics.
- For presenting materials symbolically.
- For summarizing information.
- For showing continuity in process.
- For presenting abstract ideas in visual form.
- For showing development of structure.
- For creating problems and stimulating thinking.
- For encouraging utilization of other media of communication.
- For motivating the students.

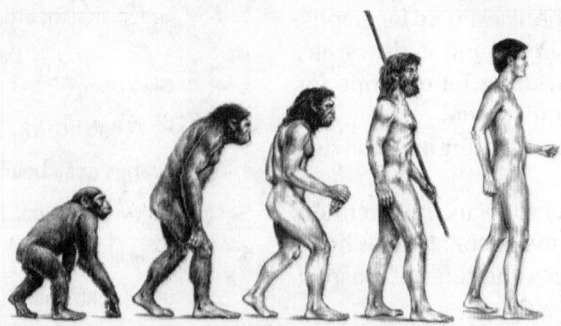

Fig. 5.6: Evolution chart.

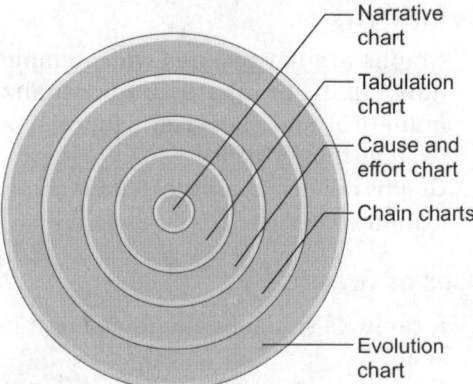

Narrative chart

Tabulation chart

Cause and effort chart

Chain charts

Evolution chart

Fig. 5.7: Types of chart.

How to use Charts Effectively?

- Teacher made charts should be preferred.
- Students should be involved in preparation of charts.
- Charts should be so large that every detail depicted should be visible to every pupil in the class whatever he is sitting.
- Charts should display information only about one specific area in a subject.
- A chart should not contain too much written material.
- A chart should not contain too many details.
- A chart should give a neat appearance.
- When a chart is to be used in the classroom, the teacher should make sure that there is provision for hanging the chart at a vantage point.
- The teacher should have a pointer to point out specific factors in the chart.
- Straight pins, staples. Pegboards clips, gummed hangers, paper-clips, folded making tapes may all be used for fastening charts without damaging them.
- Charts should be carefully stored and preserved for use in future.

Types of charts: The following is a list of basic types of charts in term of arrangements and the kinds or ideas which they may express—
- **The narrative chart:** An extended left—to right arrangement of facts and ideas for expressing
  a. The events in a process, such as shoe-making, oil cracking or the like.

  b. The events in the development of a significant issue to its point of resolution or to present status (sometimes a time limit). Examples—the events leading to the separation of the Bangladesh from Pakistan, the events leading to the establishment of the ideas that an individual should be free and that be should have a voice in his own government and events leading to increasing regulation of business by government.
  c. Technological improvement over a period of years, such as improvement over a period of years, such as improvement in transportation, communication, manufacturing, etc.
- **The tabulation chart:** A left to right, top to bottom arrangement of facts and ideas for expression
  a. Numerical data for making compartments.
  b. List of products, mountains, rivers, or the like in selected areas.
- **The cause and effort chart**, usually a limited left-to-right arrangement of facts and ideas for expressing.
  a. Relationship between standard of living and such factors as economic system, availability of natural resources, level of technological advancement.
  b. Relationship between a culture and neighboring cultures.
  c. Relationship between rights and responsibilities.
  d. Relationship between a complex of conditions and change or conflicts.
  e. Relationship between the elected and electors
  f. Relationship between community workers and the community which support them.
- **The chain charts**: A circular or semicircular arrangements of facts and ideas for expressing—
  a. Transitions, such as transition from raw materials to useful products.
  b. Cycles, such as the water cycle.
- **The evolution chart:** A left to right arrangement of facts and ideas for expressing—

a. Changes in specific items from beginning to data to data, perhaps with projections into the future. For example—origin of the automobile and its subsequent development early basic homes and changes in basic homes to date
b. Change in standard in food consumption, length of wok, weak purchasing power of a rupee, or the like.

GRAPH

Graphs are flat pictures which employ dots, lines or pictures to visualize numerical and statistical data to show relationships or statistics. Graphs defined as a visual representation of numerical data. Graphs is fundamentally a tool for expressing number relationship, which is much carrier to visualize then can be done if the statement were made only in words and figures.

Graphs are useful for showing quantitative data in a visual form. Graphs are quite effective in covering complicated facts and showing comparisons and contracts these may area graph, bar graph, pie graph, line graphs and pictographs.

Definitions

- Graphs are flat pictures-which employ dots, lines or pictures to visualize numerical and statistical data to show relationships or statistics.
- Graphs defined as a visual representation of numerical data.

Uses of Graphs

- It captures student's attention and thinking.
- Conveying information in a condensed form.
- Presenting information efficiently.
- Concretizing abstract ideas.
- Stimulating interest.

Types of Graphs

- **Bar graph:** It is a graphic presentation which extends the scale horizontally along the length of the bar. The vertical dimensions does not have a scale, but merely provides space for serious of items and for a bar to measure each.
- **The column bar:** It looks like a bar graph turned on end; it has 2 scales, 1 measuring across the graph (usually time) and 1

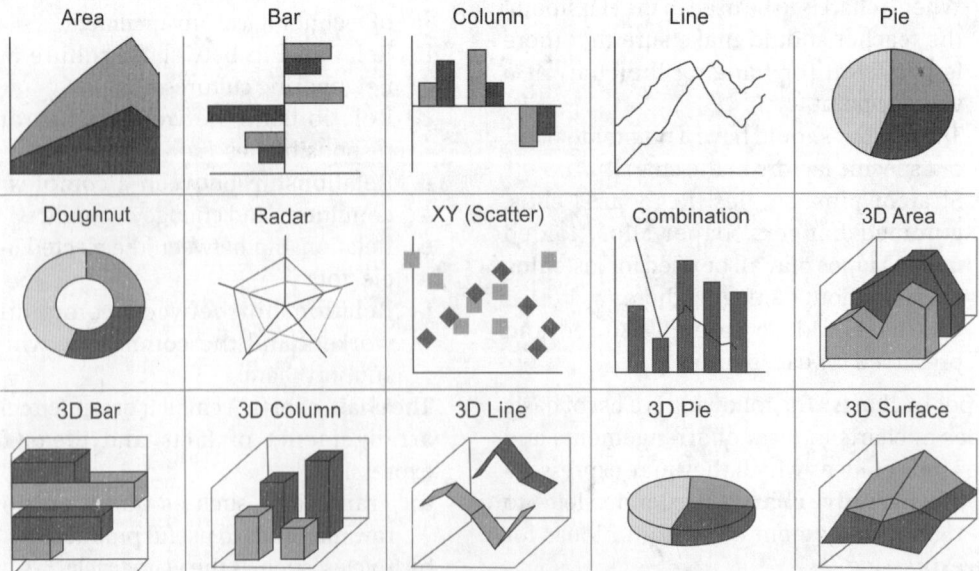

Fig. 5.8: Types of graphs.

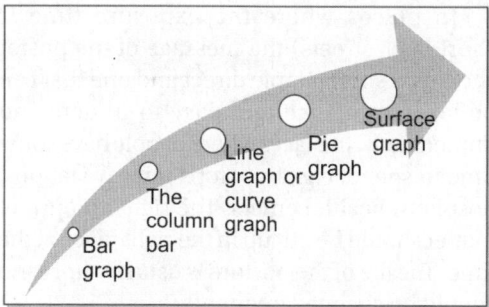

Fig. 5.9: Commonly used graphs.

measuring up or down (usually quantity). This means that every point of such a graph is measured for both scales.

- **The line graph or curve graph** is a form of graph in which the plotted points are connected to one another instead of to the base, thus producing the curve that gives the graph its name. In a line graph, data is represented with the help of simple lines horizontally or vertically drawn. For increasing the interest and readability of concepts, pictorial illustrations and cartoons are occasionally used on the line graph.
- **Pie graph:** It is a circle divided into sectors, the scale is the circumference divided into suitable scale units, such as percentages.

- **Surface graph:** Connects each plotted point to the next; such as column graphs, they join each point to the base.

POSTERS (FIG. 5.10)

A poster helps the extension works to get across one idea to the audience. It is a visual which has to catch the attention of the audience and pass on to them a simple message at a glance. The guidance should become aware of the events, practices or ideas you want to communicate. Poster has to be bold in design, simple to understand and attractive in color.

Uses of Poster

- To make an instant appeal.
- To convey single idea or few ideas.
- To be understood at a glance.
- Comprehensive at a distance and sufficiently clear.
- Suitable for patient education, presenting scientific facts, showing safety measures and many other facets relating to health.

The Components of Poster (Fig. 5.11)

- **Picture or illustration:** It should be such as to bring out clearly at a glance. If it is a drawing, the actual thing to be shown it

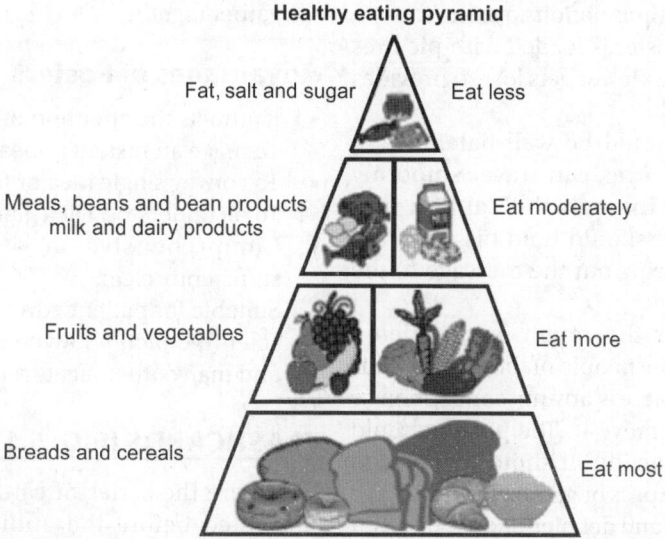

Fig. 5.10: Posters.

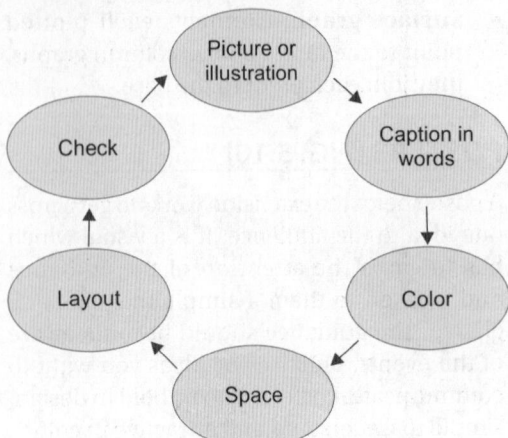

Fig. 5.11: Components of poster.

should be thought out in bold relief. Avoid unnecessary details so that the viewer's attention is not confused. If you use a photograph avoid unwanted surrounding and being out the point promptly.

- **Caption in words:** As small as possible all five caption is the best. Never write the caption vertically as it creates difficulty in reading. As not break the caption.
- **Color:** Use bright attractive colors. The center core can be highlighted with a more prominent color. Even in the captions some prominent word can be given a different color. Do not use more than three colors. Otherwise, it may be confusing. Do not use odd combinations of colors.
- **Space:** If a poster is loaded with pictures and words the viewer gets lost so provides adequate space.
- **Layout:** It should be well balanced so that viewer's eyes can travel smoothly and quickly through the caption and illustration. It should hold his attention and clearly bring out the message to the viewer.
- **Cheek:** After the rough is completed show it to some people of the level of your audience. If there is any misconception or ambiguity, remove it. The poster should recommend action. It should be placed where people pass or gather. It should give only one idea and detailed should be given through other media.

In places where the exposure time is short (e.g., streets) the message of the poster should be short simple direct and one that can be taken at glance and easy-to-understand immediately. In places where people have some time to spend, e.g., bus stops railway stations, hospitals, health centers. The right amount of matter should be put up in the right place at the time. The life of the posture is usually short and should be changed frequently.

Rules to Prepare Poster

- To do a special job.
- To promote one point.
- To support local demonstration and local exhibits.
- Planned for the specified people.
- It should stop the people and make them to look.
- Tell the message in a single glance.
- Use bold letters (20" x 301)
- Use simple, few words which conveys one idea.
- Use pleasing colors.
- Must be timely.
- **It contains:**
  - 1st division—announces the purposes of the project.
  - 2nd division—set out conditions.
  - 3rd division—recommends actions.
- It should be placed, where people pass or gather together.

Advantages of Posters

- It attracts the attention of the audience.
- To make an instant appeal.
- To convey single idea or few ideas.
- To be understood at a glance.
- Comprehensive at a distance and sufficiently clear.
- Suitable for patient education, presenting scientific fact, showing safety measures and many other facets relating to health.

FLASHCARDS (FIG. 5.12)

These are the series of cards which can be presented before the audience in proper sequence, tell a complete story, in size of the

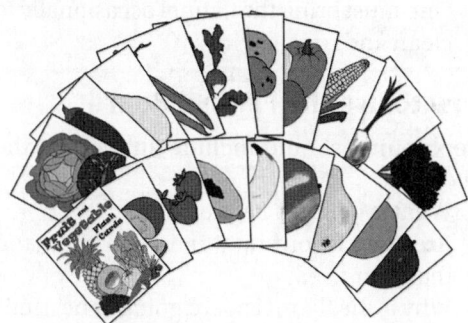

Fig. 5.12: Flashcards.

flashcard is 10 inch x 12 inch and it contains a picture or diagram. Each individual card is flashed before the audience accompanied by the verbal commentary, the extension worker or the student who wants to use thins holds them in hand and flashes the card one after another.

Uses of Flashcards

- Enable the audience to look, listen and learn.
- It gives information regarding subject.
- It captures the attention of the audience.
- It makes learning interesting and profitable.
- Fosters/develop the knowledge.
- It stimulates curiosity.
- It increases and sustains attention and concentration.

Preparation of Flashcards

A brief story should be written. The story should end with suggestions or a morale that leads to action. A suitable title should be selected for the story. The story should be divided into a number of scenes which are to be presented a number of individual cards.

The cards are numbered in sequence every set of cards should have a title. There should be a commentary written on the reverse of each cards so that the person who presents it to the accidence can easily read the commentary from the reverse. Attractive lettering increases the effectiveness of the flashcards.

How to use a Flashcard

- They should be familiar to the students or person who presents the card.
- He should use simple words and local expressions.
- He must hold cards in a way that the audience can see clearly, better against the body—and should point out the pictures on the card.
- Some important points may be jolted down by the back side of the cards to help in the telling story.
- The cards should be stacked in order, as one card is finished it may be slid behind the other. In this way, they will remain in order for the next time.

Instructions for the Teacher to use Flashcards

To teach well with flashcards, the teacher should follow certain points:
- A series or set of cards can be prepared on a single topic, put in sequential order, before starting the explanation.
- The story on each card must be familiar.
- Must use simple words and local terminology.
- Hold the cards at chest level where people can see clearly hold against body and not in air, face different parts of the groups, to show cards to all.
- Glance down at cards, as you are ready to explain and make sure to given correct information.
- Use pointer. Do not cover the matter with hand.
- Be enthusiastic and enjoy explaining the matter.

FLANNEL BOARD (FIG. 5.13)

The advantages are a type of cloth board that consists of piece of flannel cloth tightly stretched over the surface and then glued to a piece of play wood or even a very thick card boards. Because the pieces of flannel will adhere to each other, letters, figures or symbols cut from the same material can be

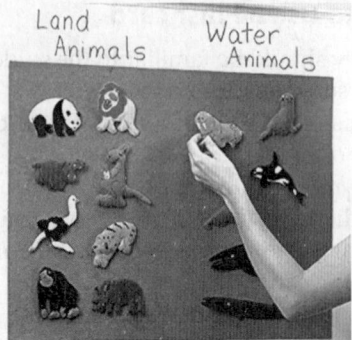

Fig. 5.13: Flannel board.

fixed on to the flannel board where they will stay without the use of tapes, pins, pictures, cards or similar other materials can also be coarse sand paper are glued to their backs.

Flannel graph can be designated as a picture-drama. The story should be simple and should not involve too many characters,. It should have good beginning, the subject matter and an ending with definite suggestions. Place the board high on a firm table or stand so that it can be seen easily by every one of the audience. Number the several objectives and place them in order.

To aid memory, make brief notes on a piece of paper and identify it on the picture or material to be put on the flannel board. Do not block the view and give sufficient time to the audience to see and understand each part.

Purpose

- To save time during class presentation.
- To encourage visual presentation of ideas.

Advantages of Flannel Board

- It can be prepared beforehand.
- It permits quickly back and forth adjustments.
- It can use a variety of visuals.
- To facilitate the attention factors.

Disadvantage

The flannel board cannot be used as a chalkboard in the class.

Holding Tips

- One must plan in advance the exact appearance of the board.

- One must bring the flannel occasionally to clean and roughen it.

How to use the Flannel Board

Preplanning should include answers to the following:

- What is going to be prepared?
- Are the cut out materials prepared and ready for use?
- Why is the flannel board going to be used?
- How is the information going to be presented?
- What will the audience get out of it?

Selecting tool: A piece of flannel, terry cloth or felt cloth attached to a rigid surface on which cut out fingers will adhere of backed with flannel or felt cloth sand paper or cotton.

BULLETIN BOARD (FIG. 5.14)

The bulletin board display is one of the in expensive instructional devices used for teaching. It may be used for informational and educational purposes. It can be used effectively in connection with every learning situation and it properly used, can motivate, supplement and enrich learning. It is a board with a background of colored cloth. It can be covered with glass or a plane board.

The material for display may be news sheets, announcements, booklets, circular letters, newspaper netting, cartoons, pictures, charts, posters, maps, graphs, subject outlines, etc. They can perform useful educational functions in all levels and fields, elementary, secondary and colleges can be used in

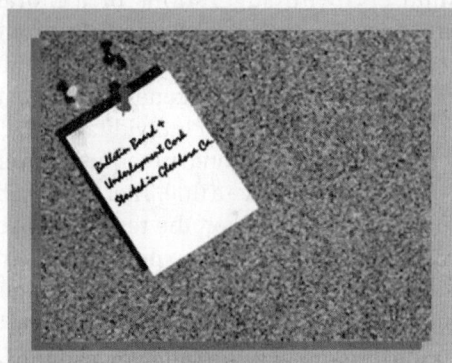

Fig. 5.14: Bulletin board.

industrial, commercial and governmental training and communication.

Purposes

- To motivate the learner, for example, it could be used in learning projects by a group of students to shave learning experiences.
- To broader the sensory experience of the learner and provide experience out scale the student environment.
- To add variety to the classroom activity.
- To promote information.
- To supplement and correlate instruction the material may be used in a unit plan as integral part of the curriculum.
- To save time, material that cannot be presented during the class hour can be used on the bulletin board.

As an aid to classroom teaching to display the unit plans in the corridor, the recreation room and the library for educational purpose. In outpatient clinics, patient education may be facilitated by appropriate use of bulletin boards. The clinical conferences room in the hospital, ward, as a correlation between class room and clinical learning experience.

Special Things to Note About Bulletin Board

- There are certain things which have an interest for a day only and these must be removed from the bulletin board at the end of the day.
- Results of sports extends, new projects undertaken individually or collectively should always be put on the bulletin board.
- Achievement of the individual pupil and that the school may be advertised.
- New arrival in the library may be exhibited on the notice board.

How to use Bulletin Board

- Teacher must collect suitable instructions for instructional projects.
- Teacher must also classify and file the material beforehand.

- Arrange the material in an interesting manner.
- Teacher must put a title and give a brief description.
- Use color harmony.
- Teacher must encourage the pupils to observe as well as to contribute to the bulletin board.
- It always serves as a place for displaying some outstanding work of the pupil.

General Care to be Taken

- Material that is going to be displayed on the bulletin board should be selected with care.
- Material that is going to be displayed on the bulletin board should be correlated with regular class activity.
- Materials displayed must be changed frequently and in time.

Characteristics of the Bulletin Board

- The board should be at a place where it will be seen by most of the people for whom it is meant.
- The type and size used will depend on the purpose for which it is used.
- The size of the board should be a little longer in length than in width.
- The highest point of the bulletin board should be only a little above the eye level of the average individual.
- Several types of bulletin boards can be used depending on the purpose as well as the money available.
- The fixed type is attached to the wall whereas the movable type is unattached and sufficiently light weight to be transported from room to room.

Item used in Bulletin Board

- Photographs
- Cut-outs
- Illustrations
- Publications
- Drawings
- Specimens
- Posters

- Newspapers
- Pasting up of announcements, assignments, distinctions, achievements.

Principles in the Use of Bulletin Board

- The board for posting notices should be kept separate from those for current events and study.
- A suggested plan for placement of bulletin boards is to have on near educational administrator's office notices, another near library, third group in each of clinical conference rooms on the hospital wards and fourth group in the classrooms.
- The contents of the board should be organized around a central theme of content; materials should be dated to ensure that it does not remain no longer than desired.
- The appearance should be neat, orderly and attractive.
- Material should be changed frequently and systematically.
- The contributions should be well labeled. A false first impression is difficult to rectify.
- Student contributions should be encouraged and used.
- Responsibility for editing the board should be placed on one person. Appoint a bulletin board committee to provide material.
- Everyone should be held responsible for reading and knowing what is on the board.
- All material should be appropriate classified and labeled for further reference.
- An interval of a day or two should be allowed to elapse during which the board is left bare in order to stimulate interest.

Use of Bulletin Board in Nursing Education

As an aid to classroom teaching to display the unit plans in the corridor, the recreation room and the library for educational purpose. In outpatient clinics, patient education may be facilitated by appropriate use of bulletin boards. The clinical conferences room in the hospital, ward, as a correlation between classroom and clinical learning experience.

Uses of Bulletin Board

- To provide information.
- To communicate the ideas.
- To motivate the learner.
- To add variety to the classroom activity.
- To describe the ways of doing a particular item.
- To follow-up instructions on thinks demonstrated and emphasized.
- To save time, material that cannot be presented during the class hour, nevertheless can be on bulletin board.
- To supplement and correlate instruction.

CARTOON (FIG. 5.15)

A cartoon is humorous caricature which gives a suitable message. In a cartoon, the features of objects and people exaggerated along with generally recognized symbols. Cartoon has an instantaneous visual appeal and tickling message. Many times cartoon in newspapers can be sarcastic and ridiculing. The main source of cartoons is periodicals.

Sources of Cartoon

- Mains sources of cartoon are periodicals.
- Newspapers carry cartoons daily which are either political or social in nature.
- Special periodicals and magazines carry cartoons on science, management, economics and education.

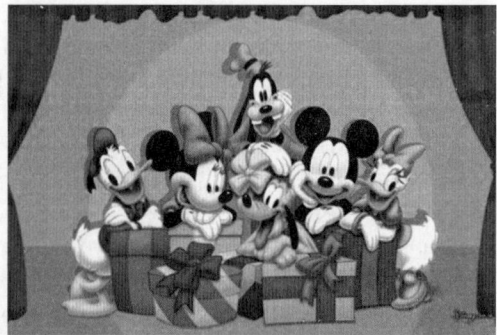

Fig. 5.15: Cartoon.

Instructional Advantages of Cartoons

- A cartoon can be effectively used to initiate certain lesson.
- A cartoon can be used to motivate students to start a discussion.
- A cartoon can be used for making lesson lively and interesting.

Uses of Cartoons

- A cartoon makes learning more interesting and effective as it creates a strong appeal to the emotions.
- A cartoon is simple, clear which tells the story without too much explanation.
- Cartoons are very good attention, capturing devices and motivate the students to learning more permanent.
- Cartoons are helpful for providing opportunity for self-expression and creativity among students.
- Cartoons are helpful in modifying behavior and developing positive attitude, interests of learners.

Preparation/Technique of Using the Cartoon

- Should be simple.
- Should give information and adequate knowledge about various subjects and current issues in an interesting way.
- Teachers should prepare cartoons according to classroom needs.
- Students should involve in the process of preparation to maximize learning experiences.

PUPPETS

Puppets are derived from Latin word *puppa* which means doll. The word puppet today means a figure which fits over the hand, such as a glove and is operated from behind below by the fingers.

Types of Puppets (Fig. 5.17)

1. **Hand puppet:** These are the simplest of all puppets. They are operated from below by fingers.

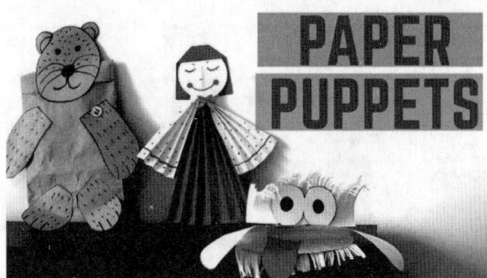

Fig. 5.16: Paper puppets.

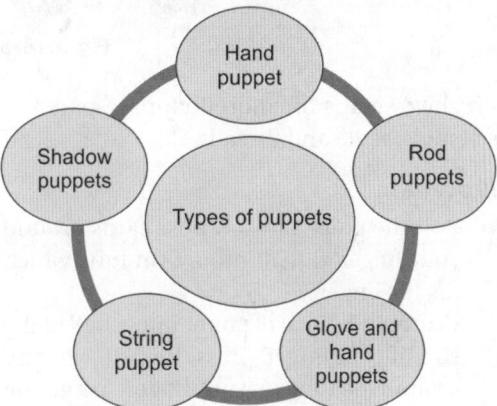

Fig. 5.17: Types of puppets.

2. **Rod-puppets:** These are operated from below the stage by a combination of rods and springs. These have jointed bodies made with stiff wires or wooden sticks attached to arms and legs.
3. **Glove and hand puppets:** This is like three fingered glove which fits on the hand. The first finger is inserted inside the hand and moves it, when we tell a story. The middle finger and thumb fit in the hands and move them.
4. **String puppet:** These are fingers with movable limbs and are operated from above by means of strings **(Fig. 5.18)**.
5. **Shadow puppets:** The shadow of hands and dolls are used as puppets against the lighted screen.

How to Prepare a Hand Puppet

Material Required

A used post cards, old newspapers, glue, two pieces of string, Indian ink, color box pins,

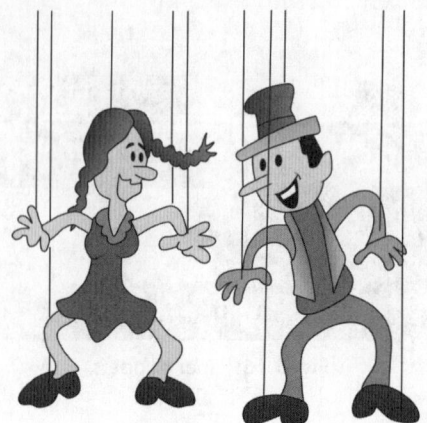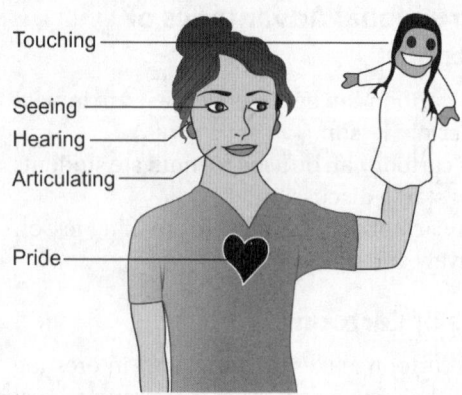

Touching

Seeing
Hearing
Articulating

Pride

Fig. 5.18: String puppets.

brushes, scraps of colored cloth, a pad and scissors needle and threads.

Procedure

- Roll the piece of used post cards around your finger glue it into a firm tube which fits the finger.
- Crumple a piece of paper into a ball of the size of your finger, press the ball over and around the tube on your finger and give at the sharp of a head.
- Tie a piece of plain paper and use Indian ink to put on eyes, hair, nose, lips and, etc., put red and black colors as needed to size it an attractive appearance.
- Take a piece of bright colored cloth and sent it into a long tube and tie the cloth on the neck and then turn it.
- Some puppets may be prepared to play roles of females, some of males or children. They may have moustaches, turbans, salwars, kurtas, etc., depicting the life and characters you want to show to audience.
- The stages further show of puppets can be prepared by using a wooded frame, two chairs, one cot, and two pillars of verandah.
- The puppets should not see with the hands or body of the puppeteers. Song or speech from the back or recorded talk is used. Usually to puppeteers are behind the stage and so only 4 characters can be on the stage at a time. The actual voices of man, women, children can be imitated.

- Before the show, a brief description of the dialogue is given. There should not be silent pauses. The dialogue should be quick and speeches and scenes should be short. There should be lot of actions wit and humor.
- Everyday people and familiar situations should be used which have relationship with village problems.

Principles of Puppets

- Does not use puppet for plays text can be done just as well as better by other dramatic means?
- Puppet plays must be based on action rather than words.
- Keep the plays short, puppet must be skillfully manipulated.
- Do not omit the possibilities of music and dancing as part of the puppet show.
- Adapt the puppet show in all respect to your audience. The age, background and tasks of the pupils must be related to the types of puppet used and to the play itself.
- Do not hesitate to adopt the puppet play. There is no value in sticking to the text. If by departing from it you can add interest and points to the play.

Advantages of Puppets

- The craft of puppetry is an effective aid to learning.
- It develops cooperation among children.

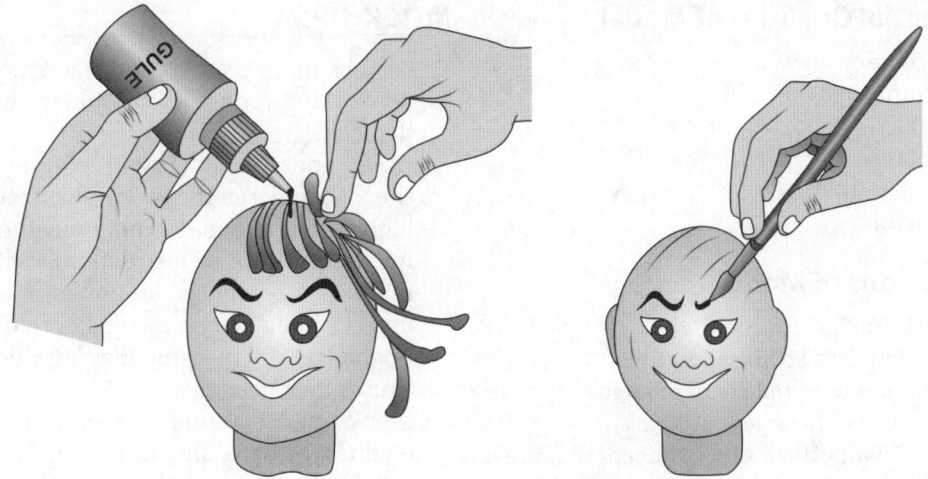

Fig. 5.19: Puppet preparation.

- Children develop their imagination by providing the puppets with speech.
- Children increase their manual dexterity through manipulation.
- Puppet playing helps timid children express themselves more freely because they are separated from the audiences by a screen.

Disadvantages

- It needs special training for manipulation of puppets and marionettes to convey ideas.
- Ideas convey through puppets show can be misinterpreted by the audience.
- It requires to keep on mind the age, background and tasks of the student.
- Puppets plays with too much action take away the attention of the audience.

MODELS (FIG. 5.20)

Models are the replicas or copies of the real object. Models are usually of three types— solid, cross-sectional, and working. Models are concrete objects, some considerably larger than the real object. Sectional models explain clearly the structure or functions of the original. In some cases, working models of the original are used where the specific function of the original is duplicated and could be explained easily.

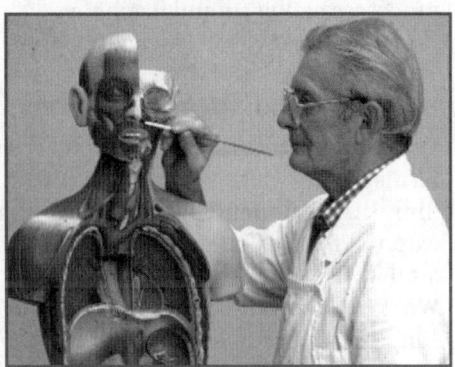

Fig. 5.20: Models.

Important Functions of Models

- Models simplify readily.
- Models concretize abstract concepts.
- Models enable us to reduce or enlarge objects to an observable size.
- Models provide the correct concepts of an industrial unit or a bride or a dam like, the Bhakra Dam, etc.
- A working model explains the various processes of object and machines.
- Preparation of models could from a topic for project work. This is very helpful to create interest in creative activity in pupils.

Cardboards, plastic, plaster of Paris, wood, thermocole and metal, etc., can be used in the preparation of a model.

Essential Qualities of Model

- Accuracy
- Simplicity
- Utility
- Solidity
- Ingenuity
- Useful

Functions of Model

- It simplifies reality
- Concretizes abstract concepts
- Enables us to reduce or enlarge objects to an observable size.
- It provides the correct concept of an real object like dam/bridge, etc.
- A working model explains the various processes of objects and machines.
- Promotes creative interest among pupils.

Types of Model (Fig. 5.21)

- **Scale model:** Correct idea of an object can be displayed.
- **Simplified model:** Gives an ideal of an external form of an object. For example, animal, fish, etc.
- **Working model:** To demonstrate in a simple way of an operation or process. For example, fetal circulation.
- **Cross-section model:** Inside of an object in visible, immense value will be observed in sciences. For example, cross-section of blood vessel.

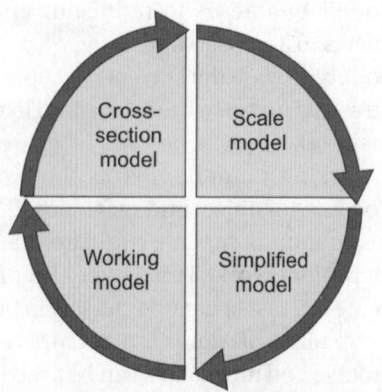

Fig. 5.21: Types of model.

MOCK-UPS

- A mock-up refers to a specialized models or working replica of the object being depicted.
- In a mock-up, a certain element of the original reality in emphasized or highlighted to make it more meaningful for the purpose of instruction. While a model is a recognizable limitation of an object (though larger or smaller than the original one), a mock-up may/may not be similar in appearance.
- Mock-ups of aeroplanes, automobile engines, bridges, ship and tunnels, etc., may be demonstrated for explaining their structure and actual working.
- Mock-ups are often used in technical instructions for training purposes.

Advantages

- To recreate things from the past or the future.
- To reduce the size of things.
- To **make model** of things too small to examine.
- To made model of things from faraway places.
- To explain difficult concepts.
- To show working parts.
- To attract interests attention.
- To promote increased **learner** participation.
- To show some selected aspect of the whole in a simple **elemental** way.
- To present an immediate sensation.

OBJECT AND SPECIMEN

A specimen is a part of an object (**Fig. 5.22**). It may be a sample that shows quality or structure. Examples would be a section of a long bone, a dissected lens from an animal's eye, a sample of a crude drug. An object is the thing itself in its entirely brought from its natural setting into the classroom to supply the type of sensory experience that will make instruction meaningful. An object might be a thermometer, a splint, a forceps, a calf's

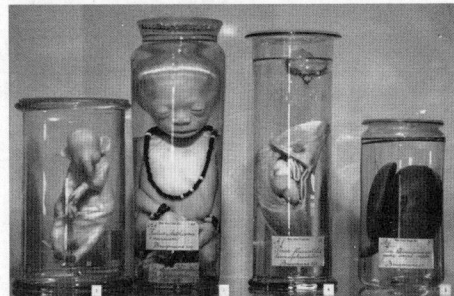

Fig. 5.22: Specimens.

heart or any such thing which pertains to the subject being taught.

Sources of Objects and Specimens

- Local markets
- Manufacturers and factories
- Discarded material from the house
- Specimen found in the nature can be collected by students from field trips and nature hunt
- Plasters casts can be purchased
- Wild flowers, leaves shells, stones butterflies moths, insects can also be procured.

Mounting the Objects and Specimens

Objects and specimens should be mounted in shallow boxes in an artistic way and the boxes should be covered with cellophane paper. Also label each object or specimen using self adhesive paper.

Advantages of Objects and Specimens

- Collection of objects and specimens by students requires interaction with others leading to development of social skills and values.
- Students when collect and display objects and specimens derive satisfaction of contributing to the school and teacher something worthwhile.
- Student's power of observation and first hand experiences is enhanced by collection of objects and specimens

- Student's personal collection of objects and specimens can be good source of doing investigatory projects.
- Collection of objects and specimens become an interesting educational pursuit of the teacher and students alike.
- It arouse some interest among students in learning
- Objects and specimens involve all the five senses in the process of learning
- It heighten the reality in the class room
- It makes teaching lively.

General Instructions

- A specimen is a sample of the real object or a material.
- Using objects and specimens—while using the specimen and objects as teaching aids, a teacher must **keep the following points in her mind**.
- Plan your teaching with certain simple and direct observations of the object or specimen being referred to.
- Ask questions from the students to elicit more details of the features of the object or specimen under observation.
- Clarify and emphasize important structural details of the object or specimen under observation
- Provide review and practice to make learning permanent.

MOULAGE

- A moulage is a mold made of plastic material (one of a diversified group of plastic suitable for this purpose) to stimulate some life object, such as a part of the body which shows evidence of trauma, infection, surgical intervention or disease.
- Phillips describes an excellent moulage developed by the medical illustration serve at the armed forces institute of pathology, which would be very useful in teaching nursing students.
- It is a colostomy moulage set, with double-barreled and single-barreled types of colostomy with skin, which may be placed on a chase doll or a live model for teaching colostomy care.

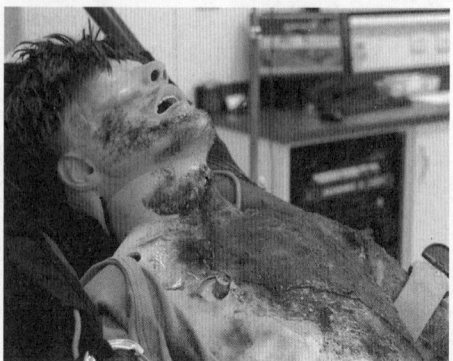

Fig. 5.23: Moulage shows evidence of trauma.

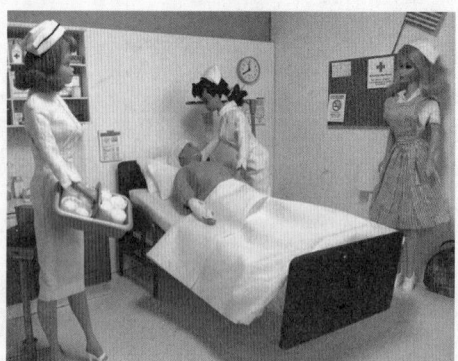

Fig. 5.24: Dioramas: Three-dimensional visual aids.

DIORAMAS

Dioramas are three-dimensional visual aids which are used to exhibit and display the reality in miniature. The desire for realism, i.e., observe and learn from the actual things and real situations, is generally present in large number among the learners and dioramas prove to be valuable means for meeting such a desire.

Definitions

- "A diorama is a scene in perspective, using three-dimensional models to depict the activity, e.g., activities at the airport, life in Sahara desert, etc." Hence, one can easily display some real life actual scene with the help of an appropriate diorama by making use of small objects, modeled figures and backgrounds in perspective, against an appropriate setting.   —**Michaelis (1976)**
- A diorama, thus, may be defined as a three-dimensional visual representation of a scene in a miniature form represented with the help of miniature objects and with backgrounds in actual perspective.
  —**SL Ahiuwaila (1967)**

Types of Diorama

The objects in diorama, such as figures, building, trees, man and animals are shown in a miniature form. However, for giving the displayed diorama the needed vividness and realism, all the necessary measures should be attempted. For example, a building or tree is made to look smaller at the far end in order to demonstrate that it lies at a greater distance. In this way, considerable attention is being paid for creating appropriate illusion of depth and distance in a relatively small space of the displayed diorama. Sometimes, the lightening effects are being used for serving the desired purpose to a dioramic display.

Educational Use

- As the dioramas can display the reality in miniature form, they can be very useful visual aids in teaching and learning of many concepts related to the school curriculum. For example, take the case of teaching of a lesson 'scene at the village fair', 'social and religious festival' or 'railway station'. Such themes can be affectively taught by the display of appropriate diorama depicting all what is usually visible at such occasions.
- Similarly, the teachers can make use of different dioramas depicting historical, social and geographical aspects, such as scenes of the battlefields, life in ancient cities, such as Mohenjodaro and Harappa, life in a modern Indian village, life of the Eskimos, distribution of natural wealth in a countryside, etc.
- Concepts related to physical surroundings and economic aspects which needs three-dimensional exhibit of places, such as man-made or nature made developments, material or manpower resources, stages of a process, functioning of a system,

historical evolution, inventions, and description of an imaginary situation can be very well explained to the students with the help of useful and appropriate dioramas.

- For the purpose of deriving maximum educational benefits, these dioramas should be constructed with the cooperation of a group of pupils using the easily available and inexpensive material, such as cardboard, wooden pieces, paper, poster, colors, brushes, stitching and stapling tools, scissors, taps and other adhesive material.

OPAQUE PROJECTOR (FIG. 5.25)

Opaque projector is the only projector on which you can project a variety of materials, for example, book pages, objects, coins, postcards, or any other similar flat material that is non-transparent. The opaque projector will project and simultaneously enlarge, directly from the originals, printed matter, all kinds of written or pictorial matter in any sequence derived by the teacher. It requires a dark room, as projector is large and not reality movables.

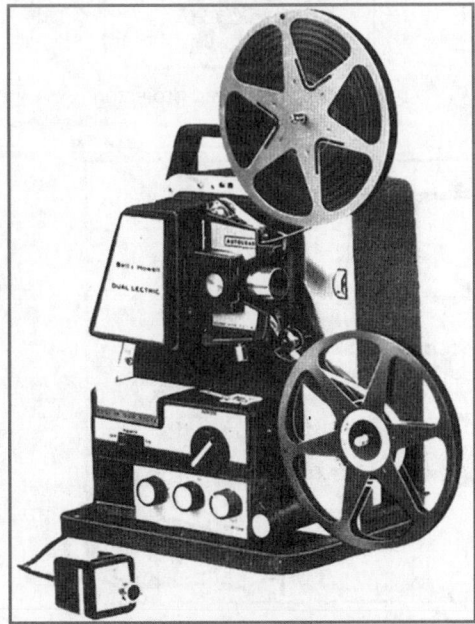

Fig. 5.25: Opaque projector.

It is very useful means for using reflected light to pick-up the image or for projection of flat pictures, diagrams, maps to a screen in enlarged form so that the entire group can see them. The opaque projector will project and simultaneously enlarge, directly from the originals, printed matter, all kinds of written or pictorial matter in any sequence derived by the teacher. It requires a dark room, as projector is large and not readily movable; therefore their usefulness is limited.

- On large screen for normal instruction.
- An approach to reading.

Advantages

The opaque projector is a wonderful teaching device with the help of which it is possible to make vivid enlarged projections of objects from the size of a postage stamp of practically that of a quarto page. In an ordinary classroom, the projections can be made visible to anyone, even to a student sitting in the remote corner or on the rearmost bench.

- Stimulates attention and arouses interest.
- Can project a wide range of materials, such as stamps, coins, specimen, when one copy is available.
- Can be used for enlarging drawings, pictures and maps.
- Does not require any written or typed materials, hand-written material can be used.
- Helps students to retain knowledge for longer period.
- Review instructional problems.
- Test knowledge and ability.
- Simple operation.

Disadvantages

- Costly equipment
- Needs to use it with care
- Needs a dark room for projector

The Opaque Projection in Teaching

The opaque projector serves many educational purposes. In procedures, the teacher may use it for the following purposes, according to his needs and teaching situations:

- Charts, diagrams and graphs can be projected on large screen for normal instruction.
- Picture stories from any source are projected and used as an approach to reading.
- Original drawings are projected to the screen, to the delight of the young artists responsible for them.
- Written composition-stories, poems, essays, letters—may be projected. This is an effective system of sharing a student's doubt. Darkness in the room focuses attention.
- The fundamentals of arithmetic, handwriting, spelling and composition are illustrated by use of the opaque projector.
- Written or types outlines of new units of study may be projected.

OVERHEAD PROJECTOR (FIGS. 5.26 AND 5.27)

Overhead projector is the projecting medium on which, with the help of transparencies or overhead transparency film (OHP film), group education can be given. While using OHP, the teacher can maintain eye contact with the students. This can be used in a well-lighted room. Transparencies can be prepared using acetate sheet with specially made marker pens. Complicated diagrams can be transferred to the acetate from the original material by Xeroxing.

Important Points in using OHP

- Transparencies are plastic sheets, readily available in A4 size on which we can write information.
- The transparency is then used with an overhead projector to show the written material on a screen.
- This instructional medium is probably next to the chalkboard and handouts in frequency of use.
- OHP is used to demonstrate visually important points, show diagrams, highlight issues, build up information as to teach, and to support other methods of visual communication.

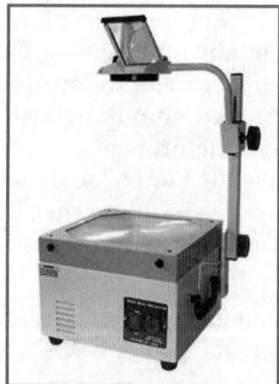

Fig. 5.27: Overhead projector.

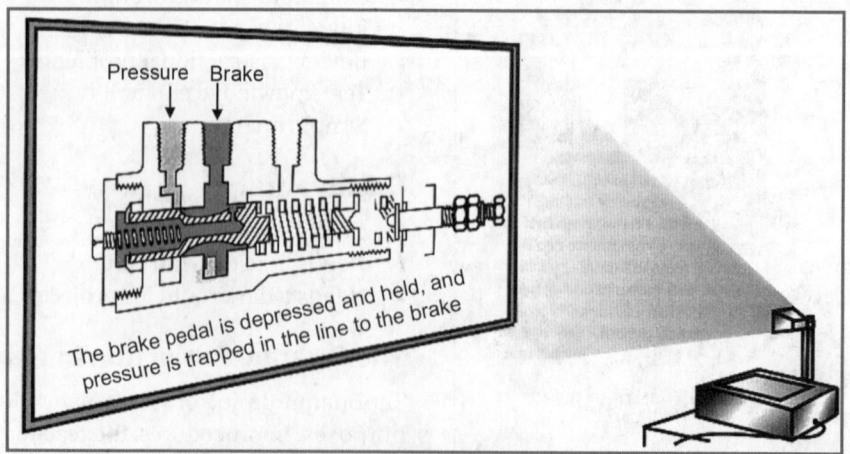

Fig. 5.26: Teaching with overhead projector (OHP).

- Transparencies can be done by using special OHP pens. There are basically two kinds of pen, such as:
  a. Spirit-based pens whose images are permanent.
  b. Water-based pens whose images can be erased with plain water.
- Use large bold letters and clear simple drawings with as few lines and tables as possible.
- Apart from pens, photocopies, laser printers, dot matrix printers and plotters can also be used to make transparencies. These may be black and white or inkjet color.
- The principle involved here is that text or diagrams can be transferred from paper to paper by a variety of means.
- Instead of paper, the information is transferred to transparencies to be used for presentation in a lecture, seminar, conference or workshop.

Useful Steps in Preparing OHP Transparencies

- Leave a margin at the slides, top to bottom. This will ensure that all information can be displayed at once.
- Plan the text and diagrams carefully. Try to summarize the main points.
- Teachers should not attempt to convey your entire talk on the OPH.

Advantages

- No dark room required.
- Pictures and letters can be projected in large size.
- Facts can be masked as per the requirement and immediate correction in the subject matter is possible.

Disadvantages

- The picture does not come clear due to wrong selection of projection sites, power interruption or true of incorrect angle.
- In the absence of white wall or screen, this is not useful.
- This is expensive and its use is impossible, if the project goes out of order.

INTERNET

Internet is a new means of computer-based communication system has opened vast capacity of transfer of knowledge and has made it possible to get into direct and instant communication across the world by means of e-mail and even a on-line chat. This is a fast growing communication media and holds very large potential to become a major health education tool. Already a fairly large number of persons in India are using this media, and the numbers are growing every day.

Vast number of health-related literature from WHO and other health agencies

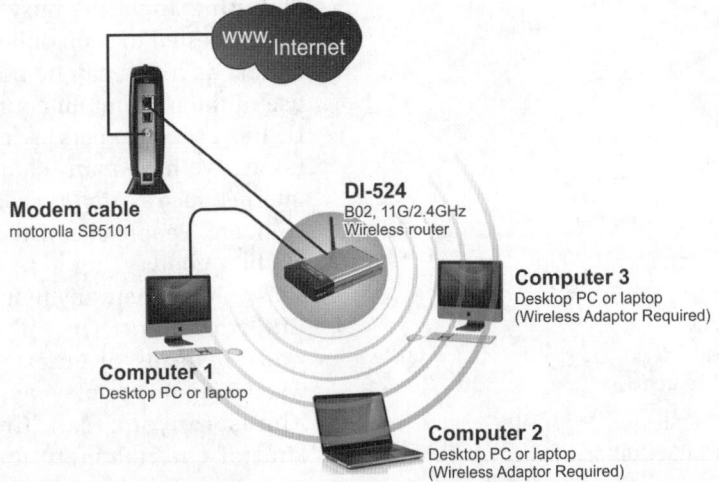

Fig. 5.28: Internet communication.

are available on line. The health-related information from the Ministry of Health and Family Welfare Government of India is also available on other website. The first recorded description of the social interactions that could be enabled through networking was a series of memos written by JCR Licklider of MIT in August 1962 discussing his "Galactic Network" concept. He envisioned a globally interconnected set of computers through which everyone could quickly **access data** and programs from any site. In spirit, the concept was very much like the Internet of today. Licklider was the first head of the computer research program at DARPA, starting in October 1962. While at DARPA he convinced his successors at DARPA, Ivan Sutherland, Bob Taylor, and MIT researcher Lawrence G. Roberts, of the importance of this networking concept.

Uses of internet (Fig. 5.29): Here is the list of some common uses of internet

- **Email:** By using internet now we can communicate in a fraction of seconds with a person who is sitting in the other part of the world. Today for better communication, we can avail the facilities of Email. We can chat for hours with our loved ones. There are plenty messenger services and email services offering this service for free. With help of such services, it has become very easy to establish a kind

of global friendship where you can share your thoughts, can explore other cultures of different ethnicity.

- **Information:** The biggest advantage that internet offering is information. The internet and the World Wide Web has made it easy for anyone to access information and it can be of any type, as the internet is flooded with information. The internet and the World Wide Web has made it easy for anyone to access information and it can be of any type. Any kind of information on any topic is available on the Internet.

- **Business:** World trade has seen a big boom with the help of the internet, as it has become easier for buyers and sellers to communicate and also to advertise their sites. Now a days most of the people are using online classified sites to buy or sell or advertising their products or services. Classified sites save a lot of money and time so this is chosen as medium by most of people to advertise their products. We have many classified sites on the web, such as craigslist, Adsglobe.com, Kijiji, etc.

- **Social networking:** Today social networking sites have become an important part of the online community. Almost all users are members use it for personal and business purposes. It is an awesome place to network with many entrepreneurs who come here to begin building their own personal and business brand.

- **Shopping:** In today's busy life most of us are interested to shop online. Now a days almost anything can be bought with the use of the internet. In countries, such as US most of consumers prefer to shop from home. We have many shopping sites on internet, such as Amazon.com, Dealsglobe. com, etc. People also use the internet to auction goods. There are many auction sites online, where anything can be sold.

- **Entertainment:** On internet, we can find all forms of entertainment from watching films to playing games online. Almost anyone can find the right kind of entertainment for themselves.

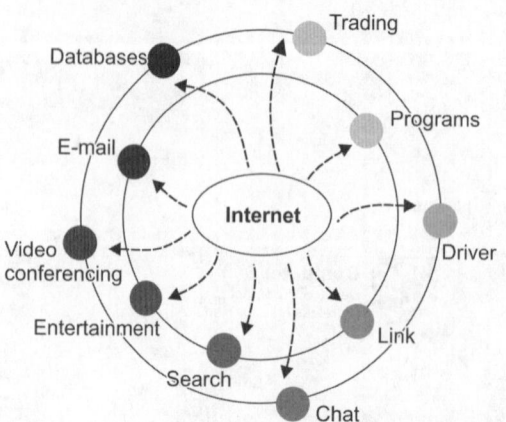

Fig. 5.29: Uses of internet.

When people surf the Web, there are numerous things that can be found. Music, hobbies, news and more can be found and shared on the Internet. There are numerous games that may be downloaded from the Internet for free.

- **E-Commerce:** E-commerce is the concept used for any type of commercial maneuvering, or business deals that involves the transfer of information across the globe via internet. It has become a phenomenon associated with any kind of shopping, almost anything. It has got a real amazing and range of products from household needs, technology to entertainment.

- **Services:** Many services are now provided on the internet, such as online banking, job seeking, purchasing tickets for your favorite movies, and guidance services on array of topics in the every aspect of life, and hotel reservations and bills paying. Often these services are not available offline and can cost you more.

- **Job search:** Internet makes life easy for both employers and job seekers as there are plenty of job sites which connect employers and job seekers.

- **Dating/Personals:** People are connecting with others though internet and finding their life partners. Internet not only helps to find the right person but also to continue the relationship.

COMPUTERS

Computers are being used in classroom as teaching techniques and they are unique in individualization of instruction. Computer-assisted instruction (CAI) in the form of tutorial mode, drill mode, stimulation mode and animation technique offers tremendous possibilities for teaching.

- Computers are being used in classroom as teaching techniques and they are unique in individualization of instruction.
- Computer assisted instruction (CAI) in the form of tutorial mode, drill mode, stimula-

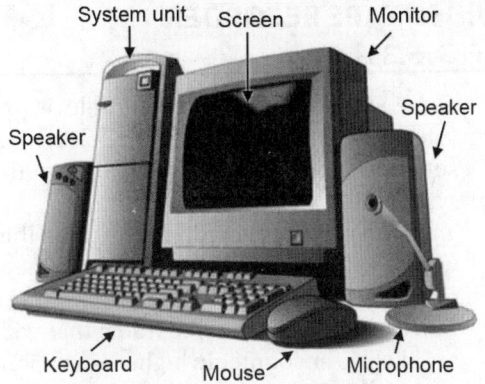

Fig. 5.30: Computer and its parts.

tion mode and animation technique offers tremendous possibilities for teaching.

- Teaching is being mechanized and reutilized in this technique. The teacher will be needed only for preparing the software program.

- Computers can also be used for strong a large number of questions and objective test items in a hard disk/CD which can serve as a question bank.

Advantages of Computer Instructions

- It allows the student to interact in the learning situation.
- Computers can also individualize learning to an extraordinary degree.
- It can also enhance a student's self-esteem in several ways.
- The computer can reply to the student's answer with statement.
- The nonjudgmental nature and endless patience of the computer are also important advantage.
- Records of student's performances on simulations or practice tests can be kept on the computer.
- Computer can also be available to students for more hours than the instructor.
- Computers can also be used for strong a large number of questions and objective test items in a hard disk/CD which can serve as a question bank.

VIDEO TAPE RECORDER (FIG. 5.31)

- There are different formats for television sets and video recorder. Some television sets and video recorders have a multi-system.
- They can play tapes made anywhere in the world, but they cost about 50% more than regular one-system ones.
- Video tapes and video recorders that you are likely to encounter in higher education are classified according to tape width, into VHS—the commonest one.
- The institution can produce video films with the help of experts.

LCD PANELS (FIG. 5.32)

This aid has been largely superseded by data projectors. Since many smaller teaching and training rooms may not be fitted with data projectors, the following guidance is provided. A Liquid Crystal Display (LCD) panel connected to a computer and placed on an overhead projector will enable to project computer generated images onto a display screen for the whole class to read. To be effective LCDs, an overhead projector which contains a very powerful lamp than is available in the usual type of projector usually need to be placed on.

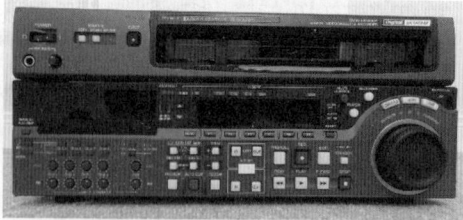

Fig. 5.31: Video tape recorder.

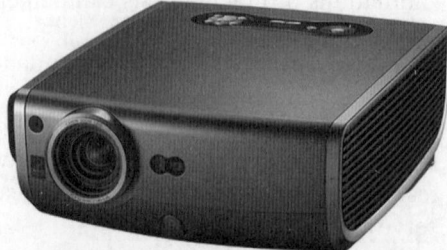

Fig. 5.32: LCD panel.

Guidelines for PowerPoint Presentations

PowerPoint is an extremely popular presentation and an alternative to using overhead transparencies for the production of interesting and visually attractive presentations.

The main advantage in using PowerPoint is the flexibility, both in terms of the content of the presentation and the way in which the information is displayed. Graphs, drawings, tables and organizational charts make presentation more interesting, but as a general rule keep presentations simple and clear. PowerPoint is most effectively used to emphasize the main features of the topic.

Guidelines for PowerPoint Presentations

- Limit the number of slides, to not more than 12 for a ten-minute presentation
- Ensure text contrasts with the background, but avoid patterned backgrounds
- Comply with copyright law when pictures, charts, tables or diagrams are used
- Standardize position, colors and styles
- Use only one or two animation or transition effects

Advantages

- The sequence of content can be interspersed with summary screens listing for example, search steps.
- It is less susceptible to last minute technical difficulties or unexpected events.

Disadvantages of a PowerPoint Presentation

- The teacher cannot interact with the content to illustrate points raised by students.
- PowerPoint can take up to a minute to load a presentation.
- It is time-consuming to prepare for teachers.
- Technical faults can raise and if the computer is not supported by UPS, it cannot be used during power failure.
- A floppy may not open or the file can get corrupted by the viruses.

SLIDE PROJECTOR (FIG. 5.33)

A slide is a small piece of transparent material on which a single pictorial image or scene or graphic image has been photographed or reproduced otherwise.

Molded slides range in size from 2 × 2 or 4.5 × 4 inches. Slides can be made from photographs and pictures by the teachers and pupils taking photographs and snapshots when they go on field trips for historical, geographical, literary or scientific excursions.

The arrangement of slides in proper sequence, according to the topic discussed, is an important aspect of teaching with them.

A teacher needs to use imaginatively and creatively to make the best use of them.

Advantages of Slides

- Help in retention of the material taught in the minds of the pupils
- Attract attention
- Arouse interest

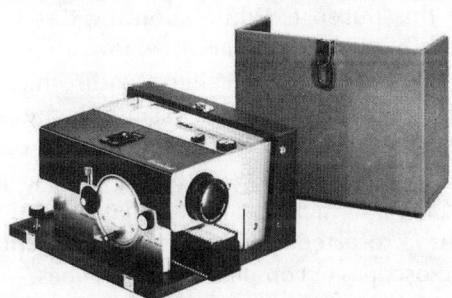

Fig. 5.33: Slide projector.

- Assist lesson development
- Test student understanding
- Review instruction
- Facilitate student-teacher participation

SLIDES

Slides are transparent pictures projected by shining light through them. The commonly used sizes of slides are 2' x 2' and 31%. The slides can be made from photographs and pictures by the teachers and pupils taking photographs and snapshots when they go on field trips for historical, geographical, literary or scientific excursions. The arrangement of slides in proper sequence, according to the topic discussed, is an important aspect of teaching with them.

Advantages of Slides

- Attract attention
- Arouse interest
- Assist lesson development
- Test student understanding
- Review instruction
- Facilitate student-teacher participation
- Help in retention of the material taught in the minds of the pupils

FILM STRIP (FIG. 5.34)

Filmstrip is a continuous strip of film consisting of individual frames or pictures arranged in sequence, usually with explanatory titles'. Each strip contains from 12 to 18 or more pictures.

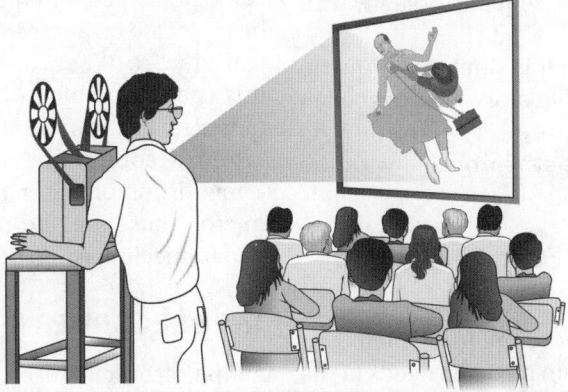

Fig. 5.34: Teaching with film strips.

It is a fixed sequence of related stills on a roll of 35 mm film or 8 mm film.

Advantages

- It is an economical visual material.
- It is easy to make and convenient to handle and carry.
- Takes up little space and can be easily stored.
- Provides a logical sequence to the teaching procedure and the individual picture on the strip can be kept before the students for a length of time.
- Filmstrip can be projected on the screen or wall or paper screen as the convenience and the teaching situation demands.

Principles of Film Strips

- Preview filmstrips before using them and selected carefully to meet the needs of the topic to be taught.
- Show again any part of the filmstrip needing more specific study.
- Use filmstrip to stimulate emotions, build attitudes and to point up problems.
- It should be introduced appropriately and its relationship to the topic of the study brought out.
- Use a pointer to direct attention, to specific details on the screen.

Types of Filmstrip

- **Discussion filmstrip**: It is continuous strip of film consisting of individual frames arranged in sequence usually with explanatory titles.
- **Sound slide film**: It is similar to filmstrip but instead of explanatory titles or spoken discussion recorded explanation is audible, which is synchronized with the pictures.

Instruction to be Followed while Using Filmstrips

- Preview filmstrips before using them and selected carefully to meet the needs of the topic to be taught.

- Show again any part of the filmstrip needing more specific study.
- Use filmstrip to stimulate emotions, build attitudes and to point up problems.
- It should be introduced appropriately and its relationship to the topic of study brought out. After showing the filmstrip, a follow-up discussion and summary is necessary. Pupil should develop an interest in the critical viewing and discussion of films screen. Teachers and pupils should learn to operate a film projector.
- Use a pointer to direct attention, to specific details on the screen.

MICROSCOPE (FIG. 5.35)

Science teachers want students to make accurate observations and to draw correct conclusions from what they see. Sometimes, live insects and specimens in microscopic slides may have to be viewed by small group pupils.

A microscope can normally be employed for this purpose. While adopting this technique, the teacher can draw the attention of the pupils of any salient feature in the image. But the teacher is not sure whether an individual observes what he says because only one student can observe through a microscope at a time. In such situations, microprojection can be resorted to using simple dissecting microscopes or compound microscopes.

Microprojection is a technique by which the actual microscopic slides or tiny objects can be enlarged and the image of which can be projected on a screen so that a small group can view it. When dissecting microscope, it is used, live objects like mosquito larvae, tadpoles, etc., can be kept on a watch glass. When a compound microscope is used, a few drops of water may be placed on a microscope slide and microorganism, such as paramecium could be projected.

TAPE RECORDER (FIG. 5.36)

A tape recorder is used to record sounds on magnetic tape which can be reproduced

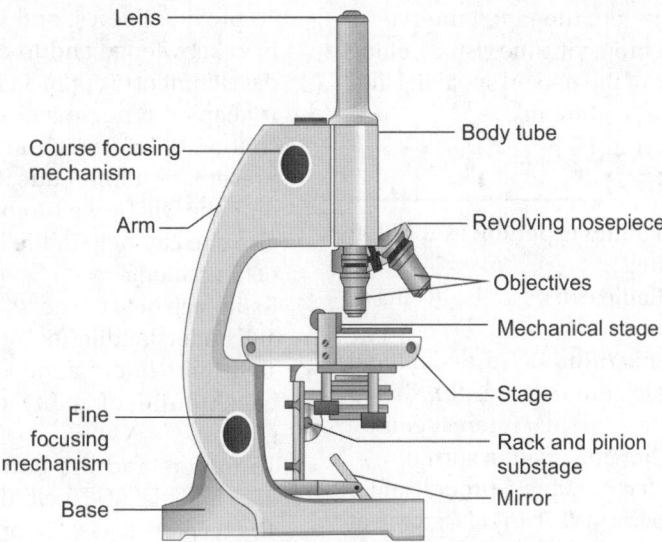

Fig. 5.35: Microscope.

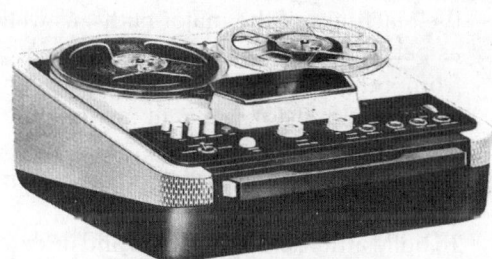

Fig. 5.36: Tape recorder.

at will as many times as required. Tape recordings are not easily damaged and can be replayed many more times. If any scratches or damages, repair can be made on the spot.

- It enables one to listen and hear recording previously made.
- Provides for the pupil to hear their own voice and event which occur in their own school.
- Language learning is facilitated by the use of tapes.
- The class can tape their own singing or discussion programs and listen into them in order to improve them later on.

Educational Uses of Tape Recorder

- It can be used to record educational broadcasts and for replay at suitable and convenient times.

- Tape recorder can be used to record music and other sound effects for use during staging of dramas in schools and cultural performances.
- It can be used to record the talk of important visitor to the institution and this can be effectively used later.
- Tape recorders are very largely used in language laboratories for giving speech training and for correction of pronunciation defects.
- It can be used for appreciation of and for teaching music.
- It will provide the necessary feedback for discussions to improve the lesson.

Functions of Tape Recorder

The tape recorder has two functions in the operation of an AV program: to rehearse a presentation; and to record "live" interviews. A tape recorder is an excellent device to use for rehearsing a talk, especially when using overhead transparencies, slides or a 35 mm. filmstrip. By replaying a tape, the planner becomes aware of how he sounds and can decide where he'll want greater or less emphasis. The planner may want to take a tape recorder out in the field and tape "live" interviews to learn people's opinions about a current issue. Later on, the taped interviews can be used when projecting the visuals, along with photographs of the person speaking and of the subject of his comments.

RADIO (FIG. 5.37)

Characteristics of audio experiences through radio and recordings:

- **Immediacy:** Radio can describe events as they happen.
- **Emotional impact:** Through the combined effect of voice, environmental sound and music, the student's interest can be captured and her imagination stirred.
- **Authenticity:** It is possible, (through audio media) for experts to visit any classroom at any time. Students' knowledge of a subject can be enriched by listening to an expert. Discuss the topic understudy on the radio. In this way, radio can bring the outside world into the classroom.
- **Conquest of time and space:** Through simulated programs, audio-media actually can overcome the barriers of time and space.
- **One-way communication:** No possibility of students' feedback.
- **Audition:** Cannot be auditioned, to determine their educational value.

Uses

- To develop increased skills in listening participation and evaluating what is heard.
- To set the stage for student discussions by presenting opinions of outside experts from remote sources.
- To provide interest and varied sources of new knowledge and to contribute to the development of appreciation and attitudes.
- It keeps the nurse well-informed on all sources of information relating to health preservation and education, so that not only she will be well-informed herself but also she can help in the health education of her patients.
- Radio, can help the nurse with background and understanding for listening attentively.
- To acquire information about the cultural background of many different ethnic groups.
- To understand the patient better, their likes and dislikes, their idiosyncrasies.
- The religion, social factor which the nurse must take into consideration in her work, through radio, the student can learn about the teachings of the major faiths, as well as personally receive inspirational values from religious programmed. She can be able to assist patients in meeting the religious needs.
- To call attention to social problems, which frequently involve health.
- To build attitude, appreciation and understandings of the great medical and nursing personalities, their struggle in bettering man's health and lengthening his lifespan.
- They acquaint the student with the social effects of scientific discoveries.
- To keep well-informed in literature, history and current events, to develop a complete well-rounded personality increased understanding, and appreciation of them.

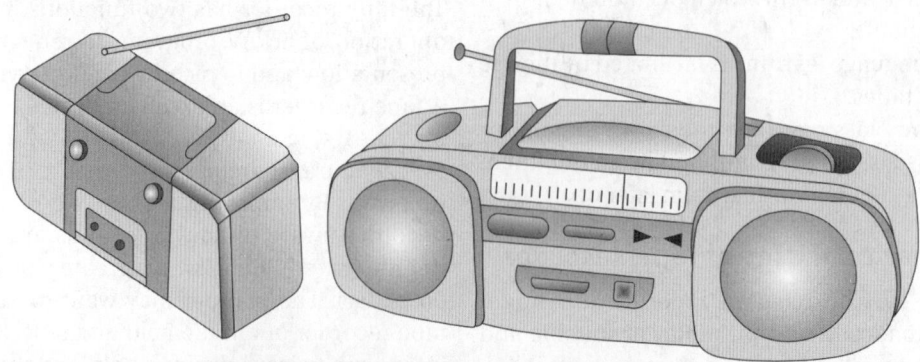

Fig. 5.37: Types of radios used as AV aids.

- Bringing the school into virtual contact with the world around timely. Presenting and interpreting events, while they are either happening and thus keeping students well-informed about what is taking place all over the world.
- It is one of the mass-media that can be used to inform the public of the objectives and the needs of nursing, nursing education.
- Public shall be informed, permitted and encouraged to participate in maintaining and raising health standards.
- Enrichment of the school program.
- Developing critical thinking, leisure time interest and appreciation.
- Broadcasts are effective means of presenting music, drama, and discussions for study and appreciation.
- These are actually team-teaching demonstrations.

MOTION PICTURES

Communicating through sound and sight simultaneously, the motion pictures blends pictures, words, objects, motion and even color to make impact on the children's minds. The viewer sees motion that can be recreated. The time factor can be controlled in any series of events, objects can be enlarged or reduced; processes hitherto a mystery may now be visualized. By the use of straight photography and special effects, motion pictures may transport the viewer into another world. Thus, this medium can bring to the student a realistic portrayed of the trials.

Education Value of Motion Picture

- It enriches the learning process and leads to greater all round achievement.
- It directly modifies beliefs in desirable directions and causes students seek additional information about subject studied.
- It helps in the improvement of educational achievement by different subjects.
- It compels attention.
- It makes the experience almost first hand.
- It is an edited version of reality.
- Motion picture can control the time factor in any operation or series of events.
- Motion picture can make distant past and the present relieve in the classroom.
- Motion picture can provide an easily reproduced record of an event or an operation.
- It offers common denominator of experience.
- It can influence and even change attitudes.
- Motion picture can be based on assist the pupils in their understanding of abstractions, in encouraging thinking and thus leading them to further reflect on human relationships.
- Motion picture brings variety to instructional materials.
- Motion picture offers a satisfying experience.

Uses of Motion Picture

- Films can teach factual materials effectively over a wide range of subject matter, ages, abilities, and conditions of use.
- Films can be effective in teaching perceptual-motor skills.
- Films can be made more effective as learning tools through the use of various teaching techniques.
- Films can modify motivations, interests, attitudes and opinions if they are designed

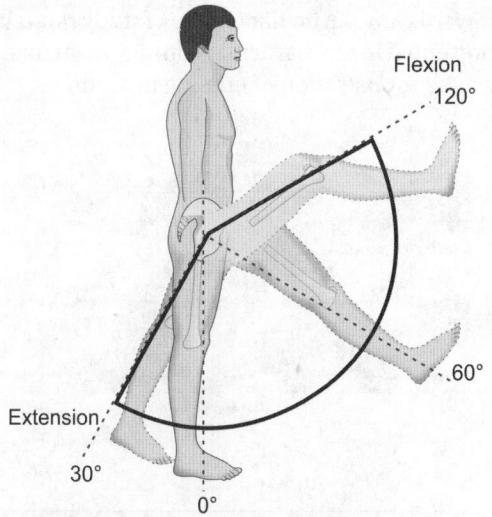

Fig. 5.38: Motion pictures.

to stimulate or reinforce existing beliefs of the audience.

- Films are greatly influenced in their effectiveness by audience-learner characteristics.

Purposes for which Films may be used

- To provide a background of sensory experience.
- To provide concrete experiences which serve as a basis for thinking, reasoning and problem-solving?
- To provide an easily accessible fund of knowledge which stimulates interest and motivates the students to further study and learning activities.
- To present a large amount of information in a short period of time.
- To increase the amount of initial learning and permanency of learning.
- To develop attitudes, appreciation and better social relationships.
- To promote unitary learning.
- To review.
- To introduce a unit by presenting a whole range of problems to students to attack.
- To demonstrate a process.
- To emphasize and bring out the underlying principles of nursing procedures.
- To supplement laboratory instructions.

EDUCATIONAL TELEVISION

Television is the electronic means by which sound and light energy are transmitted from one place to another. Technically, it is an electromechanical system of converting the energy contained in sound and light patterns into electrical and electromagnetic energy when it is then reconverted back into sound and light.

Television is the electronic blackboard of the future, which is, brought to life. It offers vitality and newness, which attracts attention, creates interest and stimulates a desire to learn. Television is a multidimensional and general medium of communication. It is an instrument of encoding, transforming,

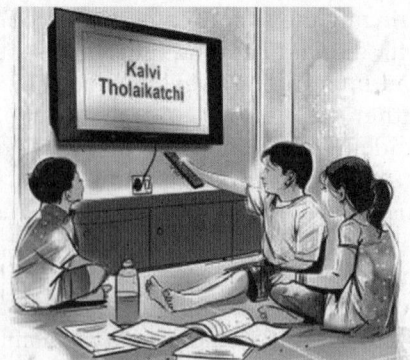

Fig. 5.39: Educational televisions.

transmitting or projecting or re-transforming and then presenting the encoded patterns of meaningful information. These processes are performed so that the information input has correspondence with the information output.

Two kinds of licensed television stations: (1) Commercial, (2) Educational.

Educational television: a) Instructional television. b) Enrichment television.

Instructional television: Broadcasts designed to aid instruction i.e., it is planned in relation to educational objectives and is presented in an orderly and sequential arrangement of learning experiences.

Enrichment television: Designed towards enriching learning, but is not directed towards any particular course of study nor is it presented in any particular learning sequence, e.g., demonstration of nursing procedures.

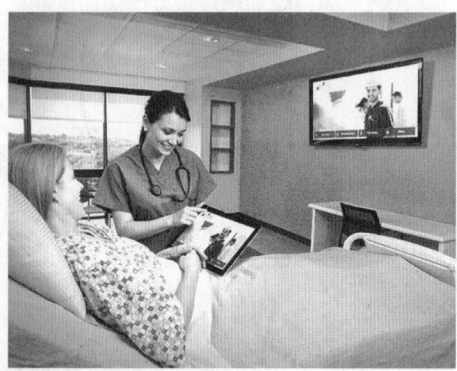

Fig. 5.40: Televisions used in health education.

Role of Teacher in the Stages of Television Programs

There are five main stages and it is essential that teacher should be associated with each stage. The stages are the following:

1. **Planning and preparation of television program:** A thorough knowledge of the educational objectives, suitability of materials, the sequence and contents are very important and it can be achieved by the teacher. A teacher can contribute effectively in this area if he/she has good grounding and is skillful with the mechanics of a good television lesson.

2. **Teacher in the production of television program:** Production is a technical thing but the knowledge about the mechanics of production must be known to the teacher if he/she is to appreciate a good lesson by identifying its strong and weak points and suggest improvement.

3. **Teacher in the presentation of television program:** It is executed by the teacher who should be initiative, imaginative and is competent in subject. The presentation involves only a selected number of teachers but the scope of selection involves all the teachers of a subject. A good selection can be possible only from a television trained group.

4. **Utilization of television program and teacher:** Utilization is the area where the teacher is the master of the situation. It may be emphasized that no television lesson is complete without introduction and follow-up exercises in the classroom. The teachers have to inspire the student, prepare lesson and arouse their curiosity before the telecast of the lesson and subsequently has to clarify their doubts, thus providing the missing links and reinforcement in the follow-up.

5. **Teacher in the evaluation of television program:** Evaluation is another important aspect which is possible only with the involvement of the teacher. This can be performed by providing the exercise sheets to the students and get it completed. The feedback helps to recognize the attainment of educational objectives and can help in improving programs.

VIDEO CASSETTES (FIG. 5.41)

The potential of video cassettes exists for providing basis for learning a wide range 01 motor, intellectual, cognitive and interpersonal skills and affective skills as well. These are significant aspects which printed materials cannot deal with adequately. The facility could be particularly useful where distance education programs are involved with updating skills and techniques of workers in the field.

Advantages

Besides the advantages of educational television, there are added advantages.

- The control of equipment and the learning process is placed in the hands of the learner through control over the mechanics of the machine.
- The capacity to order the sequence of events controls the rate of learning and facilitates practice sequences.

Disadvantages

- Equipment costs cannot always be kept down by using lower quality equipment.
- Video production for educational purposes calls for new techniques different from the entertainment modes. Producers, script writers and directors should be knowledgeable about teaching and learning.

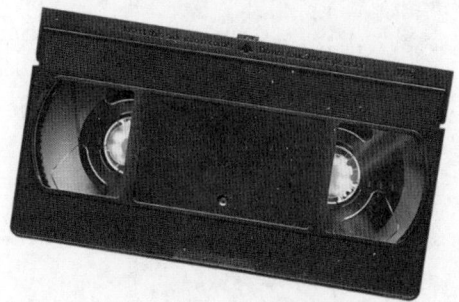

Fig. 5.41: Video cassettes.

PAMPHLETS

A pamphlet is an unbound booklet without a hard cover or binding. It may consist of a single sheet of paper that is printed on both sides and folded in half, in thirds, or in fourths, or it may consist of a few pages that are folded in half and stapled at the crease to make a simple book.

Definition

Pamphlet is a small booklet or leaflet containing information or arguments about a single subject.

Criteria for Pamphlet

- The words written should be clear, concise, understandable and short.
- The sentence formed should not be too clumsy and crowded.
- The background color and the colors used for printing the letters should be contrast.

- The letter style should be attractive and bright.
- The size of the paper should be less than 20–30 cm in length, 10–20 cm in breath.
- Both the sides can be used to print the letters.
- The sentence used should be elicited in the form of points.
- The letter size of the heading should be slightly bigger than the points that are included.

Styles for Organizing a Pamphlet

- **The tutorial style:** The first and most basic style that can be chosen is the tutorial style for pamphlets. This style basically involves easing into the topic of pamphlets so that a reader reading it can gradually understand the content. Initially, the readers should be explained with the basic concepts by providing the key definitions of the hardest words that they

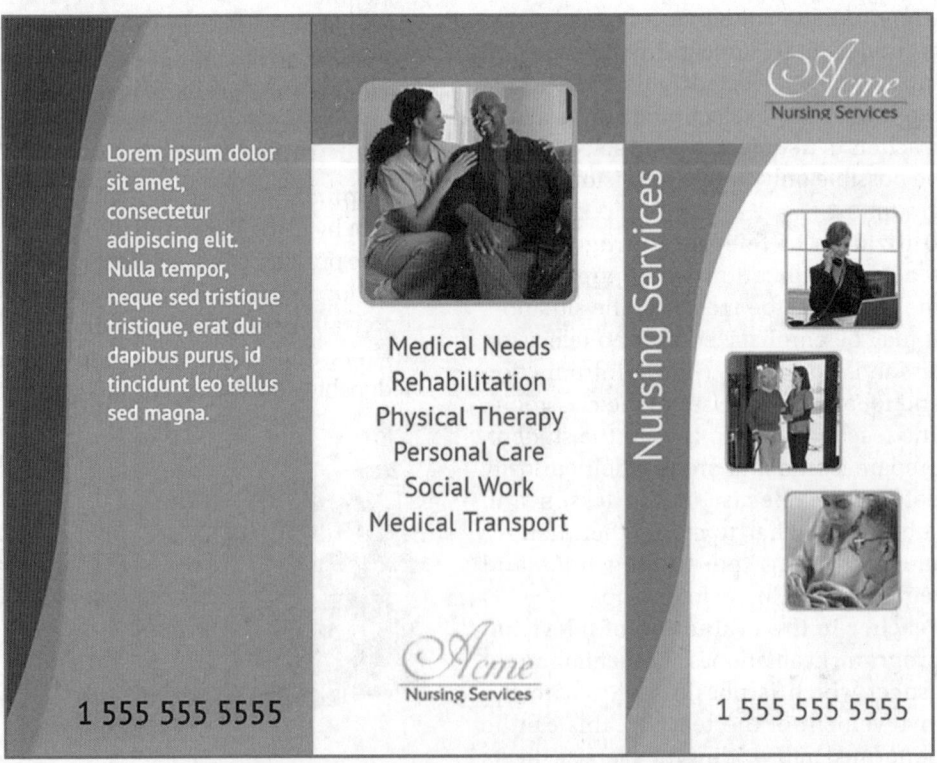

Fig. 5.42: Sample pamphlet.

have to tackle in the pamphlet. Then, delve further into pamphlet topic by adding in the relationships of these concepts and its overall meaning. It can be done using different sections explaining every step of the way until hopefully.

- **Using the frequently asked question style:** Another style the pamphlets can be prepared is frequently asked questions format. This format involves listing down the frequently asked questions about pamphlet topic. Typically, these are the information that most of the readers are curious about. Each question is listed as different sections and answers are provided to it afterwards. This is a very effective technique since usually readers want an answer to their question fast. In this format, they can just center on to the area of the pamphlet with their question and read the information that they want.
- **The testimonial style:** This style is basically like a story telling mode for pamphlets. A story is narrated about pamphlet issue and concepts are introduced one by one historically. This makes the learning process easier for most learners as they see how all the concepts are united together. Therefore, it can be a very effective method especially if a human element is included into pamphlet message.

LEAFLETS

Definition: Leaflet is a printed sheet of paper containing information or advertising and usually distributed free.

Concepts of Leaflet

- Leaflet is a small book usually having a paper cover. A leaflet is commonly referred to as any piece of printed information.
- Leaflets include fact sheets, guides, small booklets, brochures, and distributed without charge. A printed sheet that is printed, folded, and mailed as part of a direct mail campaign or handed to customers.
- Leaflet is used for propaganda message printed on substantial material is a relatively permanent document.
- Once printed and delivered, it can be retained and readily passed from person to person without distortion.

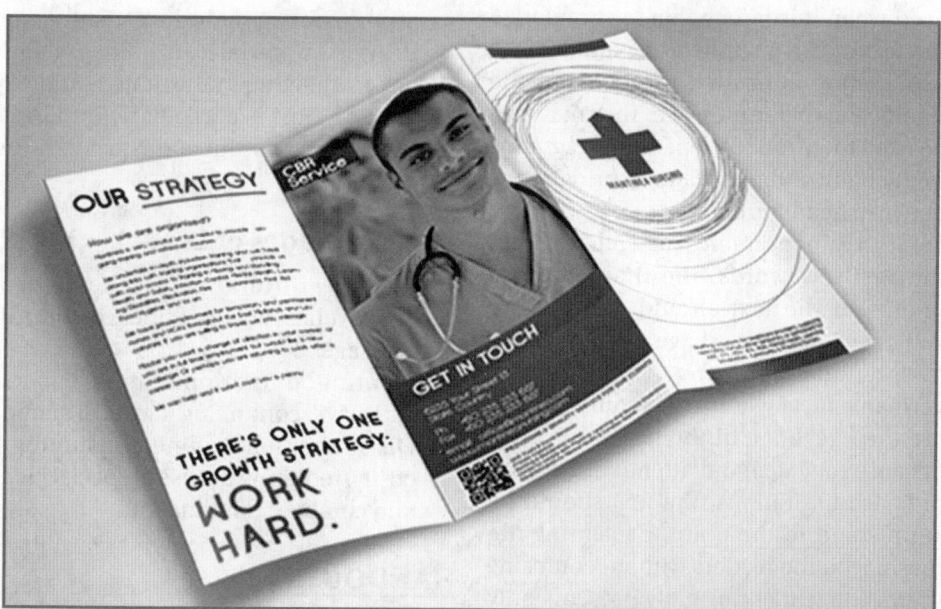

Fig. 5.43: Leaflet.

Categories of Leaflets

- Leaflets may be categorized as persuasive, informative, and directive. The persuasive leaflet attains its objective through use of reason.
- Facts are presented so that the reader is convinced that the conclusions reached by the propagandist are valid.
- The informative leaflet is factual. In presenting facts previously unknown to the reader, it attracts a reading public by satisfying curiosity.
- The directive leaflet directs action when intelligence indicates the target is receptive. It is used to direct and control activities of underground forces.

Guide to Organize the Content of a Leaflet

- **Heading:** The leaflet heading is normally the most important part of the leaflet because it is the part that first catches the eye. In composing the heading, the propaganda writer must be brief, summarizing the theme by using short, forceful words.
- **Subheading:** Leaflet subheadings are used when it is impossible to summarize the text in the main heading and further explanation is needed to point out the significance of the message. They may also be used to introduce separate paragraphs in the body of the text and to bridge gaps between headline and text.
- **Text:** To gain the interest of readers within the first few words, the first sentence or two of the text should contain the substance of the message, with the facts and details following. Credible and verifiable facts whether favorable or not, are the backbone of the leaflet message because they demand attention. Because of space limitations, the text should be simple and to the point, presenting the message to the readers without confusing them. The leaflet normally presents only one theme. A leaflet which presents two or more unrelated or vaguely related themes confuses the readers and detracts from the relative persuasive strength of each theme. If more than one theme is used, they should be closely related.
- **Pictures:** When pictures, preferably photographs, are used, the picture and the text must complement each other—convey the same idea to the readers, each expanding the ideas of the other.

Advantages of Leaflet

- The printed word has a high degree of acceptance, credibility, and prestige.
- Printed matter is unique in that it can be passed from person to person without distortion.
- It allows for the reinforcing use of photographs and graphic illustrations which can be understood by illiterates.
- It is permanent and the message will not change unless it is physically altered.
- It can be disseminated and read or viewed by a larger, widespread target audience. It can be reread for reinforcement.
- Complex and lengthy material can be explained in detail. It can be hidden and read in private.
- Messages can be printed on almost any surface, including useful items. Printed material can gain prestige by acknowledging authoritative and expert authors. This is particularly important in those societies where the printed word is authoritative.

Disadvantages of Leaflet

- A high illiteracy rate reduces the effectiveness and usefulness of the printed message.
- Printing operations require special, extensive, continuing logistical support.
- Dissemination is time-consuming and costly, requiring the use of special facilities and complex coordination.

HANDOUTS

Handouts are printed materials that are distributed to students before the presentation. It is used principally to reduce the amount of time students spend copying notes or diagrams from a board or screen.

Uses in a Variety of Ways

- Directly related to the lesson content
- **As an information sheet:** Presenting complex, rare or hard to find information
- As a reading list
- As a worksheet/quiz sheet /proforma/ workbook
- As a permanent source of reference
  Whatever type of handout is used, it should be well structured, well designed and checked rigorously for errors. It is good practice to get a colleague to check it too. It is good practice to make handouts interactive by providing space for annotation, and to inform students that they will find it useful to annotate the information as the session progresses. The layout and content of a handout is very much a matter for the individual teacher to decide.

Guidelines for Preparing Handout

A well-designed handout will:
- Be typed; use at least 12 point font
- Use headings and page numbering consistently

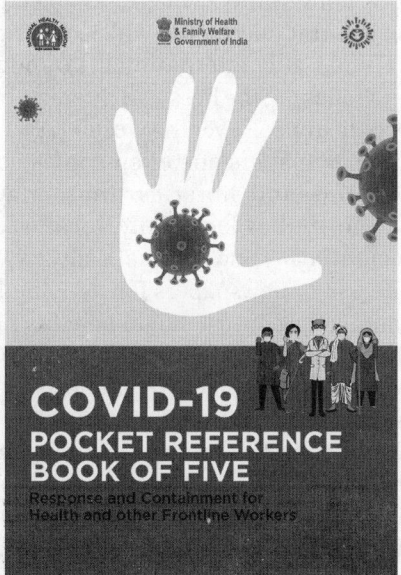

Fig. 5.44: Handouts.

- Use bullet points rather than continuous prose
- Make good use of space
- Keep lines left justified with a ragged right edge
- Avoid excessive use of capital letters and underlining
- Leave plenty of space between columns of text
- Avoid starting a sentence at the end of a line
- Avoid using glossy paper

Preparation of Handouts

Handouts should never be repetitious of the material provided in the textbook or given in live lectures. To be used effectively, handouts should be carefully planned. Necessary information should be typed neatly and concisely.

Instructions for the Preparation of Handouts

- Decide on the type of the handout. The type and purpose can be different for different lectures in order to create variety.
- Record only those items which are directly relevant to the subject of the lesson and for the desired objectives.
- Recognize the key-words and catch-words and emphasize them in the handout by underlying them.
- Use simple and clear language. Make short sentences.
- Draw sketches and graphs labeled or unlabeled. Remember 'one sketch may be worth a thousand words'.
- Draw graphs. Write point-wise, wherever possible.
- Give titles and subtitles suitably.
- Use visual symbol and easy-to-recognize nomenclature
- Use colors appropriately, if possible. Alternatively ask the students to color the black and white handouts
- Underline some words and place some key-equations and statements in boxes to emphasize them.
- If possible, prepare enlarged transparencies to match the handouts. The teacher

can project the transparencies to aid filling in the blanks, labeling the parts, etc. This is a very effective method.

Giving out Handouts

Teacher should explain the purpose of the handout and how it should be used. Handouts may be given out to the learners at one of the following points of time:

- Much in advance of the presentation.
- Just before the start of the session.
- During the progress of the session, as necessary.
- Just after the completion of the session.

Giving out handouts much in advance is only like textbooks. It is advantageous to do so if books are not available or if prior reading/working is necessary before attending the class. Handouts given out at the commencement of a lesson draw attention of the class to the objectives and the contents of the lesson. This is generally satisfactory.

Handouts provided at appropriate timings; either just before a discussion, sometimes just after a series of points have been raised or just after viewing a video and at more than one point of time, maintain high level of attention, motivation and interaction.

Giving out handouts just after the completion of a lesson leaves a record for the lesson which the student may or may not read depending upon the follow-up by the teacher. Handouts given out much too late for the requirements have no academic purpose. It is a mere formality and may well be avoided.

NEWSPAPERS

The newspaper furnishes many examples which can be used to introduce lessons. Health messages can be published in local languages which can reach to the public easily. The information will be available in low cost, easy to read and understand simple language. The people may learn to read and interpret the contents along with pictures (use adequate and sufficient suitable pictures) to enhance easy grasping.

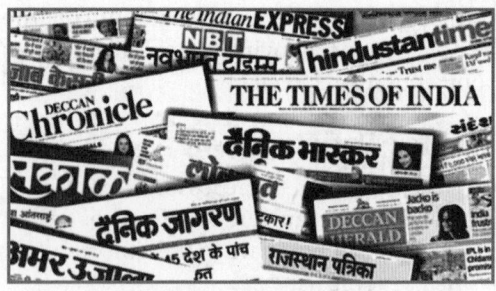

Fig. 5.45: Newspapers.

- Newspapers carry a big mass appeal for educating and influencing the opinion of the masses.
- Being a source of latest information and treasure of knowledge on the local and global issues related to each and every aspect of the social life, a newspaper can potentially become an effective aid in the process of teaching-learning.
- In its simple meaning, newspapers are known as the papers or written documents containing the news of varying general and specific interests concerning people and places.
- Their scope and area of circulation may be too limited as happens in the case of local newspapers related to the lives and interests of the people belonging to a community, village, town, city or region or it may be too wide covering the national and international boundaries and touching the lives and interests of the people from all over the world.
- The newspapers one often comes across at home and libraries, thus, may be categorized as local daily, local weekly, regional daily and national daily, etc.
- The use of newspapers for deriving educational and instructional benefits needs their reading as well as comprehension of the inherent information and ideas. It is, thus, a visual device requiring the pre-skills of reading and comprehension on the part of its users. However, pre-readers may also be exposed to and learn from the use of newspapers as an instructional aide.

Educational Advantages

Educational advantages drawn through the use of newspapers as instructional aids may be summarized as follows:

- Newspapers can be a valuable source for generating necessary interest in reading. They may also help in developing specific reading interests related to specific subjects and issues among the children from the very beginning.
- As an instructional aid, newspapers may help in the proper development of essential language and communication skills, such as reading, writing, listening, speaking, comprehending, summarizing, reporting, editing, commenting, critically evaluating, criticizing, etc.
- Newspapers are, in fact, a storehouse of current information and treasure of knowledge related to personal as well as social and local and global issues. Hence, they may prove a source of vast information and knowledge for the students of varying age and grades in all the areas of the school curriculum.
- Newspapers as an inexpensive instructional aid may also help in reinforcing and developing higher order cognition abilities and skills, such as thinking skills, reasoning and problems solving ability, analyzing, synthesizing and evaluating and application skills, etc.
- Creative abilities and expressions may also be well nurtured and developed through the help of newspapers as an instructional aide.
- Newspapers may be the source of endless learning experience adaptable to any subject of the school curriculum. Therefore, they may become a big helping hand for gaining

MAGAZINES (FIG. 5.46)

Magazines offer advertisers extensive choices of readership and frequency. Consumer magazines cover a wide range of interests, including sport, hobbies, fashion, health,

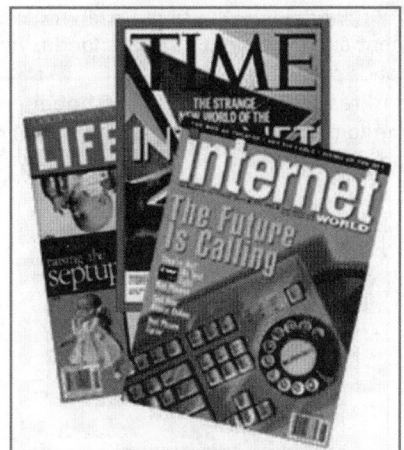

Fig. 5.46: Magazines.

current affairs and local topics. Many business and trade magazines provide coverage of specific industries, such as finance or electronics.

Others cover cross-industry topics, such as communications or human resources, while still others focus on job-specific areas, such as publications for executives, marketing professionals or engineers. Publishing frequency is typically weekly, monthly or quarterly. As with newspapers, advertisers can take advertising spaces from classified ads to full page ads in black and white or color.

BIBLIOGRAPHY

1. Barrow R. Giving teaching back to teacher—A critical introduction to curriculum theory Brighton. Wheat sheaf books, 1984.
2. Bhatia K, Bhatia BD. The Principles and Methods of Teaching: Delhi. Doaba House, 1977.
3. Bloom BS. Taxonomy of Educational Objectives, Handbook I: The Cognitive Domain. New York: David McKay Co. Inc, 1956.
4. Bloom BS. Taxonomy of Educational Objectives-The Classification of Educational Goals. New York: Susan Fauer Company, 1956.
5. Chauhan SS. Principles and Techniques of guidance. 2nd revised edition, New Delhi: Vikas Publishing House Private Limited, 2001.
6. Gaberson BK, Oermann HM. Clinical teaching strategies in nursing. 2nd edn, New York: Springer Publishing Company, 2006.

7. George KA. Principles of curriculum development and evaluation, Tirunchengodu: Vivekananda press, 2002.

8. Harkreader H, Hogan AM, Thobaben M. Fundamentals of nursing caring and clinical judgment. 3rd edn, Saunders Elsevier, 2007.

9. Hartley LC, Ellis RJ. Nursing in today's world, 5th edn, Philadelphia: JB Lippincott Company, 1995.

10. Heidgerkein EL. Teaching and learning in schools of nursing, 3rd edn. Lippincott Company, Philadelphia, 1987.

2

SECTION

Nursing Research

TERMINOLOGY

Research: Research is a systematic inquiry of discovers facts or test theories in order to obtain valid answers to questions raised or solutions for problems identified.

Sample: Sample is a selection of individuals from the total population of a particular class of intervals.

Scientific method: Scientific method is a systematic method employed in study or research in which a problem is identified, a hypothesis is made and data are gathered, systematically arranged and interpreted in order to test the hypothesis empirically.

Data: Facts of phenomena, in research, the term commonly refers to the facts observed or obtained in some systematic way.

Empirical: Name given to a method of testing or verifying a hypothesis by means of observation or experience. In empirical research, the observations are systematically controlled.

Assumptions: Beliefs that are held to be true but have not necessarily been proven; assumptions may be explicated or implicit.

Assent: Agreement to participate in research by someone, especially a child older than 7 years, who is not capable cognitively of giving informed consent.

Attrition: Study participant withdraws from a study.

Beneficence: Research participants should be protected from harm.

Abstract: Brief summaries of research studies; generally contain the purpose, methods and major findings of the study. A short (less than 200 words long), one-page summary of a research.

Anonymity: The identity of research subjects is unknown, even to the study investigator.

Case study: An in-depth study involving only one subject; occasionally used in qualitatively nursing research. Research studies that involve an in-depth examination of a single person or a group of people. A case study might also examine an institution.

Conceptual: It provides the reader with clear description of the meaning of the variable. It is similar to a dictionary definition.

Bivariate study: A research study in which the relationship between two variables is examined.

Blind review: Manuscript reviewers are not made aware of the author's identity before the manuscript is evaluated.

Bracketing: A process in which qualitative researchers put aside their own feelings or beliefs about a phenomenon that is being studied to keep from biasing their observations.

Clinical nursing research: Nursing research studies involving clients or that have the potential for affecting clients.

Clinical trial: Research studies conducted to evaluate new treatment, new drugs, and new or improved medical equipment.

Cohort study: A special type of longitudinal study in which subjects are studied who have been born during particular period or who have similar backgrounds.

Comparative studies: Studies in which intact groups are compared on some dependent variable. The researcher is not to manipulate the independent variable, which is frequently some inherent characteristic of the subjects, such as age or educational level.

Complex hypothesis: A hypothesis that concerns relationship where two or more independent variables, two or more dependent variables or both are being examined.

Clinical nurse researcher (CNR): An advanced practice nurse who is doctorally prepared and directs and participates in clinical research.

Clinical nurse specialist (CNS): An advanced practice nurse who provides direct care to clients and participates in health education and research.

Clinical practice guideline (CPG): An evidence-based guide to clinical practice developed by experts in a particular field for direct application in clinical environments.

Control group: Subjects in an experiment who do not receive the experimental treatment and whose performance provides a baseline against which the effects of the treatment can be measured. When a true experimental design is not used, this group is usually called a comparison group.

Data collection: The process of acquiring existing information or developing new information.

Empirical: Having a foundation based on data gathered through the senses (e.g., observation or experience) rather than purely through theorizing or logic.

Ethnography: A qualitative research method for the purpose of investigating cultures that involves data collection, description, and analysis of data to develop a theory of cultural behavior.

Evidence-based practice: The process of systematically finding, appraising, and using research findings as the basis for clinical practice.

Experimental design: A design that includes randomization, a control group, and manipulation between or among variables to examine probability and causality among selected variables for the purpose of predicting and controlling phenomena.

Generalizability: The inference that findings can be generalized from the sample to the entire population.

Basic research: Research that seeks to advance scientific knowledge by establishing new knowledge or facts and developing fundamental theories or principles. The findings of basic research may not be immediately applicable in the solution of problems but may lead to further research. Research that is conducted to generate knowledge rather than to solve immediate problems.

Experimental research: Future-oriented research that tests a hypothesis or hypothesis by setting up a controlled situation and then manipulating it to determine the effect of the manipulation. The design for experimental research consists of control groups and experimental groups that are tested before and after the manipulation of the experimental group or groups.

Descriptive research: Present-oriented research that seeks to accurately describe what is and to analyze the facts obtained in relation to the problem understudy. It may lead to theories or hypothesis to be tested experimentally.

Exploratory study: A preliminary study designed to help refine the problem, develop or refine hypothesis or test and refine the data collecting methods.

Historical research: Past-oriented research that seeks facts that will help one to interpret and understand past events and their influences. The methods used are systematic documentation of the evidence and evaluation of its authenticity.

Qualitative research method: Organization and interpretation of observations that provide a more holistic view of the subjects experiences without limiting questions or responses.

Sampling: Sampling is the process of selecting a portion of the population to represent the entire population.

Population: Everybody (or thing) of a defined type, which could possibly be surveyed. Often the number of adults in a defined geographical area or market. It is also known as universe.

Sample: It is a part of population- everybody (or everything) from who (or which) data was gathered.

Sample size: The number of questionnaires completed in a survey. Usually equals the number of people interviewed. Often shown in computer printouts as **N**.

Sampling unit: that is that element considered for selection in some stage of sampling (same as the elements, in a simple stage sampling), in a multistage sample, the sampling unit could be blocks, household and individuals within household.

Sampling design: The formal plan specifying a sampling method, a sample size and procedures of recruiting subjects.

Probability: Chance, expressed as a percentage or decimal, e.g., a 50-50 chance is a probability of 50%, or 0.50. **Odds** of 3 to 1 correspond to a probability of 25%.

Target population: The target population is the entire group a researcher is interested in; the group about which the researcher wishes to draw conclusions.

Independent sampling: Independent samples are those samples selected from the same population, or different populations, which have no effect on one another. That is, no correlation exists between the samples.

Random sampling: Random sampling is a sampling technique where we select a group of subjects (a sample) for study from a larger group (a population). Each individual is chosen entirely by chance and each member of the population has a known, but possibly non-equal, chance of being included in the sample.

Simple random sampling: Simple random sampling is the basic sampling technique where we select a group of subjects (a sample) for study from a larger group (a population). Each individual is chosen entirely by chance and each member of the population has an equal chance of being included in the sample. Every possible sample of a given size has the same chance of selection; i.e. each member of the population is equally likely to be chosen at any stage in the sampling process.

Stratified sampling: There may often be factors which divide up the population into sub-populations (groups / strata) and we may expect the measurement of interest to vary among the different sub-populations. This has to be accounted for when we select a sample from the population in order that we obtain a sample that is representative of the population. This is achieved by stratified sampling.

Cluster sampling: Cluster sampling is a sampling technique where the entire population is divided into groups, or clusters and a random sample of these clusters are selected. All observations in the selected clusters are included in the sample.

Convenience sample: Using a sample of people who happen to be handy or easy to survey. May be OK in preliminary research, but not guaranteed to be representative of the population.

Quota sampling: Quota sampling is a method of sampling widely used in opinion polling and market research. Interviewers are each given a quota of subjects of specified type to attempt to recruit, for example, an interviewer might be told to go out and select 20 adult men and 20 adult women, 10 teenage girls, and 10 teenage boys so that they could interview them about their television viewing.

Spatial sampling: This is an area of survey sampling concerned with sampling in two (or more) dimensions. For example, sampling of fields or other planar areas.

Sampling variability: Sampling variability refers to the different values which a given function of the data takes when it is computed for two or more samples drawn from the same population.

Standard error: Standard error is the standard deviation of the values of a given function of the data (parameter), over all possible samples of the same size.

Sampling error—because the survey used one sample of respondents rather than another. As long as the sample was chosen at random, the amount of sampling error is predictable, e.g., "there's a 95% chance that the average height of all people is within 3cm of the average of our sample".

Data: A set of values recorded on one or more observational units. Facts or phenomenon, in research, the term commonly refers to the facts observed or obtained in some systematic way (the singular of data is datum). Collected and recorded information which are either in numerical form or otherwise. As such they do not give any meaning.

Data analysis: It is a process of transforming raw data into usable information, often presented in the form of a published analytical article in order to add value to the statistical output.

Data encoding: It is activity aimed at detecting and correcting errors (logical inconsistencies) in data.

Data element: A data element is a unit of data for which the definition, identification, representation, and permissible values are specified by mean of a set of attributes.

Data format: Usually refers to a specific, possibly, proprietary, set of data structures within a software system.

Data item: A data item is an occurrence of a data element.

Data presentation: Description of the way how the data are presented.

Data set: any organized collection of data.

Data structure: Implementation of a data model consisting of file structures used to represent various features.

Data type: Data type is a set of distinct values, characteristized by properties of those values and by operations on those values.

Data validation: Data validation is an activity aimed at verifying, whether the value of a data item comes from the given set of acceptable values.

Database: A logical collection of information that is interrelated and managed and stored as a unit, for example, in the same compute file. The terms database and data set are often used interchangeably.

Electronic data processing: Pertains to data processing equipment that is predeterminantly electronic, such as electronic digital computer.

Attributes: qualitative observations of elementary units are attributes.

Qualitative data: Non-numberic features or experimental units.

Quantitative data: Data with numerical properties.

Observation: An event and its measurements, such as BP (events) and 120 mmhg (measurement).

Variable: variables are any characteristics that can take on different values, such as height, age, temperature, or test scores.

Dependent variable: The variable under observation by the investigator, who wishes to note the effect on it of the introduction of an independent variable. Sometimes called the criterion variable.

Delphi technique: A special kind of survey using a panel of experts obtained a consensus on a special topic. Opinions are solicited by mail rather than by the usual group discussion method. It has the advantage of fostering expression of independent opinion.

Critical incident technique: A method of obtaining data from study subjects written reports of previous experiences or incidents in their lives that are related to the matter under study.

Correlation survey: A survey used to collect data from a group on two or more variables to estimate the relationship between the variables.

Convenience sample: Choosing the most easily and readily accessible people (or places) to be subjected (or units) in a study.

Contingency table: A table that visually displays the relationship between sets of nominal data.

Contingency questions: Questions that is relevant for some respondents and not for others.

Content analysis: A data collection method that examines communication messages that is usually in written form.

Constant comparison: Data gathered in qualitative study are constantly or continually compared to data that have already been gathered.

Computer-assisted database: A compilation of information that can be retained by computer.

Attitude scale: Self-report data collection instrument that ask respondents to report their attitudes or feelings on a continuum.

Cells: Boxes in a table that are formed by the intersection of rows and columns.

Class-interval: A group of scores in a frequency distribution.

Analysis: The process of organizing and synthesizing data so to answer research questions and test hypothesis.

Basic attribute: Basic attribute is an attribute of a metadata item commonly needed in its specification.

Confidential data: These are data, which are subjected to confidentiality clauses.

Continuous variable: It is a potential data which occur in an infinite number of possible values in any interval.

Data: Collected and recorded information which are either in numerical form or otherwise. As such they do not give any meaning.

Discrete variable: The measurements that occur as integers. It can have only a finite number of values in any given interval.

Health information system: It is a tool for management and monitoring of health activities. It describes mechanisms and procedures for acquiring and analyzing specified information.

Health policy: A set of decision and statements defining priorities and directions to attain the goal.

Information: By reducing, consolidating, summarizing and adjusting the data, we get information which is data transformed to a format.

Qualitative data: When variables take quality into consolidation, we get qualitative data.

Quantitative data: When variables take quantity into consideration we get quantitative data.

Reliability: Inherent performance of a procedure is measured by reliability.

Sensitivity: It is a measure of correct diagnosis in terms of true positiveness.

Specificity: It is a measure of correct diagnosis in terms of true negatives.

Validity: A measurement is valid if it measures what it is supposed to measure.

Vital registration: The formal recording of events of human life like, birth, death, marriage, divorce.

Cross table: Two dimensional tables in which two variables are cross classified.

ICD: It is a system of disease classification, where systematic grouping of illness are done according to selected common characteristics. International classification of diseases helps in statistical study and is acceptable in international comparative studies.

Master table: Initial recording is transformed to a big master table which contains every detail of observation designed in the study. All units and all characteristics are taken into account in master table.

Tabulation: It is a process of data grouping into intervals or groups to which the range of the variable are divided and put.

Bar diagram: Diagrammatic presentation of frequency data for nominal classes by bars. Length of bars is proportional to the class frequencies.

Class interval: It is an interval to which a range of variable has been divided, e.g., "10.0 to 10.9" is a class interval.

Cumulative frequency curve: The frequency obtained by cumulating the frequencies of previous classes including the class in question. It shows the total observations up to the end of a particular class in the curve.

Frequency polygon: It is the frequency distribution of a quantitative data presented in the form of a diagram. Here class frequencies are plotted against class midpoints, later these points are joined by straight line.

Histogram: It is a diagrammatic representation of the frequency distribution of a quantitative data with areas of rectangles proportional to the class frequency.

Ogive: It is the graph obtained by the cumulative relative frequency distribution, which may be more than or less than ogive.

Pie chart: A circle is used where sectors of the circle are shown proportional to class frequencies. Very commonly used in data presentation of nominal classes.

Percentile: The position of a character or variable when they are arranged in ascending or descending order in an array of one hundred. For example, 50th percentile refers to median value or middle value when orderly arrangement is done.

Quartile: It is the value in 25th position of a cumulative class frequency.

Scatter diagram: It is a graphic presentation to show the correlation between two variables.

Semi-log line: If log values are taken and plotted at log scale axis and in another axis corresponding response is plotted we get arithmetic log line. This is just to make the line straight to the given extent. For example, log dose response line in pharmacology is an example of semi-log line.

6

CHAPTER

Introduction to Nursing Research

INTRODUCTION

The word research derives from the French recherché, from researcher, to search closely where chercher means to search. The word means "to go about seeking",. Research is a systematic process of utilising the scientific method for generating new knowledge that can be used to solve problem or improve the existing status of a system. Research uses the scientific method to discover facts and their interrelationships and then allows to the application of this new knowledge in practical settings.

DEFINITIONS OF RESEARCH

- Research is defined as the search for knowledge or any systematic investigation to establish facts. **—Chrish Jordan**

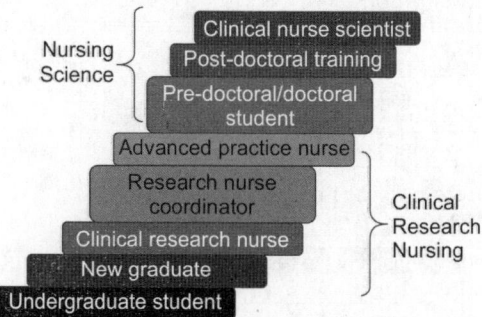

Fig. 6.1: Levels of research activities in nursing.

- Research means search for facts or ideas and to answer the questions in order to find a solution to the problem. **—Horton**
- Research is a systematic, formal, rigorous and precise process employed to gain solutions to problems and/or to discover and interpret new facts and relationships.
  —Waltz
- Research is a process of looking for specific answers to specific questions in an organized objectives reliable way.
  —Payton
- Research is a systematic, controlled, empirical and critical investigation of hypothetical propositions about the presumed relations among natural phenomena.
  —Kerlinger
- Research essentially is a problem solving process, a systematic, intensive study directed towards full scientific knowledge of subject studies. **—Ruth M French**
- Research may be defined as the systematic and objective analysis and recording of controlled observations that may lead to the development of generalizations, principles, theories relating to perdition and possible ultimate control of events.
  —JW Best
- Research is a process of systematic obtaining accurate answers to significant and pertinent questions by the use of

the scientific method of gathering and gathering and interpreting information.
—**Clover and Balsley**

- Research is a process of systematically search for new events and relationships.
—**Notter**

DEFINITIONS OF NURSING RESEARCH

- **American Nurses Association:** Nursing research develops knowledge about health and promotion of health over the full life span, care of persons with health problems and disabilities and nursing actions to enhance the ability of individuals to respond effectively to actual or potential health problems.

- **International nurses (Benolie) 1984:** Nursing research supports the need for nursing research as a means of improving health and welfare of the people. Nursing research is a way to identify new knowledge, improve professional educational practice and use of resources effectively.

- **According to Polit and Hungler:** Research is a process in which the researcher scientifically collects data to be used in the clinical administrative or instructional area in order to find solutions to nursing problems, evaluating nursing practices, procedures, policies or curriculum, assess the needs of the patients, staffs or

students and or make decisions to change or continuous various nursing process which in turn advances the scientifically knowledge in nursing field.

- **According to French-Ruth M (1968):** Research essentially in a problem solving process, a systematic, intensive study directed towards full, scientific knowledge of the subject studied.

- **According to Walls and Bauzell (1981):** Nursing research is a systematic formal, rigorous process used to give solution to problems or to discover and interact with new facts in clinical practice, nursing education and nursing administration.

MEANING OF RESEARCH

- The word research means 'to search again' or 'to examine carefully'. More specifically, research is diligent, systemic inquiry or study to validate and refine existing inquiry or study to validate and refine existing knowledge and develop new knowledge. Diligent, systematic study indicates planning, organization and persistence. The ultimate goal of research is the development of a body of knowledge for a discipline or profession such as nursing.

- Research essential to develop and refine knowledge that can be used to improve clinical practice. Nursing practice need to be able to read research reports to identify

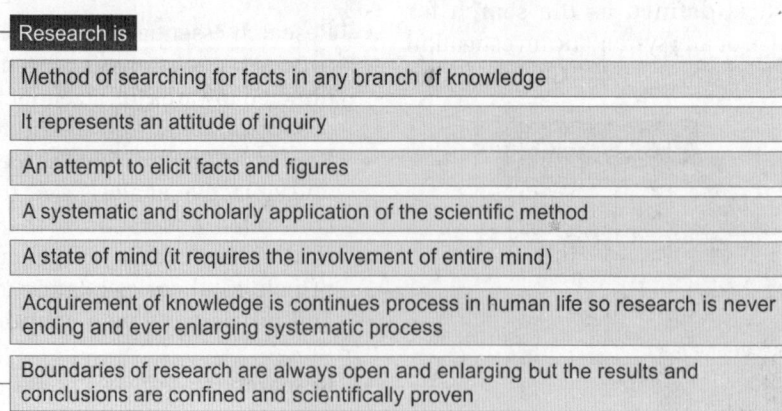

Fig. 6.2: Concept of research.

effective interventions for practice and to implement these interventions to promote positive outcomes for patients and families.

- Nursing search is also need to generate knowledge about nursing education, nursing administration, health care services, characteristics of nurses and nursing roles. The finding from the studies indirectly influences nursing practice and thus adds to nursing body of knowledge.

PURPOSE OF RESEARCH

- It unravels the mysteries of life.
- It aims to analyze interrelations between variables and to derive causal explanations.
- It aids planning and helps in national development.
- It aims at finding solutions to problems.
- It helps in the development of general laws.
- It aims at developing new tools, concepts and theories for better study of unknown phenomena.
- It extends knowledge of human being regarding social life and environment.

- It verifies existing facts and theory and these in turn help in improving our knowledge and ability to handle situations and events.

OBJECTIVES OF RESEARCH

The main of research is to find out the truth which is hidden and which has not been discovered as yet.

- To gain familiarity with a phenomenon or to achieves new insights into it. It is known as exploratory or formulation research study.
- To portray accurately the characteristics of a particular individuals, situations or a group. Such studies are known as descriptive research.
- To determine the frequency with which something occur or with which is associated with something else. Such studies are known as diagnostic research.
- To test a hypothesis of a causal relationship between variables. Studies with this object are known as hypothesis testing research.

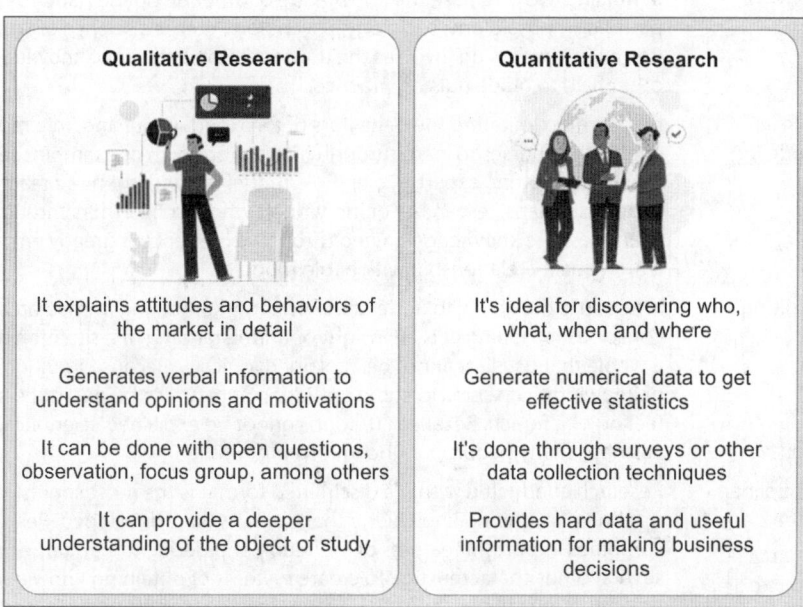

Fig. 6.3: Differences between qualitative and quantitative research.

SOURCES OF KNOWLEDGE IN RESEARCH

Sl. No.	Sources	Descriptions
1.	Tradition	Tradition offers advantages as a source of knowledge. It is efficient in the sense that each individual is not required to begin a new in an attempt to understand the world or certain aspects of it. Tradition or custom also facilitates communication by providing a common foundation of accepted truth.
2.	Authority	People with specialized knowledge are in every field, we are constantly faced with making decisions about matters with which we have had no direct experience, therefore, it seems natural to place trust in the judgment of people who are authoritative on an issues by virtue of specialized training or experience.
3.	Experience of trial and error	Our own experiences represent a familiar and functional source of knowledge. The ability to generalize, to recognize, regularize and to make predictions based on observation in an important characteristics of the human mind. Trial and error may offer a practical means of searching knowledge, but it is fallible and efficient. This method is haphazard and unsystematic and the knowledge obtained is often unrecorded and hence, inaccessible to subsequent problem solvers.
4.	Logical reasoning	Logical reasoning as a method of knowing combines experiences, our intellectual facilities and formal systems of thought. Inductive reasoning is the process of developing generalization from specific behaviour. Inductive reasoning is the process of developing generalizations from specific observations. Deductive reasoning is a process of developing specific predictions from general principles. Both system of reasoning are useful as a means of understanding and organizing phenomena, both play a role in nursing research.
5.	Borrowing	In nursing, we often use the knowledge of other disciplines (such as medicine, pathology, physiology, sociology, psychology etc) as a science of knowledge. Borrowing in nursing involves the appropriation and use of knowledge from other field to guide nursing practice.
6.	Role modeling	It is learning imitating the behaviors of an expert. In nursing, role modeling enables the nurses to learn through interactions with or examples set by highly competent, expert nurses. Role model includes admired teachers, expert clinicians, researcher or individuals who inspire others through their examples. The knowledge gained through experience is greatly enhanced by a high quality relationship with a role model.
7.	Intuition	Intuition is the ability to understand or know something immediately without conscious reasoning. It is an insight or understanding of a situation or event as a whole that usually cannot be explained logically. Because intuition is a type of knowing that seems to come unbidden, it may also be described as a gut feeling or a hunch. Because intuition cannot be explained scientifically with easiness, many people are uncomfortable with it.
8.	Disciplined research	Research conducted within a disciplined format is the most sophisticated method of acquiring knowledge that humans have developed. Research combines important features of induction and deduction. Together with several other characteristics, to create systems of obtaining knowledge that although fallible, tends to be more reliable than tradition, authority, experience or inductive or deductive reasoning alone.

SCOPE OF RESEARCH

According to Hudson Maxim, all progress is born inquiry. Doubt if often better than overconfidence as it leads to inquiry and inquiry leads to interventions.

- It promotes scientific and legal thinking.
- Operational: It is involved in solving operational problems, e.g., industries, factories, etc.
- It is also used as an aim to economic policy and has gained its importance in government and business.
- It helps in planning budget for the nation.
- It facilitates the decisions of polymaker.
- It is concerned necessary with the allocation of nation resources.
- It studies the economic and social structure of nation and gives a detailed account of the change taking place in society.
- It helps in predicting future development.
- It studies the motivation underlying the consumer behavior.
- It helps the social scientist in studying social relationship and seeking answers for various social problems.
- It helps in the attainment of high position in social structure.
- It helps in development of new ideas and insight for analysis for generation of new theories.
- It helps to identify new facts as an advancement of a profession.

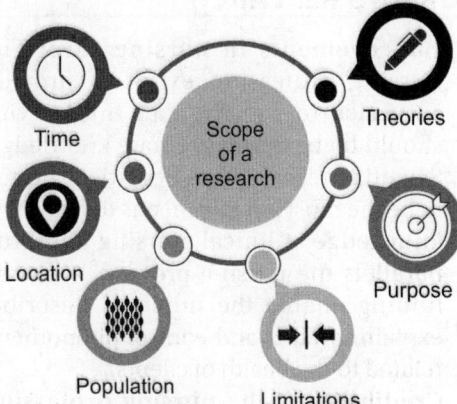

Fig. 6.4: Scope of research.

- It is a measure of means of attaining live hood for professionals.

SCOPE OF NURSING RESEARCH

- To improve the standard of nursing care.
- To redefine the existing theories and discovering new theories.
- To discover new measures for nursing practice.
- To foster a commitment to client.
- To provide basis for professional accountability.
- To impart professionalism in nursing.
- To help in decision-making.
- To improve standards in nursing education.
- To help in documentation.
- To bridge the gap between knowledge and practice.
- To build the body of knowledge in nursing profession.
- To validate improvement in nursing profession.
- To make health care efficient and cost effective.
- To act as a basis for standard setting and quality assurance.
- To find solution on immediate practical problems of nursing.
- To discover new facts about a known phenomenon.
- To discover new message for nursing practice.
- To identify the role of the nurse in changing society.

CHARACTERISTICS OF NURSING RESEARCH

According to Charles, research is a careful inquiry or examination in seeking facts or principles, a diligent investigation to ascertain something. It can also express as follows:

- R-Rational way of thinking
- E-Expect and exhaustive treatment
- S-Search for solution
- E-Exactness
- A-Analytical analysis of adequate data

- R-Relationship of facts
- C-Careful recording and critical observation
- H-Honesty and hard work
1. Research strives to be objective and logical.
2. Research emphasizes the development of generalization, principles or theories.
3. Research demands accurate observation and description.
4. Research is characterized by patience and unhurried activity.
5. Research is directed to solution of problem.
6. Research is carefully and scientifically recorded and reported.
7. Research requires expertise.
8. Research sometimes requires courage.
9. Research emphasizes the development of generalization, principles or theories.

IMPORTANCE OF NURSING RESEARCH

Nursing profession is accountable to society for providing high-quality care patients and families. The health care provided by nurses must be constantly evaluated and improved based on new information. Nursling's scientific knowledge base is expanding rapidly with the generation of new findings by nurses and other health professional using a variety of research methods. The knowledge generated through research is essential to provide a scientific basis for description, explanation prediction and control of nursing practice.

- **Descriptive descried** involves identifying the nature and attributes of nursing phenomena and sometimes the relation-

Importance of Nursing Research

- To adopt an evidence-based nursing practice (EBP)
- To improve competent nursing practice
- To increase body of knowledge
- To develop new ideas and approaches
- To improve personal and professional development
- To improve patient outcomes

Fig. 6.5: Importance of nursing research.

ship among these phenomena (Chinn and Kramer 1995). These studies are often called descriptive or explanatory. This descriptive research is essential ground work for studies that will focus on explanation, prediction and control of nursing phenomena.

- **Explanation:** Relationship among variables is clarified and the reasons why certain events occur are identified. Explanation determining relationships among variables provides a basis for conducting studies for the purpose of predicting and controlling patient outcomes.
- **Prediction:** Through prediction, one can estimate the probability of a specific outcome in a given situation (Chinn and Kramer 1995). Health promotion research is being conducted to predict the effects of healthy behaviors, such as exercising regularly, eating a balanced diet and not smoking on health status and longevity.
- **Control:** It can be described as the ability to write a prescription to produce the desired results. Control involves imposing condition on the research situation so that biases and confounding factors are minimized. Based on the research of Meek (1993), nurses could prescribe slow stroke back massage to promote comfort and relaxation in hospice patients.

OBJECTIVES OF CONDUCTING NURSING RESEARCH

- **Improvements in nursing care:** The nursing profession exists to provide a service to society, and this service should be based on accurate knowledge. Scientific research has been determined to be the most reliable means of obtaining knowledge. Clinical nursing research parallels the nursing process. Research finding enable the nurse to describe, explain, predict and control phenomena related to the health of clients.
- **Credibility of the nursing profession nursing** has traditionally borrowed

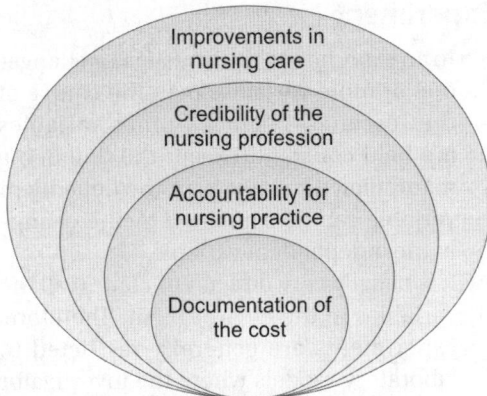

Fig. 6.6: Objectives of conducting nursing research.

knowledge that is distinct from the natural and social sciences, and only in recent years have nurses concentrated on establishing a unique body of knowledge that would allow nursing to be clearly identified as a distinct a unique body of knowledge that would allow nursing to be clearly identified as a distinct profession. The most valid means of developing this knowledge base is scientific research.

- **Accountability for nursing practice:** As nurses have become more independent in making decisions about the care of clients, their independence has brought about a greater need for accountability. Nurses must have sound rationales for their actions, based on knowledge that is gained through scientific research. Nurses have the responsibility of keeping their knowledge base current, and one of the best sources of current knowledge is the scientific literature.
- **Documentation of the cost-effectiveness of nursing care:** Nursing services can consume a large percentage of a hospital's budget. With prospective payment systems determining the amount of reimbursements that hospitals receive, nursing care services are being closely examined. There are many studied in the literature that demonstrates the cost- effectiveness of nursing care. Ventura *et al.* (1985)

conducted a study to examine the cost saving of nursing interventions with patients with peripheral vascular disease.

METHODS OF RESEARCH

There are three basic methods of research: (1) Survey, (2) Observation, and (3) Experiment. Each method has its advantages and disadvantages.

Survey

- Survey is the most common method of gathering information in the social sciences. It can be a face-to-face interview, telephone, mail, e-mail, or web survey.
- A personal interview is one of the best methods obtaining personal, detailed, or in-depth information.
- It usually involves a lengthy questionnaire that the interviewer fills out while asking questions. It allows for extensive probing by the interviewer and gives respondents the ability to elaborate their answers.
- Telephone interviews are similar to face-to-face interviews. They are more efficient in terms of time and cost, however, they are limited in the amount of in-depth probing that can be accomplished, and the amount of time that can be allocated to the interview.
- A mail survey is more cost-effective than interview methods. The researcher can

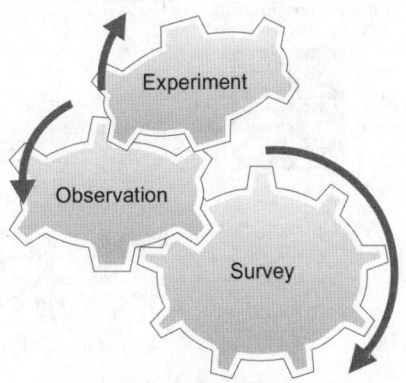

Fig. 6.7: Methods of research.

obtain opinions, but trying to meaningfully probe opinions is very difficult. Email and web surveys are the most cost-effective and fastest methods.

Observation

- The observation research monitors respondents' actions without directly interacting with them.
- It has been used for many years by A.C. Nielsen to monitor television viewing habits.
- Psychologists often use one-way mirrors to study behavior. Anthropologists and social scientists often study societal and group behaviors by simply observing them.
- The fastest growing form of observation research has been made possible by the bar code scanners at cash registers, where purchasing habits of consumers can now be automatically monitored and summarized.

Experiment

- In an experiment, the investigator changes one or more variables over the course of the research. When all other variables are held constant (except the one being manipulated), changes in the dependent variable can be explained by the change in the independent variable.
- It is usually very difficult to control all the variables in the environment. Therefore, experiments are generally restricted to laboratory models where the investigator has more control over all the variables.

TYPES OF RESEARCH

There are many types of research studies and there are also a number of ways in which they can be classified. A more widely applied way of classifying research studies is to define the various types of research according to the kinds of information that they provide.

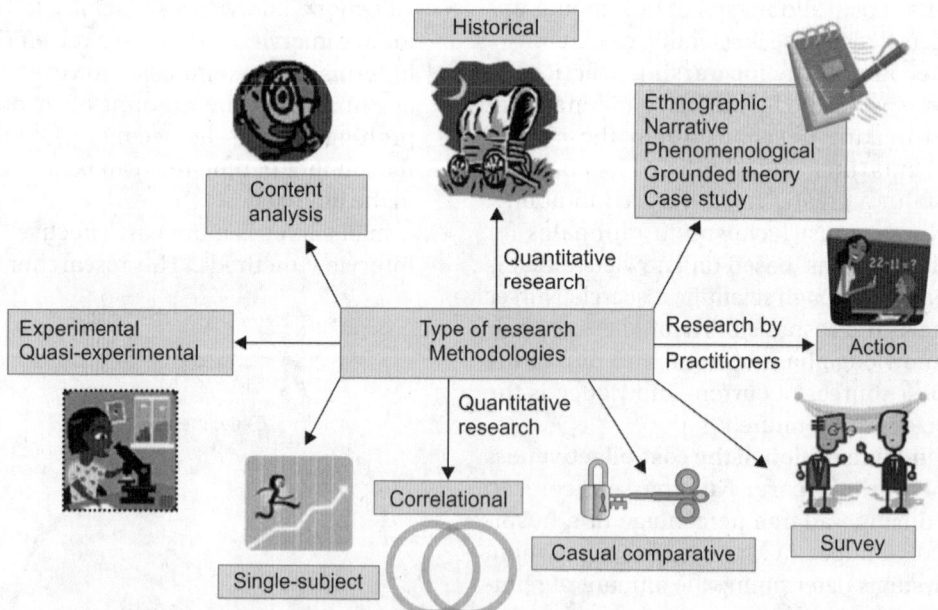

Fig. 6.8: Types of research.

Sl. No.	Types	Descriptions
1.	**Pure research**	• Also called as the fundamental or the theoretical research. • Is basic and original. • Can lead to the discovery of a new theory. • Can result in the development or refinement of a theory that already exists. • Helps in getting knowledge without thinking formally of implementing it in practice based on the honesty, love and integrity of the researcher for discovering the truth
2.	**Applied research**	• Based on the concept of the pure research. • Is problem-oriented? • Helps in finding results or solutions for real life problems. • Provides evidence of usefulness to society. • Helps in testing empirical content of a theory. • Utilizes and helps in developing the techniques that can be used for basic research. • Helps in testing the validity of a theory but under some conditions. • Provides data that can lead to the acceleration of the process of generalization.
3.	**Exploratory research**	• Involves exploring a general aspect. • Includes studying of a problem, about which nothing or a very little is known. • Follows a very formal approach of research. • Helps in exploring new ideas. • Helps in gathering information to study a specific problem very minutely. • Helps in knowing the feasibility in attempting a study.
4.	**Descriptive research**	• Simplest form of research. • More specific in nature and working than exploratory research. • It involves a mutual effort. • Helps in identifying various features of a problem. • Restricted to the problems that are describable and not arguable and the problems in which valid standards can be developed for standards. • Existing theories can be easily put under test by empirical observations. • Underlines factors that may lead to experimental research. • It consumes a lot of time. • It is not directed by hypothesis.
5.	**Diagnostic study**	• Quite similar to the descriptive research. • Identifies the causes of the problems and then solutions for this problems. • Related to causal relations. • It is directed by hypothesis. • Can be done only where knowledge is advanced.
6.	**Evaluation study**	• Form of applied research. • Studies the development project. • Gives access to social or economical programmes. • Studies the quality and also the quantity of an activity.
7.	**Action research**	• Type of evaluation study. • Is a concurrent evaluation study.

RESEARCH AS PROBLEM SOLVING PROCESS

Research is considered to be the more formal, systematic and intensive process of carrying on a scientific method of analysis, for purpose of discovery and development of an organized body of knowledge.

Definition: Problem solving "may be a formal application of problem identification, hypothesis formulating, observation, analysis and conclusion".

Problem solving approach is meaningful, development, sequential, based on discovery of generalizations.

Research essentially is problem solving process, a systematic, intensive study directed towards full, scientific knowledge of the subject studied". **—French Ruth M (1968).**

Major Approaches in Problem Solving

- Inductive approach
- Deductive approach
- Analytic approach
- Synthetic approach

Steps in Problem Solving Process

- Discovering, considering, discussing, selecting and stating the specific problem or question.
- Specify the relevance of background facts and theories.
- Collecting, organizing, comparing and judging significant information in the light of the defined problem.
- Exploring the problem and framing some possible solution. (Data collection)
- Analyzing and interpreting and synthesis of collection of facts.
- Observation and evaluate of outcomes of action.
- Considering the summarization with the possibilities of further study.

According to John Dewey, seven steps of scientific method of problem solving.

- **Recognizing the problem:** Selecting and stating the specific problem.
- **Defining the problem:** To state exactly what is problem (i.e.) identifying the problem in definite terms.
- **Collecting relevant information data:** From all possible sources that have bearing on the problem. Appropriate tools are gathered, books and magazines collected.
- **Formulation of hypothesis or possible solutions:** One tries to think of the various possibilities for the solution of one's own problem in the light of the information and his own experiences.
- **Evaluation of the hypothesis for possible solutions:** We put into practice the course of action. We have chosen as the most appropriate and verify its rightness by the results or conclusion.
- **Verification:** Validate of the derived conclusion is tested by employing them in solution of various similar problem.
- **Choosing another action if unsuccessful:** If another action is necessary you will have to return to your test of possible solution and choose gain.

A Four-step process: Billstein, Libes kind and Lott have adopted these problem solving steps in their book "A Problem Solving Approach to Mathematics for Elementary School Teachers. They are based on the problem solving steps first outlined by George Polya in 1945.

- **Understanding the problem**
  - Can you state the problem in your own words?
  - What are you trying to find or do?
  - What are the unknowns?
  - What information do you obtain from the problem?

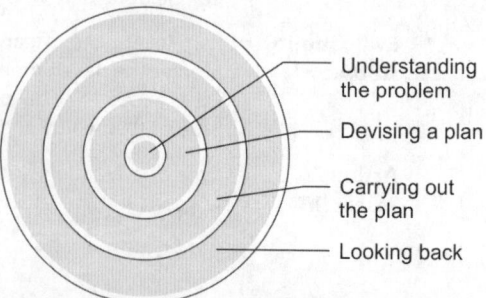

Understanding the problem

Devising a plan

Carrying out the plan

Looking back

Fig. 6.9: Steps of problem solving.

- What information, if any, is missing or not needed?
- **Devising a plan:** The following list of strategies, although not exhaustive, is very useful.
  - Look for a pattern.
  - Examine related problems, and determine if the same technique can be applied.
  - Examine a simpler or special case of the problem to gain insight into the solution of the original problem.
  - Make a table
  - Make a diagram
  - Write an equation
  - Use guess and check
  - Work backward
  - Identify a sub goal
- **Carrying out the plan:**
  - Implement the strategy or strategies in step 2, and perform any necessary actions or computations.
  - Check each step of the plan as you proceed. This may be intuitive checking or a formal proof of each step.
  - Keep an accurate record of your work.
- **Looking back:**
  - Check the results in the original problem. (In some cases this will require a proof.)
  - Interpret the solution in terms of the original problem. Does your answer make sense? Is it reasonable?
  - Determine whether there is another method of finding the solution.
  - If possible, determine other related or more general problems for which the techniques will work.

Research: Research process consists of series of actions or steps necessary to effectively carry out research and the desired sequencing of these steps.

- Define research problem
- Review of literature—review concepts and theories and review previous research finding.
- Formulating hypothesis
- Select appropriate research methodology (Research design, variables, sampling and sampling technique).

Box 6.1: Role of nurse in research activities.

These activities include the following:

- Participating in a journal club in a practice setting, which involves regular meetings among nurses to discuss and critique research articles.
- Attending research presentations at professional conferences.
- Discussing the implications and relevance of research findings with clients.
- Giving clients information and advice about participation in studies.
- Assisting in the collection of research information (e.g., distributing questionnaires to patients).
- Reviewing a proposed research plan with respect to its feasibility in a clinical setting and offering clinical expertise to improve the plan.
- Collaborating in the development of an idea for a clinical research project.
- Participating on an institutional committee that reviews the ethical aspects of proposed research before it is undertaken.
- Evaluating completed research for its possible use in practice, and using it when appropriate.

- Collect data
- Analyze the data
- Interpret the data
- Conclusion and report

ROLE OF NURSE IN RESEARCH

- **Principal investigator:** Nurses can and should serve as principal investigators in scientific investigations. To be a principal investigator, special research preparation is necessary.
- **Members of a research team:** Nurses may act as data collectors or administer the experimental intervention of the study. As nurses increasingly participate in research, it is possible that interest and enthusiasm to conduct their own investigations may grow.
- **Evaluator of research findings:** All nurses should be involved in the evaluation of research findings. As research consumers, nurses have the obligation to become familiar with research findings and

determine the usefulness of these findings in the practice area. The evaluation of research is not an easy task.

- **User of research findings:** After evaluating research findings, nurses should use relevant finding in their practice. The primary goal of nursing research, as has been mentioned, is the improved care of clients. However, nurses must be judicious in their use of research findings.
- **Client advocate during studies:** Nurses have the responsibility to act as client advocates when clients are involved in research. Nurses can help answer questions and explain a study to potential participants before the study begins. They also can be available during the study to answer questions or provide support to study participants.
- **Subject in studies:** Nurses also can act as subjects in research. Many nurses are involved in a long-term survey study that is being conducted by researcher at Harvard Medical School, with funds provided by the National Institute of Health.

LIMITATIONS OF RESEARCH

- Problems of collection of data and conceptualization may occur.
- Repetition problems.
- Outdated and insufficient information system may cause problems.
- Sometimes lack of resources becomes an obstacle.
- Non-availability of trained researchers.
- Absence of code of conduct.

CONCLUSION

Nursing research is essential of nurses are to understand the varied dimensions of their profession. Research enables nurses to describe the characteristics of a particular nursing situation about which little is known; to explain phenomena that must be considered in planning nursing care; to predict the probable outcomes of certain nursing decisions; to control the occurrence of undesired outcomes; and to initiate activities to promote desired client behavior.

BIBLIOGRAPHY

1. Donaldson, S. K. (2000). Breakthroughs in scientific research: The discipline of nursing, 1960–1999. Annual Review of Nursing Research, 18, 247–311.
2. French, P. (1999). The development of evidence-based nursing. Journal of Advanced Nursing, 29, 72–78.
3. Lindeman, C. A. (1975). Delphi survey of priorities in clinical nursing research. Nursing Research, 24, 434–441.
4. Millenson, M. L. (1997). Demanding medical evidence. Chicago: University of Chicago Press.
5. Nightingale, F. (1859). Notes on nursing: What it is, and what it is not. Philadelphia: J. B. Lippincott.

7

Research Process

LEARNING OBJECTIVES
- Definition, purpose and objectives of research process
- Steps in research process
- Quantitative research process steps
- Qualitative research process steps

TERMINOLOGY

Plan: General plan of how research questions will be answered, this includes the approach and design.

Research approach: This is the theoretical or conceptual basis for the research. For example, positivist, interpretive, realist, etc.

Research design: How data collection is organized in order to answer the research question. Basic design types are:
- Situation, 'snap-shot' or baseline (sometimes called casestudy)
- Cross-sectional comparison
- Longitudinal
- Longitudinal comparison
- Experiment.

Research strategy: It refers to a methodological practice or tradition, for example, experiment, survey research, or case studies.

Data collection techniques: How data are collected, questionnaire, interview, observation and documentary analysis.

INTRODUCTION

Nursing research is a process in which the researcher scientifically collects data to be used in the clinical administrative or instructional area in order to find solutions to nursing problems, evaluating nursing practices, procedures, policies or curriculum, assess the need of the patients, staffs or students and or make decisions to change or continuous various nursing process which, in turn, advances the scientifically knowledge in nursing field. A research study begins as a problem that a researcher would like to solve or as a question that a researcher would like to answer. Often the question or problem evolves from a broad topic area and researcher usually it is necessary to devote sometime to delimiting and explicating the problem. Nursing process is used to determine health needs and plan nursing care of clients. It is used as a basis for gaining and using information about clients to help them, restore, maintain, or promote health.

Definition

- The process of gathering information for the purpose of initiating, modifying or terminating a particular investment or group of investments.
- The research process is a process of multiple scientific steps in conducting the research work. Each step is interlinked with other steps. The process starts with the research problem at first. Then it advances in the next steps sequentially. Generally, a researcher conducts research work within seven steps.

- Research process includes following steps; identify the problem, review the literature, clarify the problem, clearly define terms and concepts, define the population, develop the instrumentation plan, collect data, and analyze the data.

MEANING OF RESEARCH PROCESS

Scientific research involves a systematic process that focuses on being objective and gathering a multitude of information for analysis so that the researcher can come to a conclusion. This process is used in all research and evaluation projects, regardless of the research method (scientific method of inquiry, evaluation research, or action research). The process focuses on testing hunches or ideas in a park and recreation setting through a systematic process. In this process, the study is documented in such a way that another individual can conduct the same study again. This is referred to as replicating the study. Any research done without documenting the study so that others can review the process and results is not an investigation using the scientific research process. The scientific research process is a multiple-step process where the steps are interlinked with the other steps in the process. If changes are made in one step of the process, the researcher must review all the other steps to ensure that the changes are reflected throughout the process. Parks and recreation professionals are often involved in conducting research or evaluation projects within the agency.

Purpose and Objectives of Research Process

Understanding the research process is an important step towards executing a thorough research or study. Let us examine the different phases in research planning as well as the stages involved in a research process. A deeper understanding of the process of research will help you identify the similar features that occur in the different fields and the variety in the purpose and approaches to some studies.

Understanding the research process will help you understand the implication of deviating from a systematic approach to research, as well as the associating consequences of ineffective and ineffectual research.

Research can be seen as a series of linked activities moving from a beginning to an end. Research usually begins with the identification of a problem followed by formulation of research questions or objectives. Proceeding from this the researcher determines how best to answer these questions and so decides what information to collect, how it will be collected, and how it will be analyzed in order to answer the research question.

STEPS IN RESEARCH PROCESS (FIG. 7.1)

Research process consists of phases or steps that can be compared and contrasted with those of the nursing process.
- **Identify the problem:** The first step and one of the most important steps in the research process is to clearly identify the problem that will be studied. This step of research process may be most difficult of all and may take a great deal of time. Study problem can be identified from personal experiences, literature sources, previous research or through the testing of theories.
- **Determine the purpose of the study:** There must be a sound rational or justification for every research project. Some studies viewed as inconsequential and wasteful of time and money. The research must take explicit the expectations for the use of the study results. If the purpose of a study is clearly presented and justified, the research will be much more likely to receive approval for the study and also will be more likely to obtain subjects for the study.
- **Review the literature:** Research should build on previous knowledge. Before beginning a study, it is important to determine what knowledge exists of the study topic. A thorough literature

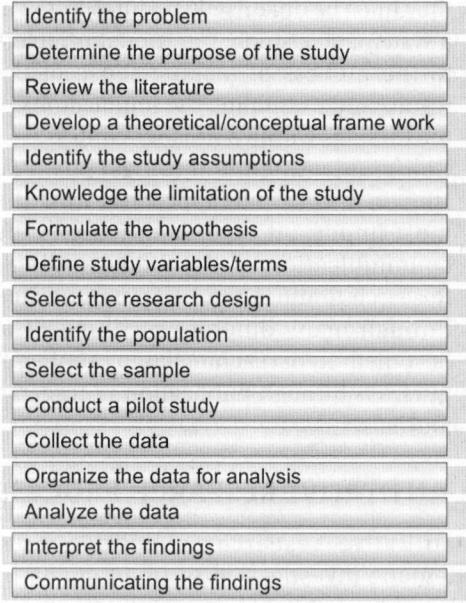

Identify the problem

Determine the purpose of the study

Review the literature

Develop a theoretical/conceptual frame work

Identify the study assumptions

Knowledge the limitation of the study

Formulate the hypothesis

Define study variables/terms

Select the research design

Identify the population

Select the sample

Conduct a pilot study

Collect the data

Organize the data for analysis

Analyze the data

Interpret the findings

Communicating the findings

Fig. 7.1: Steps in research process.

review provides a foundation on which to base new knowledge and generally is conducted well before any data are collected in quantitative study.

- **Develop a theoretical/conceptual frame work:** A theory is a systematic vision of reality that serves a scientific purpose. Research and theory are interview Research can test theories as well as help to develop and refine theories. The theoretical or conceptual frame work will assist in selection of the study variables and identifying them. The framework provides the prospective from which the investigator views the problem and is not merely 'restatement of previous research but an integration of the existing theoretical traditions and knowledge about the topic.

- **Identify the study assumptions:** Assumptions are belief that is held to be true but have not necessarily been proven. Each scientific investigation is based on assumption. It also influences the questions that are asked, the data that are gathered, the methods used to gather the data, and the interpretation of the data.

- **Knowledge the limitation of the study:** The researcher should try to identify study limitations or weaknesses. Limitations are uncontrolled variables that may affect study results and limit the generalizability of the findings. The research should openly acknowledge the limitations of a study, as much as possible, before data are collected.

- **Formulate the hypothesis:** A hypothesis predicts the relationship between two or more variables. Hypothesis in other words, is a prediction of expected out comes, it states the relationships the researcher aspects to find as a result of the study.

- **Define study variables/terms:** The definitions are usually dictionary definitions or theoretical definitions, a variable should be operationally defined. An operational definition indicates how a variable will be observed or measured. Operation definitions frequently include the instrument that will be used to measure the variables.

- **Select the research design:** It is concerned with the type of data that will be collected and means used to obtain these data. For example, the researcher must decide if the study will examine cause and effect relationship or will only describe existing situations. Research design can be categorized as quantitative or qualitative. They also can be categorized as experimental or non- experimental. Experimental design can be further divided into true experimental, quasi-experimental and pre-experimental designs. Non-experimental designs include survey studies, correlation studies, comparative studies, and methodological studies.

- **Identify the population:** The researcher must specify the broad population or group interest as well as the actual population and the second type is called the accessible population. The researcher would like to assert that study results apply to a wide target population, this population must be similar to the accessible population for such an assertion to be made.

- **Select the sample:** The sample is chosen to represent the population and is used to make generation about the population. The method of selecting the sample will determine how representative the sample is of the population. The researcher must make the determination of which sampling method to use, after considering the advantages and disadvantages of the various type of probability and non-probability sampling method.

- **Conduct a pilot study:** A pilot study involves a miniature, trial version of the planned study. People are selected for the pilot study who are similar in characteristics to the sample that will be used for the actual study. The function of pilot study is to obtain information for improving the project or for assessing its feasibility.

- **Collect the data:** The researcher should plan typically specifies procedures for collecting data for describing the study to the subjects, for obtaining the necessary informed consents, and if necessary for training those who will be involved in the collection of the data. Although the data collection step of the research may be very time consuming, it is sometimes considered to be the most exciting part of research.

- **Organize the data for analysis:** The researcher should have prepared dummy tables and graphs that could be filled in with the data once they are obtained. A statistician should be consulted in the early phase of the research process. As well as, in the data analysis phase of the study.

- **Analyze the data:** Statistical analysis cover a broad range of techniques, including some simple procedures as well as complex and sophisticated methods. Now, a researcher can sit at a computer terminal and input large amounts of data and receive the results of the analysis almost instantaneously.

- **Interpret the findings:** Before the results of a study can be communicated effectively, they must be organized and interpreted in a systematic fashion. Interpretation refers to the process of making sense of the results and examining the implications of the findings within a broader context.

- **Communicating the findings:** The final step in the research process and the most important one for nursing is the communication of the study findings. Research findings can be communicated through many different mediums. The best method of reaching large number of nurses is through publication in research journals.

QUANTITATIVE RESEARCH PROCESS

Quantitative research is defined as a systematic investigation of phenomena by gathering quantifiable data and performing statistical, mathematical, or computational techniques. Quantitative research collects information from existing and potential customers using sampling methods and sending out online surveys, online polls, questionnaires, etc., the results of which can be depicted in the form of numerical. After careful understanding of these numbers to predict the future of a product or service and make changes accordingly.

Quantitative Research Characteristics (Fig. 7.2)

Some distinctive characteristics of quantitative research are as follows:

- **Structured tools:** Structured tools, such as surveys, polls, or questionnaires are used to gather quantitative data. Using such structure methods helps in collecting in-depth and actionable data from the survey respondents.

- **Sample size:** Quantitative research is conducted on a significant sample size that represents the target market. Appropriate sampling methods have to be used when deriving the sample to fortify the research objective

- **Close-ended questions:** Closed-ended questions are created per the objective of the research. These questions help collect quantitative data and hence, are extensively used in quantitative research.

- **Prior studies:** Various factors related to the research topic are studied before collecting feedback from respondents.
- **Quantitative data:** Usually, quantitative data is represented by tables, charts, graphs, or any other non-numerical form. This makes it easy to understand the data that has been collected as well as prove the validity of the market research.
- **Generalization of results:** Results of this research method can be generalized to an entire population to take appropriate actions for improvement.

Scheme of the Research Process

- **Unsuitable status:** You have an issue, which you want to find a solution for, but do not know how.
- **Hypotheses formulation:** Creation of an assumption of the current unsuitable status and method to correct this problem.
- **Selection of the research method:** Purposeful selection of the research method

based on predefined hypotheses and survey questions.

- **Data collection:** Actual process of gathering answers from respondents using chosen method of data collection.
- **Data analysis:** Processing of collected data from data gathering process.
- **Conclusion implements:** Implementation of new findings from whole survey process into the unsuitable status of the "project".

Advantages of Quantitative Research Process

If you choose this method (a questionnaire for quantitative survey), it will come back with great many responses-answers-from clients, customers, users and other groups of residents, which you or your organization have focused on. Based on statistical processing of quantitatively collected data you can use your findings to more effective decision making, more exact planning, communication with customers, etc. This method is also characterized by being faster, cheaper and manageable by individuals,

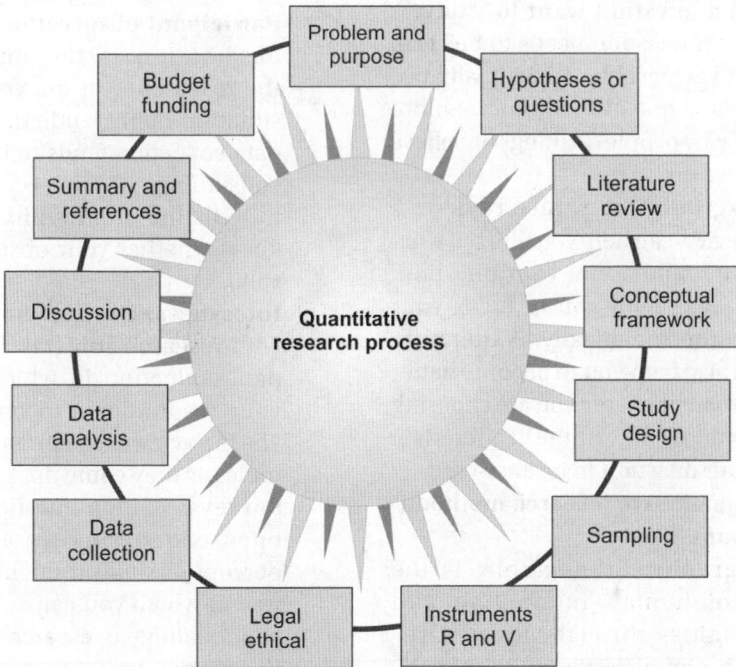

Fig. 7.2: Quantitative research process.

especially if an online questionnaire is used for data collection.

Disadvantages of Quantitative Research Process

Results of the quantitative survey may be too general. They are not always able to describe an issue in depth. A researcher can miss out the important qualities of the studied sample, because he concentrates on concrete problem and does not count in wider area of the problem.

QUALITATIVE RESEARCH PROCESS

Qualitative research is a broad field of inquiry that uses unstructured data collection methods, such as observations or documents to find themes and meanings to inform our understanding of the world. Qualitative research tends to try to uncover the reasons for behaviors, attitudes and motivations, instead of just the details of what, where, and when. Qualitative research can be done across many disciplines, such as social science, healthcare and business **(Fig. 7.3)**.

- **Decide on a question want to study:** A good research question needs to be clear, specific, and achievable. To do qualitative research, your question should explore reasons for why people do things or believe in something.
- **Do a background literature review:** A literature review can help you find out what others have found about your question. Doing this may help you to focus your question more specifically. A literature review will also help you to become better informed about the topic you are choosing and help you to determine if there is a need for your question to be answered.
- **Choose a qualitative research methodology you want to use:**
  - **Ethnography:** Ethnography is the study of human interaction and communities through direct participation and observation within the community you wish to study.
  - **Phenomenology:** Phenomenology is the study of the subjective experiences of others. It researches the world through the eyes of another person by discovering how they interpret their experiences.
  - **Grounded theory:** The purpose of grounded theory is to develop theory based on the data collected. It looks at specific information and derives theories and reasons for the phenomena.
  - **Case study research:** This method of qualitative study is an in-depth study a specific individual or phenomena in its existing context.
- **Collect your data:** There are several methods of collecting data that you can use to do qualitative research.
  - **Direct observation:** Direct observation of a situation or your research subjects can occur through video tape playback or through live observation through a one way mirror. In direct observation, you are making specific observations of a situation without influencing or participating in any way.
  - **Participant observation:** Participant observation is the immersion of the researcher in the community or situation being studied. This form of data collection tends to be more time consuming, as you need to participate fully in the community in order to know whether your observations are valid.
  - **Interviews:** Unstructured interviews with research subjects are a form of data collection in which you allow your respondents to answer freely. The interviewer can probe and explore topics as they come up.
  - **Surveys:** Written questionnaires and open-ended surveys about ideas, perceptions and thoughts is another way in which you can collect data for your qualitative research.
  - **Focus groups:** Structured or unstructured focus groups allows for

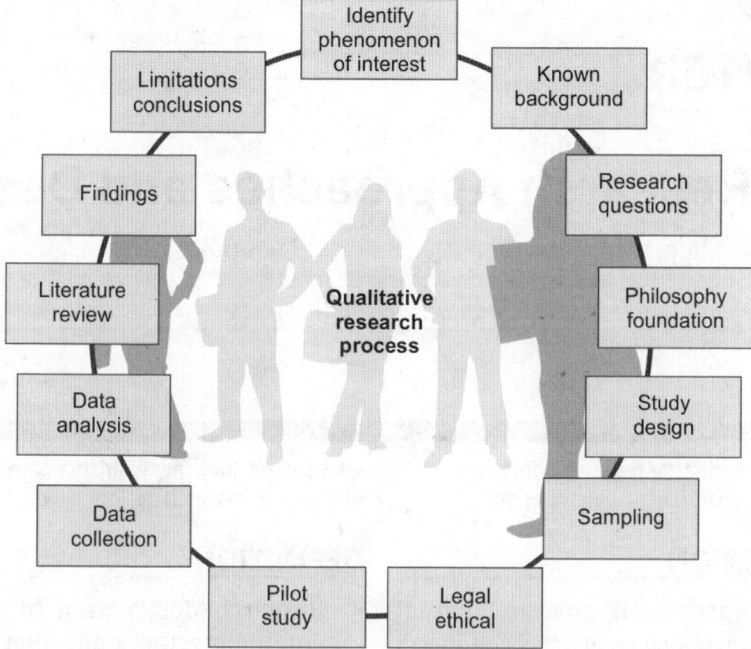

Fig. 7.3: Qualitative research process.

interaction between more participants and the interviewer about your topic. This form of data collection can be efficient as it involves more than one respondent at a time.

- **Analyze the data:** Once you have collected your data, you can begin to analyze it and come up with answers and theories to your research question.
    - **Coding:** Identify themes, ideas, and patterns in your data
    - **Statistics:** You can analyze your data using statistics. Descriptive statistics simply describe what the data is showing while inferential statistics tries to formulate conclusions beyond the data.
    - **Narrative analysis:** Narrative analysis focuses on speech and content, such as grammar, word usage, story themes, meanings of situations, the social, cultural and political context of the narrative.
    - **Content analysis:** Content analysis looks at texts or series of texts and looks for themes and meanings by looking at frequencies of words.

- **Prepare your report:** When preparing the report on your qualitative research, keep in mind, the audience for whom you are writing and also the formatting guidelines of the research journal you wish to submit your research to. You will want to make sure that your purpose for your research question is compelling and that you explain your research methodology and analysis in detail.

CONCLUSION

Research process consists of a series of actions or steps necessary to effectively carry out research and the desired sequencing of these steps. Research process is a series of closely related steps. But such steps overlap continuously rather than following a strictly prescribed sequence. The various steps involved in research process are neither mutually exclusive nor they separated from each other. They do not necessarily follow each other in any specific order and the researcher has to be constantly anticipating at each step in the research process the requirements of the subsequent steps.

8

Research Approaches and Designs

LEARNING OBJECTIVES
- Types and features of research approaches
- Need and purpose of research design
- Elements and characteristics of research design
- Types of research design

INTRODUCTION

Research approach is the conceptual structure within which research is conduced; it constitutes the blue print for the collection, measurement and analysis of data. Appropriate selection of research approach is essential because it facilitates the smooth sailing of the various research operations, thereby making research as efficient as possible yielding maximal information with minimal expenditure of effort, time and money.

MEANING OF RESEARCH DESIGN

The term research design is used in two-way some consider research design to be the entire strategy for the study from identifying the problem to final plan for data collection. The design of the study is the end result of a series of decisions made by the researchers concerning how the study will be implemented. The design is closely associated with the framework of the study and guides planning and implementing the study. As a blue print, the design is not specific to a particular study. The design is a broad pattern or guide that can be applied to many studies. Just as the blue print for a house must be individualized to the specific house being built, so must the design be made specific to a study (**Fig. 8.1**).

DEFINITION

- Research design is a blue print for conducting the study that maximizes control over factors that could interfere with the validity of the findings.
- According to Naresh Mlhotra: A research design is a framework or blue print for conducting the research project.
- According to Chris: A research design is a blue print for conducting the study that maximizes control over factors that could interfere with the validity of findings.
- According to David J Luck: A research design is the determination and statement of the general research approach or strategy adopted for the particular project. It is the heart of planning.
- According to Kerliner: Research design is the plan, structure and strategy of investigation conceived so as to obtain answer to research question and to control variance.
- According to Green and Tull: A research design is the specification of methods and procedure for acquiring the information needed. It is the overall operational pattern or framework of the project that stipulates what information is to be collected from which source and by what procedure.
- According to Russell Ackoff, research design is the process of making decisions before a situation arises in which the

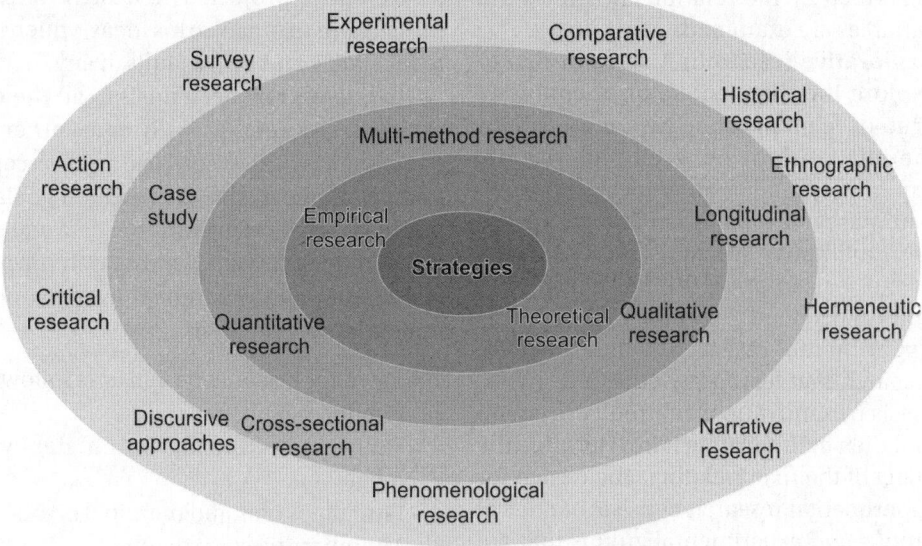

Fig. 8.1: Research designs used in research.

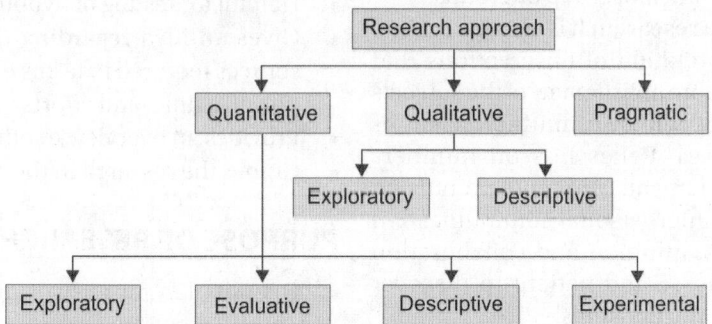

Fig. 8.2: Types of research approaches.

decision has to be carried out. It is actually a process of deliberate anticipation directed towards bringing an unexpected situation under control.

FEATURES OF RESEARCH APPROACH

- It is a plan that specifies the sources and types of information relevant to the research problem.
- It is a strategy specifying which approach will be used for gathering and analyzing the data.
- It also includes the time and cost budgets since most studies are done under these constraints.

TYPES OF RESEARCH APPROACHES (FIG. 8.2)

- **Historical research:** It is the systematic collection and critical evaluation of data relating to past occurrences – is also tradition that relieves primarily on qualitative data that has relevance for nursing. It also defined as systematic studies designed to establish facts and relationship concerning past events.
- **Descriptive research:** Research studies that have their main objective the accurate portrayal of the characteristics of person, situations or groups and/or the frequency with which certain phenomena occur. Descriptive study phenomena are

described or the relationships between variables are examined.

- **Explorative research:** A study design to explore the dimensions of phenomena or to develop or refine hypothesis about the relationships between phenomena. Exploratory studies are undertaken when a new area or topic is being investigated and qualitative methods are especially useful for exploring the full nature of a little-understood phenomenon.

- **Experimental research:** Future oriented research that tests a hypothesis or hypothesis by setting up a controlled situation and then manipulating it to determine the effect of the manipulating. The design for experimental research consists of control groups and experimental groups that are tested before and after the manipulation of the experimental group or groups.

- **Qualitative research:** It is an organization and interpretation of observations that provide a more holistic view of the subjects experiences without limiting questions or responses. Relies less on numbers and measurements and more on nursing strategies, interpersonal communication techniques, intuition and collaboration between nurse and patient to discover underlying relationships.

NEED OF RESEARCH DESIGN

Research design carries an important influence on the reliability of the results attained. It therefore provides a solid base for the whole research. It is needed due to the fact that it allows for the smooth working of the many research operations. This makes the research as effective as possible by providing maximum information with minimum spending of effort, money and time. For building of a car, we must have a suitable blueprint made by an expert designer. In a similar fashion, we require a suitable design or plan just before data collection and analysis of the research project. Planning of design must be carried out cautiously as even a small mistake might mess up the purpose of the entire project. The design helps the investigator to organize his ideas, which helps to recognize and fix his faults, if any.

In a **good research design**, all the components go together with each other in a coherent way. The theoretical and conceptual framework must with the research goals and purposes. In the same way, the data gathering method must fit with the research purposes, conceptual and theoretical framework and method of data analysis.

The need for research design is as follows:
- It reduces inaccuracy
- Helps to get maximum efficiency and reliability
- Eliminates bias and marginal errors
- Minimizes wastage of time
- Helpful for collecting research materials
- Helpful for testing of hypothesis
- Gives an idea regarding the type of resources required in terms of money, manpower, a time, and efforts
- Provides an overview to other experts
- Guides the research in the right direction.

PURPOSE OF RESEARCH DESIGN

- Overall plan for answering the research questions.
- It provides an explicit blue print of how research activities will be carried out.
- It helps to control variance by planning the study in such a way as to rule out other hypothesis and variables as causes of the study outcome. It helps to avoid bias on variables.
- It helps in identification of a research question, a search for the literature and a statement of hypothesis.
- It is a creative process of planning the empirical aspects of an investigation.
- It guides investigation in research study.

ELEMENTS OF RESEARCH DESIGN

A good research design consists of several elements **(Fig. 8.3)**.

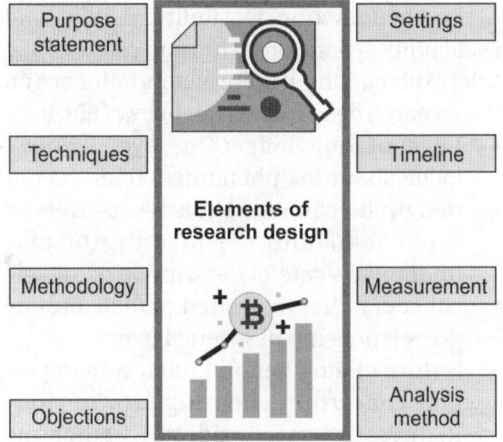

Fig. 8.3: Elements of research design.

- **Population and sample:** It refers to the subjects which are the individual who take part in study and who will be participant of study.
- **Variable:** It reflect the empirical aspects of the concepts being studied, the research measures variable. Example knowledge, attitude and practice, etc.
- **Time of data collection:** It specifies days, months or years for observation made.
- **Setting:** It measures location of study. It may be natural or laboratory setting.
- **Method of data collection:** A good research design explains method of data collection like self report methods, observation method or any other methods for the particular study.
- **Data analysis:** A good research design must also explain methods of data analysis either descriptive or inferential analysis for finding the results of the study.

CHARACTERISTICS OF RESEARCH DESIGN

Design research investigates the process of designing in all its fields. It is thus related to design methods in general or for particular disciplines. A primary interpretation of design research is that it is concerned with undertaking research into the design process. Secondary interpretations would refer to

undertaking research within the process of design. The overall intention is to better understand and to improve the design process.

- **Situational:** Good research designs reflect the settings of the investigation. This was illustrated above where a particular need of teachers and administrators was explicitly addressed in the design strategy. Similarly, intergroup rivalry, demoralization, and competition might be accessed through the use of additional comparison groups who are not in direct contact with the original group.
- **Feasible**: Good designs can be implemented. The sequence and timing of events are carefully thought out. Potential problems in measurement, adherence to assignment, database construction and the like, are anticipated.
- **Redundant:** Good research designs have some flexibility built into them. Often, this flexibility results from duplication of essential design features. For example, multiple replications of a treatment help to insure that failure to implement the treatment in one setting will not invalidate the entire study.
- **Efficient:** Good designs strike a balance between redundancy and the tendency to overdesign. Where it is reasonable, other, less costly, strategies for ruling out potential threats to validity are utilized.

IMPORTANCE OF RESEARCH DESIGN

The importance of research design in research methodology is due to the following:

- It may result in the preferred kind of study with helpful conclusion.
- It cuts down on inaccuracy.
- Allows you get optimum efficiency and reliability.
- Reduce wastage of time.
- Reduce uncertainty, confusion and practical haphazard related to any research problem.
- Of great help for collection of research material and testing of hypothesis.

- It is a guide for giving research the right path.
- Gets rid of bias and marginal errors.
- Provides an idea concerning the type of resources needed in terms of money, effort, time, and manpower.
- Smooth and efficient sailing (sets boundaries and helps prevent blind search)
- Maximizes reliability of results.
- Provides firm foundation to the endeavor.
- Averts misleading conclusions and thoughtless useless exercise.
- Provides opportunity to anticipate flaws and inadequacies (anticipates problems).
- Incorporates by learning from other people's critical comments and evaluations.

SELECTION OF RESEARCH DESIGN

While selecting a research design the researchers has to weight many considerations. The prime importance is the purpose and theory development aim of the study. Theory development usually reflects the current level of knowledge about the phenomenon and thus has guided determination of the specific research purpose. Additional influences on the study design include ethical issues related to the phenomenon, feasibility, validity, and availability of data, precision and cost, etc. The brief explanations of these factors influence on the research design are given below **(Fig. 8.4)**.

- **Level of knowledge:** Our level of knowledge about the phenomenon affects our design choices. When little is known about a phenomenon, the investigator may undertake a careful description of a single concept rather than attempt to determine the relationship of several factors.
- **Nature of the phenomena:** It is an important concern in choosing how to study it. Investigator considers whether the phenomenon can be studied in a naturalistic or non-naturalistic way. For example, certain disasters have helped to health scientists to gain better understanding of how human beings respond to crisis.
- **Nature of the purpose:** The nature of the research purposes sometimes implies the choice of a specific design.
- **Ethical consideration:** Research problems that place unethical demands on subjects may not be feasible for study. Researchers must take ethical considerations seriously. The considerations of ethics may affect the choice between an experimental design and a non-experimental design.

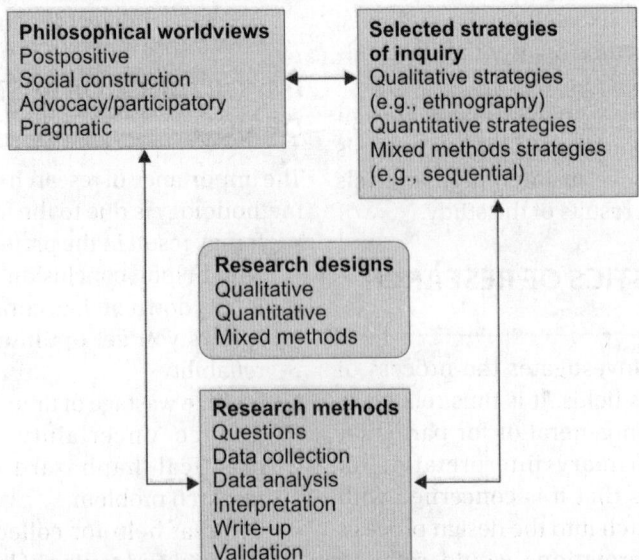

Fig. 8.4: Selection of research design.

- **Feasibility:** In some instances, feasibility is a key concern in selecting a research design. Many researches designs are elegant but not feasible. One of the feasibility considerations is the amount of time the investigator can devote to the study. The research problem must be one that can be studied within a realistic period of time. All researchers have fixed a particular time for completion of a project. It is essential that the scope of the problem be circumscribed enough to provide ample time for the completion of the entire project. Research studies generally take longer than anticipated to complete.
- **Availability of subjects:** The researcher needs to determine whether a sufficient number of eligible subjects will be available and willing to participate in the study. If one has captive audience, like students in a classroom, it may be relatively easy to enlist their cooperation. When a study involves the subject's independent time and effort, they may be unwilling to participate, when there is no apparent reward for doing so. Other potential subjects may have fears about harm or confidentiality and may be suspicious of the research process in general. Subjects with unusual characteristics are often difficult to locate. In general, people are fairly cooperative about participating, but a researcher must consider needing a larger subject poor that will actually participate. At times, when reading a research report, the researcher may note how the procedures were liberalized or the number of subjects was altered. This was probably a result of some unforeseen pragmatic consideration.
- **Availability of facility and equipment:** All research projects require some kind of equipment. The equipment may be questionnaires, telephones, stationery, stamps, technical equipment or other apparatus. Most research projects require the availability of some kind of facility. The facility may be a hospital site for data collection or laboratory space or a computer center for data analysis.
- **Validity of data:** Validity of data is another important concern in selecting a research design.
- **Precision:** An additional dimension that researchers consider when choosing a research design is precision. Precision refers to the ability to obtain the most accurate estimate of a single variable or of the effect of treatment variable on an outcome variable. Accuracy means that all aspects of a study systematically and logically follow from the identified problem statement. A design that allows researcher to account for or to control many other factors known to influence the variable of interest maximizes the precision of the estimates (e.g., orientation of patient helps in adjustment in hospital).
- **Researchers' experience:** The selection of the research problem should be based on the nurse's realm of experience and interest. It is much easier to develop a research study related to a topic that is either theoretically or experimentally familiar. Selecting a problem that is of interest to the research is essential for maintaining enthusiasm when the project has its inevitable ups and downs.
- **Cost:** Research projects require some expenditure of money. Before embarking on a study, the researcher probably itemizes the expenses and projects the total cost of the project. This provides a clear picture of the budgetary needs for items like books, stationery, postage, printing, technical equipment, telephone and computer charges and salaries.
- **Control:** A researcher attempts to use a design to maximize the degree of control over the tested variables. An efficient design can maximize results, decrease errors, and control preexisting or impaired conditions that may affect outcome. To maximize efforts the researcher should maximize control. To accomplish these tasks the research design and methods should demonstrate the researcher's efforts at control. Control is accomplished by ruling out extraneous variables that

compete with the independent variable as an explanation for a study's outcome. The means of controlling extraneous variables include the following:

- Use of a homogenous sample
- Use of consistent data collection procedures
- Manipulation of the independent variable
- Randomization.

COMPONENTS OF RESEARCH DESIGN

- Design the exploratory, descriptive and casual phase of the research.
- Define the information needed.
- Specify the measurement and scaling procedures.
- Construct and pretest a questionnaire or an appropriate form for data collection.
- Specify the sampling process and sampling size.
- Develop a plan of data analysis.

CHARACTERISTICS OF A GOOD DESIGN

- It must be flexible, appropriate, efficient and economical.

- It must minimize bias and maximize reliability of the data collected and analyzed.
- It must give smallest experimental errors.
- It must give maximum information and must provide opportunity for considering many different aspects of a problem.
- It must relate to the purpose or objective of the research problem.
- It must give weight age to the availability of time, money, skills of the research staff and the means of obtaining the information.

TYPES OF RESEARCH DESIGN

Research design is also known as a blue print that researchers select to carry out their research study; sometimes research design is used interchangeably with the term methodology. Researcher often describes a design using a concise that enables us to summarize complex design structure effectively **(Fig. 8.5)**.

FACTORS AFFECTING RESEARCH DESIGN

- Availability of scientific information
- Availability of sufficient data
- Time availability

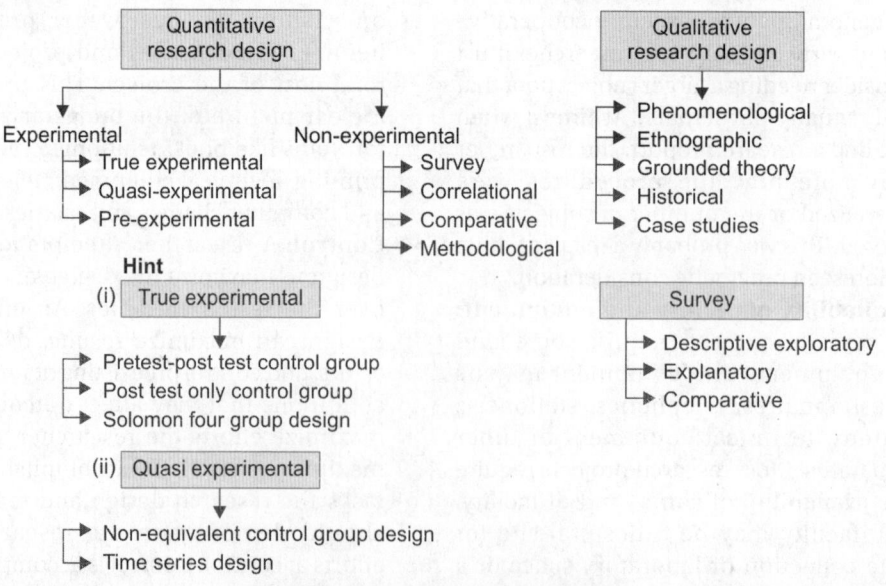

Fig. 8.5: Research design classifications.

Sl. No.	Classification	Description
I	Quantitative research	Quantitative research is a formal, objective, systematic process in which numeral data are utilized to obtain information about the world.
1	Experimental design	A design in which the researcher controls (manipulates) the independent variables and randomly assigns to different conditions.
1.1	True experimental design	Manipulation of independent variable, in the process of control group, randomization. True experimental design has following types: • Post-test only controls design. • Pretest –post-test control group design. • Solomon four group design. • Factorial design. • Randomized block design. • Cross over design.
1.2	Quasi-experimental design	Manipulation of independent variables, but absence of either randomization or control. Which has got the following two types: 1. Non-randomized control group design. 2. Time-series design.
1.3	Pre-experimental design	Manipulation of independent variables, but limited control over extraneous variables, no randomization and control group. Which has got the following two types: 1. One-shot case design. 2. One-group-pretest and posttest design.
2	Non-experimental design	A design in which the researcher collects the data without introducing an intervention.
2.1	Descriptive design	Descriptive research provides information about conditions, situations and events that occur in the present.
2.2	Correlational Design	In correlation studies the researcher examines the strength of relationships between variables by determining how changes in one variable are associated with changes in other variables.
2.3	Developmental design	Developmental research differs from the other types of research in that, rather than bringing new information to light it focuses on the interaction between research and the production and evaluation of a new product. This type of research can be formative (by collecting evaluative information about such information to modify and improve the developmental process).
2.4	Epidemiological designs	The investigation of distribution and cause of disease in a population is known as epidemiology.
2.5	Survey research design	Survey studies are the investigation in which self-report data are collected from samples with the purpose of describing populations on some variables or variables of interest. Which has got the following three types: 1. Univariant descriptive design. 2. Exploratory descriptive design. 3. Comparative descriptive design.
3	Other designs	
3.1	Methodological studies	Methodological studies are concerned with the development of testing and evaluation of research instruments and methods.
3.2	Meta-analysis	Quantitatively combining and integrating the findings of the multiple research studies on a particular topic.

Contd...

Contd...

Sl. No.	Classification	Description
3.3	Secondary data analysis	A research design in which the data collected in one research is reanalyzed by another research, usually to test new hypothesis.
3.4	Outcome research	Outcome research involves the evaluation of care practices and systems in place. It is used in nursing to develop evidence-based practice and improve nursing actions.
3.5	Evaluation studies	It is research design which involves the judgment about success of the programmes, practices or policies.
3.6	Operational research	Operational research involves the study of complex human organizations and services to develop new knowledge about institutions, programmes, use of facilities and personnel in order to improve working efficiency of an organization.
II	Qualitative research	Qualitative research is concerned with in-depth description of people or events and data are collected through such methods as unstructured interviews and participant observation. Qualitative research aims to explore, discover, understand or describe phenomena that have already been identified but are not well understood.
1	Phenomenological research	Phenomenological studies examine human experiences through the description that are provided by the people involved.
2	Ethnographic research	Ethnographic research usually consists of a description of events that occur within the life of a group with particular references to the interactions of individuals in the context of the sociocultural norms, rituals and beliefs shared by the group. The researcher generally participated in some part of the normal life the group and uses what he or she learns from his participation to understand the interactions between group members.
3	Grounded theory	Grounded theories are these studies in which data are collected and analyzed and then a theory is developed.
4	Case studies	Case study research generally refers to two distinct research approaches. The first consists of an in-depth study of a particular student, classroom or school with the aim of producing a nuanced description of the pervading cultural setting that affects education and an account of the interactions that takes place between students and other relevant persons.
5	Historical research	Historical type of research generates descriptions and sometimes attempted explanations of conditions, situations and events that have occurred in the past.
6	Action research	Action research or applied research aims at finding a solution for an immediate problem facing a society or any other organization. Research that identifies, social, medical, political trends that may affect a particular institution is example of applied research.

- Proper exposure to the data source
- Availability of the money
- Manpower availability
- Magnitude of the management problem
- Degree of top management's support
- Ability, knowledge, skill, technical understanding and technical background of the researcher
- Controllable variables
- Un-controllable variables

- Internal variables
- External variables

STEPS IN RESEARCH DESIGN (FIG. 8.6)

- **The problem:** The first step involves the proper selection and then carefully defining the problem. By this researcher will be enabled to know about what he has to search, but it should be kept in mind that the problems selected should not be unmanageable in nature and also should not be based on the desires.
- **Objective of the study:** The objective of the study should be very clear in the mind of the researcher as this will lead to the clarity of the design and proper response from the respondents.

- **Nature of the study:** The research design should be very much in relation with the nature of the study, which is to be carried out.
- **Data sources:** The various sources of the data or the information should be very clearly stated by the researcher.
- **Techniques of data collection:** For the collection of the required information, it sometimes becomes very necessary to use some especial techniques.
- **Social cultural context:** Research design based on the social cultural concept is prepared in order to avoid the various study variations.
- **Geographical limit:** This step becomes a necessity at this point of time as with the help of this step, research linked to the

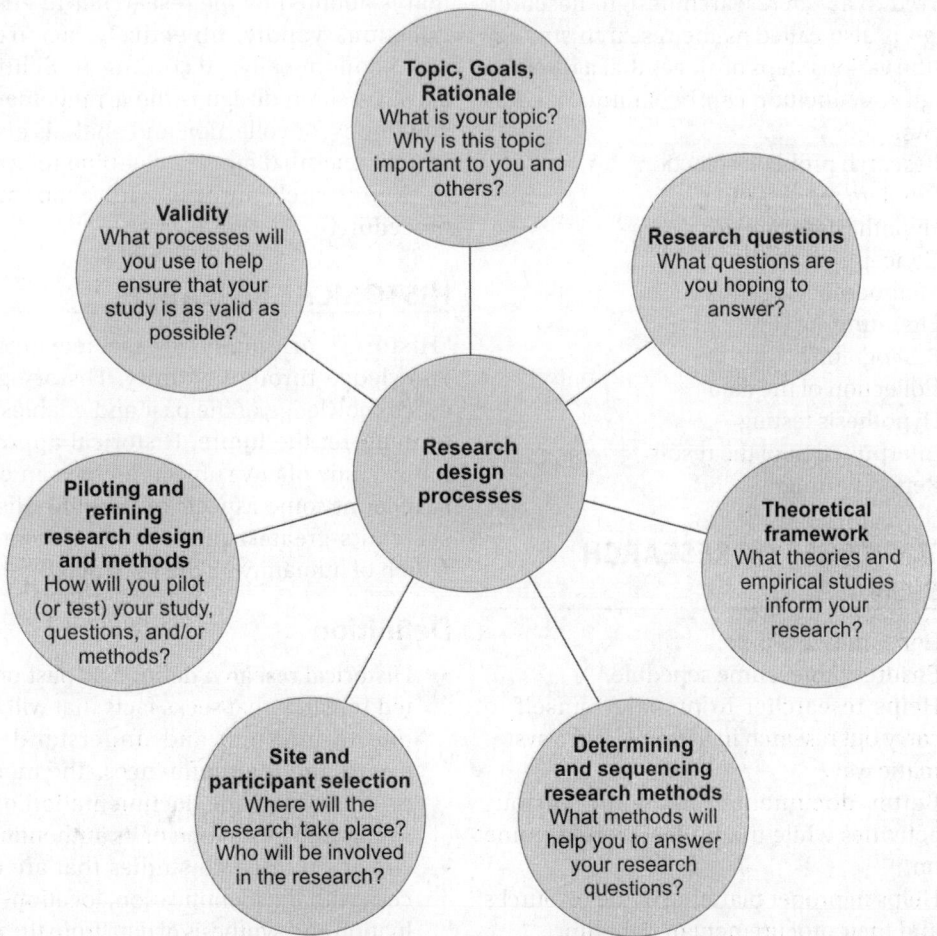

Fig. 8.6: Research design processes.

hypothesis applies only to certain number of social groups.

- **Basis of selection:** Selecting a proper sample acts as a very important and critical step and this is done with the help of some mechanics like drawing a random stratified, deliberate, double cluster or quota sample, etc.

STEPS NEED TO INCLUDE IN RESEARCH DESIGN

Like an architect prepares a blue print before he approves a construction – in the same way researcher makes or prepares a plan or a schedule of his own study before he starts his research work. This helps the researcher to save time and also save some of his crucial resources. This plan or blue print of study is referred to as the research design. Research design is also called as the research strategy and the various steps or stages that a research design may include can be summarized as follows:

- Research problem selection
- Problem presentation
- Hypothesis formulation
- Conceptual clarity
- Methodology
- Literature survey
- Bibliography
- Collection of the data
- Hypothesis testing
- Interpretation of the result
- Report writing.

ADVANTAGES OF RESEARCH DESIGN

- Consumes less time.
- Ensures project time schedule.
- Helps researcher to prepare himself to carry out research in a proper and a systematic way.
- Better documentation of the various activities while the project work is going on.
- Helps in proper planning of the resources and their procurement in right time.

- Provides satisfaction and confidence, accompanied with a sense of success from the beginning of the work of the research project.

RESEARCH DESIGNS USED IN NURSING

Designing a nursing study is the creative process of planning the empirical aspects of an investigation. A research design is a plan, structure and strategy of investigation so conceived as to obtain answers to research questions or problems. The plan is the complete scheme or program of the research. It includes an outline of what the investigator will do from writing the hypotheses and their operational implications to the final analysis of data. A research design is a procedural plan that is adopted by the researcher to answer questions validly, objectively, accurately and economically. According to Selltiz et al., 'A research design is the arrangement of conditions for collection and analysis of data in a manner that aims to combine relevance to the research purpose with economy in procedure.'

HISTORICAL RESEARCH

"Historia" originally meant learning or knowledge through enquiry. History gives exact knowledge of the past and enables one to interpret the future. Historical approach to the study of any subject denotes an effort to recount some aspects of past life. History serves its greatest purpose as a record of march of humanity on the road of progress.

Definition

- Historical research defined as past oriented research that seeks facts that will help one to interpret and understand past events and their influences. The method used is systematic documentation of the events and evaluation of its authenticity.
- Historical research studies that are concern with the identification, location, evaluation and synthesis of data from the past.

- Historical research is a systematic studies designed to establish facts and relationships concerning past events.
- Historical research is a critical investigation of events, developments and experiences of the past, the careful weighing of evidence of the validity of sources of information on the past and the interpretation of the weighed evidences. **Figure 8.7** depicts the sources of research.

Nature of Historical Research

- Historical research is the systematic collection and critical evaluation of data relating to past occurrences.
- Data for historical research are usually in the form of written records of the past, periodicals, diaries, newspapers, legal documents and reports.
- Historical approach, which refers to the organization of historical facts in support of the new concepts to be developed.
- Historical subjects, referring to biographies of great man, monographs of places and sketches of ideas, thoughts and trends.

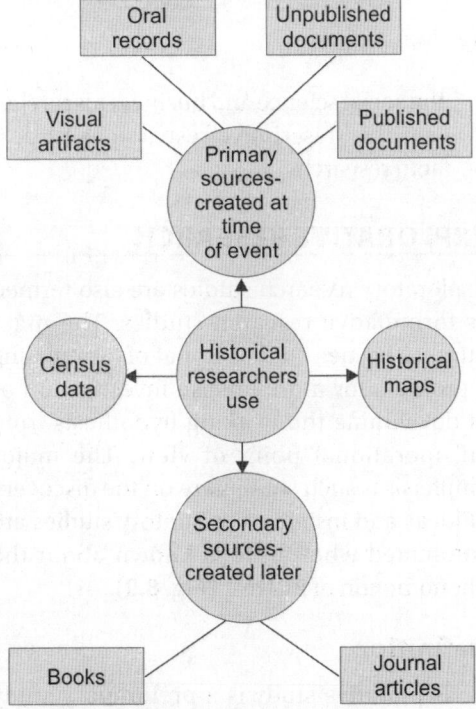

Fig. 8.7: Sources of research.

- Historical technique, which refers to research that is conducted on the basis of historical records and documents.

Importance of Historical Research

- The value of historical research is not merely that it provides a record of the past but that it also contributes to present thought and decision making regarding the future.
- According to one author, "history" value lies in its ability to help clarity the context in which today's problems exists.
- Nurses have used historical research methods to examine a wide range of phenomena. For example, Widerquist studied (1992) Florence nightingale's spirituality and its influence on the development of modern nursing through an analysis of nightingale's letters, diaries, essays and journals.

Historical Research Considerations

The historical researcher usually must evaluate the authenticity and accuracy of historical data before analyzing them.

DESCRIPTIVE RESEARCH

Descriptive research refers to the methods that describe the characteristics of the variables under study. This approach, which relies on both qualitative and quantitative methods, is appropriate when little is known about a phenomenon. Much of nursing research is descriptive **(Fig. 8.8)**.

Definitions

- Descriptive research is a present oriented research that seeks to accurately describe what is and to analyze the facts obtained in relation to the problem under study. It may lead to theories or hypothesis to be tested experimentally.
- Descriptive research studies that have as their main objective the accurate portrayal of the characteristics of person, situations or groups and/or the frequency with which certain phenomena occur.

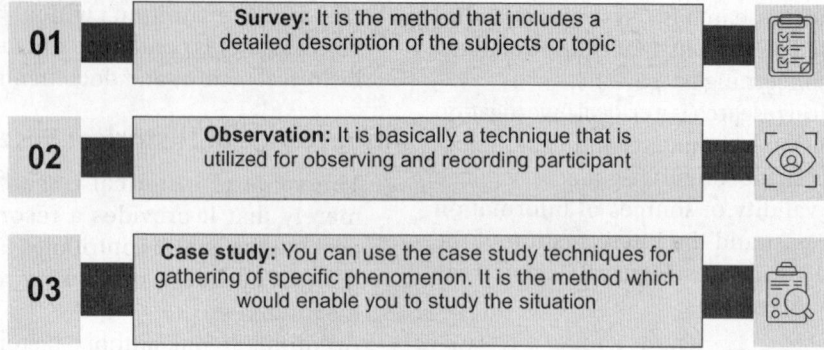

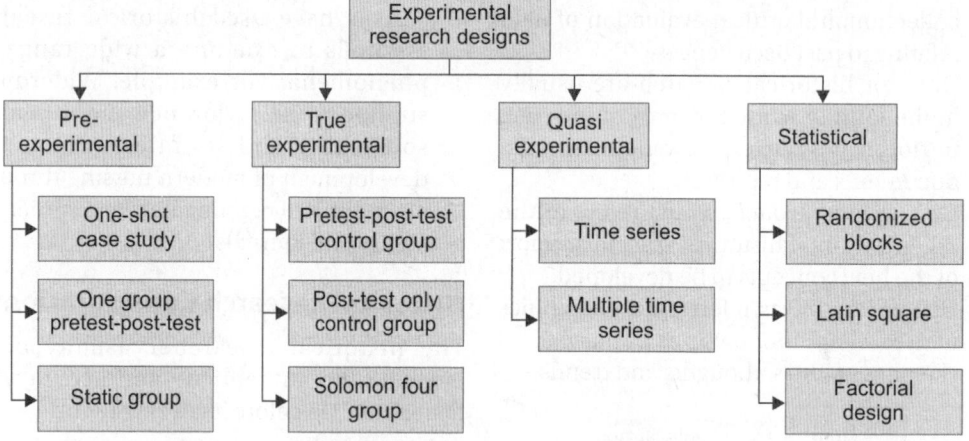

Fig. 8.8: Methods of descriptive research.

Fig. 8.9: Experimental research designs.

- Descriptive studies in which phenomena are described or the relationship between variables is examined, no attempt is made to determine cause and effect relationships.

Purpose of Descriptive Study

- To observe, describe and document aspects of a situation.
- To analyze the finding in relation to their significance.
- It is often done for the important purpose of generating hypothesis for future correlation and experimental studies.

Importance of Descriptive Research

- It is the most common type of quantitative study used in nursing research.
- Descriptive research induces surveys and fact-finding enquiries.

- The social science and business researcher uses this descriptive research as ex post facto research.

EXPLORATIVE RESEARCH

Exploratory research studies are also termed as formulative research studies. The main purpose of such studies is that of formulating a problem for more precise investigation or of developing the working hypothesis from an operational point of view. The major emphasis is such studies are on the discovery of ideas and insights. Exploratory studies are conducted when little is known about the phenomenon of interest **(Fig. 8.9)**.

Definition

- Explorative study is a preliminary study designed to help refine the problem,

Table 8.1: Exploratory vs descriptive research.

Basis for comparison	Exploratory research	Descriptive research
Meaning	Exploratory research means a research conducted for formulating a problem for more clear investigation. It is generally conducted when a little is known about a topic of interest.	Descriptive research is a research that explore and explain an individual, group or a situation.
Objective	To provide insights and understanding and develop hypothesis	To test specific hypothesis, examine relationships, and describe characteristics and functions
Overall design	Flexible	Rigid
Research process	Unstructured	Structured
Sampling	Non-probability sampling	Probability sampling
Structural design	No pre-planned design for analysis	Pre-planned design for analysis
Findings/Results	Tentative	Conclusive
Outcome	Generally followed by further exploratory or conclusive research	Findings can be used as input for decision making

develop or refine hypothesis or test and refine the data collecting methods.

- Explorative research study designed to explore the dimensions of a phenomenon or to develop or refine hypothesis about the relationships between phenomena.

Characteristics of Explorative Research

- It is likely that you would find little written on this topic.
- An exploratory research study would therefore be appropriate.
- A flexible approach rather than a structured approach to data collection would be used.
- In explorative studies, there is a greatest interest in examining the qualitative aspects of data rather than the quantitative data.

EXPERIMENTAL RESEARCH

Experiments differ from non-experiments in one important respect. The researcher is an active agent in experimental work rather than a passive observer. Experimental research is concerned with cause and effect relationship. All experimental studies involve manipulation or control of the independent variable (cause) and measurement of the dependent variable (effect).

Definition

- Experimental research is the blue print of the procedure that enable the researcher to test hypothesis by reaching valid conclusions about relationships between independent and dependent variables.
- Experimental research study in which the investigator controls (manipulates) the independent variable and randomly assigns subjects to different conditions.
- Experimental research is a future oriented research that tests a hypothesis or hypothesis by setting up a controlled situation and then manipulating it to determine the effect of the manipulation. The design for experimental research consists of control groups and experimental groups that are tested before and after the manipulation of the experimental group or groups.

Characteristics of True Experiments

- **Manipulation:** The experiments do something to at least some of the participants in the study.
- **Control:** The experimenter introduces one or more controls over the experimental situation, including the use of a control group.
- **Randomization:** The experimenter assigns participants to a control or experimental group on a random basis.

Nature of Experimental Approach

- True experimental approach is considered to be the classic form of research as experiments have the potential to provide the most evidence for strength of the association between variables.
- Experimental approach is a very strong study and greatly increases the level of internal validity that can be achieved.
- The controlled experiment is considered by many to be the ideal of science. Except for purely descriptive research the aim of many research studies is to understand the nature of relationship among phenomena.
- The strength of true experiment over other methods lies in the fact that the experiment can achieve greater confidence in genuineness and inter reliability of relationships because they are observed under carefully controlled conditions.

Types of Experimental Approach

- **True experimental:** Are those in which the researcher has a great deal of control over the research situation. There are three criteria for a true experimental research.
  1. The researcher manipulates the experimental variables.
  2. At least one experimental and one comparison group are included in the study.
  3. Subjects are randomly assigned to either the experimental or the comparison group.
- **Quasi-experimental:** Sometimes researcher are not able to randomly assign subjects to groups or for various reasons no comparison group is available for study. Generally, the researcher uses existing or intact groups for the experimental and comparison groups.
- **Pre-experimental study:** The name applied by Campbell and Stanley (1963) to experimental study that are considered very weak and in which the researcher has little control over the research. It is classified in to shot case study and the one group pretest-posttest design.

QUALITATIVE RESEARCH

The purpose of qualitative research is to explore an illuminate characteristics of human experiences about which little is known or understood in the context in which they occur using rich descriptions provided by the participants. Qualitative research, in contrast to the deductive process of quantitative research, starts from an inductive process (**Fig. 8.10**).

Definitions

- Qualitative research that is concerned with the subjective meaning of an experience to an individual.
- Qualitative research the investigation of phenomena, typically in an in-depth and holistic fashion, through the collection of rich narrative materials using a flexible research design.
- Qualitative research designs are often based on some theoretical or philosophical perspective. They attempt to preserve the wholeness of an individual's subject experience rather than reduce it to distinct variables.

Characteristics of Qualitative Research

- Qualitative design is flexible and elastic, capable of adjusting to what is being

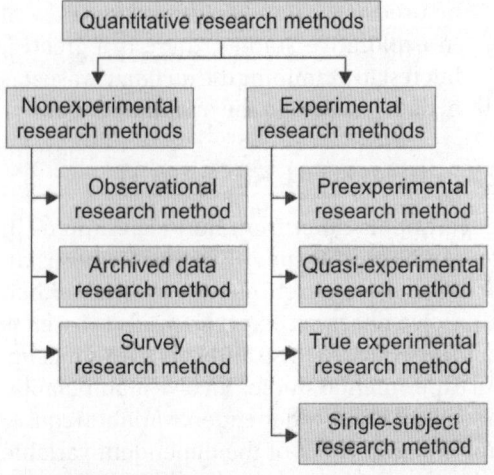

Fig. 8.10: Quantitative research designs.

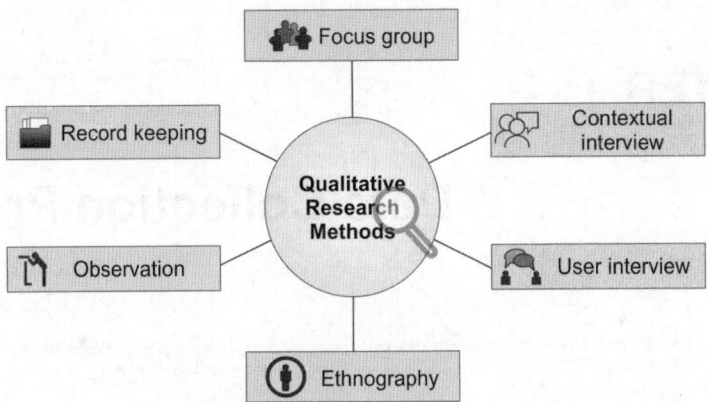

Fig. 8.11: Qualitative research methods.

learned during the course of data collection.

- Qualitative design typically involves a margin together of various methodologies.
- Qualitative design tends to be holistic, striving of an understanding of the whole.
- Qualitative design is focused on understanding a phenomenon or social setting not necessarily making predictions about the setting or phenomenon.
- Qualitative design required that the researcher become intensely involved, usually remaining in the field for lengthy periods of time.
- Qualitative design requires the researcher to become the research instrument.
- Qualitative design requires ongoing analysis of the data in order to formulate subsequent strategies and to determine when the field work is done.
- Qualitative design pushes the researcher to develop a model of what is transpiring in the social setting or what a phenomenon of interest is about.
- Qualitative design provides opportunities for description of the researcher's role as well as description of his or her own biases.

Types of Qualitative Research (Fig. 8.11)

- Field and Morse (1985) identified eight approaches – ethnography, ground theory, ethnology, ethno science, ethno

methodology, analytic sociology and phenomenology.

- Wilson and Hutchinson (1996) listed ten types of qualitative research – ground theory, ethnography, phenomenology, ethno science, hermeneutics, historical inquiry, ethical inquiry, feminist inquiry, critical social theory and case study.
- Burns and Grove (1997) presented six approaches to qualitative research–phenomenological, grounded theory, ethnographic, historical, philosophical inquiry and critical social theory.

CONCLUSION

Research design involves taking a question or problem and testing it to come up with a possible or definitive answer. There are two main types of research design: qualitative and quantitative. Additionally, there are many career options within the field of research design, including creative, scientific or a combination of both. A research design basically means the plan or technique of shaping the research or as Hakim (1987) puts it "design deals mainly with aim, purposes, motives and plans within the practical constraints of location, time, money and availability of staff". The possibilities of success of a research study are significantly improved when the "beginning" is properly defined as a precise statement of goals and justification.

9

CHAPTER

Data Collection Process

LEARNING OBJECTIVES

- Meaning of data and collection
- Sources of data
- Methods of collecting primary data
- Data collection process
- Procedure for data collection
- Selection methods of data collection
- Data collection methods

INTRODUCTION

The method that researchers use to collect information about subjects is the identifiable and repeatable operations that define the major variables being studied. After designing an approach for the research, the statistical problem begins. Collection of data is the first step in the statistical treatment of a problem. Numerical facts are the raw materials upon which the investigator is to work just as in a manufacturing concern, the quality of finished products depends. Interalia, upon the quality of the raw material, in the same manner, the validity of conclusions in a research is governed among other considerations by the quality of the data used. Assembling facts is, thus, a very important step and no pains should be spared to see that the data collected are accurate, reliable, and thorough.

DEFINITIONS

- Data is defined as the observable and measurable facts that provide information about phenomenon under study.
- Measurements are the process of assigning numbers to variables. Measurements, as used in research, imply the qualification of information that is the assigning of some type of numbers to the data.

MEANING OF DATA AND COLLECTION

- The word 'data' is a plural form of the word "datum" which means information that is systematically collected in the courses of study.
- The word "method" refers to the means of gathering data that are common to all sciences including "nursing". It is different from the word "technique", which refers to the specific tools that are used in the given method.
- Data collection is not a new intervention for nurses. Nurses use all of their senses when collecting data from the patient for whom they provide care.

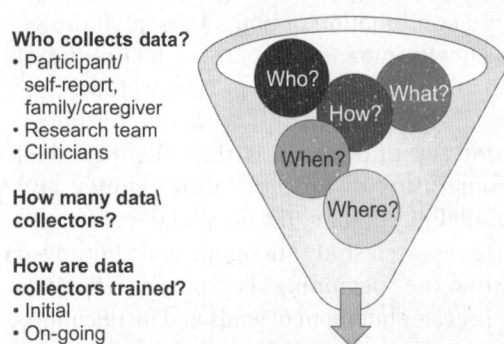

Who collects data?
- Participant/
  self-report,
  family/caregiver
- Research team
- Clinicians

How many data\ collectors?

How are data collectors trained?
- Initial
- On-going

Data collection processes

Fig. 9.1: Concept of data collection.

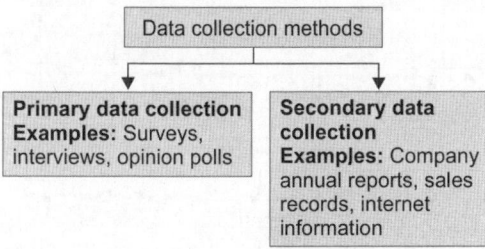

Fig. 9.2: Methods of data collection.

- Nurse-researcher, also have available many ways to collect information about their research subjects.
- The major difference between the data collected when performing patient care and the date collected for the purposes of research is that the data collection methods employed by researcher need to be objective and systematic.

NEED OF DATA

- The data serve as the bases or raw materials for analysis. Without an analysis of factual data, no specific inferences can be drawn on the questions under study.
- Inferences based on imagination or guess work cannot provide correct answers to research questions. The relevance, adequacy, and reliability of data determine the quality of the findings of a study.
- Data form the basis for testing the hypotheses formulated in a study. Data also provide the facts and figures required for constructing measurement scales and tables, which are analyzed with statistical techniques.
- Inferences on the results of statistical analysis and tests of significance provide the answers to research questions. Thus, the scientific process of measurements, analysis testing and inferences depends on the availability of relevant data and their accuracy.
- Hence, the importance of data for any research studies. The search for answers to research questions is called collection of data. Data are facts, and other relevant materials, past and present, serving as bases for study and analyses.

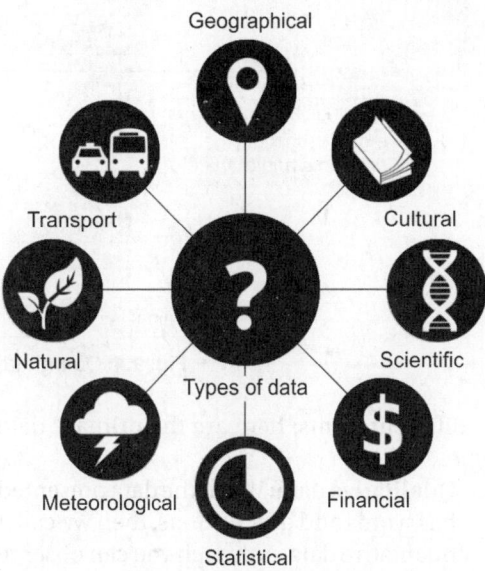

Fig. 9.3: Types of data.

Some example of data is as follows:

- The types of patients admitted in hospital or attended for OPD in hospital.
- The items of drugs and medical supplies required for the hospital management.
- The quantity of each material required for a unit of output in hospital.
- The sex, age, social class, religion, income level of respondents in a health care recipient behavior study.
- The opinions of eligible couples on birth control devices (Family Planning Survey).
- The capital expenditure proposals considered by a nursing college during a year (Financial Management).
- The marks obtained by students of BSc Nursing students in a test on a particular subject (Performances of students).
- The opinions of people on voting in a general election (Opinion Poll).
- The types of news read by newspaper readers (readership survey).

Types of Data in Research

Every kind of data has a rare quality of describing things after assigning a specific value to it. For analysis, you need to organize these values, processed and presented in a given context, to make it useful. Data can be

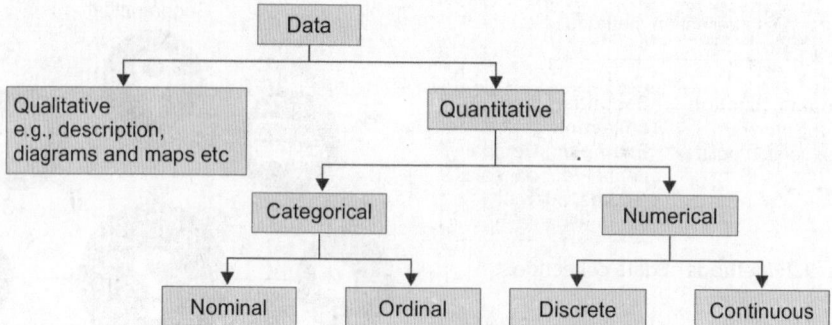

Fig. 9.4: Quantitative and qualitative data.

in different forms; here are the primary data types.

- **Qualitative data:** When the data presented has words and descriptions, then we call it qualitative data. Although you can observe this data, it is subjective and harder to analyze data in research, especially for comparison. Example: Quality data represents everything describing taste, experience, texture, or an opinion that is considered quality data. This type of data is usually collected through focus groups, personal interviews, or using open-ended questions in surveys.
- **Quantitative data:** Any data expressed in numbers of numerical figures are called quantitative data. This type of data can be distinguished into categories, grouped, measured, calculated, or ranked. Example: questions, such as age, rank, cost, length, weight, scores, etc. everything comes under this type of data. You can present such data in graphical format, charts, or apply statistical analysis methods to this data. The (Outcomes Measurement Systems) OMS questionnaires in surveys are a significant source of collecting numeric data.
- **Categorical data:** It is data presented in groups. However, an item included in the categorical data cannot belong to more than one group. Example: A person responding to a survey by telling his living style, marital status, smoking habit, or drinking habit comes under the categorical data. A chi-square test is a standard method used to analyze this data.

SOURCES OF DATA

- The task of data collection begins after a research problem has been defined and research design/plan checked out. While deciding about the method of data collection to be used for the study, the researcher should keep in mind two types of data viz., primary and secondary.
- The primary data are those which are collected afresh and for the first time, and thus happen to be original in character.
- The secondary data, on the other hand, are those which have already been collected by someone else and which have already been passed through the statistical process.
- The researcher would have to decide which sort of data would be using (thus collecting) for his study and according he will have to select one or the other method of data collection.
- The methods of collecting primary and secondary data differ since primary data are to be originally collected, while in case of secondary data, the nature of data collection work is merely that of compilation.
- The sources of data may be classified into: (a) Primary sources, and (b) Secondary sources.

Primary Sources

Primary sources are original sources from which the researcher directly collects data that have not been previously collected, e.g., collection of data directly by the researcher

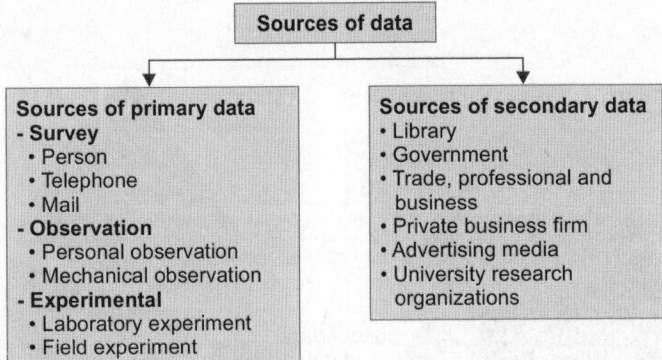

Fig. 9.5: Sources of data.

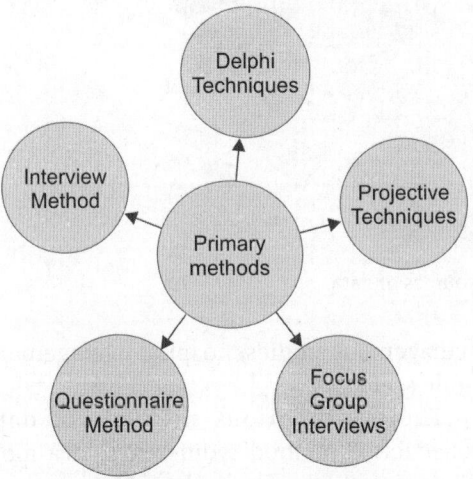

Fig. 9.6: Primary data collection methods.

on brand awareness, brand preference, brand loyalty and other aspects of consumer behavior from a sample of consumers by interviewing them. Primary data are first-hand information collected through various methods, such as observation, interviewing, mailing, etc.

Secondary Sources

These are sources containing data which have been collected and compiled for another purpose. The secondary sources consists of readily available sources and already compiled statistical statements and reports whose data may be used by researcher for their studies, e.g., census reports, annual reports and financial statements of companies, Statistical statements, Reports of Government Departments, Annual Reports on currency and finance published by the Reserve Bank of India, Statistical Statements relating to Co-operatives and Regional Rural Banks, published by the NABARD, Reports of the National Sample Survey Organization, Reports of trade associations, publications of international organizations, such as UNO, IMF, World Bank, and Financial Journals, newspapers, etc.

Secondary sources consist of not only published records and reports, but also unpublished records. The latter category includes various record and registers maintained by firms and organizations, e.g., accounting and financial records, personnel records, register of members, minutes of meetings, inventory records, etc. Though secondary sources are diverse and consist of all sorts of materials, they have certain common characteristics.

- They are readymade and readily available, and do not require the trouble of constructing tools and administering them.

- They consist of data over which a researcher has no original control over collection and classification. Both the form and the content of secondary sources are shaped by others. Clearly, this is a feature which can limit the research value of secondary sources.

- Secondary sources are not limited in time and space. That is, the researcher using them need not have been present when and where they were gathered.

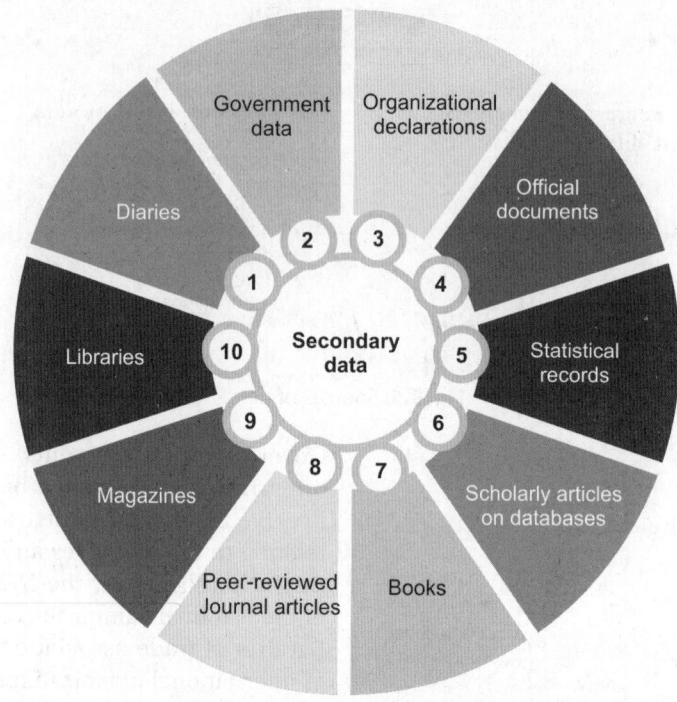

Fig. 9.7: Secondary sources of data.

METHODS OF COLLECTING PRIMARY DATA

Primary data are directly collected by the researcher from their original sources. In this case, the researcher can collect the required data precisely according to his research needs, he can collect them when he wants them and in the form he needs them. But the collection of primary data is costly and time consuming. Yet, for several types of social science research required data are not available from secondary sources and they have to be directly gathered from the primary sources.

In such cases, where the available data are inappropriate, inadequate or obsolete, primary data have to be gathered. They include: socio-economic surveys, social anthropological studies of rural communities and tribal communities, sociological studies of social problems and social institutions, nursing research, leadership studies, opinion polls, attitudinal surveys, readership, radio listening and T.V. viewing surveys, knowledge-awareness practice (KAP) studies, nursing

management studies, hospital management studies, etc.

There are various methods of data collection. A 'method' is different from a 'tool.' While a method refers to the way or mode of gathering data, a tool is an instrument used for the method. For example, a schedule is used for interviewing. The important methods are: (a) Observation, (b) Interviewing, (c) Mail survey, (d) Experimentation, (e) Simulation, and (f) Projective technique. To collect primary data during the course of doing experiments in an experimental research but in case we do research of the descriptive type and perform surveys, whether sample surveys or census surveys, then we can obtain primary data either through observation or through direct communication with respondents in one form or another or through personal interviews.

This, in other words, means that there are several methods of collecting primary data, particularly in surveys and descriptive researches.

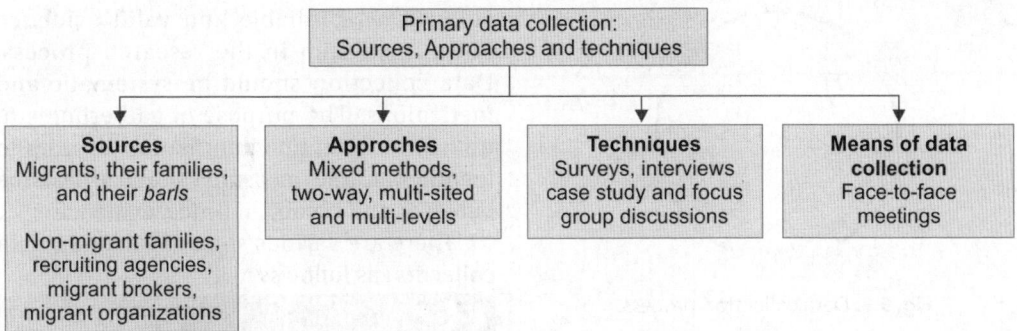

Fig. 9.8: Primary data collection techniques.

Important ones are:

- Observation method
- Interview method
- Through questionnaires
- Through schedules
- Other methods which include:
    - Warranty cards
    - Distributor audits
    - Pantry audits
    - Consumer panels
    - Using mechanical devices
    - Through projective techniques
    - Depth interviews
    - Content analysis.

Observations involves gathering of data relating to the selected research by viewing and or listening.

Interviewing involves face-to-face conversation between the investigator and the respondent. Mailing is used for collecting data by getting questionnaires completed by respondents. Experimentation involves a study of independent variables under controlled conditions. Experiments may be conducted in a laboratory or in field in a natural setting. Simulation involves creation of an artificial situation similar to the actual life situation. Projective methods aim at drawing inferences on the characteristics of respondents by presenting to them stimuli. Even method has its advantages and disadvantages.

Steps for Data Collection

- **Identify issues and opportunities for collecting data:** Every tool for collecting

data has its own pros and cons. Thus, for deciding the best method, it is important to identify issues and opportunities for collecting data according to the method. It might be helpful to engage in a pilot study to review our tools and sample size.

- **Setting goals and objectives:** The researcher uses data to address his/her research questions and must design his/her methodology accordingly. Thus, every tool used by the researcher must have certain objectives which could be used for addressing these questions after analysis.

- **Planning approach and methods:** Researcher would make decisions pertaining to who will be surveyed, how data will be collected, sources and tools for data collection, and duration of the project.

- **Collect data:** While planning the data collection, it is important to understand logistical challenges and prepare accordingly.

DATA COLLECTION PROCESS

There are five important questions to ask when the researcher is in the process of collecting data: What?, How?, Who?, Where? and When?

- **What data will be collected?** This question calls for a decision to be made about the type of data that is being sought. The type of data needed to answer the research questions or to test the research hypothesis should be the main consideration in data collection.

- **How will the data be collected?** Some type of research instrument will be

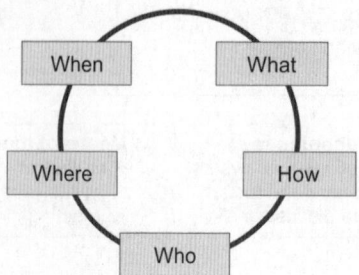

Fig. 9.9: Data collection process.

needed to gather the data. This can vary from a self-report questionnaire to the most sophisticated of physiological instruments. Choosing a data collection instrument is a major decision that should be made only after careful consideration of the possible alternatives.

- **Who will collect the data?** If the researcher is going to collect all the data, this question is easy to answer. The people outside the research team may also be used in the data – collection phase. But training will be needed for the data collections and checks should be made on the reliability of the collected data.
- **Where will the data be collected?** The setting for data collection must be carefully determined. Optimum conditions should be sought. If the questionnaires are being used, a researcher might ask respondents to complete the questionnaires while the researcher remains in the same immediate or general area.
- **When will the data be collected?** the determination will need to be made of the month, day and sometimes even one hour, for data collection. Also, how long will data collection take? if questionnaires will be used, they should be protested with people similar to the potential research subjects to determines the length of time for completion of the instruments.

PROCEDURE FOR DATA COLLECTION

Once the problem has been decided and methodology is planned, the systematic collection of reliable and valid evidence is the next step in the research process. Data collection should be systematic and meticulous. The purpose of gathering is to transform them into information in order to identify variable, measure variables, describe behavior and obtain empirical evidence.

There are various steps involved in data collection as follows:

Sl. No.	Types	Descriptions
1.	Step 1: Define your needs	The first step in any data collection project is simply to assess the needs. Try writing down your overall goal and objectives for collecting data as succinctly as possible. Just this process putting the words on paper will force you to think critically about your needs and help you refine what you are trying to do.
2.	Step 2: clearly define the project	Before you begin any data collection project, you should have a few details clearly defined, preferably written out on paper.
3.	Step 3: Identify the data sources	After clearly defining the project objectives and goals, it is time to start thinking about where to get the data you will need for your project.
4.	Step 4: Plan how to store the data	When collecting the data, you need to have an idea of how the data you collect will be stored (usually on a computer) and how someone may use the collected data to analyze it.
5.	Step 5: Choose your project design	Based on the goals of your project, you will need to select an appropriate study design. There are three main categories of the study design as follows: 1. Descriptive design, 2. Retrospective design, 3. Prospective design.

Contd...

Contd...

Sl. No.	Types	Descriptions
6.	Step 6: Eliminating bias and confounding variables	In this step, it is pointed out that a few principles that is watched carefully before conducting your research or collecting data
7.	Step 7: Participant selection	When you want to gather information about a group of people

DATA COLLECTION METHODS AND INSTRUMENTS

- There are many alternatives to choose from when selecting a data collection method. These methods include questionnaires, interviews, physiological measures, attitude scales, psychological tests, and observational measures.
- The data collection methods are governed by several factors including the research questions or hypothesis, the design of the study and the amount of knowledge available about the variable of interest.
- Many studies use more than one data collection method; in fact, nursing studies are increasingly reporting the use of more than one method of measuring the variables of interest. When several types of data collection methods produce similar results, greater confidence in the study findings will occur.
- Data collection instruments also called research instruments or research tools are the devices used to collect data. The type of instruments used in a study will be determined by the data collection methods selected.
- **Developing an instrument:** If no instrument can be discovered that is appropriate for a particular study, the researcher is faced with developing a new instrument. It may be possible to revise an existing instrument. Causation must be exercised when this approach to instrument developing is used.

- **Pilot study:** A pilot study is a small-scale, trial run of the actual research project. A pilot study should be conducted whenever a new instrument is being developed or when a pre-existing instrument is being used with people who have different characteristics from those for whom the instrument was originally developed.

SELECTION METHODS OF DATA COLLECTION

Methods of data collection should be selected for a proposed research project is one of the questions to be considered while designing the research plan. One or more methods have to be chosen. The choice of a method of a method depends upon the following factors:

- **Nature of the study of the subject-matter:** If it is a study of opinions/preferences of persons, interviewing or mailing may be appropriate depending on the educational level of the respondents. On the other hand, an impact study may call for experimentation; and a study of behavioral pattern may require observation.
- **Unit of enquiry:** The unit of enquiry may be an individual, household institution, or community. To collect data from households, interviewing is preferable. Data from institutions may be collected by mail survey and studies on communities call for observational method.
- **Size and spread of the sample:** If the sample is small and the area covered is compact interviewing may be preferable, but a large sample scattered over a wider area may require mailing.
- **Scale of the survey:** A large scale may require mailing or interviewing through trained investigators.
- **Educational level of respondents:** For a simple survey among educated persons concerned with the subject-matter of study, a mail survey may be appropriate. But for a survey of less educated/illiterate persons like industrial workers, slum dwellers, rural people, interviewing is the only suitable method.

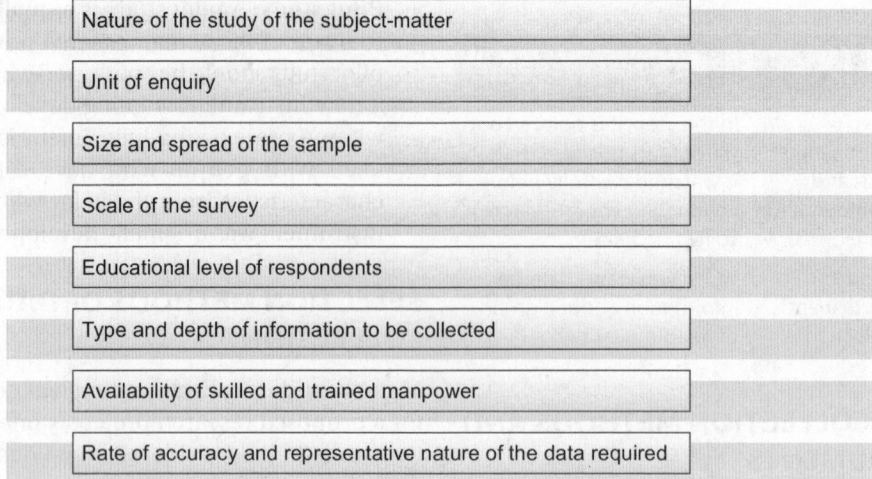

Nature of the study of the subject-matter

Unit of enquiry

Size and spread of the sample

Scale of the survey

Educational level of respondents

Type and depth of information to be collected

Availability of skilled and trained manpower

Rate of accuracy and representative nature of the data required

Fig. 9.10: Selection methods of data collection.

- **Type and depth of information to be collected:** For collection of general, simple, factual and non-emotional data, interviewing or mailing is appropriate. For an in-depth survey of personal experiences and sensitive issues, in-depth interview is essential. For collection of data on behavior, culture, customs, life style, etc., observational method is required.
- **Availability of skilled and trained manpower:** In this case, even for a large general survey entailing many complicated questions, interviewing can be adopted.
- **Rate of accuracy and representative nature of the data required:** Interviewing is the most appropriate method for collecting accurate data from a representative sample of population. Interviewing can achieve a higher response rate.

A researcher can select one or more of the methods keeping in view the above factors. No method is universal. Each methods unique features should be compared with the needs and conditions of the study and thus the choice of the methods should be decided.

SELECTION CRITERIA FOR DATA COLLECTION METHOD

There are several criteria to be considered when deciding on a data collection instrument;

these include the practicality, reliability, and validity of the instrument.

Practicality of the Instrument

The practicality of the instrument concerns its cost and appropriateness for the population.

Reliability of the Instrument

The reliability of an instrument determines its consistency and stability.

- **Stability reliability:** The consistency of a research instrument over time, test-retest procedures and repeated observation are methods to test the stability of an instrument.
- **Equivalence reliability:** The degree of an instrument to which two forms of an instrument obtain the same results or two or more observers obtain the same results when using single instruments to measure a variable.
- **Internal consistency reliability:** (Scale homogeneity) The extent to which all items of an instrument measure the same variable.

Validity

Validity concerns the ability of the instrument together the data that it is intended to gather. The types of validity are face, content, criterion, and construct.

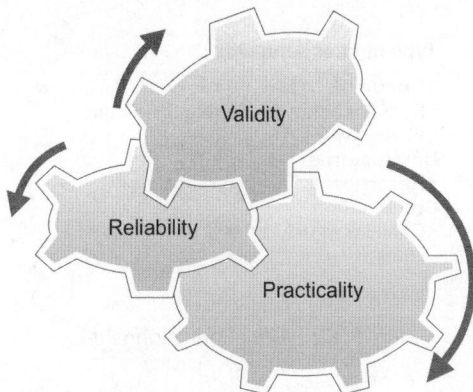

Fig. 9.11: Selection criteria for data collection method.

- **Face validity:** It measures the degree to which an instrument appears, on the surface, to measure the variable of interest.
- **Content validity:** It is concerned with the scope or range of items used to measure the variable.
- **Criterion validity:** It considers the degree to which an instrument correlates with some criterion measure on the variable of interest. Two types of criterion validity are concurrent and predictive.
  1. **Concurrent validity:** It compares an instrument measurement of a variable with a criterion measure of the same variable.
  2. **Predictive validity:** It examines the ability of an instrument to predict behavior of subjects in the future.
- **Construct validity:** It concerns the measurement of a variable that is not directly observable but rather is closely associated.

EVALUATION OF DATA COLLECTION METHOD

The appropriateness of a method of data collection may be evaluated on the basis of the following criteria:
- The efficiency, i.e., the speed and cost of data collection
- Data quality and adequacy, i.e., response rate, accuracy, and objectivity
- Naturalness of setting

- Anonymity
- Interviewer supervision
- Control of context and question order
- Ability to use visual aids
- Potential for controlling variables
- Dependence on respondent's reading and writing ability.

Primary Data

Primary data are the fresh data collected directly from the field. They are first-hand data. Since primary data are collected specially for the purpose in hand, extra care is taken to collect all the required data with appropriate degree of accuracy. Primary data are reliable, complete, and fresh.

Primary data are costly. Their collection consumes more time and labor than the collection of secondary data, especially when the population in vast. If an investigator collects information regarding births and deaths directly from the people, the data are primary data. Important methods of collecting primary data are as follows:
- Direct observation method
- Personal interview method
- Information through correspondents
- Method of questionnaire
- Method of schedule.

Secondary Data

Secondary data are the data which the investigator does not collect directly from the field. They are the data which he borrows from others who have collected them for some other purpose. Since secondary data are primarily collected for some other purpose, they may not contain all the required information. The degree of accuracy may be different. They, generally, are not as dependable as primary data. Secondary data are cheap. Especially, when the population is vast and funds available are meagre, secondary data are preferred. Collection of secondary data consumes less time and labor than collection of primary data.

If an investigator collects the required data of births and deaths from the city corporation office records, the data are secondary data. At the time of collection of secondary data, reliability of the source and validity of the data should be verified. The data should contain all the necessary information with essential degree of accuracy.

Important sources of secondary data are as follows:

- Published sources
    - Reports and publications of Central and State Government departments.
    - Reports and publications of International bodies, such as UNO IME, etc.
    - Publications of banks, research institutions, administrative offices, etc.
    - Magazines and news papers.
    - Websites of various organizations on the internet.
- Unpublished sources
    - Records maintained at Government offices, municipal offices, Panchayat offices, etc.
    - Records maintained by research institutions, research scholars, etc.

DATA COLLECTION METHODS

The word 'data' is a plural form of the word 'datum' which means information that is systematically collected in the course of a study. The word 'method' refers to the means of gathering data that are common to all sciences including nursing. Questionnaires and interviews are probably the most frequently used data collection methods in nursing research. Observation is also an important method of testing research hypothesis and seeking answers to research questions.

QUESTIONNAIRES

Questionnaires is a paper-pencil, self-report instrument. It contains questions that respondents are asked to answer in writing. Questionnaires can be used to measure knowledge levels, opinions, attitudes, beliefs, ideas, feelings and perceptions, as well as

Type of questionnaires

Structured
- Respondents select a response from those given

Unstructured
- Respondents create a response

Combination
- Contains structured and unstructured items

Fig. 9.12: Types of questionnaires.

to gather factual information about the respondents.

Factors to consider in constructing questionnaires are overall appearance, language and reading level, length of questionnaires and questions, wording of questions, types of questions and placement of questions.

Types of Questions

- **Ambiguous questions:** It contain word that has more than meaning.
- **Double barreled questions:** Ask two questions in one.
- **Demographic questions:** It concern subject characteristics.
- **Open-ended questions:** It allow respondents to answer questions in their own words.
- **Closed-ended questions:** Closed-ended questions are very structured and respondents are asked to choose from given alternatives.
- **Contingency questions:** Contingency questions are items that are relevant for some respondents and not for others.
- **Filler questions:** Filler questions are items in which the researcher has no direct interest but are included on a question to reduce the emphasis on the specific purpose of other question.

Advantages of Questionnaires

- It is a quick and generally, in expensive means of obtaining data from a large number of respondents.

Surveys	Questionnaires
Process of collecting and analyzing data	Instrument of data collection
Research process	Research tool
Time consuming process	Fairly quick process
Is conducted	Is delivered
Answers are subjective or objective	Answers are objective
Open-ended and close-ended questions	Close-ended questions only
Conducted for research or studies	Used to collect information on a topic

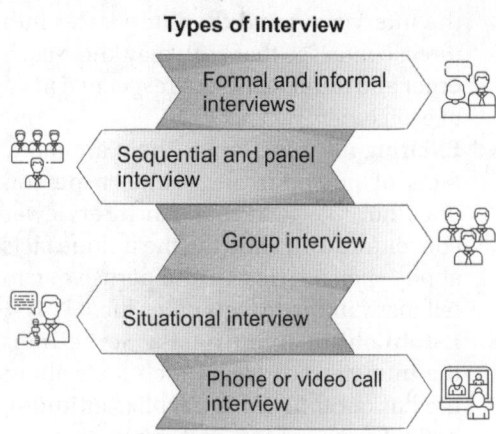

Types of interview

Fig. 9.13: Types of interview.

- It is one of the earliest research instruments to test for reliability and validity.
- The administration of questionnaires is less time consuming than interviews or observation research.
- Data can be obtained from respondents in wide – spread geographical area.
- Respondents can remain anonymous.
- If anonymity is assured, respondents are more likely to provide honest answers.

Disadvantages of Questionnaires

- Mailing of questionnaires may be costly.
- Response rate may be low.
- Respondents may provide socially acceptable answers.
- Respondents may fail to answer some of the items.
- There is no opportunity to clarify items that may be misunderstood by respondents.
- Respondents must be literate.
- The respondents may not be representative of the population.

INTERVIEWS

An interview is a data collection method in which an interviewer obtains responses from a subject in a face-to-face meeting or from telephone interviews. Interviews are frequently used in descriptive research studies and qualitative studies. Interviews are used to obtain factual data about people as well as to measure their opinions, attitudes, and beliefs about certain topics.

Definitions

- Interview is a method of data collection in which one person asks questions of another person. Interviews are conducted either face-to-face or by telephones.
- The interview constitutes a social situation between two persons, the psychological process involved requiring both individuals mutually respond though the social research purpose of the interview calls for a varied response from the two parties concerned.

Types of Interviews

- **Unstructured interviews**: It contains open-ended questions and is appropriate for exploratory studies where the researcher possess little knowledge of the study topic.
- **Structured interviews:** It uses closed-ended questions and is generally used to obtain straight forward, factual information.
- **Semi-structured interviews:** It contains both open-ended and close-ended questions. The majority of interviews are of the semi-structured type.

Aims of Interviews

- **Direct contact:** The first and the foremost aim of the interview method is to bring the interviewer and the interviewer into direct contact so that both may know each other and understand the respective need of each other.

- **Eliciting intimate facts:** There are many facts of personal life, which a person does not like to reveal. An interviewer concentrates on knowing the unique facts about a person. He can also peruse him to tell many intimate facts of his life.
- **Establishing hypothesis:** Sometimes the interviewer reveals such facts about the background of his peculiar attitudes, outlooks, aspirations, and behaviors as are not already in the comprehension of the interviewer.

Advantages of Interviews

- Responses can be obtained from a wide range of subjects.
- Response rate is high.
- Most of the data obtained are usable.
- In-depth responses can be obtained.
- Non-verbal behavior and verbal mannerisms can be observed.

Disadvantages of Interviews

- Training programs are needed for interviewers.
- Interviews are time-consuming and expensive.
- Arrangements for interviews may be difficult to make.

- Interviewer may misinterpret non-verbal behavior.

OBSERVATION METHODS

Observation research is concerned with gathering data through visual observation. Nurses are well qualified to conduct observation research because observations of clients in health care setting are an everyday experience. The researcher must decide what behaviors will be observed, who will observe the behavior, what observational procedure will be used, and what type of relationship will exist between the observer and the subjects.

Types of Observation Procedures

- **Structured observations:** Observations are carried out when the researcher has prior knowledge about the phenomenon of interest. The data collection tool is usually some kind of checklist. The

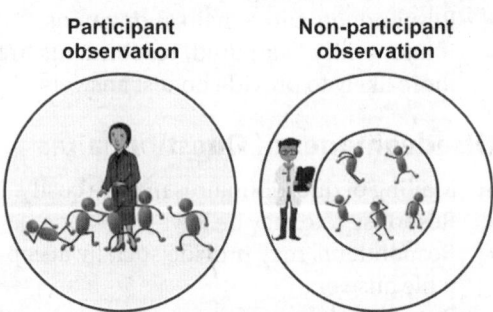

Fig. 9.14: Types of observation.

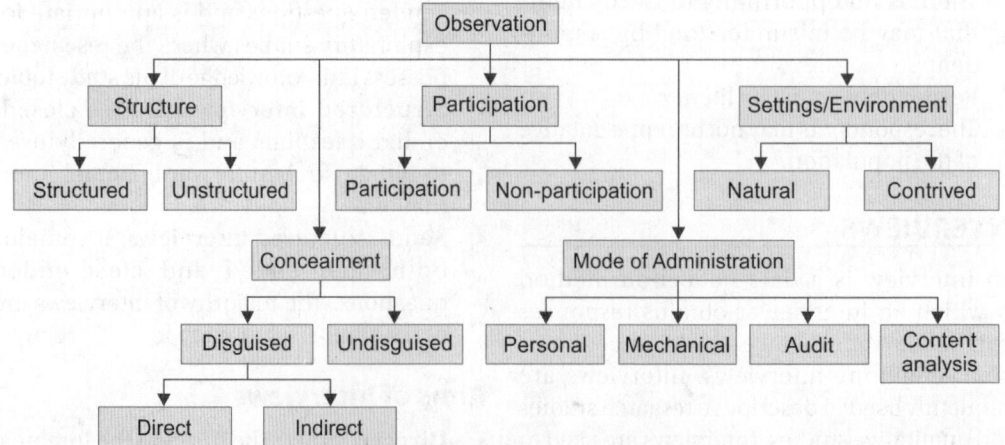

Fig. 9.15: Various types of observation methods.

expected behavior or interest has been identified on the checklist. The observer only needs to indicate the frequency of occurrence of these behaviors.

- **Unstructured observations:** The researcher attempts to describe events or behaviors as they occur, with no preconceived ideas of what will be seen. This requires a high degree of concentration and attention by the observer.

Relationship between Observer and Subjects

- Non-participant observer—overt: The observer openly identifies the research is being conducted.
- Non-participant observer—covert: Does not identify herself as a researcher. This type of observation is quite likely to be unethical.
- Participant observer—overt: Becomes involves with subjects openly and with the full awareness of those people who will be observed in their natural settings.
- Participant observer—covert: Interacts with subject's observers their behavior without their knowledge.

OTHER OBSERVATIONAL METHODS

- **Physiological measures:** Measures involve the collection of physical data from subjects. These measures are generally quite accurate. Many physiological data collection devices are available to nurses, such as thermometers, sphygmomanometers, and stethoscopes. Results of electrocardiograms, electro-encephalograms and other tests are also readily available to nurse researcher. One of the greatest disadvantages is that special expertise may be necessary to use some of these devices.
- **Attitude scale:** Attitude scales are self-report data collection instrument that ask respondents to report their attitudes or feelings on a continuum. The attitude scales are composed of a number of related items, and respondents are given a score after the item responses are totaled.

Types of Attitude Scale

- **Likert scale:** The Likert scale was named after its developer, Rensis Likert. These scales usually contain five or seven responses for each item, ranging from strongly agree to strongly disagree. An approximately equal number of positively and negatively worded items should be included on a Likert instrument.
- **Semantic differential scale:** This technique was developed by Osgood, suci, and Tannenbaum (1957) to measure the psychological meaning of concepts. They used the term semantic differential to indicate that the difference in subject's attitudes could be compared by examining their responses in "semantic space" or attitudinal space. This technique also may be used to evaluate a setting a person, a group or an educational course.

RATING SCALE METHOD

Rating is the term applied to expression of opinion or judgment regarding some situation, object, or character. The rating scale involves qualitative description of a limited number of aspects of a thing or traits of a person. When we use rating scales, we judge an object in absolute terms against some specified criteria, i.e., we judge properties of objects without reference to other similar objects.

Definition

Rating scale refers to a scale with a set of points which describe varying degrees of the dimension of an attitude being observed.

Classification

Rating scale is classified into:
- Graphic rating scale.
- Itemized rating scale/numerical rating scale.
- Comparative rating scale.
- Rank order scale.

- Self-rating scale.
- Standard scales.
- Forced choice ratings.

- **Graphic rating scale:** The graphic rating scale is quite simple and is commonly used in practice. In this type, the rater (who may be the subject himself) indicates his rating by simply marking a mark () at the appropriate point on the line of statements that runs from one extreme of the attribute or characteristic in question to the other extreme. For example, "how do you like the product?" Number one is least and highest number is most.

- **Itemized/numerical rating scale:** In this type, the rater selects one of the limited numbers of categories that are ordered in terms of three scale positions. It presents a series of statements from which a respondent selects one as best reflecting its evaluation. These statements are ordered progressively in terms of more or less some property. Scales with five or seven categories are usually employed. For example, to identify the educational level:

  - Professional education.
  - College level.
  - High school level.
  - Primary education.
  - Illiterate.

- **Comparative rating scale:** In this scale, rater is making the judgment on the basis of the individual. The rater evaluates positions in terms of relationship to other individuals or groups whose characteristics are known. We make relative judgments against other similar objects. The respondents under this method directly compared two or more objects and make choices among them. The rater/respondent, for example, may be called upon to indicate whether a problem-solving skill or some other attribute most closely resembles that of Mr X, Mr Y, and Mr Z, etc., all of whom may be known to

Graphic Scale Rating

Employee Name...

Department...

Job title...

Performance level / Work dimension	Poor	Fairly poor	Fairly good	Good	Excellent
Attendance			✔		
Behavior towards subordinates			✔		
Sincerity				✔	
Dependability					✔

Fig. 9.16: Graphic rating scale.

him (the rater), on the matter of skill and attitude.

- **Rank order scale:** Here the rater is required rank subjects/persons specifically in relation to one another. Ranking is the placement of a series of variables in ascending or descending order or the placement of an item in a category of more or less than some other item-one individual may rank higher than another in a language exam. In rating, an item is given a measure worth. When we rate a variable we are assigning a value to it. Ranking and rating technique differs in that ranking requires the judge to compare products against each other while rating requires the judge to compare products against an absolute scale. A rank in relation to all other units in the system is being measured. Rank is meaningless, unless it is given in relationship to the total. Ranking is used as an ordinal scale only. It simply says that one is higher than the other although it does not specify how much.

- **Self-rating scale:** The rater himself is the subject for the rating-it is called self-rating. Self-rating has certain typical advantages. The individual (the rater himself) is often in a better position to observe and report his feelings, opinions, etc. than anyone else. But if the individual is not aware, as is not unusual, of his biases, beliefs or feelings or is aware of such feelings but does not wish to express them for certain reasons (such as fear or image conservation) then self-rating procedure may prove to be of little value.

- **Standard scales:** In the standard scales, a set of standards is presented to the rater. The standards are of the same kind to be rated with pre-established scale values, e.g., scales for judging the quality of handwriting. The scales of handwriting provides several standard specimens that have previously been spread over on a common scale by the methods of equal-appearing intervals or pair comparisons. A new sample of handwriting can be equated to one of the standards or judged as being between two standards.

- **Forced choice ratings:** In this method, the rater is asked not to say whether the rater has a certain trait or to say how much of a trait the rater has but to say essentially whether he has more of one trait than other of a pair. Descriptions are analyzed into simple behavior quality stated in very short sentences or by trial names. For example, two pair's statements, one pair with high preference value and one with low preference value is combined in a tetrad to form an item.

LIKERT SCALES

The Likert scale is an ordinal psychometric measurement of attitudes, beliefs, and opinions. In each question, a statement is presented in which a respondent must indicate a degree of agreement or disagreement in a multiple choice type format. The advantageous side of the Likert scale is that they are the most universal method for survey collection, therefore they are easily understood. The responses are easily quantifiable and subjective to computation of some mathematical analysis. Since it does not require the participant to provide a simple and concrete yes or no answer, it does not force the participant to take a stand on a particular topic, but allows them to respond in a degree of agreement; this makes question answering easier on the respondent.

Likert Scale/Summated

- Rensis Likert developed the summated scale as a measurement device and thus named Likert.
- Likert scale consists of several statements expressing viewpoints on a topic.
- Responders indicate the degree to which they agree or disagree with each statement.
- The Likert scale usually contains as few as 4 or 5 scales. It is scored by running the numerical.
- We find these five points constitute the scale. At one extreme of the scale, there is

strong agreement with the given statement and at other strong disagreement and between lie intermediate points. Each point on the scale carries a score. Response values attached to the scale anchors. Positive and negative items are scored differently and compared and concluded accordingly to know the findings, i.e., a particular item is evaluated on the basis how well it discriminates between those persons whose total score is high and whose score is low.

Strongly agree	Agree	Undecided	Disagree	Strongly disagree
(i)	(ii)	(iii)	(iv)	(v)

The Likert scale consists of items reflecting extreme positions on a continuum, items with which people are likely either to agree or disagree. The items are typically presented in a graphic format that includes end points labeled "agree" and "disagree".

In Likert scale, the respondent is asked to respond to each of the statements in terms of several degrees, usually five degrees (but at times 3 or 7 may be used) of agreement or disagreement. For example, when asked to express opinion whether one considers his job quite pleasant, the respondent may respond in any one of following ways. i. Agree, ii. Undecided, iii. Disagree, and iv. Strongly disagree.

It can be illustrating this as under. Indicating the least favorable degree of job satisfaction is given the least score (1) and most favorable is given the highest score. If this instrument consist of 30 statements the following score values would be revealing.

Procedure

- Write a thought the scaled.
- Select a sample of respondent's represen-tation of the population on, which the scale will be used.
- Code all responses so that a higher score on a particular item indicates a stronger agreement with the attitude being scaled. Compute a scale score for each person by summating her or his course on all questions. Example: Strongly agree, agree undecided, disagree, and strongly disagree.
- Analyze responses and select for the scale the item most clearly differentiating between the highest and lowest scores. Each item can be correlated with the

Response set	1	2	3	4	5
Frequency	Never	Rarely	Sometimes	Often	Always
Quality	Very poor	Poor	Fair	Good	Excellent
Intensity	None	Very mild	Mild	Moderate	Severe
Agreement	Strongly disagree	Disagree	Neither agree or disagree	Agree	Strongly agree
Approval	Strongly disapprove	Disapprove	Neutral	Approve	Strongly approve
Awareness	Not at all aware	Slightly aware	Moderately aware	Very aware	Extremely aware
Importance	Not at all important	Slightly important	Moderately important	Very important	Extremely important
Familiarity	Not at all familiar	Slightly familiar	Moderately familiar	Very familiar	Extremely familiar
Satisfaction	Not at all satisfied	Slightly satisfied	Moderately satisfied	Very satisfied	Completely satisfied
Performance	Far below standards	Below standards	Meets standards	Above standards	Far above standards

total scores or with other items that discriminate well between the highest and lowest qualities of scores and items that do not correlate can be eliminated.

Advantages

- It is relatively easy to construct this scale in comparison to Thurstone type and can be performed without a panel of judges.
- It is considered as more reliable because under it respondents answer each statement included in the instrument. As such, it also provides more information and data than does the Thurstone scale.
- Each state is given an empirical test for discriminating ability and as such, unlike Thurstone, Likert permits the use of statements that are not manifestly related to the attitude being studied.
- It can easily be used in respondent-centered and stimulus-centered studies. By this, we can study how respondents differ between people and respondent between stimuli.
- It requires less time to construct, it is frequently used by the students of research.

Disadvantages

- Results are easily faked where individuals want to present a false impression of their attitudes (this can be offset somewhat by developing a good level of rapport with the respondents and convincing them that honest responses are in their best interests).
- Intervals between points on the scale do not present equal changes in attitude for all individuals (i.e., the differences between "strongly agree" and "agree" may be slight for one individual and great for another).
- Internal consistency of the scale may be difficult to achieve (care must be taken to have one-dimensional items aimed at a single person, group, event, or method).
- Good attitude statements take time to construct (it is usually best to begin by constructing several times as many attitude statements as you will actually

need, then selecting only those that best assess the attitude in question).

PSYCHOLOGICAL TESTS

- **Personality inventories:** They are self-report measures used to assess the differences in personality traits, needs, or values of people. These inventories seek information about a person by asking questions or requesting responses to statements that are presented. Scores are then derived for each person for the trait being measured. Some of the commonly used personality inventories are the Minnesota multiphasic personality inventory (MMPI) and Edwards personal preference schedule (EPPS).
- **Projective techniques:** A data collection method that is believed to be more accurate in gathering psychological data is the projective method. In the various projective techniques, a subject is presented with stimuli that are designed to be ambiguous or to have no definite meaning. Then the person is asked to describe the stimuli or to tell what the stimuli appear to represent. The response reflects the internal feelings of the subjects that are projected onto the external stimuli. The commonly used projective test is the thematic appearance test.

Other Methods

- **Q-methodology:** Also called Q-sort, is a means of obtaining data in which subjects sort statements into categories, according to their attitudes forward or rating of, the statements. The statements are written on card or pieces of paper and respondents are asked to arrange the items in piles according to the intensity of their attitudes or beliefs about the items.
- **Delphi technique:** It uses several rounds of questionnaires to seek consensus on a particular topic from a group of experts. This procedure is appropriate for examining the opinions, beliefs or future predictions of knowledgeable people on a topic of interest.

- **Visual analog scale (VAS):** It represents subjects with a straight line drawn on a piece of paper, and subjects are asked to make a mark on the line at the point that corresponds to their experience of pain, for example.
- **Pre-existing data:** Are data from records of agencies, such as hospitals, the governments and public health departments that have not been collected for research purposes.

CONCLUSION

Data collection would begin after a researcher has clearly defined and articulated his/her research problems. Data can be collected in two ways: By using primary sources, and by using secondary sources. The primary data is collected after visiting the field. Thus, it acts as a first-hand information to address a specific research problem. The secondary data has been collected by someone else and it has been through a rigorous statistical process. For collecting data, the researcher must decide which kind of data he/she would be using for the study. The methods of collecting primary and secondary data differ as primary data is collected originally, while in case of secondary data, the data collection work is merely about compiling the given data.

10

Analysis of Data: Classification and Tabulation

LEARNING OBJECTIVES

- Classification of data
- Tabulation
- Data classification

- Data analysis process
- Data analysis in quantitative research
- Data analysis in qualitative research

INTRODUCTION

Data analysis is a process of inspecting, cleansing, transforming, and modeling data with the goal of discovering useful information, informing conclusions, and supporting decision-making. Data analysis has multiple facets and approaches, encompassing diverse techniques under a variety of names, and is used in different business, science, and social science domains. In today's business world, data analysis plays a role in making decisions more scientific and helping businesses operate more effectively

DEFINITION

- Data analysis is a process of inspecting, cleansing, transforming, and modeling data with the goal of discovering useful information, informing conclusions, and supporting decision-making.
- Definition of research in data analysis: According to LeCompte and Schensul, research data analysis is a process used by researchers for reducing data to a story and interpreting it to derive insights. The data analysis process helps in reducing a large chunk of data into smaller fragments, which makes sense.

CLASSIFICATION OF DATA

Data classification is broadly defined as the process of organizing data by relevant categories so that it may be used and protected more efficiently. On a basic level, the classification process makes data easier to locate and retrieve. Data classification is of particular importance when it comes to risk management, compliance, and data security.

Definition

- Data classification is the process of analyzing structured or unstructured data and organizing it into categories based on file type, contents, and other metadata.
- **Array:** The raw data can be arranged in an ascending or descending order of values. This arrangement is called arraying, the format of arraying the data called an array.
- **Frequency:** It is defined as number of times each values of variable occurs in the series. It requires to the number of repetitions of a particular value of variables. It is shown with the help of counting against the particular value of class.
- **Class interval:** Class interval is defined as the size of each group of the data beginning with the lower limit and end with the

upper limit. So it is a group constitute by two limits.

Objectives of Data Classification

The primary objectives of data classification are:

- To consolidate the volume of data in such a way that similarities and differences can be quickly understood. Figures can consequently be ordered in sections with common traits.
- To aid comparison.
- To point out the important characteristics of the data at a flash.
- To give importance to the prominent data collected while separating the optional elements.
- To allow a statistical method of the materials gathered.

Reasons for Data Classification

Data classification has improved significantly over time. Today, the technology is used for a variety of purposes, often in support of data security initiatives. But data may be classified for a number of reasons, including ease of access, maintaining regulatory compliance, and to meet various other business or personal objectives. In some cases, data classification is a regulatory requirement, as data must be searchable and retrievable within specified timeframes. For the purposes of data security, data classification is a useful tactic that facilitates proper security responses based on the type of data being retrieved, transmitted, or copied.

Types

The data needed for a nursing science research may be broadly classified into:

- Data pertaining to human beings,
- Data relating to organizations, and
- Data pertaining to territorial areas, personal data or data related to human beings consist of:
  - *Demographic and socioeconomic characteristics of individuals:* Age, sex, race, social class, religion, marital

status, education, occupation, income, family size, location of the household, life style, etc.

- *Behavioral variables:* Attitudes, opinions, awareness, knowledge, practice, intentions, etc., organizational data consist of data relating to an organization's origin, ownership, objectives, resources, functions, performance and growth. Territorial data are related to geophysical characteristics, resources endowment, population, occupational pattern, infrastructure, structure, degree of development, etc., of spatial divisions like villages, cities, taluks, districts, stat and the nation. The data collected maybe for profile or prospective studies at local, state, national or international level. They are analyzed to assess changes in health or disease situations in the community or population by standard parameters. The statistical data obtained from the above sources can be divided into two broad categories **(Fig. 10.1)**:
  1. Qualitative
  2. Quantitative.

Qualitative (or Discrete) Data

- They are classified by counting the individuals having the same characteristic of attribute and not by measurement. There is only one variable, i.e., the number of persons and not the characteristic.
- Persons with the same characteristic are counted to form specific groups or classes such as attacked, escaped, died, cured, relieved, vaccinated, males, young, old,

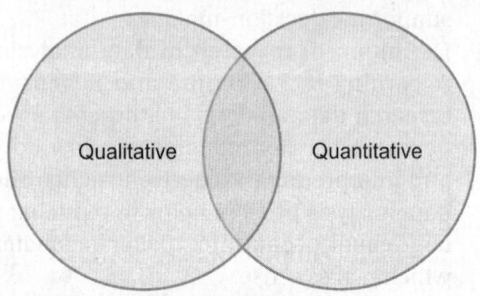

Fig. 10.1: Categories of data.

treated, not treated, on drug on placebo, etc.

- The characteristic such as being attacked by a disease or being treated by a drug is not a measurable variable, only the frequency of persons treated or diseased, varies. By one line of treatment 20 survive out of 25 while on the other line, 15 may survive out of 25. The characteristic, i.e., survival, remains the same but the number or frequency of survivors varies.
- Qualitative data are discrete in nature such as number of deaths in different years, population of different towns, persons with different blood groups in a population, and so on.
- In medical studies such data are mostly collected in pharmacology to find the action of a drug, in clinical practice to test or compare the efficacy of a drug.
- Vaccine, operation or line of treatment and in demography to find births, deaths, stillbirths, etc.
- The results thus obtained are expressed as a ratio, proportion, percentage or a rate.
- The statistical methods commonly employed in analysis of such data are standard error of proportion and chi-square tests as discussed in later chapters.

Quantitative (or Continuous) Data

- In statistical language any character, characteristic or quality that varies is called variable.
- In qualitative data as explained above the characteristics such as births, attacked or died do not vary, only the frequency, i.e., the number born or attacked varies.
- The quantitative data have a magnitude. The characteristics are measured either on an interval or on a ratio scale. In such classification, there are two variables: The characteristics such as height and the frequency, i.e., the number of persons with the same characteristic and in the same range.
- Height varies from person to person, it may be 150 cm in one and 160 cm in another person of the same age and sex.

- Number of persons with 150 cm, or in the range of 150 to 152 cm, may be 10 while those with height 160 cm or in the range of 160 to 162 cm, may be 20. Thus, we find the characteristic as well as the frequency both vary from person to person as well as from group to group.
- The quantitative data obtained from characteristic variable are also called continuous data as each individual has one measurement from a continuous spectrum or range such as body temperature from 35 to 42°C, height 150 to 180 cm, pulse rate from 68 to 84 per minute, and so on.
- The observations ascend or descend from 0 or any starting point in the range of spectrum, such as systolic blood pressure of 100 individuals rising from lowest 90 mm of Hg to the highest 150 mm of Hg.
- The characteristic may be measurable in whole numbers and fractions such as chest circumference 33 cm, 34.5 cm, 35.2 cm, 36 cm, 37.3 cm, and so on or it may be measurable or countable in discrete whole numbers only, such as pulse rate; cholesterol; blood pressure; erythrocyte sedimentation rate (ESR); blood sugar; etc.
- In medical studies, such statistics are mostly collected in anatomy and physiology, i.e., in health, to define the normal or to find the limits of deviation from the normal in healthy persons.
- When the measurement or counting crosses the normal limits, it becomes unusual and may indicate pathology.
- Some of the statistical methods employed in analysis of such data are mean, range, standard deviation, coefficient of variation and correlation coefficient.

Types of Data Classifications (Fig. 10.2)

The data can be classified on the basis of following four criterias:

Geographical

In this type of classification data are classified on the basis of geographical or vocational

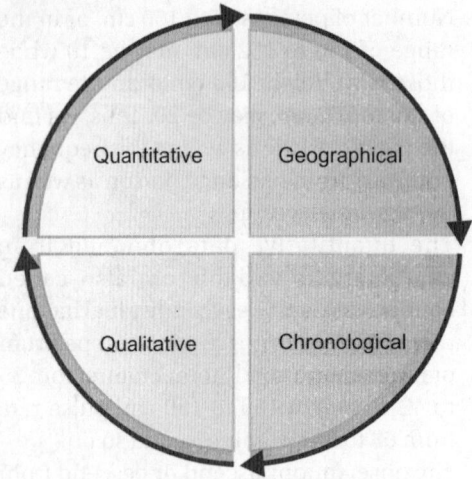

Fig. 10.2: Types of data classification.

differences between the various item like states, cities, regions, zones, etc.

Chronological

When data are observed over a period of time the type of classification is known as chronological classifications.

Sl. No.	Year	Population (in crores)
1.	1941	31.87
2.	1951	36.11
3.	1961	43.92

Qualitative

In other type classification data are classified on the basis of some attribute or quality such as sex, color of hair, literacy, religion, etc., here the attribute cannot be measured, one can only find out whether it is present or absent in the units of the population understudy. *Example:* If the attribute under study is population one can find how many people are living in urban areas and how many in rural areas.

Quantitative

Quantitative classification refers to the classification of data according to some characteristics that can be measured, such as height, weight, income, sales, production, etc. *Example:* 150 patients of a hospital may be classified according to weight as follows:

Wt. in kg	45–55	55–65	65–75	75–85	85–95
No. of patients	45	32	36	24	13

Formation of statistical services

In the process of organizing the data pertaining to a quantitative phenomenon. The following four series are considered.
1. Individual series
2. Discrete series
3. Grouped series
4. Continuous series.

Frequency distribution

Presentation of values of variables arranged according to their magnitude either individuality or in group or classes. It depicts the different values of variable in one column and their respective frequencies in another. It is also called as frequency table, frequency chart and frequency series. There are three types of frequency distribution. They are as follows:

1. **Discrete (discontinuous) frequency distribution:** The variables which can take only definite or particular integers are called discrete frequency distribution. While constructing the discrete frequency distribution we count the number of times each value of variable occurs in the series. This is facilitated through the techniques or tally bars or tally marks method.
   - *Tally mark method:* Tally bars are small vertical lines or bars scored parallel to each other. They are put opposite to a particular value or class to facilitate the counting of the frequencies. Usually a block of five bars is used in the counting processes. This procedure makes the counting process easier in the form of a unit of five frequencies.

2. **Grouped frequency distribution:** When the number of observations and the number of values of variables both are large in size, the discrete frequency distribution is not suitable. The entire range of the values of variables is to be considered by dividing it into a suitable groups or classes. Each class is having two limits: upper limit and lower limit.

As the values of variables are integers or whole numbers (not functional) inclusive method of classes are prepared. Both the limits are included while counting the number of observations against the particular class. However, there is a gap of one between the upper limit of the proceeding class interval and the lower limit of the succeeding class interval.

3. **Continuous frequency distribution:** When the number of observation and number of values of variables both are large in size and the values of variable are both integral and fractional, the grouped frequency distribution is not suitable. The entire range of values is to be considered by dividing it into suitable groups or classes. Each class is having two limits: Upper and lower limit. Exclusive method of classes is prepared. There will not be a gap of 1 between the upper limit of the proceeding class and the lower limit of the succeeding class.

TABULATION

The collected data and classified data can be presented in a tabular form. Tabulation stands for the systematic and scientific presentation of quantitative date in such a form as to elucidate the problem under consideration. Thus tabulation in an orderly arrangement of data in columns and rows systematically in a tabular form. In fact tabulation is the first step before the data is used for analysis or interpretation. By tabulation the data becomes simple for a lot of collection of statistical data.

Definition

Tabulation is the first step before the data is used for analysis of interpretation. A table can be simple or complex. Both qualitative and quantitative data may be presented in numerical form through tables.

Objectives of Tabulation

- To summarize the data systematically.
- To classify the data in a simple form.
- To facilitate the data for a comparative study.
- To present the data in a minimum space.

Meaning of Tabulation

The collected and classified data can be presented in a tabular form. Tabulation stands for the systematic and scientific presentation of quantitative data in such a form as to elucidate the problem under consideration. Thus, tabulation is an orderly arrangement of data in columns and rows systematically in a tabular form. In fact tabulation is the first step before the data is used for analysis or presentation. By tabulation the data becomes simple for a lot of collection of statistical data.

Classifications of Tabulation

- **Simple table:** Only one type of data or characteristics is presented.
- **Frequency distribution table:** In this, the data is first split up into convenient groups (class intervals) and the number of items (frequency) which occur in each group in the adjacent column.

Frequency Distribution Table

It is the method by which data of a long series of observations are systematically organized and recorded. Each one of the observations should fall into one and only one of the categories and there should be at least one category for each observation, i.e., categories should mutually exclusive and exhaustive.

Steps for presentation of a frequency distribution table

- Determine the range between the highest and lowest observation.
- Settle upon either number or size of the groupings (class intervals) for making classification. Estimate the other (number of classes or size! width) by using the relationship. W = R/K; where W is width or size of the class K is no. of class intervals R range (difference between the smallest and the largest observation). A commonly followed rule of thumb states that there should be no fewer than six intervals and

no more than 15. Those who wish to have more specific guidance in the matter of deciding how many class intervals are needed may use the formula which gives K = 1 + 3.322 log (N); where, K stands for the no. of class intervals and N is the no. of values in the data set under consideration. Class intervals generally should be of the same width, this is essential for comparison of different class frequencies.

- Tally the observations in their proper class. (Give four straight and one oblique line to make a bundle of five).
- Count tallies and present the classification in tabular form with a suitable heading.

Basic Principles for Tabulation of Data

- The tables should be numbered like table: Table 1, Table 2, so on.
- Title of the table must be brief and self-explanatory.
- The heading of the columns and rows should be clear and concise, e.g., height in cm, weight in kg, age in years, etc.
- The data must be presented according to size or importance.
- If percentage or averages are to be compared they should be placed as close as possible to the actual numbers in the data.
- The table should not be too large or too small. 10–20 rows are allowed in a table. Ideal is 20 rows.
- The class interval should be the same throughout the table except in case of age.
- Groups should be tabulated in ascending or descending order from the lowest value in the range to highest value.
- If certain data is omitted or extended details should be given.

Components of a Table

The various components of a table may vary from case to case depending upon the given data. But a good table must contain at least the following components:
- Table number
- Table heading

- Caption
- Stub
- Body of table
- Head note
- Footnote

Let us throw some light on these components one by one.

Presentation of Table

Tables are orderly arrangement of data. Following are the different parts of table necessary for preparation of a table:

- **Table number:** When a number of tables are used in a report, each table should be numbered for the purpose of identification and reference.
- **Title:** A table should have suitable title which is placed at the top with bold letters. The title should be complete and unambiguous as regard the subject matter of the data. It should be clear, properly worded and self-explanatory.
- **Captions:** They refer to the heading of the information shown at the top of the vertical column. Under the captions, there may be subheading which is written in small letters.
- **Body:** It refers to the numerical information that are present in the caption and status. It covers the major portion of the table.
- **Head note:** It is a brief note preferably placed in brackets just below the title. It is a preparatory or supplementary note to the title.
- **Footnote:** It is a brief note given at the foot of the table. It meant to clarify certain terms in details. They can be attached to any part of the table by using the asterisk to show that explanation is given below.
- **Source note:** A source note is given at the bottom of the table, the foot note which contains the name of the publication and the journal from which the data are collected.

Mechanical Tabulation

- Edge punch cards are also called as Cope-chat cards, McBee cards; these are cards of standard size having a row of holes along each edge at fixed positions.

- Here cards of 5" X 8" are employed. Coded information is transferred to these cards.
- In the simplest case a single hole is assigned and only two alternatives are permitted for any item, say yes or no. For any one specified alternative a V-shaped notch is cutout of the card so as to obliterate any desired hole by means of a punch similar to an ordinary ticket punch.
- A diagonal cut across one corner of each of these cards provide a check that the edges of all cards in the pack are placed in the right position.
- If more than 2 alternatives for an item, a group of holes can allotted for that item and each alternative assigned a punch against a specific hole.

Disadvantages

- They are more expensive than ordinary cards.
- If any mistake is made, a new card will have to be prepared or a special pasting is required.
- While scoring, cards have to be thoroughly checked to see that all cards punched against the hole have fallen and this process because laborious when the cards are in use for sometimes.

DATA ANALYSIS PROCESS

The analysis process consists of five key stages **(Fig. 10.3)**. We will cover each of them more in detail later in the post, but to start providing the needed context to understand what is coming next; here is a rundown of the five essential steps of data analysis.

1. **Identify:** Before you get your hands dirty with data, you first need to identify why do you need it in the first place. The identification is the stage in which you establish the questions you will need to answer. For example, what is the customer's perception of our brand? Or what type of packaging is more engaging to our potential customers? Once the

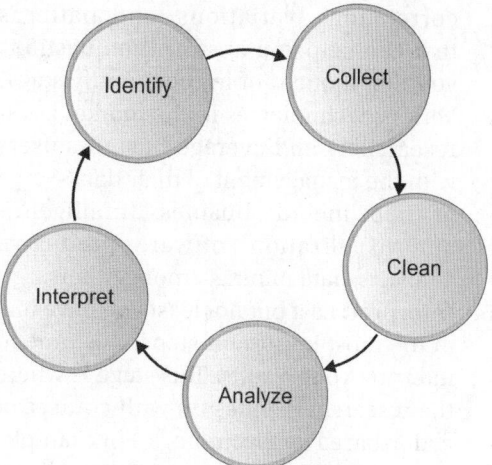

Fig. 10.3: Data analysis process.

questions are outlined you are ready for the next step.

2. **Collect:** As its name suggests, this is the stage where you start collecting the needed data. Here, you define which sources of information you will use and how you will use them. The collection of data can come in different forms such as internal or external sources, surveys, interviews, questionnaires focus groups, among others. An important note here is that the way you collect the information will be different in a quantitative and qualitative scenario.

3. **Clean:** Once you have the necessary data it is time to clean it and leave it ready for analysis. Not all the data you collect will be useful, when collecting big amounts of information in different formats it is very likely that you will find yourself with duplicate or badly formatted data. To avoid this, before you start working with your data you need to make sure to erase any white spaces, duplicate records, or formatting errors. This way you avoid hurting your analysis with incorrect data.

4. **Analyze:** With the help of various techniques such as statistical analysis, regressions, neural networks, text analysis, and more, you can start analyzing and manipulating your data to extract relevant conclusions. At this stage, you find trends,

correlations, variations, and patterns that can help you answer the questions you first thought of in the identify stage. Various technologies in the market assist researchers and average business users with the management of their data. Some of them include business intelligence and visualization software, predictive analytics, data mining, among others.

5. **Interpret:** Last but not least you have one of the most important steps: it is time to interpret your results. This stage is where the researcher comes up with courses of action based on the findings. For example, here you would understand if your clients prefer packaging that is red or green, plastic or paper, etc. Additionally, at this stage, you can also find some limitations and work on them.

DATA ANALYSIS IN QUANTITATIVE RESEARCH

Preparing Data for Analysis

The first stage in research and data analysis is to make it for the analysis so that the nominal data can be converted into something meaningful. Data preparation consists of the below phases.

Phase I: Data Validation

Data validation is done to understand if the collected data sample is per the preset standards, or it is a biased data sample again divided into four different stages

1. **Fraud:** To ensure an actual human being records each response to the survey or the questionnaire.
2. **Screening:** To make sure each participant or respondent is selected or chosen in compliance with the research criteria.
3. **Procedure:** To ensure ethical standards were maintained while collecting the data sample.
4. **Completeness:** To ensure that the respondent has answered all the questions in an online survey. Else, the interviewer had asked all the questions devised in the questionnaire.

Phase II: Data Editing

- More often, an extensive research data sample comes loaded with errors.
- Respondents sometimes fill in some fields incorrectly or sometimes skip them accidentally.
- Data editing is a process wherein the researchers have to confirm that the provided data is free of such errors.
- They need to conduct necessary checks and outlier checks to edit the raw edit and make it ready for analysis.

Phase III: Data Coding

Out of all three, this is the most critical phase of data preparation associated with grouping and assigning values to the survey responses. If a survey is completed with a 1,000 sample size, the researcher will create an age bracket to distinguish the respondents based on their age. Thus, it becomes easier to analyze small data buckets rather than deal with the massive data pile.

Methods Used for Data Analysis in Quantitative Research

After the data is prepared for analysis, researchers are open to using different research and data analysis methods to derive meaningful insights. For sure, statistical techniques are the most favored to analyze numerical data. The method is again classified into two groups. First, 'descriptive statistics' used to describe data. Second, 'Inferential statistics' that helps in comparing the data.

Descriptive Statistics

This method is used to describe the basic features of versatile types of data in research. It presents the data in such a meaningful way that pattern in the data starts making sense. Nevertheless, the descriptive analysis does not go beyond making conclusions. The conclusions are again based on the hypothesis researchers have formulated so far. Here are a few major types of descriptive analysis methods.

Measures of frequency

- Count, percent, frequency
- It is used to denote home often a particular event occurs.
- Researchers use it when they want to show-case how often a response is given.

Measures of central tendency

- Mean, median, mode
- The method is widely used to demonstrate distribution by various points.
- Researchers use this method when they want to showcase the most commonly or averagely indicated response.

Measures of dispersion or variation

- Range, variance, standard deviation
- Here the field equals high/low points.
- Variance standard deviation = difference between the observed score and mean
- It is used to identify the spread of scores by stating intervals.
- Researchers use this method to showcase data spread out. It helps them identify the depth until which the data is spread out that it directly affects the mean.

Measures of position

- Percentile ranks, quartile ranks
- It relies on standardized scores helping researchers to identify the relationship between different scores.
- It is often used when researchers want to compare scores with the average count.

Inferential Statistics

Inferential statistics are used to make predictions about a larger population after research and data analysis of the representing population's collected sample. For example, you can ask some odd 100 audiences at a movie theater if they like the movie they are watching. Researchers then use inferential statistics on the collected sample to reason that about 80–90% of people like the movie.

Here are two significant areas of inferential statistics.

1. **Estimating parameters:** It takes statistics from the sample research data and demonstrates something about the population parameter.

2. **Hypothesis test:** It is about sampling research data to answer the survey research questions. For example, researchers might be interested to understand if the new shade of lipstick recently launched is good or not, or if the multivitamin capsules help children to perform better at games.

These are sophisticated analysis methods used to showcase the relationship between different variables instead of describing a single variable. It is often used when resear chers want something beyond absolute numbers to understand the relationship between variables.

Here are some of the commonly used methods for data analysis in research.

- **Correlation:** When researchers are not conducting experimental research where-in the researchers are interested to under-stand the relationship between two or more variables, they opt for correlational research methods.

- **Cross-tabulation:** Also called contingency tables, cross-tabulation is used to analyze the relationship between multiple varia-bles. Suppose provided data has age and gender categories presented in rows and columns. A two-dimensional cross-tabulation helps for seamless data analysis and research by showing the number of males and females in each age category.

- **Regression analysis:** For understanding the strong relationship between two variables, researchers do not look beyond the primary and commonly used regression analysis method, which is also a type of predictive analysis used. In this method, you have an essential factor called the dependent variable. You also have multiple independent variables in regression analysis. You undertake efforts to find out the impact of independent variables on the dependent variable. The values of both independent and dependent variables are assumed as being ascertained in an error-free random manner.

- **Frequency tables:** The statistical procedure is used for testing the degree to which two or more vary or differ in an experiment. A considerable degree of variation means research findings were significant. In many contexts, ANOVA testing and variance analysis are similar.

- **Analysis of variance:** The statistical procedure is used for testing the degree to which two or more vary or differ in an experiment. A considerable degree of variation means research findings were significant. In many contexts, ANOVA testing and variance analysis are similar.

Considerations in Research Data Analysis

- Researchers must have the necessary skills to analyze the data, getting trained to demonstrate a high standard of research practice. Ideally, researchers must possess more than a basic understanding of the rationale of selecting one statistical method over the other to obtain better data insights.
- Usually, research and data analytics methods differ by scientific discipline; therefore, getting statistical advice at the beginning of analysis helps design a survey questionnaire, select data collection methods, and choose samples.
- The primary aim of data research and analysis is to derive ultimate insights that are unbiased. Any mistake in or keeping a biased mind to collect data, selecting an analysis method, or choosing audience.
- Irrelevant to the sophistication used in research data and analysis is enough to rectify the poorly defined objective outcome measurements. It does not matter if the design is at fault or intentions are not clear, but lack of clarity might mislead readers, so avoid the practice.
- The motive behind data analysis in research is to present accurate and reliable data. As far as possible, avoid statistical errors, and find a way to deal with everyday challenges like outliers, missing data, data altering, data mining, or developing graphical representation.

DATA ANALYSIS IN QUALITATIVE RESEARCH

Data analysis and qualitative data research work a little differently from the numerical data as the quality data is made up of words, descriptions, images, objects, and sometimes symbols. Getting insight from such complicated information is a complicated process. Hence, it is typically used for exploratory research and data analysis.

Finding Patterns in the Qualitative Data

Although there are several ways to find patterns in the textual information, a word-based method is the most relied and widely used global technique for research and data analysis. Notably, the data analysis process in qualitative research is manual. Here the researchers usually read the available data and find repetitive or commonly used words.

For example, while studying data collected from African countries to understand the most pressing issues people face, researchers might find "food" and "hunger" are the most commonly used words and will highlight them for further analysis.

Methods Used for Data Analysis in Qualitative Research

There are several techniques to analyze the data in qualitative research, but here are some commonly used methods.

- **Content analysis:** It is widely accepted and the most frequently employed technique for data analysis in research methodology. It can be used to analyze the documented information from text, images, and sometimes from the physical items. It depends on the research questions to predict when and where to use this method.
- **Narrative analysis:** This method is used to analyze content gathered from various sources such as personal interviews, field observation, and **surveys**. The majority of times, stories, or opinions shared by

people are focused on finding answers to the research questions.

- **Discourse analysis:** Similar to narrative analysis, discourse analysis is used to analyze the interactions with people. Nevertheless, this particular method considers the social context under which or within which the communication between the researcher and respondent takes place. In addition to that, discourse analysis also focuses on the lifestyle and day-to-day environment while deriving any conclusion.

- **Grounded theory:** When you want to explain why a particular phenomenon happened, then using grounded theory for analyzing quality data is the best resort. Grounded theory is applied to study data about the host of similar cases occurring in different settings. When researchers are using this method, they might alter explanations or produce new ones until they arrive at some conclusion.

CONCLUSION

Data analysis is the process of systematically applying statistical and/or logical techniques to describe and illustrate, condense and recap, and evaluate data. According to Shamoo and Resnik (2003) various analytic procedures "provide a way of drawing inductive inferences from data and distinguishing the signal (the phenomenon of interest) from the noise (statistical fluctuations) present in the data".

BIBLIOGRAPHY

1. Shamoo AE, Resnik BR. Responsible Conduct of Research. Oxford University Press; 2003.
2. Shepard RJ. Ethics in exercise science research. Sports Med. 2002; 32 (3): 169-83.
3. Silverman S, Manson M. Research on teaching in physical education doctoral dissertations: A detailed investigation of focus, method, and analysis. Journal of Teaching in Physical Education. 2003; 22(3): 280-97.
4. Smeeton N, Goda D. Conducting and presenting social work research: some basic statistical considerations. Br J Soc Work. 2003;33: 567-73.
5. Thompson B, Noferi G. Statistical, practical, clinical: How many types of significance should be considered in counseling research? Journal of Counseling and Development.2002; 80(4):64-71.

11

CHAPTER

Data Presentation

LEARNING OBJECTIVES

- Importance of data presentation
- Quantitative data presentation
- Qualitative data presentation

INTRODUCTION

Presentation of data is generally done by either of these two methods:
1. Tabular presentation
2. Graphical presentation

Tabulated data will give some information and also allow for further analysis. The columns and rows in a table make eye strain and there are chances of poor visual impression of data presented in a tabular form. In such circumstances data can be presented in the form of picture, diagram or figure which will help in good comparison through good visual impression. Hence graphs and diagrams are of utmost importance in creating interest from the observational data. One should take care to select major data presentable in graph or diagram. The presentation of data by diagram proves a very considerable aid and has much to commend it, if certain basic principles are not forgotten. Main objective of diagram is to help the eye to grasp series of numbers and to grasp the meaning of series of data and also to assist the intelligence **(Fig. 11.1)**.

DEFINITION

- Presentation of data is refers to the organization of data into tables, graphs or charts, so that logical and statistical conclusions can be derived from the collected measurements.

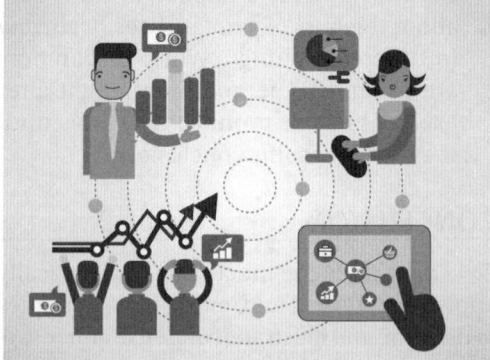

Fig. 11.1: Data presentation in research.

- Presentation of data refers to an exhibition or putting up data in an attractive and useful manner such that it can be easily interpreted.

NEED OF DATA PRESENTATION

Raw data should be presented in a correct manner so that it:
- Arouses interest in the reader.
- Makes the data sufficiently concise without losing important details.
- Enables the readers to form quick impression and to draw some conclusion directly or indirectly.
- Facilitates further statistical analysis.
- It facilitates good communication.

IMPORTANCE OF DATA PRESENTATION

Data presentation could be both, can be a deal maker or deal breaker based on the delivery of the content in the context of visual depiction. Data presentation tools are powerful communication tools that can simplify the data by making it easily understandable and readable at the same time while attracting and keeping the interest of its readers and effectively showcase large amounts of complex data in a simplified manner.

If the user can create an insightful presentation of the data in hand with the same sets of facts and figures, then the results promise to be impressive. There have been situations where the user has had a great amount of data and vision for expansion but the presentation drowned his/her vision. To impress the higher management and top brass of a firm, effective presentation of data is needed.

Data presentation helps the clients or the audience to not spend time grasping the concept and the future alternatives of the business and to convince them to invest in the company and turn it profitable both for the investors and the company. Although data presentation has a lot to offer, the following are some of the major reason behind the essence of an effective presentation:

- Many consumers or higher authorities are interested in the interpretation of data, not the raw data itself. Therefore, after the analysis of the data, users should represent the data with a visual aspect for better understanding and knowledge.
- The user should not overwhelm the audience with a number of slides of the presentation and inject an ample amount of texts as pictures that will speak for themselves.
- Data presentation often happens in a nutshell with each department showcasing their achievements towards company growth through a graph or a histogram.
- Providing a brief description would help the user to attain attention in a small amount of time while informing the audience about the context of the presentation.
- The inclusion of pictures, charts, graphs and tables in the presentation help for better understanding the potential outcomes.
- An effective presentation would allow the organization to determine the difference with the fellow organization and acknowledge its flaws. Comparison of data would assist them in decision making. Presentation of data is shown in **Figure 11.2**.

QUANTITATIVE DATA PRESENTATION

- **Tabulation:** Tabulation is the first step before the data is used for analysis of interpretation. A table can be simple or complex. Both qualitative and quantitative

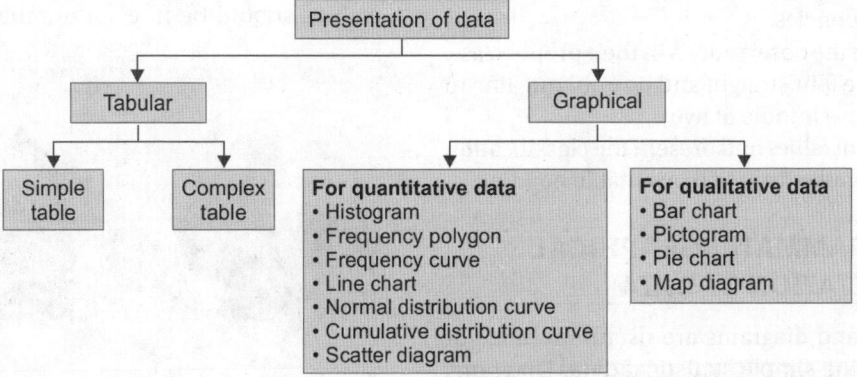

Fig. 11.2: Presentation of data.

data may be presented in numerical form through tables.

- **Tabular presentation:** Frequency distribution table—it is the method by which data of a long series of observations are systematically organized and recorded. Each one of the observations should fall into one and only one of the categories and there should be at least one category for each observation, i.e., categories should mutually exclusive and exhaustive.

Steps for Presentation of a Frequency Distribution Table

- Determine the range between the highest and lowest observation.
- Settle upon either number or size of the groupings (class intervals) for making classification. Estimate the other (number of classes or size width) by using the relationship. W = R/K; where W is width or size of the class K is no. of class intervals R range (difference between the smallest and the largest observation).

  A commonly followed rule of thumb states that there should be no fewer than six intervals and no more than 15. Those who wish to have more specific guidance in the matter of deciding how many class intervals are needed may use the formula which gives K = 1 + 3.322 log (N); where, K stands for the no. of class intervals and N is the no. of values in the data set under consideration. Class intervals generally should be of the same width, this is essential for comparison of different class frequencies.

- Tally the observations in their proper class. (Give four straight and one oblique line to make a bundle of five).
- Count tallies and present the classification in tabular form with a suitable heading.

DIAGRAMMATIC/GRAPHICAL PRESETATION OF DATA

Charts and diagrams are useful methods of presenting simple statistical data. Diagrams are better retained in the memory than statistical tables. Diagrams are attractive and easy to understand, at the same time they free us from the burden of figures, comparison is made easy, time and energy is saved and they become more effective and useful in research **(Fig. 11.3)**.

General Principles

- It should be simple and attractive.
- It should be of proper size.
- Minimum use of words and figures.
- It should present the reality.
- Symbolic presentation and its explanation are essential.
- The facts should be clearly classified in the diagram.
- Every diagram or chart should have a heading.
- The diagram should be absolutely neat and clean.

General Rules of Constructing Diagrams

The following general rules should be followed while constructing diagrams:

- **Title:** Every diagram must be given a suitable title. The title should convey in as few words as possible the main idea that the diagrams intend to portray.
- **Proportion between width and height:** A proper proportion between the height and width of the diagram should be maintained. If the height and width is too short or too long in proportion, the diagram would give an ugly look.
- **Selection of scale:** The scale showing the values should be in even numbers or in

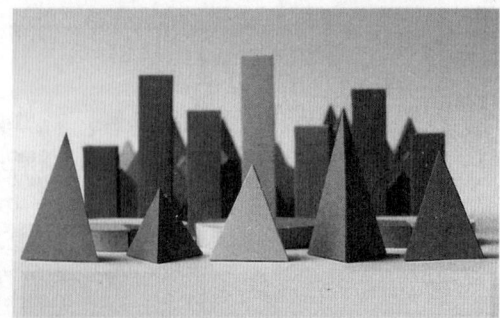

Fig. 11.3: Data presentation.

Table 11.1: Types of graphical presentation of data.

Type	Primary uses	What to keep in mind
Pie chart	• Synthesize quantitative or qualitative data. • Display relative proportions of several classes of data. • Provide visual check and proportional relationship without a lot of explanation.	You can show large amounts of data in total and compare against each other in easily understandable charts. You may want to ensure that you do not have too many "small" categories as these can make the pie chart too busy and difficult to visualize.
Line graph	• Present the relationship between two variables (independent and dependent) over time. • Demonstrate trends and predictions visually to support discussion.	You can map the relationship between variables of interest to you over time in the past and also use for forecasting purposes. Check that the scale on the axis makes sense and is consistent; otherwise, the line graph may be unclear.
Frequency distribution table	• Summarize large amounts of data into groupings. • Present frequency of occurrence of a characteristic within the dataset. • Identify population characteristics to be compared.	This format uses a very intuitive approach; however, values on the extreme (that may be "surprises" and of interest to you) may be hidden within the larger classifications. Very large data sets should typically be segmented into intervals classes to make the table easier to read and understand.

multiplies of five or ten, e.g., 25, 50, 75 or 20, 40, 60. Odd values like 1,3,5,7 should be avoided.

- **Footnotes:** In order to clarify certain points about the diagram, footnotes may be given at the bottom of the diagram.
- **Index:** An index illustrating different types of lines or different shades. Colors should be given so that the reader can easily make out the meaning of the diagram.
- **Neatness and cleanliness:** Diagram should be absolutely neat and clean.
- **Simplicity:** Diagram should be as simple as possible so that the reader can understand their meaning clearly and easily.

Advantages of Diagrammatic Presentation

The most important advantages of diagrammatic presentation of data is that diagrams are very attractive and interesting so far as the common man is concerned. Since no efforts are necessary in understanding diagrams they may save time which is otherwise needed in drawing inferences from set of figures.

- To compare two or more numbers (bar, pictogram)
- To express the distribution of individual objects or measurements into different categories (histogram and pie chart)
- To express the change in some quantity over a period of time (line graph)
- To express the relationship between two measurements in it situation where they occur in pairs (scatter diagram).

Presentation of quantitative, continuous or measured data is through graphs.

The common graphs in use are:

- Histogram
- Frequency polygon
- Frequency curve
- Line chart or graph
- Cumulative frequency diagram
- Scatter or dot diagram

HISTOGRAM

It is a pictorial diagram of frequency distribution **(Fig. 11.4)**. It consists of a series of blocks. The class intervals are given along the horizontal axis and the frequencies along the vertical axis. They are of each block or rectangle is proportion to the frequency. It is a graphical

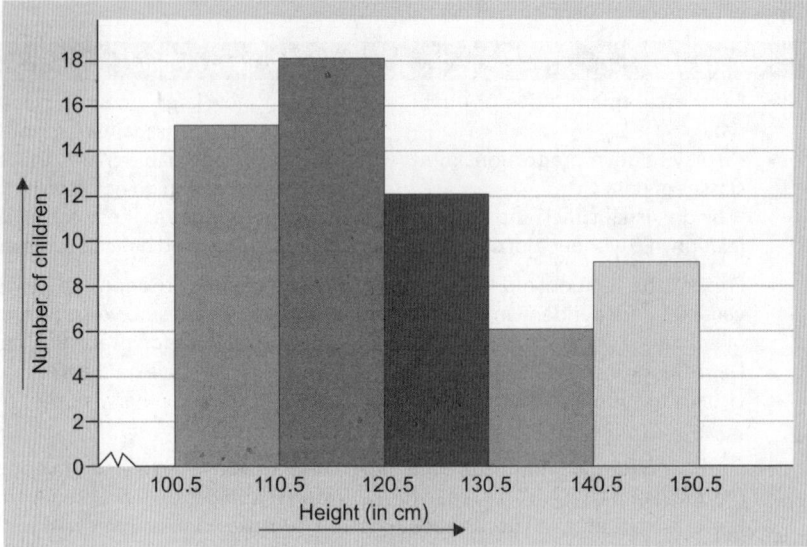

Fig.11.4: Histogram.

presentation of frequency distribution. Variable characters of the different groups are indicated on the horizontal line (X-axis) called abscissa while frequency, i.e., number of observations is marked on the vertical line (Y-axis) called ordinate.

Frequency of each group will form a column or rectangle. Such a diagram is called 'histogram' and is made use of in presenting any quantitative data, obtained after Mantoux test. If the class intervals are different in certain groups then area of the rectangle alone indicates the frequency, e.g., the frequency of the persons in group with size of Mantoux reaction from 16 to 24 mm may be presented as one rectangle only. In this case to plot the frequency for this group, divide the total frequency by 4 (40 ÷ 4). Now the horizontal line will start opposite 10 on the vertical line. It would have given an erroneous idea if the horizontal line would start opposite 40 on the vertical line, instead of 10.

FREQUENCY POLYGON

A frequency distribution may also be represented diagrammatically by the frequency polygon **(Fig. 11.5)**. It is obtained by joining the midpoint of the histogram blocks. It has more than four sides. It is

particularly effective comparing two more frequency distribution. It is again an area diagram of frequency distribution developed over a histogram. Join the midpoints of class intervals at the height of frequencies by straight lines. It gives a polygon, i.e., a figure with many angles.

Types

There are two ways in which a frequency polygon may be constructed.

1. Draw a histogram of the give data and then join by straight lines the midpoints of the upper horizontal side of each rectangle with the adjacent ones. The figured formed is called frequency polygon.

2. Another method is to take the midpoints of the various class intervals and then plot the frequency corresponding to each point and to join all these points by straight lines. Here there will be no histogram.

Steps in Drawing Frequency Polygon

- First take the first group with the lowest class interval, then take the midpoint of these class interval. So place a point corresponding to OX-axis and on OY-axis.
- The same way all the frequencies are marked.

Frequency Polygon

Draw a frequency polygon to represent this data

Key points....

- Firstly, find the midpoints of the groups in the table (same as before)

- Then, plot the midpoints against the frequency on your graphs ***You must be accurate, use a pencil and check the scale !!!**

- Finally, join up your points with a **Ruler** and **Pencil**, starting at the first point, stopping at the last

The frequency table gives information about the times it took some office workers to get to the office one day

Time (t minutes)		Frequency	
$0 < t \le 10$	5	4	(5,4)
$10 < t \le 20$	15	18	(15,18)
$20 < t \le 30$	25	24	(25,24)
$30 < t \le 40$	35	16	(35,16)
$40 < t \le 50$	45	6	(45,6)
$50 < t \le 60$	55	12	(55,12)

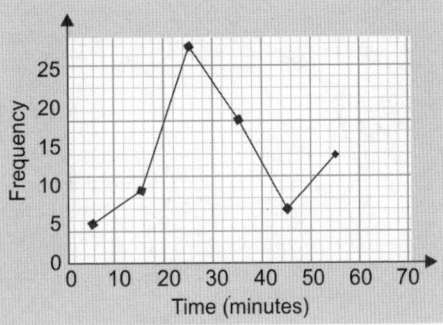

Fig. 11.5: Representation of frequency polygon.

- Then connect the points with straight line.
- Rather than leaving the graph incomplete assumes that there is another interval above or below which is having frequencies of zero. So correct the curve to this zero line. The graph is allowed to meet X-axis on both ends.

Advantages

- Easy to construct and interpret.
- Useful in portaging more than two distributions on same graph with different colors.
- Useful to compare two or more distributions.

FREQUENCY CURVE

When the number of observations is very large and group interval is reduced, the frequency polygon tends to lose its angulation giving place to a smooth curve known as frequency curve. This provides continuous graph giving the relative frequency for each value of an attribute such as that of height in **Figure 11.6** of a normal curve. Such a curve is obtained in normal distribution of individuals in a large sample or of means in population or of differences in pairs of sample means.

A frequency table arranges all data collected in ascending order, showing the number of time a data item or value occurs. Tally marks can be used to record the number of times a value occurs in the data set. It is difficult to construct frequency tables for large sets of data, which makes it necessary for you to classify the data into class intervals or groups, which can help in interpreting, organizing and analyzing the data. Frequency tables are normally used to illustrate nominal and interval data, although they can also be used for representing ordinal data as well. There are merits and demerits associated with using frequency tables for data representation.

Simple to Interpret

Frequency tables are simple to understand and read since they mostly have three columns showing the value, tally and frequency. Other columns such as cumulative frequencies and percentages can also be calculated from the frequencies. The values in the rows and columns are linearly related showing a direct relationship between the data value and the corresponding frequency or percentage. Comparison between different data sets or frequencies can be made when frequency tables are used.

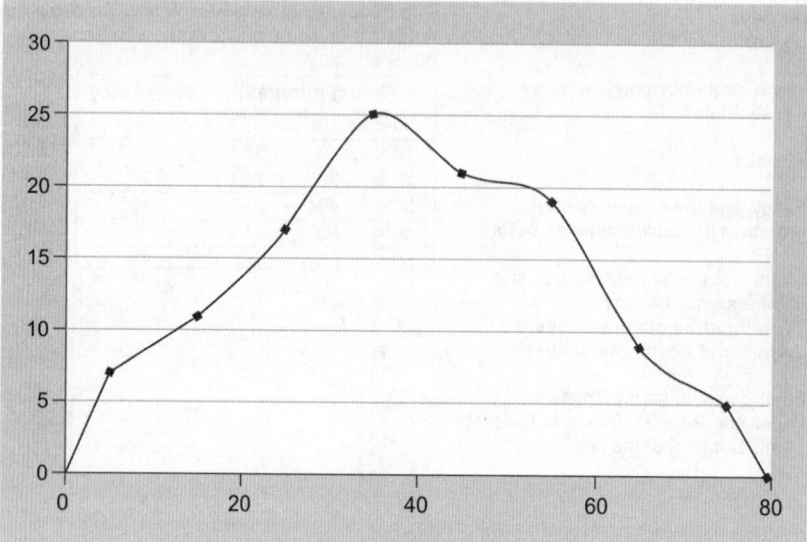

Fig. 11.6: Frequency curve.

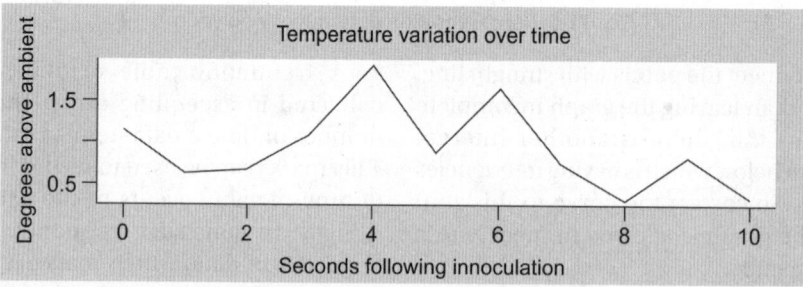

Fig. 11.7: Temperature variations in frequency curve.

LINE GRAPH

Line diagrams are used to show the trend of events with the passage of time. The data is presented with the help of horizontal line and the paths of line show the trend of incidents. This is a frequency polygon presenting variations by line. It shows the trend of an event occurring over a period of time rising, falling or showing fluctuations such as of cancer deaths, infant mortality rate, birth rate, death rate, etc., say from year 1900 to 1960.

Uses of Line Graph

- To show the trend of one or more data sets over time or another continuous scale.
- With lines to suggest a gradual flow between data points.

- With symbols to clarify the position of individual data points.
- With symbols alone (no lines) to downplay an impression of flow between data points.
- With vertical sticks to reinforce the grid and to highlight the value of data points.

Advantages

- Can compare multiple continuous data sets easily.
- Interim data can be inferred from graph line.
- Good way to look at how something changes usually over time.

Disadvantage

Use only with continuous data.

CUMULATIVE FREQUENCY DIAGRAM OR OGIVE

Ogive is a graph of the cumulative relative frequency distribution **(Fig. 11.8)**. To draw this, an ordinary frequency distribution table in a quantitative data has to be converted into a relative cumulative frequency table. Cumulative frequency is the total number of persons in each particular range from lowest value of the characteristic up to and including any higher group value. It is obtained by cumulating the frequency of previous classes including the class in question.

Methods of Constructing Ogive

There are two methods of constructing Ogive, namely: The less than method and the more than method.

1. **Less than method:** In this method we start with the upper limits of the classes and go on adding the frequencies. When these frequencies are plotted we get a rising curve.
2. **More than method:** In this method we start with the lower limit of the classes and from the frequencies we subtract the frequencies of each class. When these frequencies are plotted we get a declining curve.

Application of Ogive

- By using Ogive we can locate any percentile that will divide the series into two parts.
- Comparison of one percentile values of a variables of one sample with that of another sample drawn from some population or different population.
- To study growth in children.
- As a measure of dispersion (interquartile range of semi-quartile range) it is also useful.

SCATTER OR DOT DIAGRAM

Scattered or dot design otherwise called statistical maps. When statistical data refer to geographical or administrative areas; it is presented either as shaded maps or dot maps **(Fig. 11.9)**.

According to suitability: Scatter diagram shows the relationship between two variables. It is also a simple way of diagrammatic representation of a bivariate distribution by which we can ascertain the correlation between the two variables.

Uses of Scatter Graph

- To view actual measurements or observations on a grid, possibly revealing patterns and trends in those data.

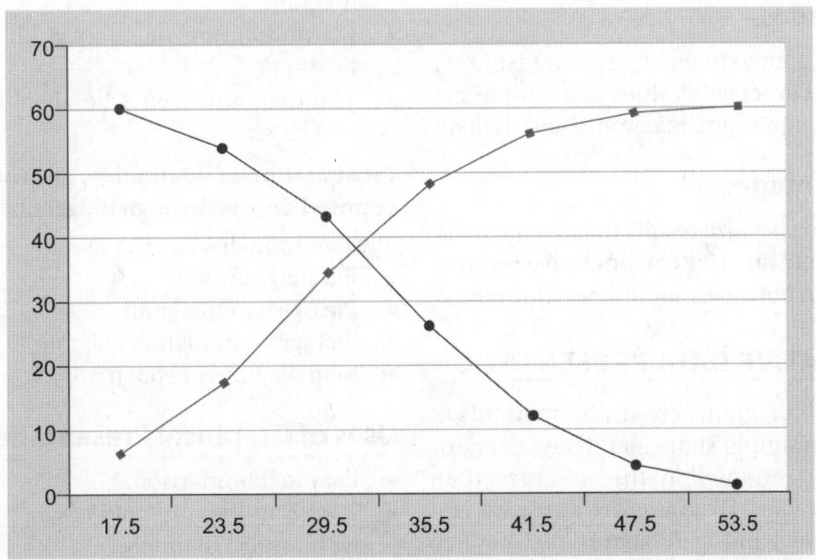

Fig. 11.8: Ogive.

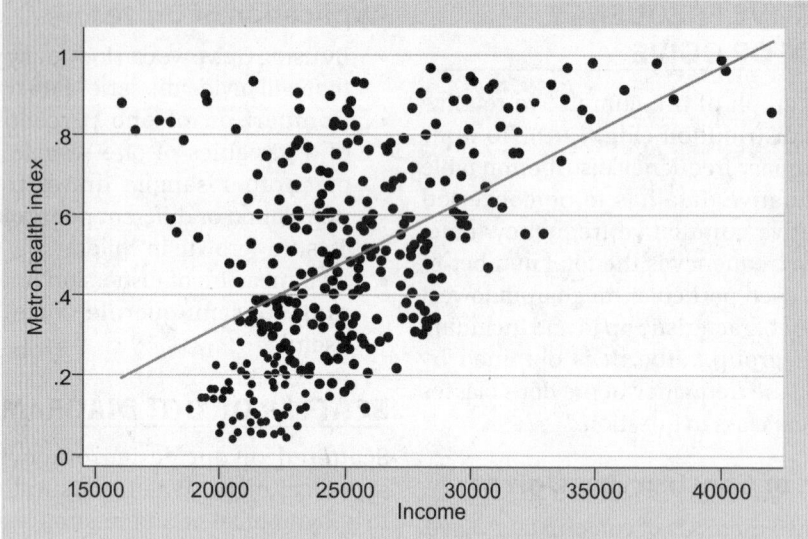

Fig. 11.9: Scatter or dot diagram.

- With plotted points alone when you want to show the data empirically, without suggesting a relationship between the X and Y variables.
- With a curve alone when you want to show the relationship between the X and Y variables as suggested by the data, irrespective of the actual data points.
- With both plotted points and a curve when you want to show the empirical data as well as suggest trends.

Advantages

- Shows a trend in the data relationship
- Retains exact data values and sample size
- Shows minimum/maximum and outliers

Disadvantages

- Hard to visualize results in large data sets
- Flat trend line gives inconclusive results
- Data on both axes should be continuous.

QUALITATIVE DATA PRESENTATION

Charts and diagrams are useful methods of presenting simple statistical data. Diagrams are better retained in the memory than statistical tables. Diagrams are attractive and easy to understand, at the same time. They free us from the burden of figures, comparison is

made easy, time and energy is saved and they become more effective and useful in research.

General Principles

- It should be simple and attractive.
- It should be of proper size.
- Minimum use of words and figures.
- It should present the reality.
- Symbolic presentation and its explanation are essential.
- The facts should be clearly classified in the diagram.
- Every diagram or chart should have a heading.
- The diagram should be absolutely neat and clean.

Presentation of qualitative, discrete or counted data is through diagrams

The common diagrams in use are:

- Bar diagram
- Pie or sector diagram
- Pictogram or picture diagram
- Map diagram or spot map.

Uses of Graphical Presentation

- Easy for comparison.
- Trends in the observation can be noticed with respect of time.
- Lay people can understand it.

- Median, percentile, quartile, etc., can be calculated.
- When lot of fluctuations is seen, then semi log or double log graphs can be good representations. Here, by double log graphs, irregularities (that are seen in arithmetic scale) is smoothened out.

BAR DIAGRAM

Bar charts are merely a way of presenting a set of numbers by the length of a bar— the length of the bar is proportional to the magnitude to be represented. Bar charts are a popular media of presenting stationary data because they are easy to prepare and enable values to be compared visually. The types of bar charts are simple bar chart, multiple bar charts and component bar chart. From frequency table, data on variable is represented on "X" axis and the frequency on "Y" axis. The rectangles drawn are called bars **(Figs. 11.10 A and B)**.

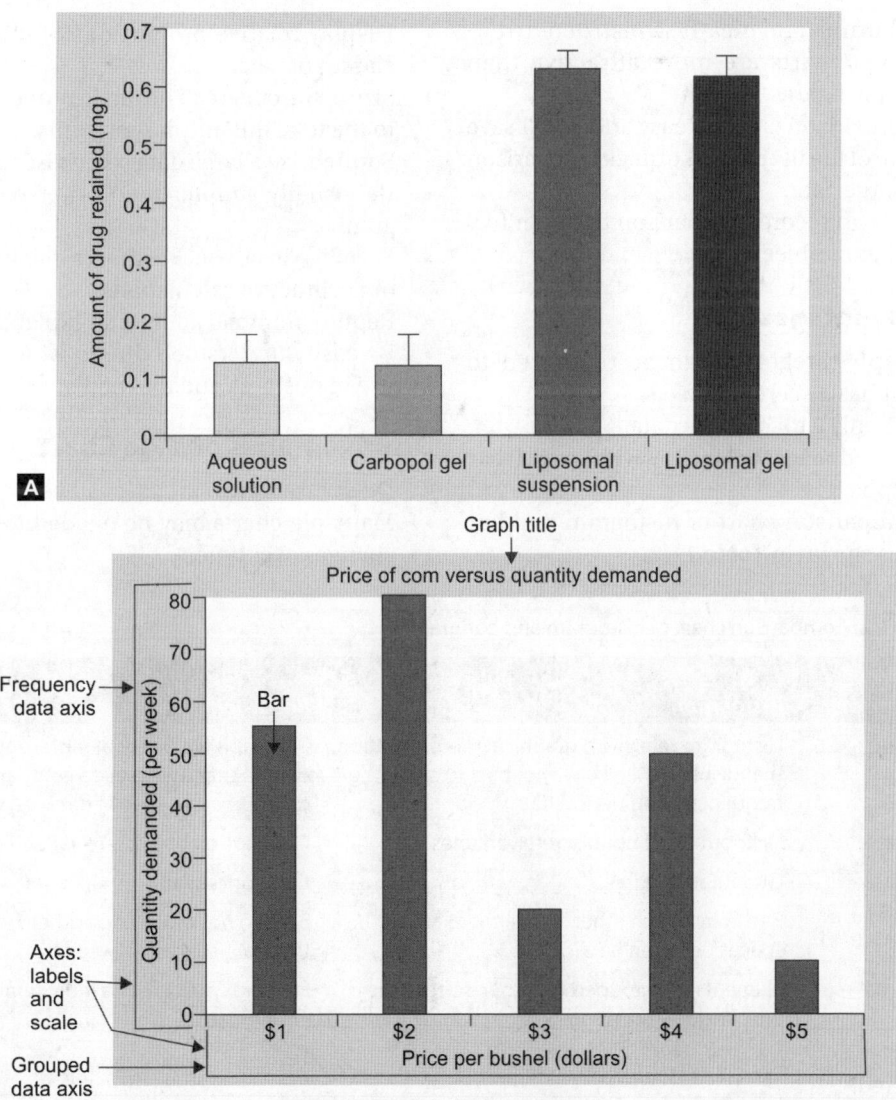

Figs. 11.10A and B: Bar diagram.

Method of Drawing Bar Diagram

Bar graphs are a great way to visually display your data in order to compare items or show how they change over time. Making a bar graph and plotting your data is a simple process once you understand the basic components of all bar graphs. All bar graphs have four basic elements. The first is a title, which is a critical component of the bar graph because it clarifies the overall significance of the data.

Advantages

- Beautiful and neatly constructed diagrams/charts are more attractive than simple figures
- Comparison is made easy and it will save time of the user to make quick comparison of large data.
- You can record comparison between two things or objects.

Disadvantages

- Graph categories can be reordered to emphasize certain effects.
- Use only with discrete data.
- Limited space for labeling with vertical bar graphs.

Comparison chart of histogram and bar graph is shown in **Table 11.2**.

PIE OR SECTOR DIAGRAM

Pie charts are extremely popular with the laity, but not with statistician who considers them inferior to bar charts. It is often necessary to indicate the percentages in the segments. The pie chart can be made more attractive by giving three-dimensional effects to it. The pie diagrams are useful for depicting the relative frequency of disease by system or part of the body affected by place or by season of occurrence (**Fig. 11.11**).

Advantages of a Pie Chart

- Display relative proportions of multiple classes of data.
- Size of the circle can be made proportional to the total quantity it represents.
- Summarize a large data set in visual form.
- Be visually simpler than other types of graphs.
- Permit a visual check of the reasonableness or accuracy of calculations.
- Require minimal additional explanation.
- Be easily understood due to widespread use in business and the media.

Disadvantages of a Pie Chart

- Do not easily reveal exact values.
- Many pie charts may be needed to show changes over time.

Table 11.2: Comparison chart of histogram and bar graph.

Basis for comparison	Histogram	Bar graph
Meaning	Histogram refers to a graphical representation, that displays data by way of bars to show the frequency of numerical data	Bar graph is a pictorial representation of data that uses bars to compare different categories of data
Indicates	Distribution of nondiscrete variables	Comparison of discrete variables
Presents	Quantitative data	Categorical data
Spaces	Bars touch each other, hence there are no spaces between bars	Bars do not touch each other, hence there are spaces between bars
Elements	Elements are grouped together, so that they are considered as ranges	Elements are taken as individual entities
Can bars be reordered?	No	Yes
Width of bars	Need not to be same	Same

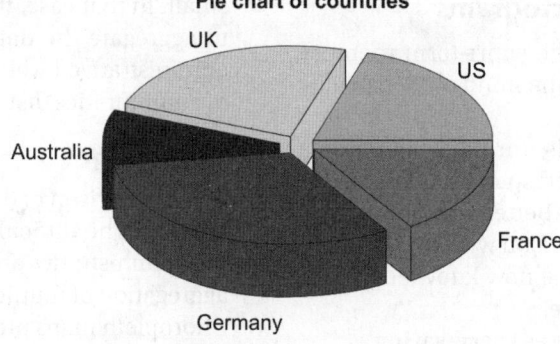

Pie chart of countries

Fig. 11.11: Pie chart.

- Fail to reveal key assumptions, causes, effects, or patterns.
- Be easily manipulated to yield false impressions.

PICTOGRAM OR PICTURE DIAGRAM

Pictogram, the data's are made clear with the help of pictures or symbols. Pictograms are a popular method of presenting data to the "man in the street" and to those who cannot understand orthodox charts. The fractions of the picture can be used to represent numbers smaller than the value of a whole symbol. It is a popular method to impress the frequency of the occurrence of events to common man such as attacks, deaths, and number operated, admitted, discharged, accidents, etc., in a population.

Uses for a Pie Graph

To graph a single data set when your primary message is the relationship of the parts to the whole.

Pointers for a Pie Graph

- Each pie chart can graph only one data set, with each data point represented by a pie slice.
- To keep your graph readable and allow easy comparisons, avoid dividing pies into more than six slices.
- Negative data points are ignored and not shown.

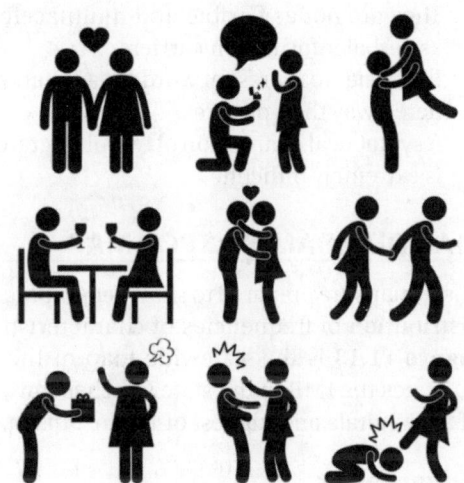

Fig. 11.12: Pictograms.

- You can highlight any slice by "exploding" it (moving it slightly away from the center of the pie).

Features of Pictogram

- Universally understandable with regard to crossing language as well as culture boundaries.
- Supply clear messages together with minimal detail.
- Easily readable.
- Reduce the quantity of control elements which clutter up person interfaces.
- There is a global standard for a few pictogram.

Advantages of Pictograms

- Pictograms free the short-term memory and thereby offer the mind more capacity to solve problems.
- Semantic contents, through pictograms onscreen, can be grasped immediately.
- Pictograms make better use of memory capacity in comparison with words.
- Pictograms link the new knowledge with existing knowledge.
- Pictograms feature as space-saving.

Disadvantages of Pictograms

- They are not as flexible and multifaceted as verbal information carriers.
- It is easier to represent words in a differentiated way than pictures.
- A syntactical connection of two pictograms is extremely difficult.

MAP DIAGRAM OR SPOT MAP

These maps are prepared to show geographical distribution of frequencies of characteristic. **Figure 11.13** is the statewide map of India indicates the IMR in the state which is lowest of 23 in Kerala and highest of 126 in Odisha.

Advantages

- The graphical visualization of statistic data can be realized relatively easy and fast, due to the fact that the statistic data usually is related to political areas.
- Choropleth maps with administrative structures are applicable to any scale, provided that the areas do not become too

small. In that case, there is the possibility to aggregate the date to the next higher administrative level: per example instead of communities districts are used.

Disadvantages

- The comparison of datasets from different years can be difficult, for example when the administrative areas change due to the aggregation of municipalities.
- Choropleth maps presume that the object density within a reference area is constant. In case that the real object density varies within an area the map falsifies reality. You can observe this effect for instance in mountainous regions where the populated part of the communities is much smaller than the effective community areas. The following example shows the problem: The most dense section does not appear in the map because it is compensated by the less dense part.

COMPARISON BETWEEN DIAGRAMS AND GRAPHS

- Graph represents mathematical relationship between two variables whereas a diagram does not.
- Diagrams are more attractive to the eyes but not very much useful for further statistical analysis.
- For presenting frequency distribution and time series graphs are more appropriate than diagram.

DIFFERENCE BETWEEN HISTOGRAM AND BAR DIAGRAM (FIG. 11.14)

Bar diagrams is one-dimensional, i.e., only the length of the bar is material and not the width, a histogram is two-dimensional, i.e., both the lengths as well as the width are important. Histograms represents continuous data, adjacent rectangles are shown touching one another.

When the class intervals of the frequency distribution are all equal area is a constant multiple of the length and the rectangles in

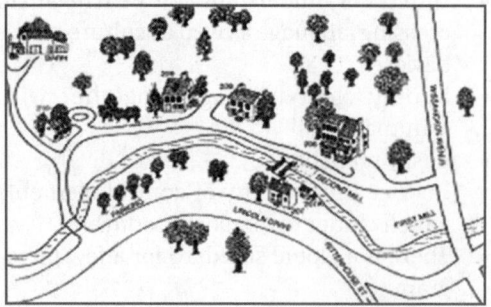

Fig. 11.13: Map diagram or spot map.

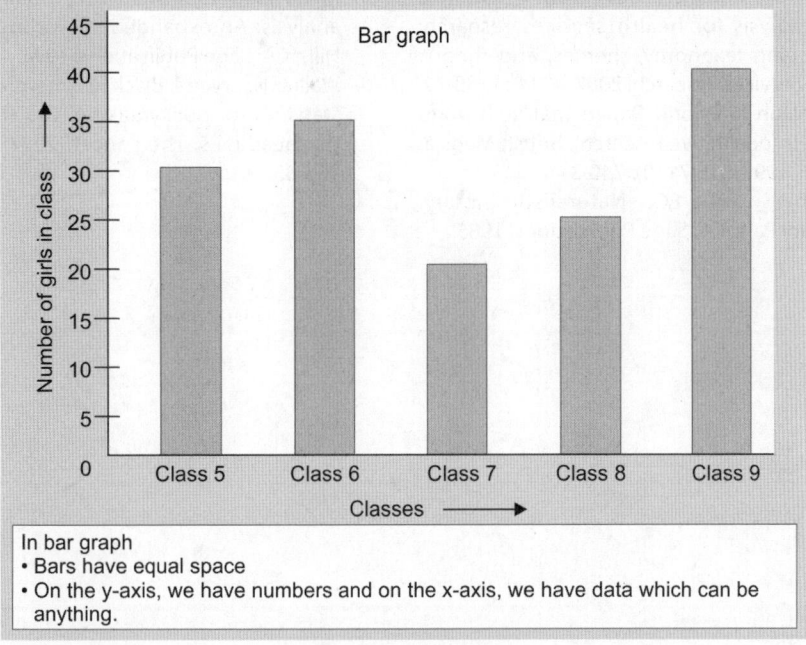

In bar graph
• Bars have equal space
• On the y-axis, we have numbers and on the x-axis, we have data which can be anything.

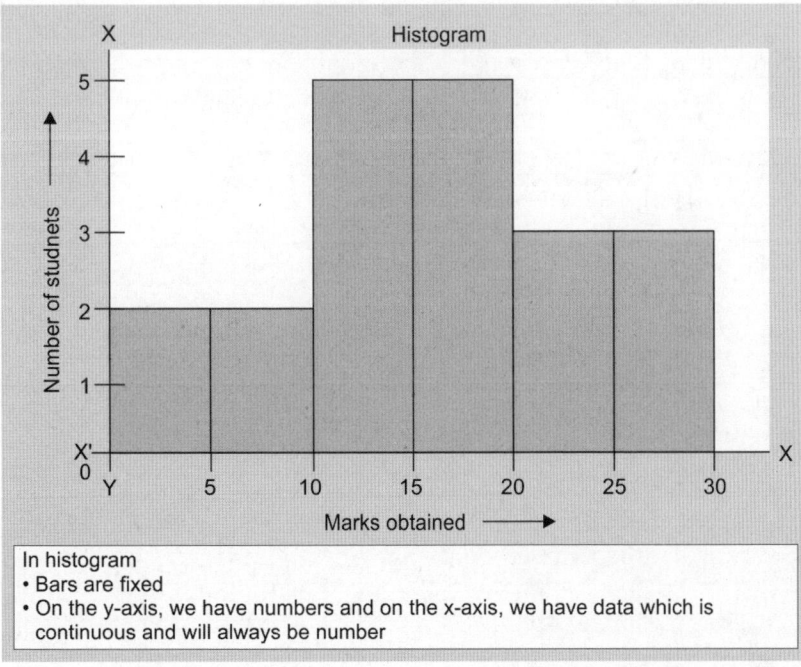

In histogram
• Bars are fixed
• On the y-axis, we have numbers and on the x-axis, we have data which is continuous and will always be number

Fig. 11.14: Difference between histogram and bar diagram.

the histogram can be drawn exactly as for the bar charts. When the class intervals are not all equal than the width of the rectangles will certainly not all be the same.

BIBLIOGRAPHY

1. Atkinson S, Abu el Haj M. Domain analysis for qualitative public health data. Health Policy and Plan. 1996; 11(4): 438-42.

2. Bradley EH, Curry LA, Devers KJ. Qualitative data analysis for health services research: Developing taxonomy, themes, and theory. Health Services Research. 2007; 42 (4): 1758-72.

3. Greenhalgh T, Taylor R. Papers that go beyond numbers (qualitative research). British Medical Journal. 1997; 315(7110): 740-3.

4. Lincoln YS, Guba EG. Naturalistic inquiry. Newbury Park, CA: Sage Publications; 1985.

5. Miles MB, Huberman AM. Qualitative data analysis: An expanded sourcebook. Beverly Hills, CA: Sage Publications; 1994.

6. Walker N, Bryce J, Black RE. Interpreting health statistics for policymaking: The story behind the headlines. The Lancet. 2007; 369(9565): 956-63.

12

CHAPTER

Data Summarization

LEARNING OBJECTIVES

- Meaning of data summarization
- Tools used in data summarization
- Data analysis and reporting
- Data preparation for analysis

- Data summarization and visualization
- Data analysis and modeling
- Data distribution

INTRODUCTION

Summarization is a key data mining concept which involves techniques for finding a compact description of a dataset. Simple summarization methods, such as tabulating the mean and standard deviations are often applied for data analysis, data visualization and automated report generation. Clustering is another data mining technique that is often used to summarize large datasets. Data summarization in very large multi-dimensional datasets as in the case of data warehouses is a very challenging work.

DEFINITION

Data summarization summarizes evaluation of data included both primitive and derived data, in order to create a derived evolutional data that is general in nature. Since the data in the data warehouse is of very high volume, there needs to be a mechanism in order to get only the relevant and meaningful information in a less messy format. Data summarization provides the capacity to give data consumers generalize view of disparate bulks of data.

MEANING OF DATA SUMMARIZATION

Data summarization is quite a common thing but may require a very powerful and time consuming approach in order to analyze ultra large datasets. This can be presented in a compact summary with a plotting of the average salary level against educational level. But some other data consumers may have more requirements such the inclusion of

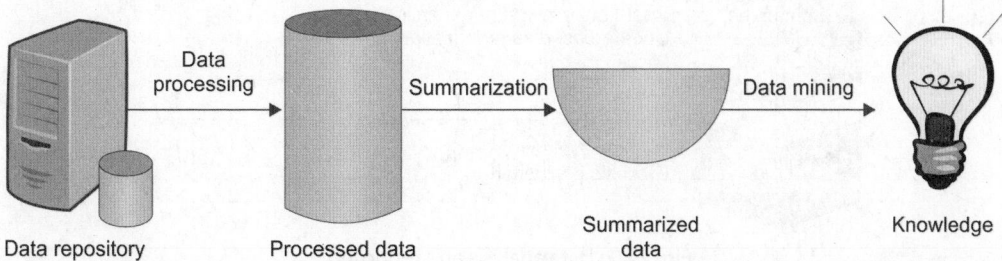

Fig. 12.1: Data summarization process.

Data processing — Summarization — Data mining

Data repository — Processed data — Summarized data — Knowledge standard deviation information along with the averages. Yet some other data consumers may require breaking down the average salaries by age group or excluding outlying salaries. In addition, there may be those who will require the salary and education level relationship in the men and women, or by race or geography. Effective data summarization involves identifying overall trends and substantial exceptions to them. Data summarization can also be done with a simple spreadsheet application, such as Microsoft Excel.

TOOLS USED IN DATA SUMMARIZATION

- There are many tools available in the market to make data summarization a lot easier by making it in visual environment. These tools may help a data consumer produce a data summary of the data one at a time and they can also allow the end user to explore the dataset manually.
- While the end user only clicks and drags, the computer is performing the exhaustive search at the back while informing the end user about where further investigation is warranted.
- Data summarization makes it easy for business makers to spot trends and patterns in the industry where the business operates as well as trends and patterns in the internal operations of the business organization.
- This way, the decision makers can get accurate pictures of the strong and weak points in the operation. When they get the details of these areas, the decision makers can make moves on how to optimize the strong points and how to innovate and improve products in order to overcome the problems associated with the weak points.
- Large amounts of data are often compressed into more easily assimilated summaries, which provide the user with a sense of the content, without overwhelming him/her with too many numbers.
- There a number of ways data can be presented. We will consider two here one is to present the data in a distribution, and the other is to provide summary statistics that capture key aspects of the data.

DATA ANALYSIS AND REPORTING

Data analysis comprises of a collection of methods to deal with data/information obtained through observations, measurements, surveys or experiments about a phenomenon of interest. The aim and purpose of data analysis is to extract as much information as possible that is pertinent to the subject under consideration.

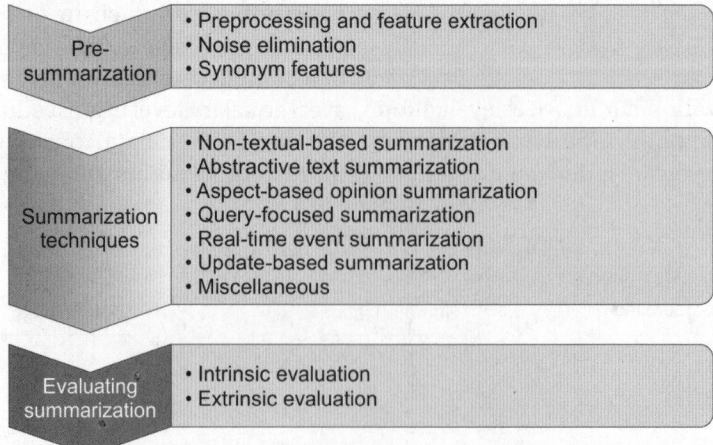

Fig. 12.2: Data analysis and reporting.

The nature of the subject and also the purpose of analysis may vary greatly. The subject could be physical, social or economic and the purpose of the analysis could be purely academic or practical. Due to the great diversity of statistical data, the methods of analysis and the manner of application differ significantly from situation to situation. One cannot possibly expect a single unified system of techniques to be applicable to all cases. However, we have several formal methods of analysis are more or less mutually related and have been successfully applied to most, if not all statistical data.

We can classify data into several types according to some few criteria; qualitative or quantitative in line with the property of the observation or measurement, univariate or multivariate according to whether one or more observations or measurements are taken per subject respectively and finally cross-sectional or longitudinal according to whether measurements are taken at a point in time or over a period of time. Thus each different type of data will require a different type of analysis technique. Reporting of the results will be largely guided by the purpose of the study undertaken and also the audience to which the results are targeted. Data analysis, modeling and reporting is generally carried out through a set of steps. These steps are however interrelated and the process of data analysis reviews each step on the basis of both the previous and the subsequent step. We can list the steps under four headings as follows;

1. Data preparation for analysis
2. Data summarization and visualization
3. Data analysis and modeling
4. Discussion and report writing

Data Preparation for Analysis

- **Firstly,** before any analysis is carried out, data is entered into a computer system (if not done already) and has to be checked, updated and validated. Next, it is crucial to read and re-read your data in order to know it inside-out. Get completely

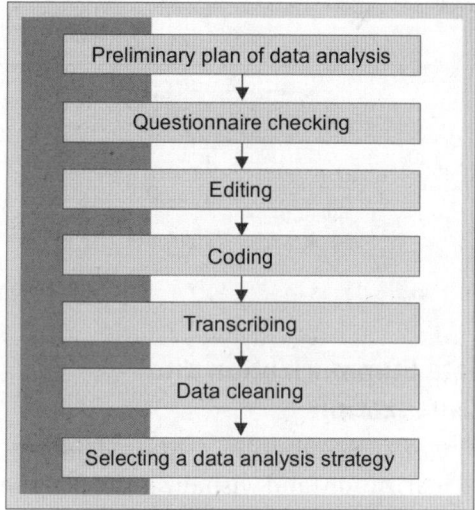

Fig. 12.3: Data preparation process.

familiar with your data before start of any analysis.

- **Secondly,** there follows data manipulation into a structural form suitable for analysis and which the software to be used in the analysis can upload easily. This could involve copying, selecting subsets of the data, transforming and merging the data at various levels. Transforming and deriving new variables from existing ones. This might involve coding and categorizing existing variables. Coding can simply be defined as a process

- **Thirdly,** it is crucial to identify the data structure, sometimes known as data layers of the data/information to be analyzed. For example, you may have farms, plots within farms or farms, animals within farms or forests, species within forests, etc.

- **Fourthly,** the unit of measurement has to be clearly defined. For example in a survey that involves farms, information taken will be at individual or at farm level. At the farm level, we may record number of trees, number of persons, and size of the farm in acres and at persons level we could record their ages. Further, we should consider which of our data are quantitative and which are qualitative.

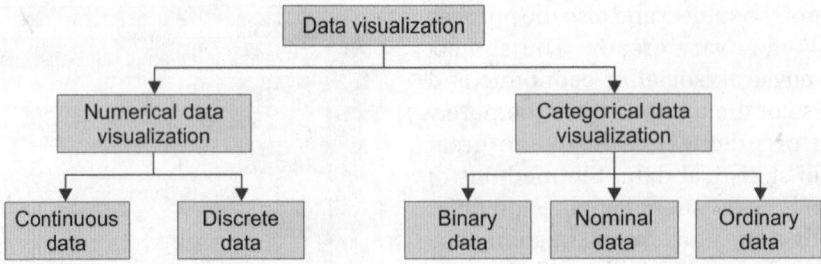

Fig. 12.4: Data visualization process.

Data Summarization and Visualization

- Various methods to achieve data summarization and visualization include; tabulations, X-Y scatter plots, box plots, category-value plot, normal probability plots and density estimates among others.
- The aim of data summarization and visualization is to bring about the main features of the data and to guide in choosing the appropriate statistical techniques.
- Furthermore, these procedures will help in spotting errors and unusual values in the data matrix allowing corrective steps to be taken early in the analysis.
- The process of data summarization and visualization can be appropriately linked to the concept of exploratory data analysis (EDA) whose approach and philosophy is to allow the data to dictate the process and techniques of analysis to be employed.
- EDA is carried out through a variety of mostly graphical techniques. It allows the data analyst to obtain maximum insight into a set of data by revealing the underlying structure, spotting outliers and anomalies as well as testing underlying assumptions among other things.

Data Analysis and Modeling

- Following data exploration through descriptive statistics and data visualization that are guided by objectives of the study, we identify appropriate statistical analysis techniques (if any) needed to do further data investigation that will assist in answering the objectives of the research study in order to draw sound conclusions.
- Assumptions associated with the identified statistical techniques require to be confirmed that they are met.
- Data may arise in the context of two broad areas of statistical inquiry, experimentation and surveys. Methods of analysis chosen usually reflect the kind of inquiry from which the data arose.
- Furthermore the type of measurements (ordinal, nominal, continuous and ratio) taken during data collection dictate the kind of statistical techniques and models to be employed in the analysis.

Discussion and Report Writing

- It is important that the results of analysis are conveyed or communicated to other parties in clear and unambiguous manner.
- Technical jargon should be avoided as much as possible. Almost always, results of an analysis are used to make decisions, such as to repeat the study (with modifications), to perform another study altogether or even to influence other actions, (e.g., policy).
- Report writing is the process through which we share the findings and/or results of data analysis; of course we can also share the same verbally. Ideally, the report should begin with a brief outline of the main point of the study or experiment that was conducted and its purpose.
- It is also advisable to indicate time and place where the research was carried out. A systematic outline of the procedures undertaken during the data analysis including modeling should be stated clearly.

- The report should also capture the main findings of the study and should point out the next course of action.

DATA DISTRIBUTION

- When presented with thousands of pieces of information, you can break the numbers down into individual values (or ranges of values) and indicate the number of individual data items that take on each value or range of values. This is called a frequency distribution.
- If the data can only take on specific values, as is the case when we record the number of goals scored in a soccer game, you get a discrete distribution.
- When the data can take on any value within the range, as is the case with income or market capitalization, it is called a continuous distribution.
- The advantages of presenting the data in a distribution are twofold. For one thing, you can summarize even the largest data sets into one distribution and get a measure of what values occur most frequently and the range of high and low values.
- The second is that the distribution can resemble one of the many common ones about which we know a great deal in statistics.
- A normal distribution is symmetric, has a peak centered around the middle of the distribution, and tails that are not fat and stretch to include infinite positive or negative values.
- Not all distributions are symmetric, though. Some are weighted towards extreme positive values and are called positively skewed, and some towards extreme negative values and are considered negatively skewed.

AUTOMATIC SUMMARIZATION

Automatic summarization is the process by a computer program creates a shortened version of text. The product of the process contains the most important points from the original text. Search engines, such as Google use automatic summarization to produce key phrase extractions in search results. Automatic summarization helps to reduce large text documents to a short set of words or a paragraph that conveys the meaning of the full text.

There are two methods used in automatic summarization:

1. The extractive method selects a subset of existing words, phrases or sentences in the original text to form summaries.
2. The abstractive method builds an internal semantic representation and uses natural language generation techniques to create summaries that resemble the ones created by humans. This summary may have words that are not present in the original document.

There are also two main types of automatic summarization:

1. Key-phrase extraction selects individual words or phrases to tag documents.
2. Document summarization selects whole sentences to create short paragraph summaries.

Technologies that produce coherent summaries of any type must take document length, writing style and syntax into account to make useful summaries.

ANALYSIS STYLES

- **Quasi-statistical style:** That begins with a pre-established code book of themes or words and that tends itself to basic descriptive statistical analysis.
- **Template analysis style:** That involves the development of an analysis guide used to sort the data.
- **Editing analysis style:** That involves an interpretation of the data on which a categorization scheme is based.
- **Immersion/crystallization style:** That involves the analyst's total immersion in and reflection of text materials.

Use a strategy that is best characterized as an editing synthesizing theorizing and recontextualizing.

QUALITATIVE ANALYSIS PROCESS

- **Comprehending:** The research is able to prepare a thorough and rich description of the phenomenon under study, and new data do not add much to that description. In other words, comprehension is completed when saturation has been attained.
- **Synthesizing:** Synthesizing involves a "sifting" of the data and putting pieces together. At the end of the synthesis process, the researcher can begin to make some generalized statements about the phenomenon and about the study participants.
- **Theorizing:** Another important process in qualitative analysis is theorizing which involves a systemic sorting of the data. During the theorizing process, the researcher develops alternative explanations of the phenomenon under study. The theorizing process continues to evolve until the best and most parsimonious explanation is obtained.
- **Recontextualizing:** The process of re-contextualization involves the further development of the theory such that its applicability to other setting or groups is explored.

QUALITATIVE DATA MANAGEMENT AND ORGANIZATION

- The first major step in analyzing qualitative data is to organize the materials according to some plan, so that portions of the data can be readily retrieved.
- Qualitative researchers usually develop a categorization scheme based on a reading of a portion of the data and then code the content of the data based on this system.
- Traditionally, researchers have developed conceptual files for organizing their data. In using this system, researcher first code their data in the margins of the printed narrative materials cut out the coded excerpts. And finally place each excerpt into files corresponding to each of the topics covered in the coding scheme.

- Then researcher can retrieve all of the information on a topic by going to a single file. However, the widespread availability of personal computers and appropriate software has tasseled the burden of indexing, organizing and retrieving qualitative materials.
- There are now a wide variety of programs that perform not only basic indexing functions, but also offer various enhancements that can facilitate analysis of data.

ANALYTIC PROCEDURES

- The actual analysis of data begins with search for themes. The search for themes involves not only the discovery of commonalities across subjects but also of natural variation in the data.
- The next step generally involves a validation of the thematic analysis.
- Some researchers use quasi–statistics, which involves a tabulation of the frequency with which certain themes or relations are supported by the data.
- In a final step, the analyst tries to weave the thematic strands together into an integrated picture of the phenomenon under investigation.

GROUND THEORY ANALYSIS

Analytic induction refers to an approach in which the researcher alternates back and forth between tentative definition of emerging hypothesis and tentative explanation.

- **Open coding (level I coding):** The development of a categorization scheme and subsequent initial coding of the data.
- **Axial coding (level II coding):** It is a reconstructive process that puts data back together in new ways by connecting categories and subcategories. The analyst begins the process of integration by reviewing and sorting the memos that have been used to document conceptual ideas throughout the data collection and data analysis process.

- **Selective coding (level III coding):** The ground theory analyst searches for the core category—the central phenomenon used to integrate all others. This phase results in an emergency theory of a basic social process that is grounded in the data.

CONCLUSION

Statistics summarize and provide information about your sample data. It tells you something about the values in your data set. This includes where the mean lies and whether your data is skewed.

13

CHAPTER

Data Interpretation and Communication

INTRODUCTION

The interpretation of research findings, an activity in which both producers and consumers of research engage, basically is a search of the broader meaning and implications of the results of an investigation. The results of the data analysis need to scrutinized and reflected on with consideration to the conceptual framework, the specific questions that were addressed or the hypothesis that were tested, prior research findings and the short comings of the methods used to answer the research questions. Data analysis and interpretation is the process of assigning meaning to the collected information and determining the conclusions, significance, and implications of the findings. The steps involved in data analysis are a function of the type of information collected; however, returning to the purpose of the assessment and the assessment questions will provide a structure for the organization of the data and a focus for the analysis.

Definition

- Data interpretation refers to the process of using diverse analytical methods to review data and arrive at relevant conclusions. The interpretation of data helps researchers to

categorize, manipulate, and summarize the information in order to answer critical questions.
- Data interpretation is the process of reviewing data through some predefined processes which will help assign some meaning to the data and arrive at a relevant conclusion. It involves taking the result of data analysis, making inferences on the relations studied, and using them to conclude.

OBJECTIVES OF DATA INTERPRETATION

- Analyzing the accuracy and believability of the results.
- Searching for the underlying meaning of the results.

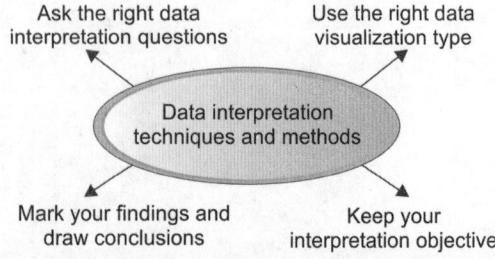

Fig. 13.1: Data interpretation techniques and methods.

- Considering the importance of the findings.
- Analyzing the generalizability and transferability of the finds.
- Assessing the implications of the study in regard of theory, nursing practice and future research.

PRESENTATION OF FINDINGS

- The findings of a study are the presentation of the study results in the form of empirical data. The methods of presenting findings include narrative presentation, tables and figures.
- The findings of a study should be clearly and concisely presented in the narrative text of the study report. The results of hypothesis should contain the statistical test used, the test results, the degrees of freedom and the obtained probability level.
- Tables are a means of organizing data to make study findings more easily understood and interpreted. Tables should never appear in a report unless they have been discussed in the text and should appear as soon as possible in the report after they have been referred to in the text.
- The word "figure" is the term used to indicate any visual presentation of data, other than a table. Figure includes graphs, diagrams, line drawing and photographs.
- The researcher makes interpretations of the findings in light of the theoretical framework and in the context of the literature review.
- An important aspect of the findings of a study is the discussion of the hypothesis testing.
- The research should distinguish between statistical and clinical significance.
- The study conclusions are based on the findings and take into consideration the study problem, purpose, hypothesis and theoretical framework.
- Recommendations for future research should be contained in each research report.

Data interpretation

Things to consider when interpreting your data:
• Interpret findings based on the purpose and objectives of your study
• Relate the findings to real life context
• Use persuasive language to convince your readers to see the research from your point of view
• Organize your interpretation to highlight the most important findings
• Include limitations to your research
• Use simple, clear language

Fig. 13.2: Data interpretation.

Importance of Data Interpretation

The importance of data interpretation is evident and this is why it needs to be done properly. Data is very likely to arrive from multiple sources and has a tendency to enter the analysis process with haphazard ordering. Data analysis tends to be extremely subjective. That is to say, the nature and goal of interpretation will vary from business to business, likely correlating to the type of data being analyzed. While there are several different types of processes that are implemented based on individual data nature, the two broadest and most common categories are "quantitative analysis" and "qualitative analysis".

COMMUNICATION OF NURSING RESEARCH REPORTS

There are many different ways for researchers to communicate the results of their studies. They might begin by presenting the results to peers in school or in the agency where they work. Next they might attend a research conference at which they present their study results in an oral presentation or in a poster session. As a next step, they might publish their results in a journal article.

The researcher have the first responsibility of communicating the findings of their studies, other nurses and nursing organizations also bear the responsibility of seeing that research findings are distributed inside the nursing profession to other healthcare disciplines and even to general public.

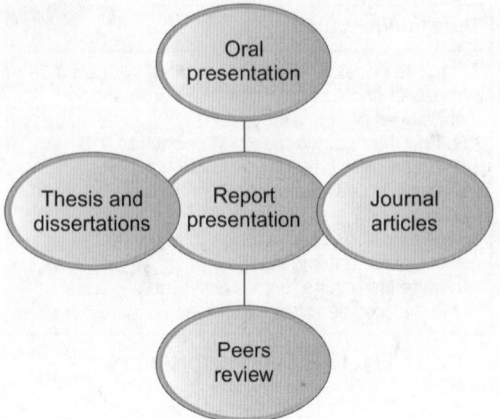

Fig. 13.3: Report presentation.

Interpretation:

Interpretation is the relationship amongst the collected data with analysis. Interpretation looks beyond the data of the research and includes researches, theory and hypothesis.
Interpretation in a way act as a tool to explain the observations of the researcher during the research period and it acts as a guide for future researches

Why interpretation?

- The researcher understands the abstract principle underlying the findings.
- Interpretation links up the findings with those of other similar studies
- The researcher is able to make others understands the real importance of the research findings

Fig. 13.4: Need of data interpretation.

METHODS OF RESEARCH REPORT PRESENTATION

- **The oral presentation** of a research report at a conference is referred to as a paper presentation.
- **Journal articles:** Research is generally published in journal articles. A referred journal is one that uses subject experts to review manuscripts. Non-referred journals use editorial staff members or consultants to review manuscripts.
- **Peers review:** The process involves the review of a manuscript by professional colleagues who have content and methodological expertise in the area of the study discussed in the manuscript.
- **Thesis and dissertations:** They are a means of communicating results of research studies that are conducted in conjunction with educations requirement.

COMMON ERRORS OF INTERPRETATION

- Failure to see the problem in proper perspective.
- Failure to appreciate the relevance of various elements.
- Failure to recognize limitations in the research evidence.
- Misinterpretation due to unstudied factors.
- Ignoring selective factors.
- Inadequate attention to individual cases.

COMMON BARRIERS IN UTILIZATION

- Nurses lack of knowledge of research findings.
- Nurses negative attitude towards nursing research.
- Inadequate means of disseminating nursing research findings
- Lack of institution support
- Study findings that are not ready for use in nursing programs

NUMERICAL DATA INTERPRETATION

The analysis of numerical (quantitative) data is represented in mathematical terms. The most common statistical terms include:

- **Mean:** The mean score represents a numerical average for a set of responses.
- **Standard deviation:** The standard deviation represents the distribution of the responses around the mean. It indicates the degree of consistency among the responses. The standard deviation, in conjunction with the mean, provides a better understanding of the data. For example, if the mean is 3.3 with a standard deviation (StD) of 0.4, then two-thirds of the responses lie between 2.9 (3.3–0.4) and 3.7 (3.3 + 0.4).
- **Frequency distribution:** Frequency distribution indicates the frequency of each response. For example, if respondents answer a question using an agree/disagree

scale, the percentage of respondents who selected each response on the scale would be indicated. The frequency distribution provides additional information beyond the mean, since it allows for examining the level of consensus among the data. Higher levels of statistical analysis [e.g., t-test, factor analysis, regression, analysis of variance (ANOVA)] can be conducted on the data, but these are not frequently used in most program/project assessments.

QUALITATIVE DATA PRESENTATION

Qualitative data interpretation tends to be more subjective in nature and many times can be influenced by the researcher's biases. Effort must be put into the data collection process to eliminate bias including collecting more than one kind of data, get many different kinds of perspectives on the events being studied, purposely look for contradicting information, and acknowledging your biases that relate to your research report.

- Qualitative data analysis is time consuming and complex because a lot of data can be created that is both useful and not useful. There is no "correct way" to analyze qualitative data.
- Efforts can be made to make your data presentation and interpretation more credible and less biased by using the above methods.
- The analysis of narrative (qualitative) data is conducted by organizing the data into common themes or categories.
- It is often more difficult to interpret narrative data since it lacks the built-in structure found in numerical data.
- Initially, the narrative data appears to be a collection of random, unconnected statements. The assessment purpose and questions can help direct the focus of the data organization. The following strategies may also be helpful when analyzing narrative data.

Focus Groups and Interviews

Qualitative data analysis can be summed up in one word—categorical. With qualitative analysis, data is not described through numerical values or patterns, but through the use of descriptive context (i.e., text). Typically, narrative data is gathered by employing a wide variety of person-to-person techniques.

Steps

- Read and organize the data from each question separately. This approach permits focusing on one question at a time (e.g., experiences with tutoring services, characteristics of tutor, student responsibility in the tutoring process).
- Group the comments by themes, topics, or categories. This approach allows for focusing on one area at a time (e.g., characteristics of tutor—level of preparation, knowledge of content area, availability).

Techniques

- **Observations:** Detailing behavioral patterns that occur within an observation group. These patterns could be the amount of time spent in an activity, the type of activity, and the method of communication employed.
- **Focus groups:** Group people and ask them relevant questions to generate a collaborative discussion about a research topic.
- **Secondary research:** Much like how patterns of behavior can be observed, different types of documentation resources can be coded and divided based on the type of material they contain.
- **Interviews:** One of the best collection methods for narrative data. Inquiry responses can be grouped by theme, topic, or category. The interview approach allows for highly-focused data segmentation.

The analysis of the data via statistical measures and/or narrative themes should provide answers to the assessment questions. Interpreting the analyzed data from the appropriate perspective allows for determination of the significance and implications of the assessment.

QUANTITATIVE DATA INTERPRETATION

If quantitative data interpretation could be summed up in one word (and it really can't) that word would be "numerical." There are few certainties when it comes to data analysis, but you can be sure that if the research you are engaging in has no numbers involved, it is not quantitative research. Quantitative analysis refers to a set of processes by which numerical data is analyzed. More often than not, it involves the use of statistical modeling, such as standard deviation, mean and median. Let us quickly review the most common statistical terms:

- **Mean:** A mean represents a numerical average for a set of responses. When dealing with a data set (or multiple data sets), a mean will represent a central value of a specific set of numbers. It is the sum of the values divided by the number of values within the data set. Other terms that can be used to describe the concept are arithmetic mean, average and mathematical expectation.
- **Standard deviation:** This is another statistical term commonly appearing in quantitative analysis. Standard deviation reveals the distribution of the responses around the mean. It describes the degree of consistency within the responses; together with the mean, it provides insight into data sets.
- **Frequency distribution:** This is a measurement gauging the rate of a response appearance within a data set. When using a survey, for example, frequency distribution has the capability of determining the number of times a specific ordinal scale response appears (i.e., agree, strongly agree, disagree, etc.). Frequency distribution is extremely keen in determining the degree of consensus among data points.

Typically, quantitative data is measured by visually presenting correlation tests between two or more variables of significance. Different processes can be used together or separately, and comparisons can be made to ultimately arrive at a conclusion. Other signature interpretation processes of quantitative data include:

- **Regression analysis:** Essentially, regression analysis uses historical data to understand the relationship between a dependent variable and one or more independent variables. Knowing which variables are related and how they developed in the past allows you to anticipate possible outcomes and make better decisions going forward.
- **Cohort analysis:** This method identifies groups of users who share common characteristics during a particular time period. In a business scenario, cohort analysis is commonly used to understand different customer behaviors.
- **Predictive analysis:** As its name suggests, the predictive analysis method aims to predict future developments by analyzing historical and current data. Powered by technologies, such as artificial intelligence and machine learning, predictive analytics practices enable businesses to spot trends or potential issues and plan informed strategies in advance.
- **Prescriptive analysis:** Also powered by predictions, the prescriptive analysis method uses techniques, such as graph analysis, complex event processing,
- **Conjoint analysis:** Typically applied to survey analysis, the conjoint approach is used to analyze how individuals value different attributes of a product or service. This helps researchers and businesses to define pricing, product features, packaging, and many other attributes.
- **Cluster analysis:** Last but not least, cluster analysis is a method used to group objects into categories. Since, there is no target variable when using cluster analysis, it is a useful method to find hidden trends and patterns in the data.

DATA INTERPRETATION METHOD

- **Descriptive statistics** provide a description of what the data look like. They provide a means to describe the points of central tendency (mean, mode, median, etc.) and dispersion (standard deviation, variance, interquartile range, etc.).

- **Inferential statistics** allow the researcher to make inferences about populations from smaller samples of the population. Statistics of the sample are used to estimate parameters of the population. A parameter is a constant value representative of the population (such as population mean and standard deviation) while a statistic is any calculation performed on the sample being tested (Leedy and Ormrod, 2001). Inferential statistics also allow the researcher to test their research hypotheses. Some measures used in inferential statistics include the standard error of the mean, estimators, and the p-value. The way that the data is interpreted can have varying effects on your conclusions. Absolute honesty in recording and interpreting data is required to maintain the credibility of research. All of the conditions of a situation should be considered and that we make inferences in strict accordance with the data obtained.

Using statistics to determine relationships is paramount to the success of good research. Using tools, such as ANOVA, correlations, Fisher Exact Tests, regression, etc., can predict whether or not your research hypothesis is satisfied. But, remember to select your p-value before you begin your research project. Doing this will add credibility to your research.

BASIC PRINCIPLES IN INTERPRETING THE DATA

Methods of statistical inference (statistical tests, confidence intervals) are sometimes misused or interpreted incorrectly in practice. Also, the methods should be used consistently with statistical assumptions (including independence assumptions).

Statistical Significance

In general, a statistical test has the following components.

- A **null hypothesis** is formulated. This is usually a probability model that assumes no effect of interest, any apparent effects being attributable to chance.

- A **test statistic** is chosen, which will be computed from results of the experiment to quantify how strongly the results contradict the null hypothesis.

- Once the study has been conducted, the p-value is the probability of any result that contradicts the null hypothesis as strongly as the results actually obtained, based on the value of the test statistic. The p-value from a test is not the probability of truth or untruth of a hypothesis. It is the probability of data that contradict the null hypothesis as strongly as the data actually obtained, if the null hypothesis is true.

Statistical Tests and Randomized Experiments

- Although causal assessments may be based largely on observational data, some consideration of perspectives during planning of a randomized experiment may be helpful in understanding statistical testing concepts.

- At the planning stage, a test statistic is tentatively identified that will be computed from results of the experiment and used in deciding what outcome to report for the experiment.

- In our example, the number of cups that the subject will classify correctly is used to accept or reject the subject's claim.

- A cutoff (critical) value of the test statistic is identified, such that the chance of some erroneous conclusions is acceptably low.

- Indeed, the experimenter hopes for a low chance of finding an effect, if there really is no effect, i.e., a low chance of a false positive.

- According to the null hypothesis, the treatments may be viewed simply as random labeling of experimental units.

- If the experimenter has decided to enforce a 5% chance of a false positive, use of the critical p-value of 0.05 is justified as just a matter of checking that results satisfy a pre-specified criterion, before claiming to have observed something of interest.

- In addition, the experimenter hopes that if there are substantial effects of the treatment, there will be a substantial probability of finding statistical significance, i.e., that the test will have good power.

Confidence Intervals

A 95% confidence interval has the following interpretations:
- There is a 95% chance of the true value of the parameter falling within the interval.
- Values outside the interval can be rejected on the basis of a two-sided statistical test with alpha 5%. Confidence intervals are likely to be more easily interpreted than statistical tests in some situations. A large p-value, by itself, is ambiguous, as previously noted. A confidence interval may be more informative, displaying an estimated effect along with a measure of statistical uncertainty (which will be large in case of few or variable data). Unlike statistical tests, confidence intervals are neutral regarding the relative "burden of proof" to be associated with various hypotheses about effect sizes.

General Recommendations for the Use of Statistical Tests and Confidence Intervals

- Methods that assume normality should not be applied to data that contain outliers or have heavy-tailed distributions. Rank-based or other outlier-resistant methods may be applied, without needing to exclude putative outliers from the analysis.
- Methods that assume normality may be applied to data with skew distributions if the data are transformed to correct skewness.
- Assessment of distributional assumptions should be based in part on graphical evaluation of distributions and familiarity and experience with particular types of variables, and not only on statistical tests of assumptions. It is often of interest to know in what way a distribution deviates from normality, e.g., because of outliers or skewness. The normal distribution should not be treated as a default in cases where experience indicates that, say, a particular type of variable is more likely to have a lognormal distribution.
- Possible effects of and remedies for autocorrelation or pseudoreplication should be considered.
- When focusing on effects of one variable, possible effects of other variables should be taken into account. It is desirable to consider methods that minimize confounding. Some standard methods for evaluating the effects of a single variable on a response, while ignoring others may not be suitable for ecological data.
- In a regression context, tests of assumptions are generally applied to regression residuals (differences between observed values of the Y variable, and values predicted by the model).
- Correct use of statistical tests and confidence intervals requires that the appropriate interpretation be kept in mind. In particular, statistical significance (a low p-value) is conceptually distinct from practical significance, i.e., from the issue of whether biological effects observed in a situation are large enough in magnitude to be of practical importance.

CONCLUSION

When interpreting data, an analyst must try to discern the differences between correlation, causation, and coincidences, as well as much other bias—but he also has to consider all the factors involved that may have led to a result. There are various data interpretation methods one can use. The interpretation of data is designed to help people make sense of numerical data that has been collected, analyzed, and presented. Having a baseline method (or methods) for interpreting data will provide your analyst teams with a structure and consistent foundation. Indeed, if several departments have different approaches to interpret the same data while sharing the same goals, some mismatched objectives can result. Disparate methods will lead to duplicated efforts, inconsistent solutions, wasted energy, and inevitably—time and money.

14

Statistics

INTRODUCTION

The word **"statistics"** came from the Italian word "**statista**" means Statesman or German word "statistik" which means a political state. The term "statistics" has been used to indicate facts and figures of any kind. It can be health statistics, vital statistics, business statistics etc. The word **"statistics"** was first used by professor Gottfried Achenwall (1719-1772). Statistics is a body of methods of obtaining and analyzing data in order to base decisions on them. Statistics also converts the mass of numbers into useful information.

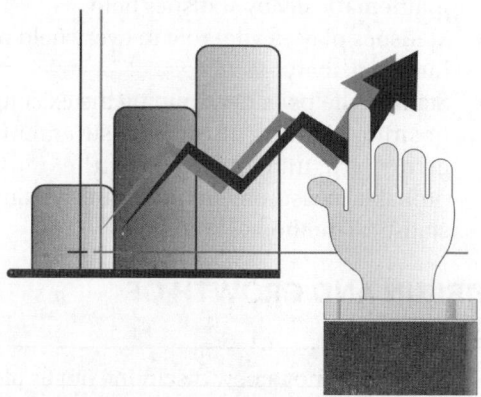

Fig. 14.1: Need of statistics in research.

DEFINITION

Statistics is a branch of mathematics dealing with the collection, analysis, interpretation, presentation, and organization of data.

- **Professor AL Bowley:** "Statistics may be called the science of counting" this definition is too narrow. It covers only one aspect of science viz, the collection of data, other aspects like analysis, presentation, interpretation, etc., are completely ignored.
- **Yule and Kendall:** "By statistics we mean quantitative data affected to a marked extent by multiplicity of causes. This definition is not exhaustive and it fails to provide for comparative study of the figures and their arrangement.
- **Berenson and Levin:** "The science of statistics can be viewed as the application of the scientific method in the analysis of numerical data for the purpose of making rational decisions".
- **Croxton and Cowden:** "Statistics may be defined as the collection, organization, presentation, analysis and interpretation of numerical data".
- Statistics can be defined as a part of applied mathematics that is concerned with the collection, classification, interpretation,

analysis or the numerical and categorical data and facts, and drawing conclusions, so as to present the same in a systematic manner.

MEANING OF STATISTICS

Statistics is the study of the collection, organization, analysis, interpretation and presentation of data. It deals with all aspects of data including the planning of data collection in terms of the design of surveys and experiments. When analyzing data, it is possible to use one of two statistics methodologies **(Fig. 14.2)**: Descriptive or inferential statistics.

Statistics is a mathematical body of science that pertains to the collection, analysis, interpretation or explanation, and presentation of data or as a branch of mathematics. Some consider statistics to be a distinct mathematical science rather than as a branch of mathematics. Medical uses of statistics has served as one of the most influential works on the subject for physicians, physicians-in-training, and a myriad of healthcare experts who need a clear idea of the proper application of statistical techniques in clinical studies as well as the implications of their interpretation for clinical practice. Statistics is the study of how to collect, organizes, analyze, and interpret

numerical information from data. Descriptive statistics involves methods of organizing, picturing and summarizing information from data. Inferential statistics involves methods of using information from a sample to draw conclusions about the population.

- Statistics may be defined as the collection, organization, presentation, analysis and interpretation of numerical data.
- The science of statistics can be viewed as the application of scientific method in the analysis of numerical data for the purpose of making rational decisions.
- It is a science of experimentation which may be regarded as mathematics applied to observational data.
- Statistics is a science and art of dealing with variation in such a way as to obtain reliable results.
- Statistics may be called the science of counting.

Statistics is the study of how to collect, organizes, analyze, and Interpret data.

SIGNIFICANCE OF STATISTICS

- Statistics is the science of collecting, analyzing and making inference from data. It is important for researchers and also consumers of research to understand statistics so that they can be informed, evaluate the credibility and usefulness of information, and make appropriate decisions.
- Statistics are important because today we live in the information world and much of this information's are determined mathematically by statistics help.
- Statistics plays a vital role in every field of human activity.
- Statistics helps in determining the existing position. During these measurements errors are unavoidable, so the most probable measurements are found by using statistical methods.

ORIGIN AND GROWTH OF STATISTICS

- Statistics is not a new discipline but as old as the human society itself. It has been

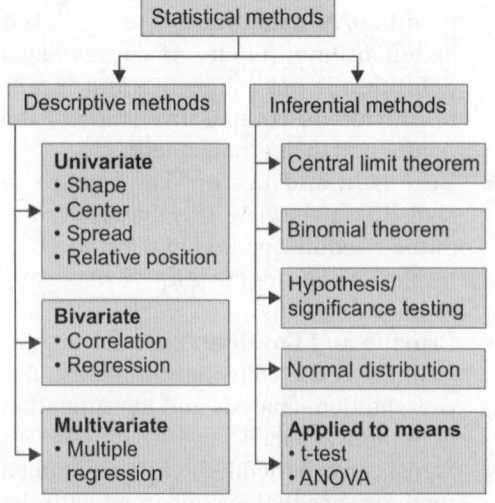

Fig. 14.2: Statistical methods.

used right from the existence of life on earth, through its use was very limited.

- In the olden days statistics was registered as the "science of statecraft" and was the byproduct of the administrative activity of the state, e.g., keeping records of population, birth, deaths, etc., counting and measuring these events may generate much kind of numerical data.
- Though in its present usage, the word statistics is barely a century old, it has been used for a much longer period. Census of population and wealth were even in the ancient times. According to a Greek historian in 1400 BC, a census of all the lands in Egypt was taken.
- The word statistics was first used by professor Gottfried Achenwall (1719–1772), a professor in Malborough in 1749 to refer to the subject matter as a whole. The science of statistics is said to have originated from government records and mathematics.
- Statistics which originated as a science of kings, there has been a phenomenal development in the use of statistics in several fields. Statistics is now regarded as one of the most important role for taking decision in the midst of uncertainty. Today, almost all the sciences including medical science utilize statistics.

CHARACTERISTICS OF STATISTICS

According to the definition given by professor Horace Secrist, the following characteristics of statistics can be noticed **(Fig. 14.3).**

Aggregate of facts
Affected to a substantial extent by a variety of reasons
Numerical expression
Enumerated and estimated as per reasonable standard of accuracy
Data collection is carried out in a systematic manner
Data must be placed in relation to one another

Fig. 14.3: Characteristics of statistics.

- **Statistics means an aggregate of facts:** Facts can be analyzed only when there is more than one fact. Single fact cannot be analyzed. Thus, the fact Mr John is 180 cm tall, cannot be statistically analyzed. On the other hand, if we know the heights of 40 students of a class, we can comment upon the average height, variation, etc. Hence, only a collection of many facts can be called statistics.
- **Statistics are affected to a marked extent by multiplicity of causes:** The facts are the results of action and interaction of a number of factors. Thus, statistics of yield of paddy, is the result of factors such as fertility of soil, amount of rainfall, quality of seed used, quality and quantity of fertilizer used, etc. These factors, in turn, are the results of many other factors.
- **Statistics are numerically expressed:** Only numerical facts can be statistically analyzed. Therefore, facts such as 'price decreases with increasing production' cannot be called statistics.
- **Statistics are enumerated or estimated according to reasonable standards of accuracy:** The facts should be enumerated (collected from the field) or estimated (computed) with required degree of accuracy. The degree of accuracy differs from purpose to purpose. In measuring the length of screws, accuracy up to a millimeter may be required, whereas, while measuring the heights of students in a class, accuracy up to a centimeter is enough.
- **Statistics are collected in a systematic manner:** The facts should be collected according to planned and scientific methods. Otherwise, they are likely to be wrong and misleading.
- **Statistics are collected for a predetermined purpose:** There must be a definite purpose for collecting facts. Otherwise, the facts become useless and hence, they cannot be called statistics.
- **Statistics are placed in relation to each other:** The facts must be placed in such a way that a comparative and analytical

study becomes possible. Thus, only related facts which are arranged in logical order can be called statistics.

DIVISIONS OF STATISTICS

The different types or branches of statistics are as follow **(Fig. 14.4)**.
- **Descriptive statistics**: It involves describing and summarizing the sets of numerical data with the help of pictures and statistical quantities. Techniques used may include averages dispersion, skewness, time series, etc.
- **Inferential statistics**: It encompasses those methods that are helpful in drawing conclusion and inferences with respect to parameters of population, based on estimates which are drawn from samples. Chi-square, F-test, t-test, etc., techniques is used.
- **Applied statistics**: Those methods and techniques are used in applied statistics which are applicable to specific problems of real-life scenarios. Techniques used may include sample survey, quality control, index numbers, etc.
- **Inductive statistics**: Those methods and techniques are covered here which are used to identify a specific phenomenon based on random observation. Techniques used may include extrapolation.
- **Analytical statistics**: Analytical statistics uses such methods and techniques that are helpful in setting up functional relationship amidst variables. In this correlation, regression, association and attributes techniques are used.
- **Mathematical statistics**: It deals with the application of different mathematical theories and techniques to develop different statistical techniques. It uses techniques like integration, differentiation, trigonometry, matrix, etc.

IMPORTANCE OF STATISTICS IN NURSING

- Statistics in nursing are very important.
- Nurses can use statistics to identify patterns in vital signs and symptoms so they can make informed decisions to better respond to a patient's changing medical status.
- Even the use data sheets or frequency charts to document the timing of medications given to patients is a way nurses can use statistics.
- Knowledge of statistics helps medical professionals evaluate studies that assess the efficacy of treatments and interventions.
- Statistics in healthcare convey valuable information about the health of a society.
- Nursing knowledge based on empirical research plays a fundamental role in the development of evidence-based nursing practice.
- The ability to interpret and use quantitative findings from nursing research is an essential skill for advanced practice nurses to ensure provision of the best care possible for our patients.
- Statistics is integral part of the nursing profession.
- It has a direct affect on patient care in a variety of settings as well as the potential to change policies and procedure on a wider scale.

TYPES OF STATISTICS (FIG.14.5)

There are two major divisions of the field of statistics. Each of these segments of statistics is important, and accomplishes different

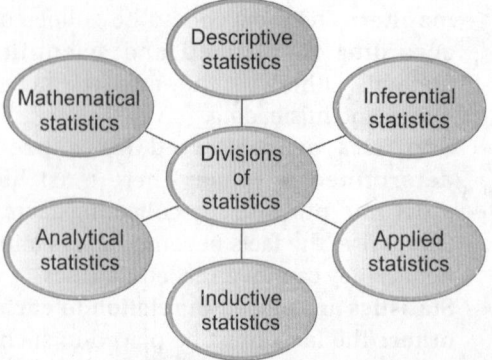

Fig. 14.4: Division of statistics.

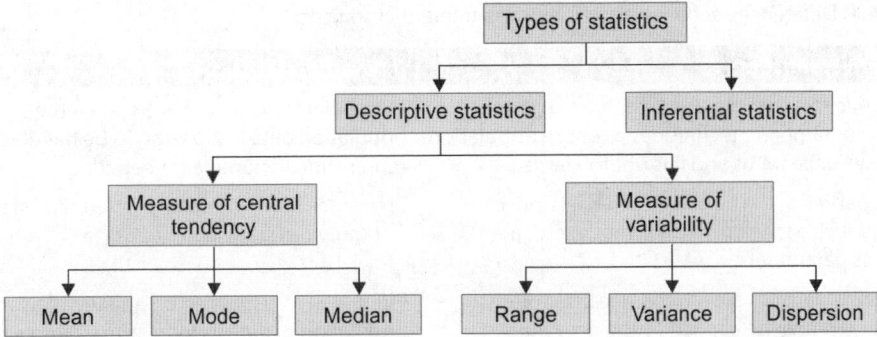

Fig. 14.5: Types of statistics.

objectives. The names of these subfields are descriptive and inferential statistics.

Descriptive Statistics

Descriptive statistics is the type of statistics that probably springs to most people's minds when they hear the word "statistics." Here the goal is to describe. Numerical measures are used to tell about features of a set of data. There are a number of items that belong in this portion of statistics, such as:

- The average, or measure of center, consisting of the mean, median, mode or midrange.
- The spread of a data set, which can be measured with the range or standard deviation.
- Overall descriptions of data such as the five number summary.
- Other measurements such as skewness and kurtosis
- The exploration of relationships and correlation between paired data.
- The presentation of statistical results in graphical form.

Inferential Statistics (Fig. 14.6)

For the area of inferential statistics we begin by differentiating between two groups. The population is the entire collection of individuals that we are interested in studying. It is typically impossible or infeasible to examine each member of the population individually. So we choose a representative subset of the population, called a sample.

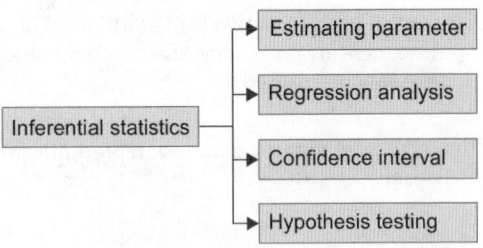

Fig. 14.6: Inferential statistics.

Inferential statistics studies a statistical sample, and from this analysis is able to say something about the population from which the sample came. There are two major divisions of inferential statistics:

1. A confidence interval gives a range of values for an unknown parameter of the population by measuring a statistical sample. This is expressed in terms of an interval and the degree of confidence that the parameter is within the interval.

2. Tests of significance or hypothesis testing tests a claim about the population by analyzing a statistical sample. By design there is some uncertainty in this process. This can be expressed in terms of a level of significance.

Difference between these Areas

- As seen above, descriptive statistics is concerned with telling about certain features of a data set. Although this is helpful in learning things such as the spread and center of the data we are studying, nothing in the area of descriptive statistics can be used to make any sort of generalization.

Table 14.1: Differences between descriptive and inferential statistics.

Descriptive statistics	Inferential statistics
Descriptive statistics are used when we don't opt for any kind of sampling techniques as entire population data is available for us and it is not too large.	Inferential statistics are used when the population data is too large to be handled and a representative sample is needed.
The properties of the population in descriptive statistics such as mean, median, mode, etc., are known as parameters.	Properties of the samples in inferential statistics are known as statistics.
Descriptive statistics are limited because the statistics can only be applied to the data that you have actually measured. They cannot be extrapolated to other groups of data.	Inferential statistics can be applied to a larger population of data as long as the sample data which is used is correct representative of the population.
Descriptive statistics are likely to be 100% accurate because there are no assumptions being made about the raw data that is used.	Inferential statistics always make inference about a large population based on a smaller sample. This system cannot be foolproof and is therefore not 100% accurate.
There is a diagrammatic or tabular representation of final result.	The final result is displayed in the form of probability.

- In descriptive statistics measurements such as the mean and standard deviation are stated as exact numbers. Though we may use descriptive statistics all we would like in examining a statistical sample, this branch of statistics does not allow us to say anything about the population.
- Inferential statistics is different from descriptive statistics in many ways. Even though there are similar calculations, such as those for the mean and standard deviation, the focus is different for inferential statistics.
- Inferential statistics does start with a sample and then generalizes to a population. This information about a population is not stated as a number. Instead we express these parameters as a range of potential numbers, along with a degree of confidence.
- It is important to know the difference between descriptive and inferential statistics. This knowledge is helpful when we need to apply it to a real world situation involving statistical methods.
- **Biostatistics:** The methods used in dealing with statistics in the fields of medicine, biology and public health and in planning, conducting and analysis data which arise in investigation in these branches.

- **Vital statistics:** It is the numerical description of birth, death, abortion, marriage, divorce, adoption and judicial separation.
- **Fertility statistics:** It relates to data about the current and future family size.
- **Health statistics:** It deals with data about health resources and diseases.
- **Demographic statistics:** It deals with demographic phenomena such as population density, movement and education level.

Table 14.1 summarizes differences between descriptive and inferential statistics.

STAGES OF STATISTICAL INVESTIGATION (FIG.14.7)

- **Collection:** One of the first and most decisive step in statistical investigation is collection of data. The data are the pieces of information or facts that are collected in scientific investigations.
- **Organization:** After the data are collected, it is necessary to organize to determine if they have been completed correctly. The collected data must be edited very carefully so that the omission, inconsistencies, irrelevant answers and wrong computation may be corrected and adjusted.

- **Presentation:** Third stage of statistical investigation is presenting the organized data in the form of diagrams and graphs.
- **Analysis:** Statistical analysis is done by using central tendency, measure of variation, correlation and regression. It helps find out useful information for decision making.
- **Interpretation:** After the data are analyzed, the findings should be interpreted in light of the study hypothesis.

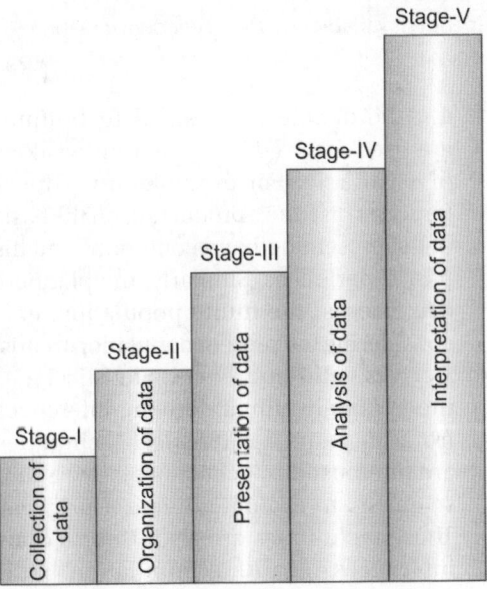

Fig. 14.7: Stages of statistical investigation.

FUNCTIONS OF STATISTICS

Statistics as a discipline is considered indispensable in almost all spheres of human knowledge. There is hardly any branch of study which does not use statistics. Scientific, social and economic studies use statistics in one form or another. These disciplines make-use of observations, facts and figures, enquiries and experiments, etc., using statistics and statistical methods. Statistics studies almost all aspects in an enquiry. It mainly aims at simplifying the complexity of information collected in an enquiry. It presents data in a simplified form as to make them intelligible. It analzses data and facilitates drawal of conclusions. Now let us briefly discuss some of the important functions of statistics **(Fig. 14.8)**.

- **Presents facts in simple form:** Statistics presents facts and figures in a definite form. That makes the statement logical and convincing than mere description. It condenses the whole mass of figures into a single figure. This makes the problem intelligible.
- **Reduces the complexity of data:** Statistics simplifies the complexity of data. The raw data are unintelligible. We make them simple and intelligible by using different statistical measures. Some such commonly used measures are graphs, averages, dispersions, skewness, kurtosis, correlation

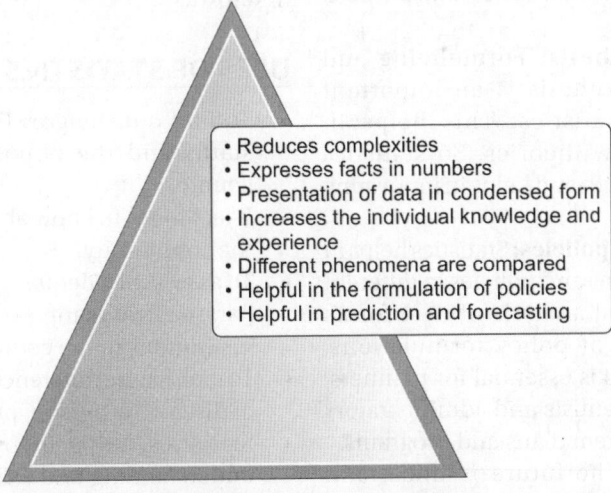

- Reduces complexities
- Expresses facts in numbers
- Presentation of data in condensed form
- Increases the individual knowledge and experience
- Different phenomena are compared
- Helpful in the formulation of policies
- Helpful in prediction and forecasting

Fig. 14.8: Functions of statistics.

Table 14.2: 7C's in functions of statistics.

Sl. No.	Functions	What it does
1.	Collection	The basic ingredient of statistics is data. It should be carefully and scientifically collected
2.	Classification	The collected data is grouped based on similarities so that large and complex data are in understandable form
3.	Condensation	The data is summarized, precisely without losing information to do further statistical analysis
4.	Comparison	It helps to identify the best one and checking for the homogeneity of groups
5.	Correlation	It enables to find the relationship among the variables
6.	Causation	To evaluate the impact of independent variables on the dependent variables

and regression, etc. These measures help in interpretation and drawing inferences. Therefore, statistics enables to enlarge the horizon of one's knowledge.

- **Facilitates comparison:** Comparison between different sets of observation is an important function of statistics. "Comparison is necessary to draw conclusions as professor Boddington rightly points out." The object of statistics is to enable comparison between past and present results to ascertain the reasons for changes, which have taken place and the effect of such changes in future. So to determine the efficiency of any measure comparison is necessary. Statistical devices like averages, ratios, coefficients, etc., are used for the purpose of comparison.
- **Testing hypothesis:** Formulating and testing of hypothesis is an important function of statistics. This helps in developing new theories. So statistics examines the truth and helps in innovating new ideas.
- **Formulation of policies:** Statistics helps in formulating plans and policies in different fields. Statistical analysis of data forms the beginning of policy formulations. Hence, statistics is essential for planners, economists, scientists and administrators to prepare different plans and programs.
- **Forecasting:** The future is uncertain. Statistics helps in forecasting the trend

and tendencies. Statistical techniques are used for predicting the future values of a variable. For example, a producer forecasts his future production on the basis of the present demand conditions and his past experiences. Similarly, the planners can forecast the future population, etc., considering the present population trends.

- **Derives valid inferences:** Statistical methods mainly aim at deriving inferences from an enquiry. Statistical techniques are often used by scholar's planners and scientists to evaluate different projects. These techniques are also used to draw inferences regarding population parameters on the basis of sample information.

Table 14.2 summarizes 7C's in functions of statistics.

USES OF STATISTICS

- To find out the growth rate, the fertility status and the population size of the country.
- It facilitates to know about health status of the community.
- To assess the adequacy of the medical and paramedical manpower and of the health institutions in the country.
- To look for the differences in the magnitude of disease by person, place and time.
- Statistics helps in providing a better understanding and exact description of a phenomenon of nature.

- Statistical helps in proper and efficient planning of a statistical inquiry in any field of study.
- Statistical helps in collecting an appropriate quantitative data.
- Statistics helps in presenting complex data in a suitable tabular, diagrammatic and graphic form for an easy and clear comprehension of the data.
- Statistics helps in understanding the nature and pattern of variability of a phenomenon through quantitative observations.
- Statistics helps in drawing valid inference, along with a measure of their reliability about the population parameters from the sample data.

SCALES OF MEASUREMENT

In statistics and quantitative research methodology, various attempts have been made to classify variables (or types of data) and thereby develop taxonomy of levels of measurement or scales of measure. Perhaps the best known are those developed by the psychologist Stanley Smith Stevens. He proposed four types: nominal, ordinal, interval, and ratio.

Normally, when one hears the term measurement, they may think in terms of measuring the length of something (e.g., the length of a piece of wood) or measuring a quantity of something (i.e., a cup of flour). This represents a limited use of the term measurement. In statistics, the term measurement is used more broadly and is more appropriately termed **scales of measurement**. Scales of measurement refer to ways in which variables/numbers are defined and categorized. Each scale of measurement has certain properties which in turn determine the appropriateness for use of certain statistical analyses. The four scales of measurement are nominal, ordinal, interval, and ratio **(Fig. 14.9)**.

Definition

Measurements are the process of assigning numbers to variables. Measurements, as

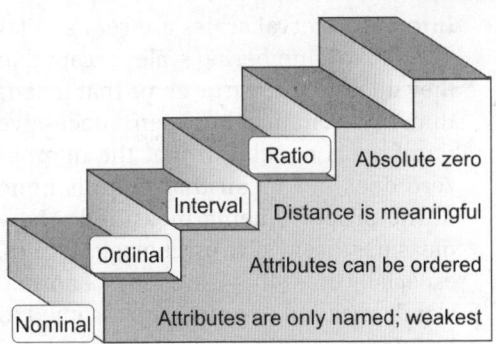

Fig. 14.9: Four scale of measurement.

used in research, imply the qualification of information that is the assigning of some type of numbers to the data.

Levels of Measurement

- **Ordinal measurements:** It involves the sorting of objects on the basis of their relative standing to each other on a specified attribute.
- **Interval measurement:** It indicates not only the rank ordering of objects on an attribute but also the amount of distance between each object. Distance between numeric values on the interval scale represents equivalent distance in the attribute being measured.
- **Nominal measurement:** Are distinguished from interval measurement by virtue of having a rational zero point. Most sophisticated statistical procedures require measures on the interval or ratio scales.

Classifications of Measurements

- **Nominal**: Nominal scales are naming scales. They represent categories where there is no basis for ordering the categories.
- **Ordinal:** Ordinal scales involve categories that can be ordered along a pre-established dimension. However, we have no way of knowing how different the categories are from one another. We state the latter property by saying that we do not have equal intervals between the items. Rankings also represent ordinal scales because we know the order but do not know how different each person is from the next person.

- **Interval:** Interval scales are very similar to standard numbering scales except that they do not have a true zero. That means that the distance between successive numbers is equal, but that the number zero does not mean that there is none of the property being measured. Many measures that involve psychological scales, especially those that use a form of normal standardization (e.g., IQ), are assumed to be interval scales of measurement.
- **Ratio:** Ratio scales are the easiest to understand because they are numbers as we usually think of them. The distance between adjacent numbers is equal on a ratio scale and the score of zero on the ratio scale means that there is none of whatever is being measured. Most ratio scales are counts of things.

Functions of Measurement

Measurements is widely used for:
- Selection of personnel in industry/institution.
- Various types of classification effectively.
- In order to compare two individuals.
- In research, it is basic part of research.
- Improving classroom instruction.

Properties of Measurement

- In the process of measurement numbers are assigned according to some rules.
- Measurements always concerned with certain attributes/features of the object.
- In measurement numerals are used to represent quantities of the attributes.

MEASURES OF CENTRAL TENDENCY

The term **central tendency** refers to the "middle" value or perhaps a typical value of the data, and is measured using the **mean**, **median**, or **mode**. Each of these measures is calculated differently, and the one that is best to use depends upon the situation. The central tendency otherwise called statistical averages. The word "average" implies a value in the distribution, around which the other values are distributed. It gives a mental picture of the central value. Measures of central tendency help to get one single value that describes the characteristics of the entire mass of unwieldy data. This single value for each group of observations tends to representative of that group. This level around which the observations serve as a cluster may vary from group to group. Several measures of central tendency can be calculated for a group of observations. The commonly used central tendency is mean, median and mode (**Fig. 14.10**).

Definition

Central tendency is defined as "the statistical measure that identifies a single value as representative of an entire distribution." It aims to provide an accurate description of the entire data. It is the single value that is most typical/representative of the collected data. The term "number crunching" is used to illustrate this aspect of data description. The mean, median and mode are the three commonly used measures of central tendency.

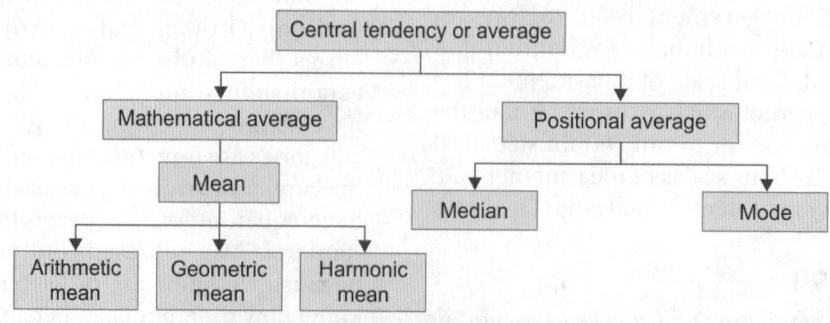

Fig. 14.10: Measures of central tendency.

Meaning of Central Tendency

A measure of central tendency is a single value that attempts to describe a set of data by identifying the central position within that set of data. As such, measures of central tendency are sometimes called measures of central location. They are also classed as summary statistics. The mean (often called the average) is most likely the measure of central tendency that you are most familiar with, but there are others, such as the median and the mode. The mean, median and mode are all valid measures of central tendency, but under different conditions, some measures of central tendency become more appropriate to use than others. In the following sections, we will look at the mean, mode and median, and learn how to calculate them and under what conditions they are most appropriate to be used.

Characteristics of Central Tendency

- **It should be rigidly defined:** If an average is left to the estimation of an observer and if it is not a definite and fixed value it cannot be representative of a series. The bias of the investigator in such cases would considerably affect the value of the average. If the average is rigidly defined; this instability in its value would be no more, and it would always be a definite figure.
- **It should be based on all the observations of the series:** If some of the items of the series are not taken into account in its calculation the average cannot be said to be a representative one. As we shall see later on there are some averages which do not take into account all the values of a group and to this extent they are not satisfactory averages.
- **It should be capable of further algebraic treatment:** If an average dose not possesses this quality, its use is bound to be very limited. It will not be possible to calculate, say, the combined average of two or more series from their individual averages; further it will not be possible to study the average relationship of various parts of a variable if it is expressed as the sum of two or more variables. Many other similar studies would not be possible if the average is not capable of further algebraic treatment.
- **It should be easy to calculate and simple to follow:** If the calculation of the average involves tedious mathematical processes it will not be readily understood and its use will be confined only to a limited number of persons. It can never be a popular average. As such, one of the qualities of a good average is that it should not be too abstract or mathematical and there should be no difficulty in its calculation. Further, the properties of the average should be such that they can be easily understood by persons of ordinary intelligence.

Table 14.3: Types of central tendency.

Term	Definition
Central tendency	• The tendency for a set of values to gather around the middle of the set • Generally measured by mean, median, and mode
Mean	• Average • $\Sigma x/n$ (sum of all values [x] over the number of values [n]) • should be applied to continuous data if normally distributed
Median	• Middle value of an ordered sample of numerical values • Extreme values do not affect the median as much as the mean. For example: Length of stay, house prices • Usually applied to numerical data (unless normally distributed)
Mode	• Value that occurs most frequently • Can be used for skewed numerical data or categorical data

- **It should not be affected by fluctuations of sampling:** If two independent sample studies are made in any particular field, the averages thus obtained, should not materially differ from each other. No doubt, when two separate enquires are made, there is bound to be a difference, in the average values calculated but in some cases this difference would be great while in others comparatively less. These averages in which this difference, which is technically called "fluctuation of sampling" is less, are considered better than those in which its difference is more.

Uses of Central Tendency

Central tendency is very useful in psychology. It lets us know what is normal or 'average' for a set of data. It also condenses the data set down to one representative value, which is useful when you are working with large amounts of data. Could you imagine how difficult it would be to describe the central location of a 1,000 item data set if you had to consider every number individually? Central tendency allows you to compare one data set to another. For example, let's say you have a sample of girls and a sample of boys and you are interested in comparing their heights. By calculating the average height for each sample, you could easily draw comparisons between the girls and boys. Central tendency is also useful when you want to compare one piece of data to the entire data set. Let's say that you received an 60% on your last Psychology quiz, which is usually in the D range. You go around and talk to your classmates and find out that the average score on the quiz was 43%. In this instance, your score was significantly higher than those of your classmates. Since your teacher grades on a curve, your 60% becomes an A. Had you not known about measures of central tendency, you probably would have been really upset by your grade and assume that you bombed the test.

Mean

The arithmetic mean is widely used in statistical calculation. They give us an idea about the centralization of the values in the central part of the distribution. To obtain the mean, the individual observations are first added together, and then divided by the number of observations.

Definition

- According to professor Bowley, mean is a statistical constant which enable us to comprehend in a single effort, the significance of the whole.
- Averages or what is typical for a group of values such as scores, grades, etc. The three major measures of central tendency are the mean, median and mode.

Uses of averages or measures of central tendency

- An average helps to find that how the normal observations lying close to central value while few of the too large or too small lie for away at both the ends.
- To find which group is better by comparing the average of one group with that of the other group.
- Mean is used when a reliable and accurate measure of central tendency is needed.
- Mean is used when the same scores are distributed symmetrically around the central point.
- Mean is used when the greatest stability is required.
- Mean is used when other statically calculation SD/MD/AD are to be completed.
- Mean is used when we are having a series with no extreme items.

Mean calculation

- The operation of adding together is called summation and is denoted by the sign Σ or S. The individual observation is denoted by the sign π and the mean is denoted by the sign X.
- The mean (X) is calculated thus: The symbol blood pressure of 10 individuals was 100, 110, 115, 120, 126, 124, 115, 110, 130, 120. The total was 1170. The mean is 1170 divided by 10 which are 117.

Mean is the arithmetic average. For example, the mean of the following group of numbers 60,70, 80, 90,100 is 80 and is calculated by dividing the sum of the values by the number of values in the group (N = 5): 60 + 70 + 80 + 90 + 100 = 400/5 = 80. The mean is the most commonly used statistical measure and is most useful in depicting what is typical for a group of values. It is also used extensively with other statistical formulae.

Merits

- Simple to understand
- Aggregate by the value of every item
- Defined by rigid formula
- Relatively reliable
- Central or gravity and balance is present
- Calculated value is not based of position.

Demerits

- It does not take into account the precise value of each observation and hence does not use all information available in the data.
- Unlike mean, median is not amenable to further mathematical calculation and hence is not used in many statistical tests.
- If we pool the observations of two groups, median of the pooled group cannot be expressed in terms of the individual medians of the pooled groups.
- Large proportion of the values, the mean may be subjected to statistical error.
- It may be unduly influenced by abnormal values in the distribution.

Median

It is a middle value in a distribution. To obtain the median, the data is first arranged in an ascending or descending order of magnitude, and then the value of middle observation is located. The median is a better measure of center than mean when the distribution is skewed.

Median is used

- When midpoint of the given distribution is to be found.
- When the series contain extreme scores.
- When there is open end distribution it is more reliable than mean.
- Mean cannot be calculated graphically, median can be calculated graphically.

- For articles that cannot be precisely measured.

Median calculation

The birth weight of 9 babies were 3.0, 2.6, 2.4, 2.8, 3.2, 2.9, 3.0, 3.4, 2.6 kg. First the data are ordered 2.4, 2.6, 2.6, 2.8, 2.9, 3.0, 3.2, and 3.4. The fifth one, which is the central value. The median birth weight of the nine babies is 2.9 kg.

Properties of median

- It cannot calculated from raw data.
- It can be found out graphically.
- It is not distorted by the presence of extreme or disproportionate values.

Merits

- It is easier to compute than mean.
- Extreme values do not affect.
- More appropriated average in dealing with qualitative data.
- The median indicated the value of middle item in the distribution.

Limitations

- It is not capable of algebraic treatment.
- In positional average, its value is not determined by each and every observation.
- The value of median is affected more by sampling fluctuations than the value of arithmetic mean.

Mode

The mode or the modal value is that the value in the series of observations which occur with great frequency. The mode is the commonly occurring value in a distribution of data. It is the most frequent item or the most "fashionable" value in a series of observations.

Mode calculation

The diastolic blood pressure of 10 individuals was 90, 98, 100, 98, 94, 96, 98, 94, 96, and 94. The mode or the most frequently occurring value is 96.

Merits

- It is the most typical or representative value of distribution.
- Mode is not unduly affected by extreme values.

- Its value can be determined the class limit.
- It can be used to describe qualitative phenomenon.
- Mode value can be determined graphically.

Limitations

- The value of mode cannot be always be determined. In some cases we may have a bimodal series.
- It is not capable of doing algebraic manipulation.
- The value of mode is not based on each and every item of the series.
- It is not rigidly defined measure.

Standard Deviation

- Standard deviation is the most widely used measure of dispersion of a series and is commonly denoted by the symbol 'sigma'.
- Standard deviation is defined as the square root of the average of squares of deviations, when such deviation for the values of individual items in a series is obtained from the arithmetic average.
- Standard summarizes average amount of deviation from mean. This is an important measure of dispersion and most commonly used in statistical analysis.
- Standard deviation is the positive square root of the arithmetic mean of the squares of deviation of the given values from arithmetic mean.

Steps of computing SD

- Calculate the mean(X).
- Find the difference of each observation from the mean (X – X).
- Square the difference (X –X)².
- Add the squared values to get the sum of squares [Σ(X–X)²].
- Divide the sum by the number of observations minus 1 to get root mean square deviation.

$$\text{Sigma square} = \frac{\Sigma\,(X{-}X)^2}{n{-}1}$$

- Find the square root of the variance to get root mean square deviation.

$$\text{Sigma} = \text{square root of } \frac{\Sigma\,(X{-}X)^2}{n{-}1}$$

Uses of standard deviation

- Standard deviation is the best measure of dispersion. It is widely used because it possess most of the characteristics of an ideal measure of dispersion.
- It is mostly used in research programs.
- It is uses in coefficient of correlation and in the study of frequency distribution and normal distribution.
- The standard deviation otherwise known as variance, which is frequently used in the context of analysis of variation.

Merits

- Standard deviation is rigidly defined.
- Standard deviation is based upon all observations.
- Standard deviation is capable of further mathematical treatment.
- Standard deviation is less affected by sampling variations.

Demerits

- Standard deviation is not simple to understand and not easy to calculate.
- Standard deviation is much affected by extreme values.
- Standard deviation cannot be calculated for open end classes without any assumptions.
- It cannot be calculated for qualitative data.

NORMAL DISTRIBUTION AND CURVE

- The normal distribution or normal curve is an important concept in statistical theory. Standard deviation measures the position of an observation with regard to mean. It defines the limits of normality and indicates changes of occurrence of an observation in a population. To know how standard deviation does all these one has to understand what is normal distribution or standard distribution.
- When a large number of observations of any variable characteristics such as height, weight, blood pressure, pulse rate, etc., are taken at random to make it a representative sample. In normal curve,

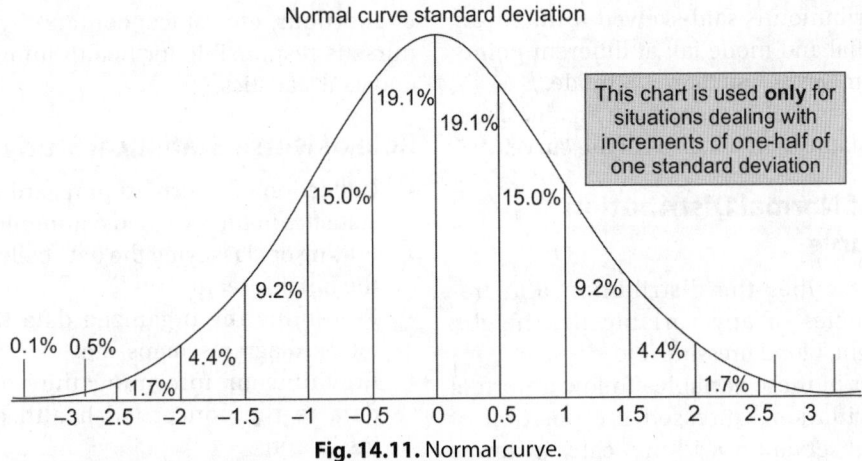

Fig. 14.11. Normal curve.

		Which of the following are characteristics of a normal distribution?
☐	A.	A normal distribution curve is bell shaped.
☐	B.	The normal distribution curve is symmetric about the standard deviation.
☐	C.	The normal distribution curve crosses the X axis.
☐	D.	The normal curve is a discrete distribution.
☐	E.	The total area under the normal distribution curve is 1.00.
☐	F.	The area under the part of a normal curve that lies within 2 standard deviations of the mean is approximately 0.95.
☐	G.	The area under the part of a normal curve that lies within 3 standard deviations of the mean is approximately 0.95.
☐	H.	The area under the part of a normal curve that lies within 1 standard deviation of the mean is approximately 0.68.
☐	I.	The normal distribution curve is unimodal.
☐	J.	The mean, median, and mode are located at the center of the distribution.

the shape depends upon the number and nature of observations.

Definition

Normal curve defined as the frequency distribution of the curve, which represents a normal symmetrical distribution of quantitative data series.

Characteristics of a Normal Curve

- The normal curve is symmetrical, smooth and bell shaped.
- The highest frequencies are concentrated in the center of the curve around the mean and lowest at the two extremes.

- All the three measures of central tendency: Mean, median and mode—at the center of the curve; their values are identical in a normal distribution series.
- It has two curves, central part is convex, when it comes down it becomes concave on both sides.
- A perpendicular from the point of inflection will cut the base at a distance of ISD from mean on either side.

Skewness and Kurtosis

- Skewness is studied to have an idea about the shape of the curve, which we can draw with the help of the given data. The distribution is said skewed if the mean, medial and mode fall at different points, i.e., mean =/= median =/= mode.

- Kurtosis enables us to have an idea about the flatness or peakness of the curve.

Uses of Normal Distribution and Curve

- It describes the distribution and frequencies of any variable like height, weight, blood pressure, etc.
- Most of these variables follow a normal distribution expressed the position of an observation arithmetically in terms of mean and SD and drawn/shown graphically as a histogram.
- Normal distribution curve is of paramount importance in applied statistics, it is fundamental to the tests of significance.

STATISTICS AND NURSING

In health research, statistics may be used to determine the prevalence and incidence of illness, or to establish if a new treatment is effective. Presenting the results from the statistical analysis of the data collected is a key part to establishing the evidence from the research undertaken. The results of studies must be examined carefully to ensure that the data collected are presented and interpreted accurately. It is also important to observe whether the results are misleading, in that there is evidence of selective reporting, or the strength of the findings is overestimated. It is important to note that statistically significant findings do not always indicate clinically significant findings.

Statistics signifies numerical information qualitative as well as quantitative. Qualitative data deals with race, religion, residence, sex, marital status, educational status, occupational status, social status, and health status. Quantitative data deals with height, weight, temperature, blood pressure, pulse rate, birth order, number of children and number of abortions, etc., since; community health nurse is responsible for health information and vital statistics.

Role of Nurse Statistical Study

- Collection of information regarding vital statistics in the assigned community.
- Editing or classifying the data collected by the nursing team.
- Presenting the organized data through tables, diagrams, maps, etc.
- Providing or informing the collected data to the concerned health officer/institutions.
- Application of nursing process steps to analyze the data.
- Creating health awareness through mass health education based on obtained data.
- Nursing diagnosis are prepared and formed based on analyzed data for providing care.
- Updating the current data and information are applied into the nursing practices.
- Utilizing and linking the health information management system effective in the community.
- Conducting and organizing nursing research at the community level based on existing statistical issues.

CONCLUSION

Statistics are the methods and techniques used to collect, analyze, interpret and present data. We are all exposed to statistics on a daily basis as the use of statistics is common place within the media, being used within political, health, financial or sports reports. Nurses also routinely use statistics within their practice, such as when they give health information to patients about their diagnosis or prognosis and in discussing the adverse effects of medication or treatment. Knowledge of basic statistics is therefore essential and will help nurses to understand and assess the credibility of the evidence presented.

15

Utilization of Research in Nursing Practice

LEARNING OBJECTIVES

- Meaning of research utilization
- Methods to promote and disseminate research findings
- Research utilization in nursing practice

- Nurses role to fill the gap
- Value of research utilization
- Evidence-based nursing research

INTRODUCTION

Research utilization is the process of synthesizing, disseminating, and using research-generated knowledge to make an impact on or change in the existing nursing practice. The research utilization process was developed years ago to address the problems of using research findings in practice. Research utilization refers to the actual systematic implementation of a scientifically sound, research-based innovation in a health care setting with an accompanying process to access the outcome(s) of the clinical change. Research utilization fosters movement from innovation into practice. The process of dissemination is intended to produce an effective utilization of information on the part of the recipient.

DEFINITION

- Research utilization is defined as "the use of **research** knowledge, often based on a single study in clinical practice."
- Research utilization is "a process of using findings from conducting research to guide practice".
- "The process by which scientifically produced knowledge is transferred to practice" (Barnsteiner and Prevost, 2002).

- Research utilization refers to the review and critique of scientific research, and then the application of the findings to clinical practice (Estabrooks, 1998).

MEANING OF RESEARCH UTILIZATION

Research utilization is the process of synthesizing, disseminating, and using research-generated knowledge to make an impact on or change in the existing nursing practice. The research utilization process was developed years ago to address the problems of using research findings in practice. Research utilization is a multi-step process that involves; critique and synthesis of findings from several studies, application of these findings to make a change in nursing practice, and measurement of the outcomes from the change in nursing practice. Research utilization has a smaller focus than evidence-based practice.

In the past two decades, professional practice development has evolved from research utilization to evidence-based practice. Evidence-based practice requires integration of best research evidence of high-quality studies in a health-related area, focusing on health promotion, illness prevention, and the assessment, diagnosis and

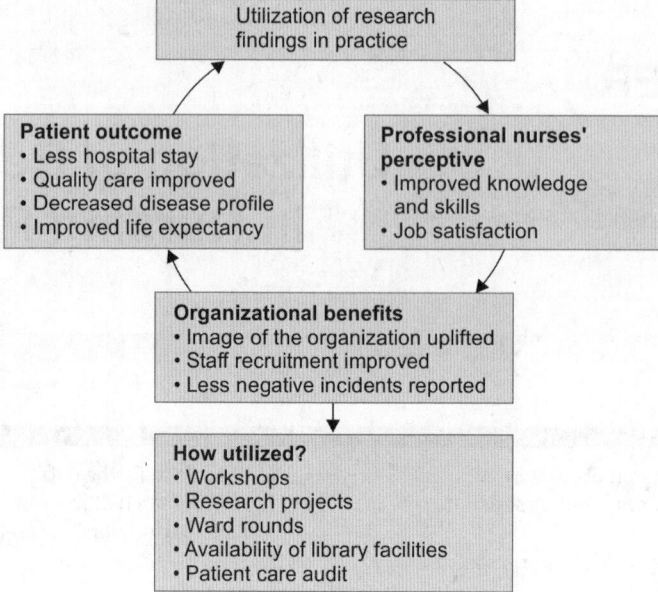

Fig. 15.1: Research utilization.

management of acute and chronic illnesses. In addition, clinical expertise, patient values and needs in the delivery of quality, cost-effective health care are essential components in the conscientious integration of evidence-based practice.

PURPOSE OF RESEARCH UTILIZATION

- Application of available knowledge to improve client outcomes.
- Validation of existing nursing procedures and intervention.

METHODS TO PROMOTE AND DISSEMINATE RESEARCH FINDINGS

Methods that promote and disseminate research findings include:
- Publication of findings in scholarly journals
- Presentations at national or local professional conferences
- Written clinical summary statements
- Poster presentations at local and national conferences

- Verbal information at local unit meetings and at various hospital committee meetings
- Presentations at journal clubs
- Dissertations
- Presentations at continuing educational in-services

Points to kept in mind before dissemination of research findings:

To be most effective, dissemination strategies must be incorporated into the earliest planning stages of a research study. In fact, the most successful dissemination processes are typically designed prior to the start of any research project.

In creating a dissemination plan, researchers should consider several key questions:

- **Goals** and objectives of the dissemination effort? What impact do you hope to have?
- **Audience**: Who is affected most by this research? Who would be interested in learning about the study findings? Is this of interest to a broader community?
- **Medium:** What is the most effective way to reach each audience? What resources does each group typically access?

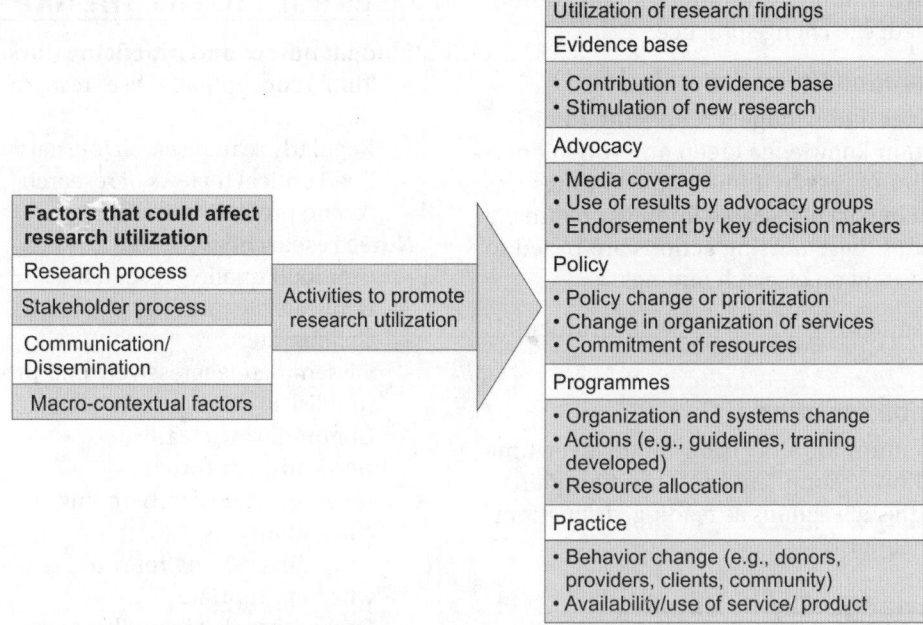

Fig. 15.2: Activities to promote research utilization.

- **Execution:** When should each aspect of the dissemination plan occur (e.g., at which points during the study and afterwards)? Who will be responsible for dissemination activities?

CHARACTERISTICS OF EFFECTIVE COMMUNICATION

Characteristics of effective communication of the research findings:
- Orient toward the needs of the audience, using appropriate language and information levels.
- **Include various dissemination methods:** Written text including illustrations, graphs and figures; electronic and web-based tools; and oral presentations at community meetings and scientific conferences.
- Leverage existing resources, relationships, and networks fully.

RESEARCH UTILIZATION IN NURSING PRACTICE

By research utilization - nurses in the clinical setting it helps the nurse in:

- Promotes critical thinking
- Enhances professional self-concept
- Ensures safe and reflective practice
- Practice based on current, scientific, sound knowledge
- Enrich nurse's self-confidence.

Utilization in Clinical Setting

- Conceptual utilization—use of findings to cognitively restructure thinking about a phenomenon, influences nurses' thinking about an issue. A continuum in terms of the specificity or diffuseness of the use of knowledge.

Conceptual ←——————→ Instrumental
        Mid-ground

Situations in which users (nurses) are influenced in their thinking about an issue based on their knowledge of one or more studies but do not put the knowledge to any specific documented used.

Instrumental Utilization

Base specific actions on research, and is discrete with clearly identifiable attempts to base some specific action on the results of research findings and direct application of knowledge to change practice.

Mid-ground Utilization

Includes knowledge creep and decision accretion knowledge creep an evolving percolation of research ideas and findings has partial impact of research findings on nursing activities these nursing actions are based to some extent on research findings.

Conceptual $\longleftarrow$ Mid-ground $\longrightarrow$ Instrumental

Decision Accretion

Momentum for a decision builds over time based on accumulated information gained through such actions as reading, discussions, and meetings.

Knowledge Gap in Nursing Production and Utilization

- A gap does exist in nursing, as well as other disciplines.
- Some gap is inevitable given the imperfection of scientific research as a means of knowing.

Possible Inflated Gap Nursing Knowledge: Production and Utilization

- **Technical changes:** Utilization studies do not always consider changes that make the knowledge irrelevant.
- **Risk/benefit analysis:** The risks for problems if the results are implemented and prove to be incorrect.
- **Non-captured utilization:** Focus of utilization studies is most often on instrumental utilization; probably mid-ground utilization of the continuum not capture.

NURSES ROLE TO FILL THE GAP

- **Student nurses and practicing nurses**
  - Think, conceptually "use" research findings
  - Regularly read research journals
  - Read critical reviews of research
  - Attend professional conferences
- **Nurse researchers**
  - Conduct "quality" research
  - Replicate
  - Collaborate
  - Disseminate aggressively and broadly (publish)
  - Communicate clearly
- **Scholars and educators**
  - Incorporate research findings into the curriculum
  - Note absence of relevant research, when appropriate
  - Encourage research utilization
  - Prepare integrative research reviews with class content
- **Administration**
  - Foster a climate of intellectual curiosity
  - Offer emotional or "moral" support for utilization reward efforts for utilization.

Planned Change

Change agent one who works to bring about a change.

Driving and Restraining Forces

- Begin the change process by analyzing the entire system involved to identify the forces for and against change.
- **Driving forces:** Push the system toward change
- **Restraining forces:** Pull the system away from change.

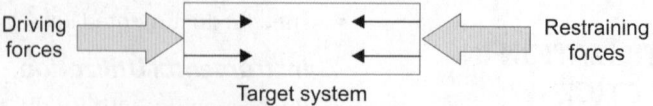

Driving forces → Target system ← Restraining forces

(Force Field Model) Adapted from Lewis, K. (1951)

Fig. 15.3: Driving and restraining forces.

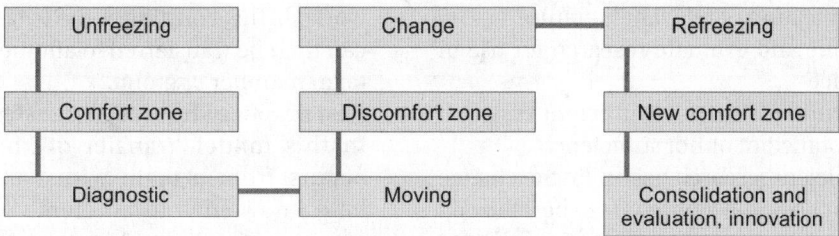

Fig. 15.4: Change process in research utilization.

Problem

Concern: When the existing restraining forces are the same or stronger than the driving forces.

Resolution

Use participative change strategies to reduce the restraining forces and increase the driving forces for change to occur.

Assessing opposing forces

Need a thorough knowledge about:
- The target system
- The environment
- The characteristics of the change
- The potential responses to change

People resist change sources

Technical, psychological needs and threats to position and power.

THE CHANGE PROCESS IN RESEARCH UTILIZATION

Change process: It occurs in four phases:
1. **Unfreezing creates disconfirmation** (feelings of discomfort or dissatisfaction)—introduces guilt and anxiety (demonstrate unmet goal or value), provides psychological safety (sufficient security to minimize risk and at completion of the unfreezing phase—people feel "off-balance", have hyper-energy and people require direction for productive action.
2. **Implementation phase of change:** The target system is unfrozen and moving towards change) the change agent—introduces new information, encourages the new behavior, continues the supportive climate, provides opportunities for ventilation, feedback and clarification of

goals and presents self as trustworthy to overcomes resistance.
3. **Refreezing:** To stabilize and integrate the change so that it becomes a regular part of target system beginning of the phase—Situation still fluid the target system could still take another course than the planned change.
4. **Change agent's action in the refreezing phase:** Continues to act as an energizer, guide new behavior, increase delegation of responsibilities for change behavior, maintain visibility and credibility of change and increases others' responsibility.

LOWA MODEL FOR RESEARCH-BASED PRACTICE

Application of LOWA model for research-based practice:

Steps

- Determine type trigger to improve practice through research that will initiate the need for change.

Problem-focused triggers
- Risk management data
- Process improvement data
- Internal/external benchmarking data
- Financial data
- Identification of clinical problem

Knowledge-focused triggers
- New research or other literature
- National agencies or organizational standards and guidelines
- Philosophies of care
- Observation from institutional standards committees

- Identification of relevant literature
- Critique and evaluate research for use in practice
- Determine if there is sufficient research base sufficient or not sufficient
- If sufficient research base pilot the change in practice: Select outcome to be achieved
  - Design nursing/multidisciplinary practice interventions
  - Implement practice changes on a pilot unit
  - Evaluate process and outcomes
  - Modify intervention as needed
- Insufficient research base:
  - Conduct research
  - Base practice on other types of evidence
    - Case reports
    - Expert opinions
    - Scientific principles
    - Theory
- Ask: Is the change appropriate for adoption in practice
- If answer is "no" continue to evaluate quality of care and new knowledge
- If answer is "yes" Institute the change in practice
- Monitor outcomes:
  - Patient family
  - Environment staff
  - Fiscal and (cost)
- Disseminate results.

KNOWLEDGE TRANSFER MODELS

Many researchers (Dixon, 2000; NCDDR, 2001) in the knowledge utilization and management area describe the appropriate choice of knowledge transfer activity to be critically linked to the leveraging of knowledge from one group to another. Some examples and descriptions of knowledge transfer models follow:

- **Serial knowledge transfer model:** In this model, transfer is leveraged from one work "team" to a very similar work team in another similar work setting. Knowledge is transferred from individual members of the team, to the team as a whole, i.e., integrated into a commonly-held perception of what

worked. This constitutes the basis of what can then be transferred to another similar team member or group.

- **Best practice knowledge transfer model:** In this model, transfer of knowledge occurs from a team with commonly-held knowledge to all elements of the organization within which the team exists. This transfer model is usually inspired within a competitive organization that is looking to increase its "edge" on the competition. Knowledge that is transferred is generally accepted as "best practices" within the organization, thus, encouraging utilization.
- **Exemplary knowledge transfer model:** In this model, the knowledge transfer is from the organizational level, and the transfer is intended to impact other organizations that may or may not be similar in scope and function. In this case, what an organization has done well is the "knowledge" subject to transfer, and generally, competitive secrets are not given away in the process.
- **Strategy–based knowledge transfer model:** In this model, the knowledge encompasses an overall strategy or approach in addressing a specific and often non–routine problem. Transfer is based around other entities that may recognize a similar problem and be in need of developing a responsive and effective strategy.
- **Expert knowledge transfer model:** In this model, individuals that may have been known to have experienced and overcome similar problems, are viewed as experts. This expertise becomes known and valued and is called upon when "problems" generally related to the original "problem" occur.

These examples of knowledge transfer models provide a conceptual framework upon which the dissemination and utilization of research results can be based. Some of these knowledge transfer models can be accomplished best through face-to-face contact. Others, however, do lend themselves to the use of electronic network and web-based information sharing techniques.

- **Building blocks of utilization modeling:** To develop the knowledge transfer base that underlies utilization, there are five common core elements that are keys to success. These core elements strongly influence whether utilization efforts will be effective:
  1. *Source*: Where does the research information come from?
  2. *Content*: What is the research information about?
  3. *Context*: How does the research information relate to existing knowledge or products?
  4. *Medium*: How can I get the research information?
  5. *User*: How can I benefit from this research information?

VALUE OF RESEARCH UTILIZATION

As nurse researcher—value of research utilization:
- Validates researcher's efforts, existing nursing knowledge re-procedures or interventions
- Provides motivation for scholars to continue to discover new knowledge
- Reinforces professional accountability
- Helps uncover new clinical problems for investigation
- To facilitate an innovative change that leads to improved client outcomes.

Evidence-based Practice

- Uses research to direct client care.
- Challenges nurses to critically examine traditional practices, procedures, and nursing rituals and question those that are not substantiated by research or other evidence.

Value of Research Utilization

- Promotes critical thinking and reflective practice
- Enhances professional self-concept

- Ensures provision of safe and effective care
- Practice is based on current, scientifically sound knowledge
- Self-confidence of the nurse is enhanced.

Value of Research Utilization to the Researcher

- Validates the efforts of the researcher
- Motivates scholars to continue to discover new knowledge
- Reinforces professional accountability
  Helps discover new clinical problems for investigation.

Value to the Health Care Agency

- Cost-effective nursing care
- High-quality care
- Improved client outcomes
- Retention and recruitment tools
- Professionally satisfied and stimulated nursing staff

Value to the Profession

- Enhanced autonomy of practice
- Positive professional image
- Strengthen professional status
- Expand the field of nursing's scientific knowledge base.

STEPS IN RESEARCH UTILIZATION PROCESS

Steps in the research utilization process to bridge the gap between research-practice through research utilization.

Select a relevant problem area that requires evidence to bring about change problem focused triggers for problem identification that is evident to nurses in the practice setting-clinical problems.

Common areas for the problem identifications are:
- Journal clubs
- Attending a professional/academic conference
- Reading a scientific paper
- Review the literature obtain the sufficient quantity and quality

- Determine if the literature findings are appropriate to apply in your setting
- Develop a written research-based protocol and/or procedure to communicate the innovation and ensure consistency in approach and show research base for it
- Implementation of the planned innovation
- Evaluation of the success of the innovation
- Dissemination of the findings.

BARRIERS TO RESEARCH UTILIZATION

- Characteristics of the nurse
- Characteristics of the setting
- Characteristics of the research
- Characteristics of the innovation.

Barriers: Nurse

- Knowledge
- Attitude
- Erroneous beliefs
- Lack of time.

Barriers: Setting

- Ethos of openness to new ideas
- Interpersonal and information linkages
- Freedom from organizational constraints
- Supportive leadership
- Trust.

Barriers: Research

- Communicate results clearly and comprehensively
- Publish widely in user-friendly journals
- Focus on problems of importance to nursing practice
- Increase the number of replicated studies.

Barriers: Innovation

- Must offer a relative advantage over the status quo
- Compatibility with current practice
- Complexity of innovation is inversely related to success
- Trial ability or pilot testing
- Observability of benefits and limitations

STRATEGIES TO FACILITATE RESEARCH-BASED PRACTICE

- Planned change (unfreezing, moving, re-freezing) phases (Lewin, 1951)
- Theory of diffusion of innovation (awareness, persuasion, decision, implementation, confirmation stages) (Rodgers, 1965, 1995)
- Deliberately expose one-self to research literature and findings
- Journal clubs
- Conference attendance
- Support research in setting
- Educators can role model utilization of research in their teaching and engage students in reflective practice
- Provide critiquing assignments and regular research reviews to students
- Researchers can conduct rigorous studies
- Identify implications of research for practice
- Replicate previous studies
- Incorporate research findings into text books.

Guidelines for evaluating implementation of research findings:

- Utility to practice
- Applicability to practice
- Replication
- Scientific merit
- Client safety
- Feasibility.

DIFFICULTIES IN RESEARCH UTILIZATION

The purpose of research is to be of use-to change current practice, or to confirm it. Yet the process of moving new understandings and new products from research to practice usually takes years, decades, or even generations. Although there are good reasons for moving carefully-new research needs to be evaluated, replicated, and refined-too often the pace of change is set, not by a rigorous process of review and refinement, but by the gap between the research community and the world of practice.

Research on dissemination, or knowledge utilization as it is sometimes called, has yielded a wealth of information about what does and does not work. But, due to this gap, those understandings for the most part have not moved from the research community-those who study the process of knowledge use—to the practice community-those responsible for adopting and applying research outcomes. As a result, most dissemination practices are still based on a mechanistic, linear conception of dissemination as a process of "getting the word out."

Approaches designed to promote knowledge utilization within the fields of rehabilitation and education traditionally have been drawn from the agricultural extension model, whose basic presumption is that people will use research-based products only if they have access to information about them. The success of the agricultural extension model, along with other experience, tells us that this presumption is true, in some cases, and under specific circumstances. However, even with its long-term funding, strong coordination, and close links with practitioners, the agricultural extension system has proved to be much less effective when the research-based outcomes to be disseminated stray from agricultural production technology into areas calling for attitudinal or behavioral changes.

Below is a list of findings from research on knowledge use that suggest a few of the complexities in identifying utilization "models" and encouraging their application by others. Researchers are frequently not addressing utilization goals with sufficient detail to overcome these complexities:

- The actual quality of a research design is less important, in terms of its likelihood of being adopted and used, than the extent to which it fits with users' established beliefs and experience.
- The source producing research outcomes is more important than the quality of the research design. People tend to trust sources with whom they have established relationships and/or for whom they have high levels of respect.

- The degree of credibility of information sources is related to two factors: Perceived expertise and perceived trustworthiness. The more intensely people are involved with an issue; the more likely they are to question both the expertise and the trustworthiness of those whose information contradicts their own current understandings.
- When research outcomes do get used in real-world settings, the resulting practices, programs, or products are often quite different from the researcher's original conception. While researchers often produce new information, they do not routinely provide demonstrations or other utilization assistance to interpret how it "fits" into real-world environments. Additionally, utilization requires that some adaptations be made to apply new models into existing contexts.
- The extent to which the intended beneficiaries of particular research are involved in the research process, the more likely a researcher will have stories, examples, and general information that is couched from the "user" perspective. This information is often critical in promoting utilization.

EVIDENCE-BASED NURSING RESEARCH

Evidence-based nursing practice was started in 1800s with Florence nightingale. It is a problem solving approach to clinical decision making. It is the process of integrating clinical knowledge, judgment, proficiency skills with the best available clinical evidence, such as nursing practice into patient care. Gaining knowledge and skills in evidence-based practice provides nurses and other clinicians the tools needed to take ownership of their practice and transform health care in a comprehensive manner.

Definition

- Evidence-based practice is an integration of the best evidence available, nursing expertise and the values and preferences of

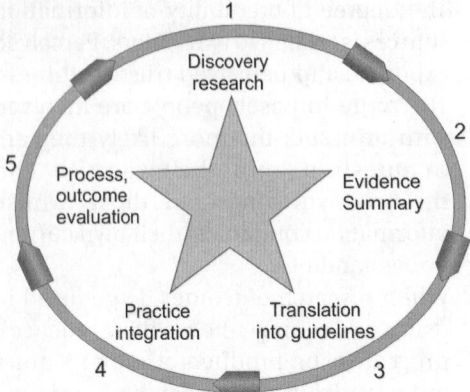

Fig. 15.5: Evidence-based nursing research.

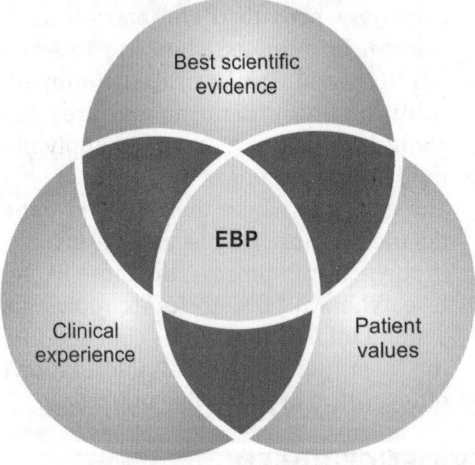

Fig. 15.6: Components of evidence-based practice.

	• **Patient, Population or Problem**
P	• How would you describe a group of patients similar to yours? What are the most important characteristics of the patient?

	• **Intervention, prognostic factor, or exposure**
I	• Which main intervention, prognostic factor, or exposure are you considering? What do you want to do for the patient?

	• **Comparison**
C	• What is the main alternative to compare with the intervention?

	• **Outcome**
O	• What can you hope to accomplish, measure, improve or affect? What are you trying to do for the patient?

Fig. 15.7: PICO model.

the practitioner systematically finds, appraises and uses the most current and valid research findings as the basis for clinical decisions. **—Mosby**

- Evidence-based practice is the conscientious use of current best evidence in making clinical decisions about patient care.

Evidence-based nursing practice (EBNP) means that nurses make clinical decisions based on the best research evidence, their clinical expertise, and the health care preferences of their patients/clients. Although EBNP may be based on factors other than research findings, such as patient preferences and the expertise of clinicians, the aim of EBNP is to provide the best possible care based on the best available research. To back up the importance of EBNP, Sigma Theta Tau International, Honor Society of Nursing and Blackwell Publishing initiated a new journal in 2004 titled World views on evidence-based nursing. It is a quarterly peer-reviewed journal. The nursing profession exists to provide a service to society, and this service should be based on accurate knowledge. Research has been determined to be the most reliable means of obtaining knowledge. As previously mentioned, there are other means of acquiring knowledge, such as through tradition, authority, and trial and

the individuals, families and communities are served. **—Chris Jordan**

- Evidence-based practice is a continuous interactive process involving the explicit, conscientious and judicious consideration of the best available evidence to provide care.

—Canadian Nurses Association

- Evidence-based practice is a problem solving approach to the delivery of health care that integrates the best evidence from studies and patient care data with clinician expertise and patient preferences and values. **—Fineout Overholt**

- Evidence-based practice nursing is the practice of health care in which

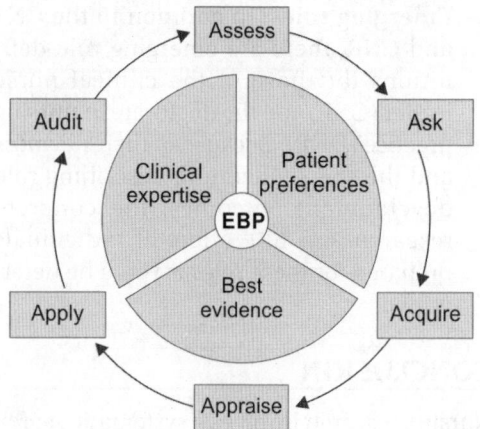

Fig. 15.8: Approaches of evidence-based practice.

error. The scientific method, however, has been determined to be the most objective, systematic way of obtaining knowledge.

Purposes of EBP

- To provide the highest quality and most cost-efficient nursing care possible.
- To advance quality of care provided by the nurses.
- To increase satisfaction of patients.
- To focus on nursing practice away from habits and tradition to evidence and research.

Steps Involved in EBP

- Select a topic and correct appropriate reviews.
- Analyze data for clinical practice and design interventions based on evidence.
- Predict and analyze outcomes and examine the pattern of behavior and outcomes.
- Identify gaps in EBP and evaluate projects to determine and implement best practices.

Limitations

- Resistant to change in nursing practice.
- Ability to critically appraise research findings in nursing.
- Poor administrative support in nursing.

- Fear of stepping on one's toes in nursing.
- Lack of continuing educational programmes in nursing.

Nurse Researcher and Evidence-based Practice Roles

Nursing roles are specifically focused on research and EBP:

Clinical nurse specialist (CNS) and the clinical nurse researcher (CNR).

1. **Clinical nurse specialist:** The CNS is a registered nurse with graduate preparation in a specialized area of nursing practice and an expert clinician with additional responsibility for education and research. A CNS is in an ideal position to link research to practice by assessing an agency's readiness for research utilization, consulting with staff to identify clinical problems, and helping staff to discover, implement, and evaluate findings that improve health care delivery (National Association of Clinical Nurse Specialists, 2003, 2004). CNSs are educated in the research process and can conduct their own investigations and collaborate with doctorally prepared nurses.

2. **Clinical nurse researcher:** The CNR should be a doctorally prepared nurse with clinical and research experience. Terminology used to refer to this type of position tends to vary among countries, settings, and agencies. One might see position postings for clinical nurse scientist, nurse scientist, director of nursing research, and others. A CNR can focus either on the conduct or facilitation of research and should possess knowledge of statistics, grantsmanship, evaluation research, and administration. Interpersonal skills, such as patience, flexibility, and approachability, are imperative. A CNR employed by a hospital or home health agency must develop relationships with staff nurses to identify the research questions that staff nurses see as most significant in the particular setting.

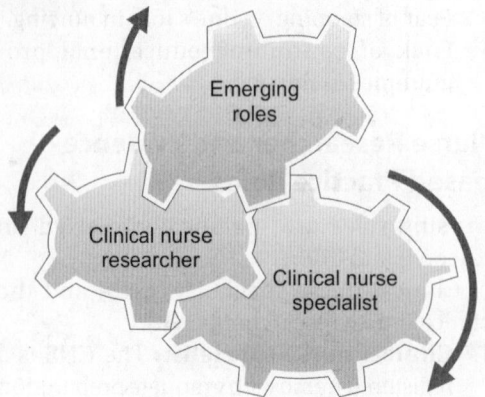

Fig. 15.9: Role of nurse in evidence-based practice.

The CNR is responsible for designing studies and assisting staff nurses with understanding the implications of the study. In addition, the CNR provides guidance to the staff regarding their role in the research process. This role could involve patient recruitment for studies or actual data collection. The CNR also is responsible for disseminating findings of the research not only to staff nurses but also to administrators of the agency so that findings can be incorporated into practice.

3. **Emerging roles:** In addition to the CNS and CNR, there are emerging role definitions for those of the clinical nurse leader (CNL) and the doctorate in nursing practice (DNP). Because of their newness and the sparse literature describing role development outcomes, the concrete research and EBP effect of individuals prepared for these roles is yet to be determined.

CONCLUSION

Nursing research involves a systematic search for knowledge about issues of importance to nurses. Nursing research also contributes to the profession by helping to define the parameters in nursing. Many nurses are engaging in research to help develop, refine and extend the base of knowledge fundamental to the practice of nursing. This expansion of knowledge is essential for continued improvement in patient care. Nurses who incorporate high quality research evidence into their clinical decisions are being professionally accountable to their clients and are also helping nursing to achieve its own professional identity.

3

SECTION

Professional Trends and Adjustment

TERMINOLOGY

Beneficence: The state or act of intentionally doing or producing good. The principle of beneficence involves duties to prevent harm, remove harm, and promote the good of another person. The obligation of health care professionals to seek the well-being or benefit of other patients. Duties of beneficence concern the welfare of others.

Arbitration: Alternative dispute resolution (ADR) performed outside of legal processes and before the trial where participation is usually voluntary, and a third party who participates can be a private judge who implements a resolution. Arbitrations, usually, occur because parties to contracts agree that any future dispute concerning the agreement will be resolved by the arbitration ADR.

Advanced directives: Advanced directives are written instructions regarding a patient's medical care and preferences. The patient's family, physician, and caregivers will consult the advanced directive if a patient is unable to make his own health care decision.

Allegation: A statement that a person expects to be able to prove.

Assault: An intentional act which is designed to make the victim fearful and which produces reasonable apprehension of harm.

Battery: The touching of one person by another without permission.

Certified legal nurse consultant (CLNC): A registered nurse who uses medical expertise in conjunction with specialized legal training and comprehensive exam toward certification which enables them to assist attorneys to research and develop medically related cases.

Common law: The legal traditions of England and the United States where part of the law is developed by means of court decisions.

Consent: A voluntary act by which one person agrees to allow someone else to do something. For medical liability purposes, consents should be in writing with an explanation of the procedures to be performed.

Decedent: A deceased person.

Deconditioning: The loss of muscle tone and endurance due to chronic disease, immobility, or loss of function brought on by inactivity or bed rest affects important body systems and results in reduced functional capacity. Elderly individuals are particularly vulnerable to becoming deconditioned.

Defamation: The injury of a person's reputation or character caused by the false statements of another made to a third person.

Defendant: In a civil suit, the party against who suit is brought demanding that he or she pay the other party for legal relief.

Deposition: The questioning under oath of a witness, expert, or party by an attorney prior to the trial.

Discovery: The procedures for obtaining information from the parties involved in the lawsuit before the trial begins.

Forensic Document Examiner (FDE): Legal professional specially trained to assess and scientifically/factually detect inaccuracies, inconsistencies, and potential tampering of a medical document.

Harm or Injury: Any wrong or damage done to another, either to the person, to rights, or to property.

2012 HIPAA (American Health Insurance Portability and Accountability Act): HIPAA is a set of rules to be followed by doctors, hospitals, and all health care providers. It helps ensure that all patient medical records, medical billing, and patient accounts meet consistent standards with regard to documentation, handling, and privacy. Any healthcare provider that electronically stores, processes, or transmits medical records, medical claims, or remittances or certifications must comply with all HIPAA regulations.

Interrogatories: A set or series of written questions directed to a party in a lawsuit requiring written responses.

Liability: An obligation one has incurred or might incur through any act or failure to act.

Living will: Written legal document spells out the types of medical treatment and life-sustaining measures the patient requests, or refuses, such as mechanical breathing, tube feeding or nutritional sustenance, or resuscitation. In some states, living wills may be called health care declarations or health care directives.

Malpractice: Professional misconduct, improper discharge of professional duties, or failure to meet the standard of care of a professional, which resulted in harm to another.

Mediation: Alternative dispute resolution (ADR) outside the legal process completed before trial where there is a third party, a mediator, who facilitates the resolution process (and may even suggest a resolution, known as a "mediator's proposal"), but does not require a resolution of the parties.

Medical or health care power of attorney (POA): The medical POA is a legal document that designates an individual-referred to as a health care agent or proxy- to make decision in the event that a patient is unable to do so.

Negligence: Carelessness, failure to act as an ordinary prudent person, or action contrary to what a reasonable person would have done.

Negotiation: Alternative dispute resolution (ADR) outside of the legal process before trial where participation is voluntary and with no third party to facilitate the resolution process or impose a resolution.

Ombuds: Third party selected by an institution— for example, a university, hospital, corporation or government agency—to deal with complaints by employees or clients or related effected parties.

Physical and mental examination: Any party who's physical or mental status in question may be required to have an appropriate examination.

Plaintiff: The party to a civil suit who brings the suit seeking damages.

Prima facie case: Plaintiff must show a duty owed (standard of care implied by law) to him by the defendant.

Privileged communication: Statement made to a physician, attorney, spouse or anyone in a position of trust. Due to the confidential nature of such information, the law protects it from being revealed, even in court. Term can occur in two distinct situations. (1) The communications between certain persons, such as physician and client, cannot be divulged without consent of the client. (2) In some situations, the law provides an exemption from liability for disclosing information where there is a higher duty to speak, such as statutory reporting requirements.

Proximate: In immediate relation with something else. In negligence cases, the careless act must be the proximate cause of injury.

Request for admission: A written statement of facts or opinions regarding the case submitted to a party where that party must admit or deny the opinions/facts under oath.

Request for production: A request to another member in the lawsuit asking that party to produce certain documents or tangible items.

Res Ipsa Loquitur: "The thing speaks for itself." A doctrine of law applicable to cases where the defendant had exclusive control of the thing which caused the harm and where the harm ordinarily could not have occurred without negligent conduct.

Respondeat Superior: "Let the master answer." The employer is responsible for the legal consequences of the acts of the servant or employee while acting within the scope of employment. (Don't be fooled by this one, the hospital can then turn around and sue you for being sued)

Stare decisis: "Let the decision stand." The legal principle indicating that courts should apply previous decisions to subsequent cases involving similar facts and questions.

Statute of limitations: A statute defining the period within which legal action may be taken.

Subpoena: It requires the individual to appear at a designated time and place to give testimony.

Subpoena duces tecum: It requires the legal party questioned (deposed) to supply any and all documents related to the deposition. Essentially, any documents discoverable and not privileged that are used for deposition preparation should be turned over.

Suit: Court proceeding where one person seeks damages or other legal remedies from another.

Tort: A civil wrong. Torts may be intentional or unintentional.

Tort-feasor: One who commits a tort.

Tort of intentional spoliation: A civil wrong pertaining to when the defense intends to destroy or conceal evidence, or fails to preserve evidence (lost records).

Voir dire: "To speak the truth" is to test the legal qualifications and preliminary examinations of the potential jury panel members by counsel. It also may be implemented during preliminary examination to determine witness competency.

Competent: A legal concept that describes people who are able to make decisions for themselves. Minors are presumed to be incompetent, except under certain specified conditions. The corollary medical-ethical term is decisional capacity.

Confidentiality: The professional-client promise not to reveal information without consent.

Durable power of attorney for health care: An advance directive that goes into effect in the event that a patient who has completed such a document loses decisional capacity. Allows an individual to name a person(s) who is empowered to make health care decisions when the individual becomes incapacitated.

Emancipated minor: A teenaged minor, who is legally, independent of parental control and who can thus give informed consent to medical treatments.

Ethics committees: An interdisciplinary group that deals with conflicts of values in patient care in acute and long-term settings. Such committees discuss policy issues (e.g., regarding withholding and withdrawing of life-sustaining treatments).

Euthanasia: The act of either permitting a person to die or intentionally ending a person's life generally rooted in motives of mercy, beneficence, or respect for patient dignity.

Informed consent: The legal and ethical requirement that no significant medical procedure can be performed until the competent patient has been informed of the nature of the procedure, risks and alternatives, as well as the prognosis if the procedure is not done. The patient must freely and voluntarily agree to have the procedure done.

Nonmaleficence: The state of not doing harm or evil; see also beneficence.

Privileged communication: Information communicated to an attorney, physician, spouse, or counselor that may not be revealed, even in court, without the consent of the person who made the statement.

Proxy consent: Voluntary informed consent given on behalf of another who is for some reason incapable of giving it for himself or herself.

Abortion: Expulsion or removal of a usually nonviable fetus. (a fetus that cannot live outside the uterus at that time).

Active euthanasia: The ending of another person's life by an aggressive method to end suffering.

Assault: A deliberate act wherein one person threatens to harm another without consent and the victim feels the attacker has the ability to carry out the threat.

Character: Collective qualities that distinguish a person or a thing.

Clinician: One who is qualified to provide care and treatment to the sick in hospitals.

Objective: Something sought or aimed at which it actually exists.

Philosophy: Use of reason and argument in seeking truth and knowledge of reality and principles governing existence/love of wisdom.

Practitioner: One who is qualified to work and practice as professional in her field.

Requisites: Required and necessary to success or needed for some purpose.

Scope: Range or opportunity.

Self-care: The practice of activities that individuals personally initiated and perform on their own behalf to maintain life, health, and well-being.

Specialist: A person who is a recognized expert in a specific occupation or branch of learning.

Accessibility: Removal of the barriers to entering and receiving services or working within any health care setting.

Assistive device: Equipment that enables an individual who requires assistance to perform the daily activities essential to maintain health and autonomy and to live as full a life as possible. Such equipment may include, motorized scooters, walkers, walking sticks, grab rails and tilt-and-lift chairs.

Assistive technology: An umbrella term for any device or system that allows individuals to perform tasks they would otherwise be unable to do or increases the ease and safety with which tasks can be performed.

Attendant care: Personal care for people with disabilities in non-institutionalized settings generally by paid, non-family carers.

Autonomy: The perceived ability to control, cope with and make personal decisions about how one lives on a daily basis, according to one's own rules and preferences.

Care The application of knowledge to the benefit of a community or individual.

Intermediate care: A short period of intensive rehabilitation and treatment to enable people to return home following hospitalization or to prevent admission to hospital or residential care.

Primary care: Basic or general health care focused on the point at which a patient ideally first seeks assistance from the medical care system. It is the basis for referrals to secondary and tertiary level care.

Secondary care: Specialist care provided on an ambulatory or inpatient basis, usually following a referral from primary care.

Tertiary care: The provision of highly specialized services in ambulatory and hospital settings.

16
CHAPTER

Nursing as a Profession

INTRODUCTION

In professional nursing today, there is an increasing emphasis on evidence-based practice. Almost all the currently used nursing theories address this issue in some way. Simply stated, evidence-based practice is the practice of nursing in which interventions are based on data from research that demonstrates that they are appropriate and successful. It involves a systematic process of uncovering, evaluating, and using information from research as the basis for making decisions about and providing client care. Many nursing practices and interventions of the past were performed merely because that was the way it was always done (accustomed practice) or because of deductions from physiological or pathophysiological information. Clients are now more sophisticated and knowledgeable about health-care issues and demand a higher level of knowledge and skill from their health-care providers.

DEFINITIONS OF PROFESSION

- Profession has been defined as that requires extensive education or a calling that requires special knowledge, skill, and preparation.
- Profession is an occupation with moral principles that are devoted to the human and social welfare. Professional nursing is a service devoted to the promotion of human and social welfare.
- Professionalism refers to professional character, spirit, or methods. It is a set of attributes, a way of life that implies responsibility and commitment.
- Professionalization is the process of becoming professional that is of acquiring characteristics considered to be professional.

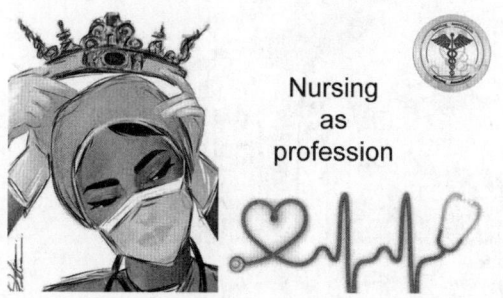

Nursing
as
profession

Fig. 16.1: Nursing as profession.

- Professional nurse is a health worker, a graduate from a recognized school who is identified by law as a registered nurse whether graduated from a baccalaureate (BSc) or a diploma program.

HISTORY OF NURSING

Evolution of nursing, like any other discipline or profession, has undergone noticeable changes. The progress in nursing had been relatively slow in the early period of independence. However, through the later part of the 20th century there has been definite growth and development in nursing education as well as nursing services. This chapter will enable you to go through the history of nursing from the early era to the present scenario. The historical overview of nursing reflects the development of nursing from early times to the modem era.

Nursing in Early Period

In the early Judeo-Christian era, women provided nursing services at home as part of their ethical and humanitarian responsibilities. No formal education or training was expected; rather a woman used her skills as a loving mother to care for the sick on a person-to-person basis. By Middle Ages (500-1500) A.D. nursing had become an organized service. Most nurses were part of religious orders. They received training from their practical experience in caring for the sick. Most of them were expected to devote their time outside the home to care for the poor and sick as an expression of Christian love. It was during this period that a rich person like Phoebe of Cenchraea dedicated her life to nursing and was called the first visiting nurse. She founded Deaconesses, an order of Christian women who served the sick and poor. Nursing continued in the same fashion for many centuries. Many religious orders were disbanded and women were expected to devote their time and energies to their own families and homes. The nurses who existed were social outcaste of the time. These women worked off jail sentences through nursing duties and had no training or preparation for the care of the sick. This period is referred to as the Dark Age of Nursing.

In ancient Egypt, physicians practiced medicine in temples and were assisted by women helpers. Though the records of nursing procedures are available, there is no indication whether these helpers were nurses or any other persons. Hippocrates, the Father of Medicine, emphasized on observation of signs and symptoms of illnesses, but nursing was still not practiced as women remained at home.

Nursing in Medieval Period (AD 1000—1450 AD)

In Europe, many nursing orders developed during the time. Clara of Assisi founded 'The Poor Clares which cared for the sick and lepers. During Renaissance to the 19th

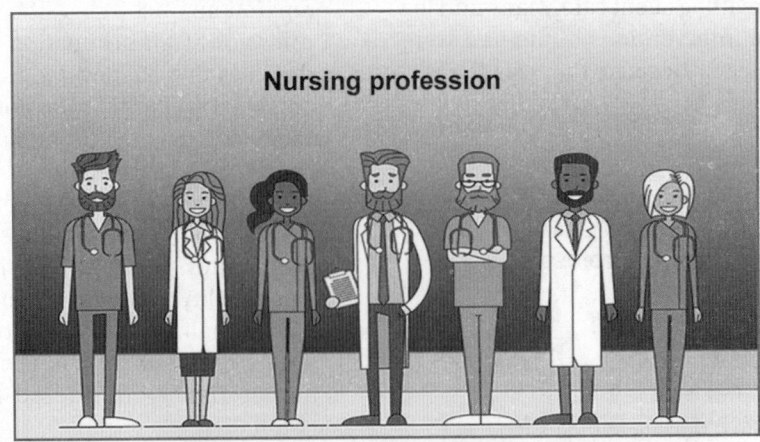

Fig. 16.2: Professional nurse as a member of health care team.

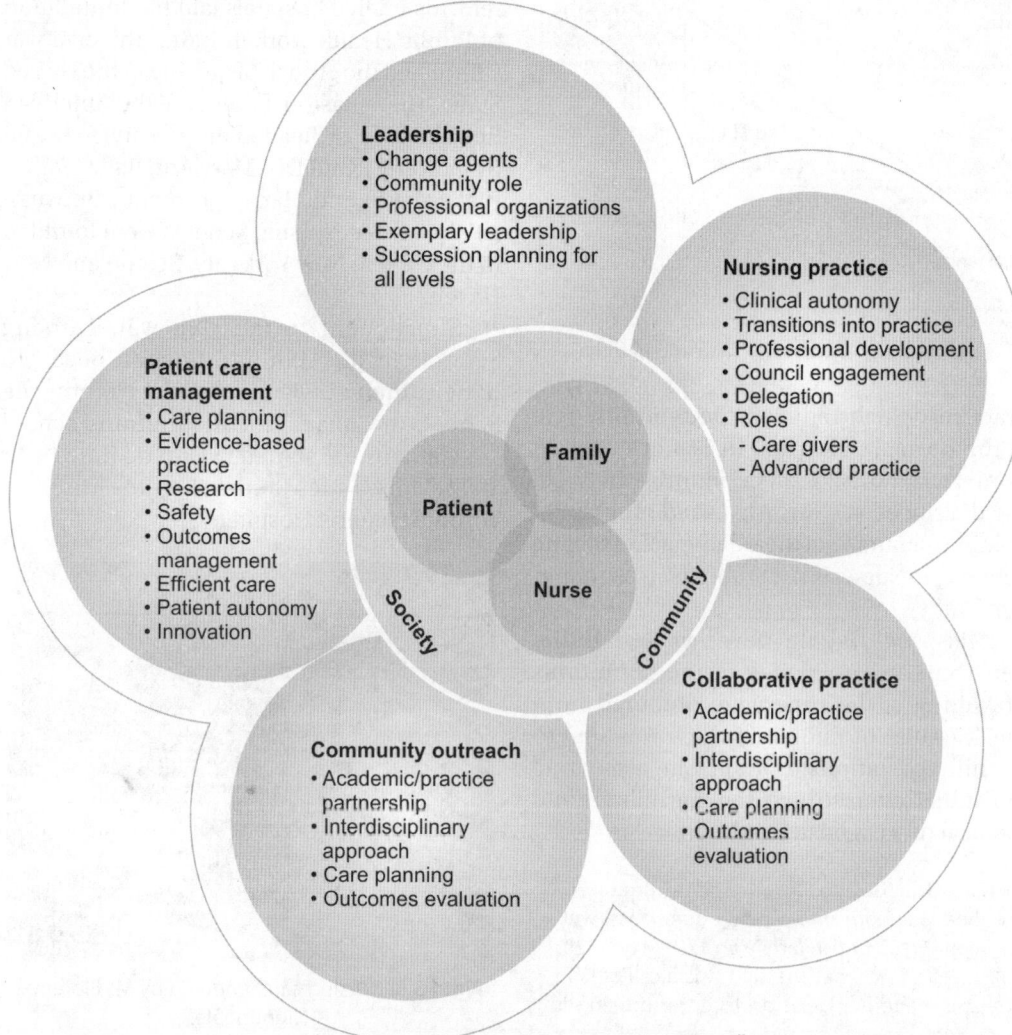

Fig. 16.3: Nursing professional practice model.

century (1450-1800 AD) there were despair, wars, plague and indifference to the poor and sick. This was a period of decline for nursing but the field of medicine was growing. During the 17th century, St. Vincent de Paul founded the Sisters of Charity who cared for the sick. This pattern continued till the Industrial Revolution (1800) until the time of Florence Nightingale of England.

Modern Nursing

Miss Florence Nightingale (1820-1910) was born in a prominent English family. With the benefits of excellent education and knowledge of social conditions and reforms of the time, she believed that nursing should be a separate career, and not part of a religious responsibility. Miss Nightingale received the Year Book of the Institution of Deaconesses at Kaiserworth in October 1846. She went to Kaiserworth in 1847 to work with the Deaconesses. She went to Paris in 1853 to study with the Sisters of Charity. She was later appointed Superintendent of the English General Hospitals in Turkey. During the Crimean war, the major reforms brought in by her were in hygiene, sanitation and nursing

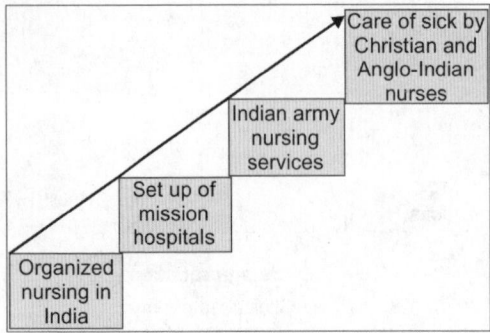

Fig. 16.4: Development of nursing in India.

practices which reduced the mortality rate at the Barracks Hospital in Scutari, Turkey, from 42.7% to 2.2% in six months. In 1860, she developed the first organized program of training for nurses, at the 'Nightingale Training School for Nurses at St. Thomas' Hospital in London'.

Miss Nightingale never visited India, her accurate knowledge of the conditions prevailing at the time were obtained from the "Circular of Enquiry" which was sent to all military stations in India. She also wrote individual letters to high-ranking military and medical officers posted in India.

An Introduction to Florence Nightingale
- She was born into a rich, upper-class, well-connected British family on 12th May, 1820.
- Inspired by what she said was a call of God, she made her decision to enter nursing in 1844.
- In this, she rebelled against the expected role for a women of her status, which was to become a wife and mother.
- Nightingale worked hard to educate herself in the art and science of nursing, in spite of opposition from her family and the restrictive societal code for affluent young English women.
- Convinced that marriage would interfere with her ability to follow her calling to nursing, she rejected politician and poet Richard Monckton Milnes, 1st Baron Houghton, who was courting her.

The Royal Sanitary Commission on the Health of the Army in India was appointed in 1859 and facts collected in 1861. The ensuing

reforms in civil hospitals laid the foundation of Public Health work in India. The civil war stimulated the growth of nursing in the United States. Clara Baston, founder of the American Red Cross, spearheaded the activity, followed by Dorothy Lyndi Dis, Mary Ann Ball (Mother Bickerdyke) and Harriet Tubman. Between 1872-73 three Nursing Schools were founded in the USA: in New York City, Boston and New Haven.

Subsequent to the civil war, Nursing Schools in the USA and Canada began to pattern their curricula after the Nightingale School. In Canada, the first training school "St. Catherine's" started in Qutario in 1874. In 1884, Mary Agnes Sninely became Director, Toronto General Hospital.

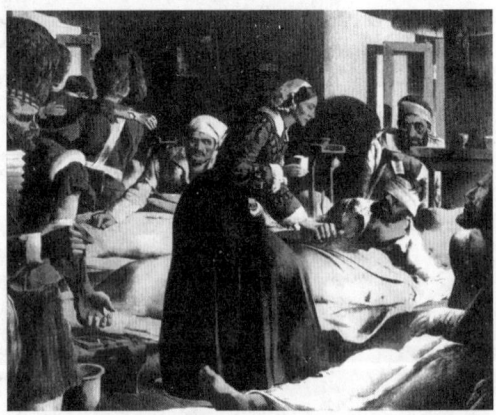

Fig. 16.5: Nursing care rendered by Ms Florence Nightingale.

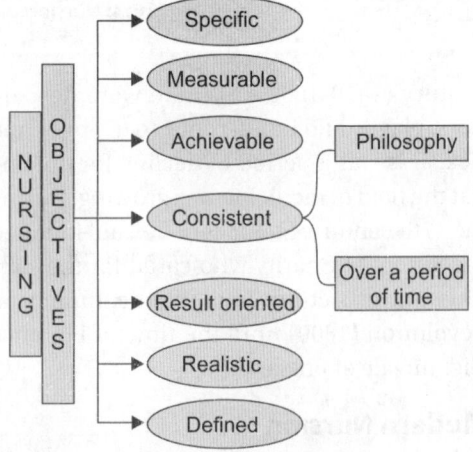

Fig. 16.6: Objectives of nursing.

HISTORICAL DEVELOPMENT OF NURSING IN INDIA

- **1905:** Association of Nursing Superintendents was constituted/formed.
- **1908:** Trained Nurses Association of India was established/formed.
- **1909:** Bombay Presidency Nursing Association was formed. Missionary Nurses North India Board, set up under Medical Missionary Association of India.
- **1911:** The South Indian Board was established INAI affiliated to International Council of Nurses.
- **1912:** The First Nurses, Registration Act was enacted in Madras Presidency.
- **1930:** The Christian Nurses Auxiliary formed by the missionary nurses.
- **1934:** The Bengal Nurses Act was enacted for the nurses, midwives and H.V. of undivided Bengal.
- **1936:** The Mid India Board of Education affiliated to Christian Nurses league, Christian Nurses Auxiliary Association was affiliated to TNAI.
- **1941:** Standardized pay scales and terms of services were established in Madras. State nursing superintendent, appointed at state level (Madras).
- **1942:** The Auxiliary Nursing Service (ANS) was established. One nursing superintendent was appointed as nursing advisor at DGHS, Government of India, to organize nursing services.
- **1943:** Establishment of School of Nursing Administration for Military Nursing Services Health Survey and Development Committees (Bhore) constituted by Government of India. Study groups worked on proposal for university education in nursing in India. CMC Vellore and Madras General Hospital started courses to train nursing tutors. Commissioned rank was given to the Indian Military Nursing sisters.
- **1946:** Bhore Committee submitted report, recommendations made on improvement of various aspects of nursing profession: Nursing education, working conditions, nursing services in hospital and community and deputing nurses for higher education to abroad, etc. Establishment of the College of Nursing at Delhi (now Rajkumari Amrit Kaur College of Nursing) under the Union Ministry of Health to start university nursing education program for the first time in India leading to Bachelor's degree in nursing, i.e., BSc (Hons.) Nursing.
- **1947:** Indian Nursing Council Act was passed (31.12.1947) on the basis of recommendations of Bhore Committee. Degree program for nursing started in Vellore.
- **1948:** The first meeting of Indian Nursing Council (INC) was held.
- **1950:** The INC took decision to establish ANM program to meet the requirement of workers in nursing.
- **1951:** Establishment of urban field teaching centre is started at College of Nursing, Delhi in collaboration with existing MCH centers of Municipal Corporation, Delhi for teaching of urban community health nursing.
- **1952:** Establishment of residential field teaching center for teaching community health nursing in the rural area under College of Nursing, Delhi in collaboration with primary health center, Najafgarh.
- **1953:** Ms Edith Buchanan, vice principal, College of Nursing (RAK), Delhi was sent to Columbia University to earn her Doctorate in Education (D. Ed.) through WHO fellowship.
- **1954:** Government of India constituted committee to review conditions of services, emoluments; etc., of nursing profession (Shetty committee). Shetty Committee Report was published, recommended nursing staff norms of hospital community and other improvements in nursing.
- **1955:** Establishment of child guidance clinic at College of Nursing. (RAKCON) for providing services and strengthening community health nursing and pediatric nursing. Ms Margaretta Craig, principal, College of Nursing, Delhi attended ICN

meeting in France, to present a paper on the need for nursing research in India.

- **1959:** Dr Edith M. Buchanan, succeeded in establishing the long cherished "Master of Nursing" degree program at (RAK) College of Nursing, New Delhi under University of Delhi (October 1959). Healthy Survey and Planning Committee (Dr LN Mudaliar) was constituted by Government of India to review the progress made in health since, Bhore committee recommendation.

- **1961:** Mudaliar Committee report published made some recommendations to improve nursing profession.

- **1963:** A WHO assisted technical project was undertaken at the INC to revise the GNM course. Dr. Buchanan, succeeded in sending Mrs Sulochara Krishnan, one of the first graduates of this newly established, M.N. degree program, to earn the D. Ed. degree from Columbia University.

- **1964:** Dr. Marie Furguson, a public health nurse came to the College of Nursing, Delhi was able to create greater appreciation and understanding of the need and value of research in planning nursing administration and education with senior leaders of the country conducted "Activity studies to define the nursing and non-nursing functions of nursing personnel.

- **1965:** A WHO publication on 'Guide for School of Nursing' in India was published.

- **1966:** TNAI established research section under the Chairmanship of Ms Margarata Craig. TNAI conducted 'Time study' with the co-operation of Ms Anna Gupta, principal, RAKCON, under the supervision of Dr Sulochana Krishnan.

- **1969-71:** INAI and VHAI, CHAP conducted study on survey on the socioeconomic status of nurses in India.

- **1973:** Kartar Singh Committee report on multipurpose workers and Health and family planning department published and recommended ANM and LHVs were redesignated and health workers (F) and

health assistant (F) to cover the required population at rural area for providing proper health services.

- **1975:** Shrivastav Committee report on 3 tier-plan of health care delivery system to rural area was recommended.

- **1976:** Dr Marie Farell and Dr Aparna Bhaduri of Rajkumari Amrit Kaur College of Nursing, New Delhi, conducted seminars on nursing research for educationists at Delhi, Mussoorie (Uttarakhand) and Yarcaid to strength the nursing research in India.

- **1978:** Government Nurses Association of Karnataka established.

- **1981:** Dr Farrel and Dr Bhaduri's book 'Health Research'-A Community based Approach' published by World Health Organization.

- **1986:** The Nursing Research Society of India (NRSI) was established to promote research within and around nursing environment. Dr (Mrs) Inderjit Walia was founder president. Mrs Uma Hunda was its secretary. M Phil in nursing program started at RAKCON, under Delhi University.

- **1987:** Reports of the expert committee on health and manpower planning, production and management (Bajaj Committee) published. This committee also dealt with nursing service conditions norms and nurse's emoluments, etc.

- **1988:** RAKCON, New Delhi was designated as World Health Collaboration Center for nursing Developments reports of the high power committee on nursing and nursing profession published. Dr Ruth Hurner book "Nursing Education in India" published on the basis of survey.

- **1991:** Author registered PhD in nursing at Bangalore University.

- **1992:** PhD in nursing program started at RAKCON, under Delhi University. Mrs Asha Sharma got registered for the Doctoral course.

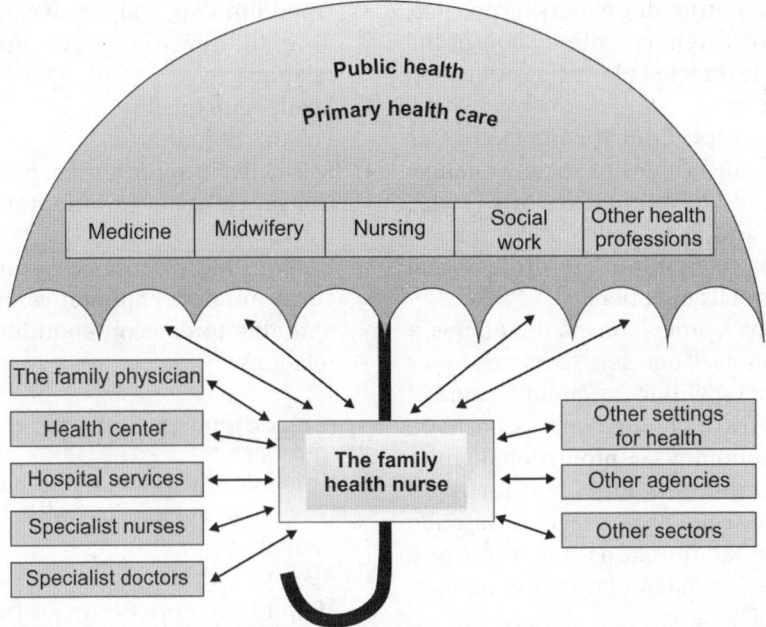

Fig. 16.7: Role of family health nurse.

CRITERIA OF PROFESSION

- **Specialized education:** Specialized education is an important aspect of professional status. In modern times, the trend in education for the professions that shifted towards programs in colleges and universities.
- **Body of knowledge:** As a profession, nursing is establishing a well-defined body of knowledge and expertise. A number of nursing conceptual frameworks contribute

to the knowledge base of nursing and give direction to nursing practice, education and ongoing research.

- **Service orientation:** Nursing as a tradition of service to others. This service, however, must be guided by certain rules, policies, or codes of ethics. Today, nursing is also an important component of the health care delivery system.
- **Ongoing research:** Since the 1970s nursing research has focused on practice related issues. Increasing research in

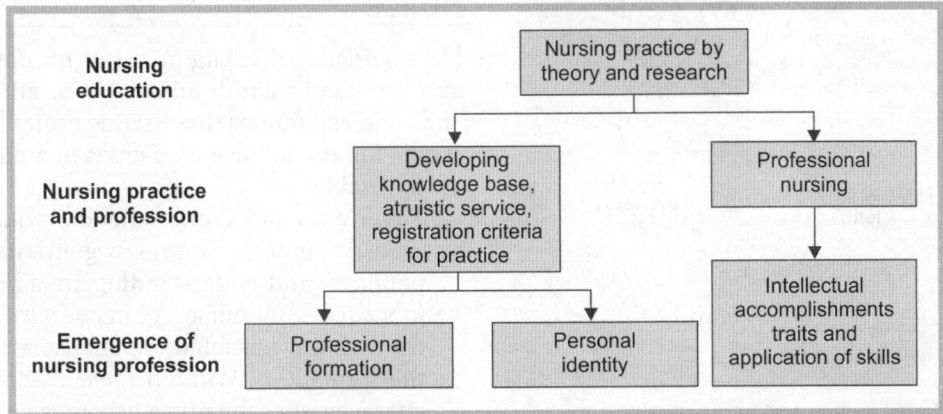

Fig. 16.8: Scope of nursing.

nursing is contributing to nursing practice. Nursing research as a dimension of the nurse's role directed to nursing education and practice.

- **Code of ethics:** Ethical code change as the needs and values of society change. Nursing has developed its own codes of ethics and in most instances has set up means to monitor the professional behaviors of its members.
- **Autonomy:** A profession is autonomous, if it regulates itself and sets standards for its members. Providing autonomy is one of the purposes of a professional association. To be autonomous, a professional group must be granted legal authority to define the scope of its practice, describe its particular functions and roles and determine its goals and responsibilities in delivery of its services.

CHARACTERISTICS OF PROFESSIONAL NURSE

- Good physical and mental health.
- Truthful and efficient in technical competence.
- Cleanliness, tidy, neat and well groomed.
- Confidence in others and self.
- Intelligence.

Occupation versus Profession	
Occupation refers to the work that a person does	Profession is a paid occupation, one that especially requires a long training and formal qualifications
Neutral, generic term	Refers to intellectual pursuit
May not need formal qualifications or training	Requires formal qualifications and training

Fig. 16.9: Occupation versus profession.

- Open minded, cooperative, responsible, able to develop good interpersonal relations.
- Leadership quality.
- Positive attitudes.
- Self-belief towards human care and cure.
- Convey co-operative attitudes towards co-worker.
- Responsible towards family and society.
- Open minded, cooperative, responsible, and able to develop good interpersonal relations.

PROFESSIONAL EQUITIES

- Be gentle and polite in your talk.
- Greet your seniors, co-workers, and your patient.
- Keep your dress neat and tidy.
- Help the seniors to carry a heavy load if you find them on the way.
- Be punctual always.
- Keep eye contact and sit face-to-face when listening to someone.
- Knock at the door and wait for the answer before you enter into others room.
- Excuse yourself before you interfere with others engaged in talking or doing some work.
- You should not give and receive any gifts or present especially from the patients and their relatives.

QUALITIES OF PROFESSIONAL NURSE

For an efficient discharging of her/his duties and for a satisfactory fulfillment of all the aims and aspirations that her/his profession stands for, the following qualities in a nurse are inevitable.

- **Love:** With all its other attendant qualities like mercy, kindness, gentleness, patience, and understanding are a must in a successful nurse. All her service for the sick and disabled are sponsored by these qualities. Without these essential characteristics the nurse becomes only a mechanical aid.

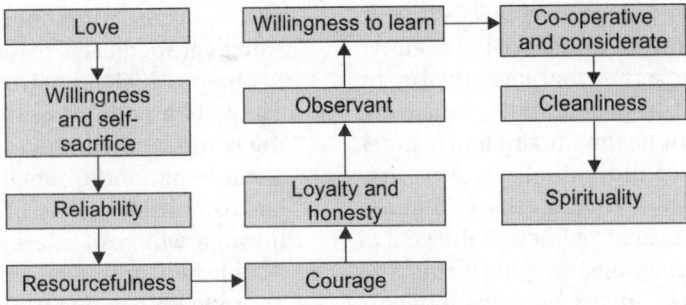

Fig. 16.10: Professional nurse qualities.

- **Willingness and self-sacrifice:** These two qualities are complimentary to each another. Because she is willing to serve under any trying situation, a nurse sacrifices her time, comfort and even material benefits, e.g., Florence Nightingale at Scutari.
- **Reliability:** A nurse is one who can be depended upon for a faithful discharging of her duties, the patients under her care, their families, doctors and members of the "health team" depend on her, for she is trust worthy and competent.
- **Resourcefulness:** In critical circumstances she uses her wisdom and knowledge and performs her duties to the best of her ability with whatever means that are at her disposal. She tackles situations with alacrity.
- **Courage:** In times of confusion, calamity or catastrophe, the nurse manages her work with compassion and is ready to meet any problem with courage. She is cool and levelheaded and does not get agitated easily.
- **Loyalty and honesty:** Her relationship with the patient, the doctor and her associates are marked by utmost loyalty and honesty.
- **Observant:** A good nurse is always vigilant. She keeps a close and constant watch on the patients, their progress, their changes and reactions to treatment, etc., and gives the doctor timely reports. A nurse should anticipate and meet the patients' needs.
- **Willingness to learn:** A nurse must keep in touch with the latest discoveries and developments in medicine and treatment and must "maintain her knowledge and skill at a consistently high level".
- **Co-operative and considerate:** A nurse learns to live in harmony with patients, doctors and other members of the health team and tries to help them in times of need.
- **Cleanliness:** A nurse is always clean and neat personally and in her work. She must be tidy and demand high standards of cleanliness from those whom she is associated within her profession.
- **Spirituality:** A nurse must learn to create a spiritual atmosphere for the patient and must try and help the patients to put their confidence and trust in a "Power" that is higher than any other power in the world.

NEW PERSPECTIVES OF NURSING PROFESSION

Historically, only medicine, law and the ministry were accepted as profession.

Criteria of a profession: Genevieve and Roy Bixler first wrote about the status of nursing as a profession in 1945. These criteria include the following:

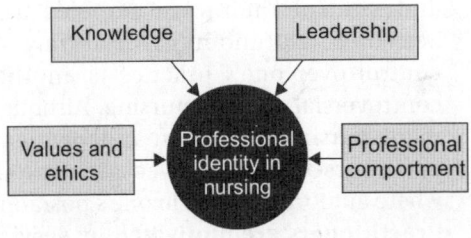

Fig. 16.11: Professional identity in nursing.

- **The services provided are vital to humanity and the welfare of the society:**. Nursing is the service that is essential to the well-being of the people and to the society. Nursing promotes, maintains and restores the health of individuals, groups and communities. Assisting others to attain the highest level of wellness is the goal of nursing. Caring, meaning nurturing and helping others are the basic components of professional nursing.
- **There is a special body of knowledge** that is continually enlarged through research. In the past, nursing was based on principles borrowed from the physical and social sciences and other disciplines. Today there is a unique body of knowledge to nursing
- **The services involve intellectual activities.** Individual responsibilities (accountability) are a strong feature. Nursing has developed and refined its own unique approach to practice. Nursing process is a cognitive activity that requires both critical and creative thinking and serves as the basis of providing nursing care. Individual accountability in nursing has become the hallmark of practice. Accountability is 'is being answerable to someone for something one has done through legal opinion and court cases, society has demonstrated that nurses are individually responsible for their actions as well as for those of personnel under their supervision.
- **Practitioners are educated in institution of higher learning.** There are basic nursing program, baccalaureate program, masters and Doctoral program in nursing.
- **Practitioners are relatively independent** and control their own policies and activities (Autonomy). Autonomy or control over one's practice is another controversial area for nursing. Although many nursing actions are independent, most nurses are employed in hospitals where authority resides in one's position.
- **Practitioners are motivated by service (altruism)** and considered their work an important component of their lives. Nurses are dedicated to the ideal of service to others, which is known as altruism.
- **There is a code of ethics to guide the decisions** and conduct of practitioners. The International Council of Nurses (ICN) has established Code of Nursing Ethics through which standards of practice are established, promoted, and refined.
- **There is an organization (Association)** that encourages and supports high standards of practice. Nursing has a number of professional associations that were formed to promote the improvement of the profession. Foremost among these, is the TNAI (The Trained Nurses Association of India). The purposes of TNAI are to foster high standards of nursing practice, promote professional and educational advancement of nurses and promote the welfare of the nurses.

CONCEPT OF PROFESSIONALISM IN NURSING

- **Art of nursing:** Professional nursing practice is grounded in the art of nursing, described as taking a holistic, client-centered focus; being caring and ethical in interactions with patients, families and colleagues; having above-average interpersonal skills; and making sound judgments based on experience and knowledge, thus averting potential problems.
- **Competence:** Professional practice demands competence in relation to knowledge and technical skills. This requires not only a broad base of knowledge, but also depth of knowledge in a chosen area of practice, a desire and ability to continue developing that knowledge base and to share it with others and critical thinking in decision-making.
- **Attributes of practice:** Professional practice reflects a particular approach to one's work, with collaboration by far most salient characteristic. Professional nursing practice means working in partnership

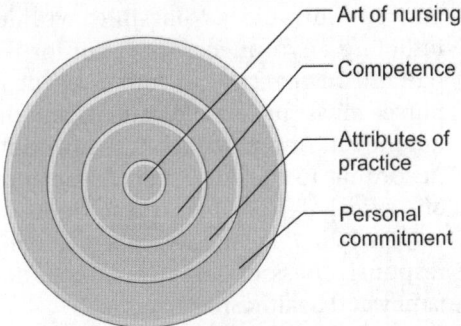

Fig. 16.12: Professional in nursing.

with other nurses and health professionals in providing client care, being highly organized in managing activities and time, having the ability to manage many complex tasks simultaneously, working autonomously as appropriate and having an open mind and nonjudgmental manner.

- **Personal commitment:** In describing this element of professional practice, respondents referred to the importance of having confidence in one's abilities and taking responsibility for one's actions, including having a sound understanding of the boundaries and limitations of nursing practice. Having a balanced lifestyle and supporting the advancement of the profession were also considered important characteristics of a professional nurse.

VALUES OF PROFESSIONAL NURSE

To be successful, nurses must be equipped with certain tools and abilities. These skills are developed over time as a nurse gains experience and confidence.

- **Confidentiality and autonomy:** Nurses have to have an awareness of legislation on patient confidentiality and the policies of their own organization. Nurses should not breach confidentiality, unless the circumstances are exceptional, for instance, if the patient is threatening harm to himself or others. Nurses must not discuss patients' details outside of the care setting, and must take care of notes,

paper and computer files. Nurses should make all efforts to promote the patient's rights to make her own decision whenever possible.

- **Protection from harm:** The nurse's conduct must protect the patient from harm. He must not undertake something he thinks might cause harm to the patient even if he has been told or asked to do so by another person. The nurse is accountable for her own actions, and might be asked' to explain these in later proceedings. If the nurse sees anything she fears may endanger the patient, she must immediately report this to management.
- **Professional development:** The nurse has a duty to keep up to date with all developments that may have an impact on his job. He must attend professional development and training activities. Part of his duty may involve training and mentoring new and junior staff. Nurses must meet training requirements and pay any fees needed to maintain licensing.
- **Dedication:** Professional nursing is a difficult profession with many stressful scenarios. Nurses must work long shifts and deal with many vastly different issues on a daily basis. The combination of long work hours, constant care of patients, and the stress of seeing death can cause nurses to unravel. Thus, professional nurses need to be calm a id level-headed, able to

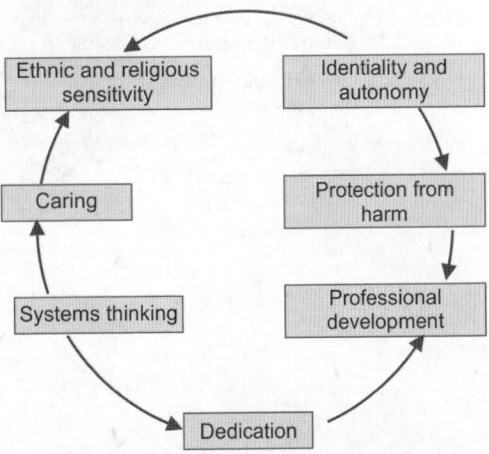

Fig. 16.13: Values of professional nurse.

quickly handle a multitude of problems effectively. Nurses are responsible for patient quality of care and the execution of the health care plan. A dedication to the job is essential for a nurse to fulfill her nursing duties.

- **Systems thinking:** A nurse is faced with a plenty of situations throughout each workday. Each patient has individual problems and requires a different approach. Nurses are expected to develop individualized decisions of care depending on the patient and the specific circumstances.

- **Caring:** Nurses are required to take care of the patient throughout the entire health care process. Their goal is to make the healing process and painless and comfortable as possible, without inflicting any unnecessary grief for the patient. In the case of imminent deal, nurses must console the patients and the families in order to ease the transition. According to the American Association of Critical Care Nurses, these duties of care include "vigilance, engagement, and responsiveness of caregivers, including family and healthcare personnel."

- **Ethnic and religious sensitivity:** Nurses take care of patients from a variety of ethnic and religious backgrounds. Professional nurses must be sensitive to the specific requirements of various cultures and religions in order to facilitate the patient's health care. Nurses must demonstrate a desire to respect various practices while

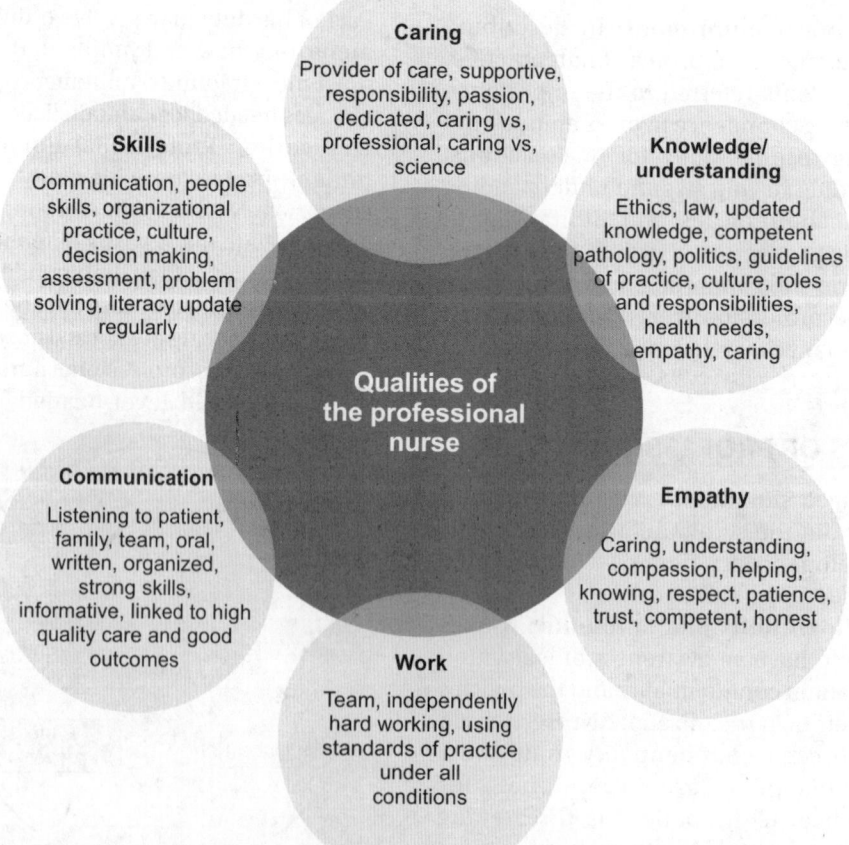

Caring
Provider of care, supportive, responsibility, passion, dedicated, caring vs, professional, caring vs, science

Skills
Communication, people skills, organizational practice, culture, decision making, assessment, problem solving, literacy update regularly

Knowledge/ understanding
Ethics, law, updated knowledge, competent pathology, politics, guidelines of practice, culture, roles and responsibilities, health needs, empathy, caring

Qualities of the professional nurse

Communication
Listening to patient, family, team, oral, written, organized, strong skills, informative, linked to high quality care and good outcomes

Empathy
Caring, understanding, compassion, helping, knowing, respect, patience, trust, competent, honest

Work
Team, independently hard working, using standards of practice under all conditions

Fig. 16.14: Professional qualities of a nurse.

continuing to adhere to professional standards.

ROLE OF PROFESSIONAL NURSE

The professional nurse occupying a position of a professional nurse accepts responsibility and accountability in:

- Provide quality nursing to the clients in their care, placing emphasis on the medical psychosocial, spiritual needs of the clients and be mindful of the needs of the relatives or attendants.
- Cooperating with the nursing units and all other departments within the hospital.
- Understanding all activities in relaxation to patient care and other assigned duties.
- Actively participating in the nursing team.
- Actively pursuing continuing self-education.
- Actively providing appropriate health education to the individuals, families and groups and community at large in various settings.

FUNCTIONS AND RESPONSIBILITIES OF PROFESSIONAL NURSE

- **Client care:** Providing safe and effective nursing care within a health care set up or community. It includes participating in the delivery of nursing care based on the best practice principles stated by statutory body, maintaining nursing standards, observing and participating in quality improvement programs, fostering congeniality between all members of the health care team, assisting with cost containment by utilizing resources effectively, participating in appropriate meetings, workshops or committees related to improving nursing care.
- **Professional practice:** In professional practice, the aspects included are

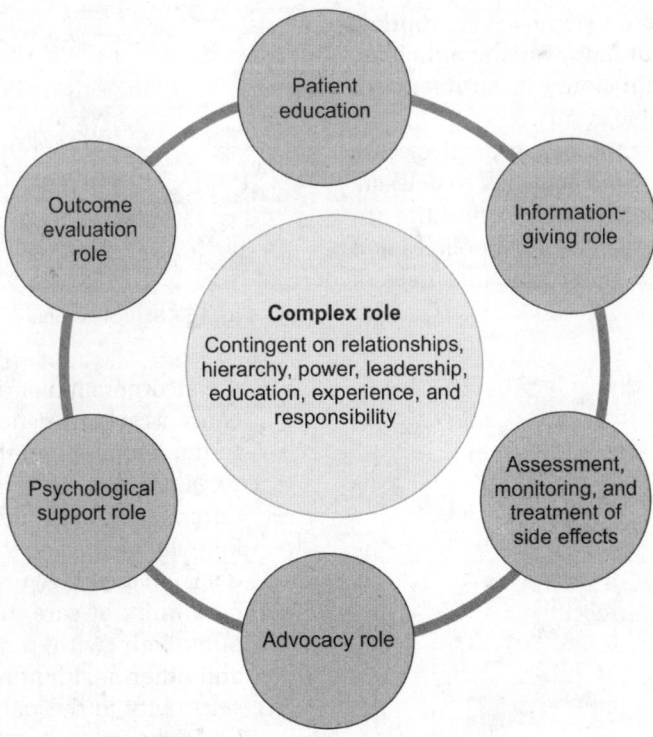

Fig. 16.15: Complex role of a nurse.

maintaining confidentiality, taking reasonable care in health and safety of persons on the unit, being familiar with the resources to be used in case of any emergency or disaster, adhering to all infection control policies and safety rules, cooperating with management for health, safety and welfare provisions, actively seeking knowledge of the diagnosis and treatment given, actively participating with a member of multidisciplinary team, complying with the professional code of ethics, demonstrating accountability and responsibility for the professional conduct, practicing with limits of own abilities and qualification, initiating and maintaining effective communication with others.

- **Management:** There are three kinds of management roles, i.e., planning, organizing, implementation and evaluation.
  - In planning, the management roles are to describe the planning process in the assigned clinical area, to assess client's needs, work environment and available resources, to set appropriate priorities for days work, to anticipate and plan for potential problems or unpredictable events.
  - In organizing, the management roles are to organize work activities, to delegate tasks and share responsibilities, to adhere to organizational policies and procedures, to describe instances of

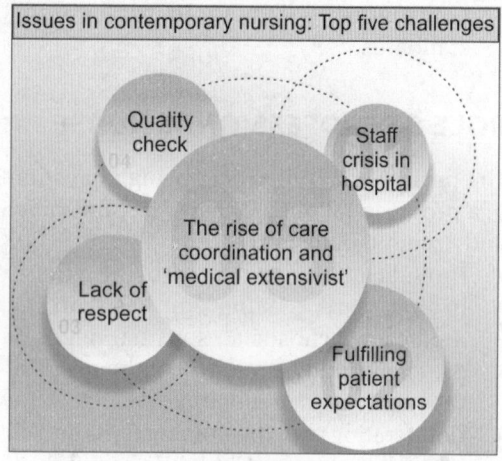

Fig. 16.17: Challenges in nursing.

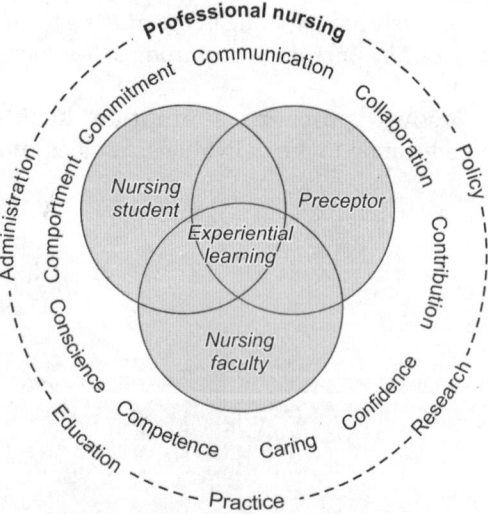

Fig. 16.18: Professional nursing areas.

the incorporation of risk management concepts in the assigned clinical setting.
  - In implementation, the management roles are to perform nursing procedures safely, accurately and scientific knowledge based, to describe the decision making process, to assure continuity of care, to communicate effectively with patients, families and other health personnel, to show sensitivity to the patients' needs, to bring change in the status quo of the organization as required.

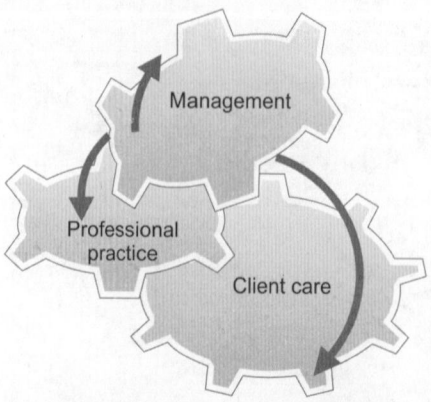

Fig. 16.16: Vital functions in nursing.

– In evaluation, the management roles are to analyze the flow of communication in the unit and within the organization, to describe the nurse manager's role as evaluator of personnel performance, to assess patient care evaluation activities that are done in clinical setting.

PROFESSIONAL CONDUCT FOR NURSING

- Act always in such a manner as to promote and safeguard the interests and the well-being of the patients and the clients.
- Ensure that no action or omission on your part or with your sphere of responsibility is detrimental to the interest, condition or safely of the patients and clients.

- Maintain and improve your professional knowledge and competence.
- Acknowledge any limitation in your knowledge and competence and decline any duties or responsibilities unless you are not able to perform them in a safe and skilled manner.
- Work in an open and co-operative manner with patients, clients and their families, foster their independence, recognize and respect their involvement in the planning and delivery of care.
- Work in a collaborative and co-operative manner with health care professionals and others involved in providing care, recognize and respect their particular contributions within the care team.
- Recognize and respect the dignity of each patient and client, and respond to their

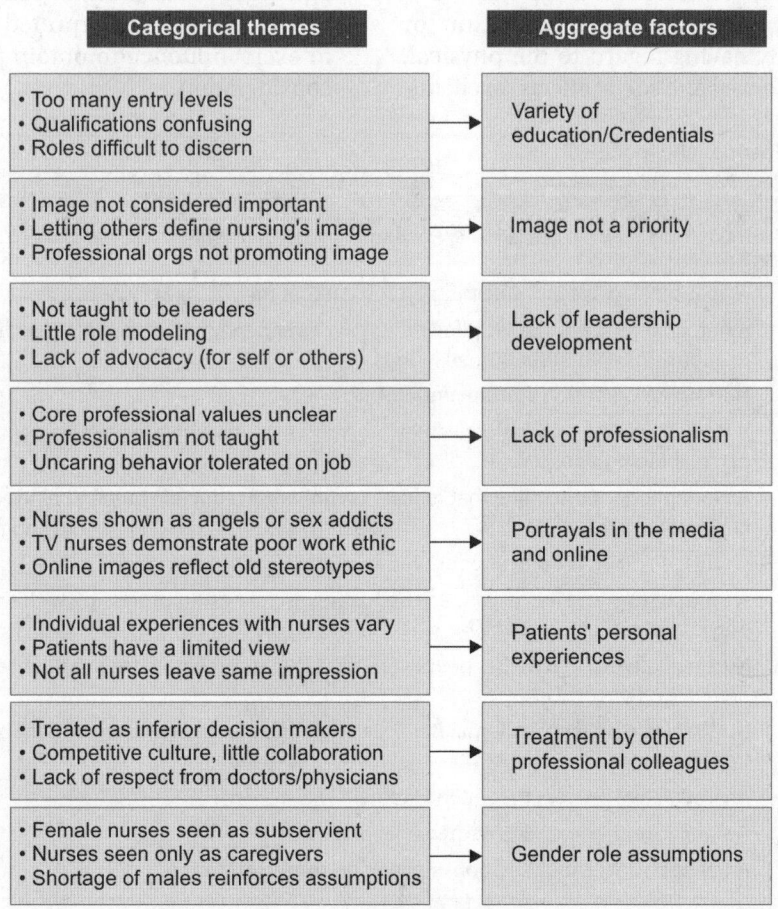

Fig. 16.19: Challenges in nursing profession.

need with care, irrespective of their ethnic origin, religious beliefs, personal attributes and the nature of their health problems or any other factors.

- Report to an appropriate person, authority, at the earliest. Any conscientious objection may be relevant to your professional practice.
- Avoid any abuse of your privileged relationship with patients and clients and of the privileged access allowed to their person, property, residency, or work place.
- Protect all confidential information concerning patients and clients obtained in the course of professional practice, and make its disclosures only with the consent or when required by the order of a court or where you can justify disclosure in the wider public interest.
- Report to an appropriate person or authority having regard to the physical, psychological and social effects on clients.

Any circumstances in the environment of care could jeopardize standard of practice.

- Report to an appropriate person or authority at any circumstance in which safe and appropriate care for the patient and clients cannot be provided.
- Report to an appropriate person or authority where it appears that the health or safety of the client is at risk, these circumstances may compromise standard of practice and care.
- Assist professional colleagues in the context of your own knowledge, sphere of responsibility to develop their professional competence and assist others in the care team including informal carriers to contribute safely and to a degree appropriate to their role.
- Refuse gifts, favors or hospitality from patients or clients currently in your care which might be interpreted as seeking to exert influence to obtain preferential consideration.

Table 16.1: Theories and models.

Theorist	Definition of nursing
Johnson	A force that supplies assistance when disturbances in system balance occur or to prevent such disturbances.
King	A goal-seeking system; a helping profession that provides a service to meet a social need.
Levine	A human interaction; a discipline rooted in dependency of the individual on his/her relationships with other human beings.
B Neuman	Nursing is prevention as intervention.
Orem	A form of assistance or help given by nurses to persons with a legitimate need for it; one person helping another.
Rogers	An independent discipline that focuses on unitary, irreducible human beings and their environments.
Roy	A science and an art that support and promote patient adaptation.
Leininger	A transcultural and humanistic scientific care discipline and profession with the central purpose to serve humankind.
M. Newman	Nursing is caring that assists people to utilize the power within them as they evolve to a higher level of consciousness.
Parse	Nursing is being with; it illuminates meaning, synchronizes rhythms, and mobilizes transcendence.
Orlando	An interactive process that intends to help.
Peplau	A significant therapeutic interpersonal process.
Watson	A transpersonal caring relationship; person-to-person caring.

Note: From Fawcett (2005).

- Ensure that your registration status is not used in the promotion of commercial products or services. Declare that any financial or other interests in relevant organizations providing such goods and services will ensure that your professional judgment is not influenced by any commercial considerations.

The code is subject for regular review and changes, any recommendations for change and improvement would be welcomed.

Roles of a Professional Nurse

- **Caregiver/care provider:**
  - The traditional and most essential role.
  - Functions as nurturer, comforter, provider.
  - "Mothering actions" of the nurse
  - Provides direct care and promotes comfort of client.
  - Activities involves knowledge and sensitivity to what matters and what is important to clients.
  - Show concern for client welfare and acceptance of the client as a person.
- **Teacher:**
  - Provides information and helps the client to learn or acquire new knowledge and technical skills.
  - Encourages compliance with prescribed therapy.
  - Promotes healthy lifestyles.
  - Interprets information to the client.
- **Counselor:**
  - Helps client to recognize and cope with stressful psychologic or social problems; to develop an improve interpersonal relationships and to promote personal growth.
  - Provides emotional, intellectual to and psychologic support.
  - Focuses on helping a client to develop new attitudes, feelings and behaviors rather than promoting intellectual growth.
  - Encourages the client to look at alternative behaviors recognize the choices and develop a sense of control.

- **Change agent:** Initiate changes or assist clients to make modifications in themselves or in the system of care.
- **Client advocate:**
  - Involves concern for and actions in behalf of the client to bring about a change.
  - Promotes what is best for the client, ensuring that the client's needs are met and protecting the client's right.
  - Provides explanation in client's language and support clients decisions.
- **Manager:**
  - Makes decisions, coordinates activities of others, allocate resource.
  - Evaluate care and personnel.
  - Plans, give direction, develop staff, monitor operations, give the rewards fairly and represent both staff and administrations as needed.
- **Researcher:**
  - Participates in identifying significant researchable problems.
  - Participates in scientific investigation and must be a consumer of research findings.
  - Must be aware of the research process, language of research, a sensitive to issues related to protecting the rights of human subjects.

Expanded Role as of the Nurse

- **Clinical specialists:** It is a nurse who has completed a master's degree in specialty and has considerable clinical expertise in that specialty. She provides expert care to individuals, participates in educating health care professionals and ancillary, acts as a clinical consultant and participates in research.
- **Nurse practitioner:** It is a nurse who has completed either as certificate program or a master's degree in a specialty and is also certified by the appropriate specialty organization. She is skilled at making nursing assessments, performing P. E., counseling, teaching and treating minor and self-limiting illness.

- **Nurse-midwife:** A nurse who has completed a program in midwifery; provides prenatal and postnatal care and delivers babies to woman with uncomplicated pregnancies.
- **Nurse anesthetist:** A nurse who completed the course of study in an anesthesia school and carries out pre-operative status of clients.
- **Nurse educator:** A nurse usually with advanced degree, who beaches in clinical or educational settings, teaches theoretical knowledge, clinical skills, and conduct research.
- **Nurse entrepreneur:** A nurse who has an advanced degree, and manages health-related business.
- **Nurse administrator:** A nurse who functions at various levels of management in health settings; responsible for the management and administration of resources and personnel involved in giving patient care.

Fields and Opportunities in Nursing

- Hospital/institutional nursing—a nurse working in an institution with patients
  Example: rehabilitation, lying-in, etc.
- Public health nursing/community health nursing—usually deals with families and communities. (no confinement, OPD only)
  Example: brgy. Health Center
- Private duty/special duty nurse—privately hired
- Industrial/occupational nursing—a nurse working in factories, office, companies
- Nursing education—nurses working in school, review center and in hospital as a CI.
- Military nurse—nurses working in a military base.

- Clinic nurse—nurses working in a private and public clinic.
- Independent nursing practice—private practice, BP monitoring, home service.

CONCLUSION

Nursing is a healthcare profession that focuses on the care of individuals and their families to help them recover from illness and maintain optimal health and quality of life. Nurses are distinct from other healthcare providers as they have a wide scope of practice and approach to medical care. In its development as a profession, nursing has struggled with its definition, its image, and its role in the health care delivery system. This is due in part to its history and the fact it has both theoretic and practical aspects. The role of the nurse in the health care delivery system has probably never been more important than it is today. Nursing is distinct from medicine. Medicine deals with diagnosis and treatment of disease and nursing is concerned with caring for the person. The position nursing occupies as a profession is often judged against sociologically developed characteristics of a profession. Not everyone agrees that nursing meets those standards. The standards of a profession typically include seven requirements: (1) Possess a well-defined and well-organized body of knowledge; (2) Enlarge a systematic body of knowledge and improve education; (3) Educate its practitioners in institutions of higher learning; (4) Function autonomously in the formulation of policy; (5) Develop a code of ethics; (6) Attract professionals who will be committed to the profession for a lifetime; and (7) Compensate practitioners by providing autonomy, continuous professional development, and economic security.

17

Professional Ethics

LEARNING OBJECTIVES

- Importance of ethics in nursing
- Nightingale pledge
- Nursing ethics
- Code of ethics

- Ethical principles involved in nursing ethics
- Statements of ethical responsibility
- Relationship of professional ethics and etiquettes
- Professional etiquettes for nurses

INTRODUCTION

The word ethics is derived from the Greek word "Ethos" which means custom or guiding beliefs. Ethics are characteristics of a profession and are called as a "code". The ethics of nursing provides professional standards for nursing activities which protect the nurse and the patient. Ethics are the rules or principles that govern right contact. Ethics are designed to protect the rights of human being. Ethics are characteristics of a healthy profession. We have a set of ethics that is used by the nursing profession **(Fig. 17.1)**.

It may be written or unwritten, but each profession has a set of ethics usually called a code. This code tells the members what kind of conduct is expected of them as they practice. It will state responsibilities of its members towards those whom they serve, their coworker, the profession and society as a whole. When a person becomes a member of a profession he/she accept the responsibility of living up to the code of ethics for that profession **(Fig. 17.2)**. It should be understood

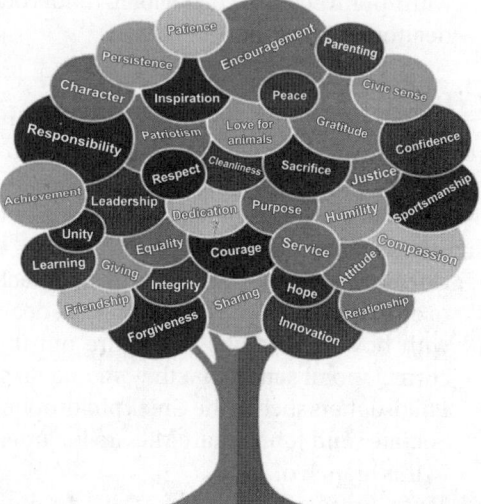

Fig. 17.2: Human values and professional ethics.

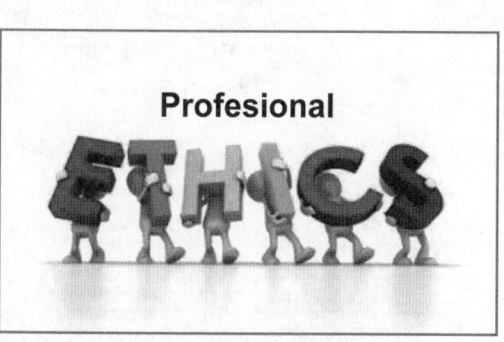

Fig. 17.1: Ethics.

that a code of ethics is not a strict set of rules. It is a guide. Although some behavior may be clearly correct or clearly wrong, other behaviors will depend upon the situation.

DEFINITION

- Ethics is defined as rules for a correct behavior. Professional ethics for nursing will state the ideal way of a nurse behaving in all professional relationships (patient, patient's relatives, coworkers, members of other professions and the public).
- Code of ethics defined what kind of conduct is expected of the members of a profession, it also used to guide professional behavior, help teachers plan education, prevent below standard practice, protect a nurse if falsely accused and guide direction for legal action.
- Ethics is a system of understanding determinations and motivations based on individual conceptions of right or wrong. It is not determined by strict rules or rigid guidelines and although it is relatively stable, it can change over time.
- Nursing ethics are the professional standard of conduct practiced by nurse practitioners related to or in accordance with approved moral behavior in rendering healthcare services.

TYPES OF ETHICS

You can study ethics from both a religious and a philosophical point of view. There are five branches of ethics, each of which offers a different perspective.

- **Normative ethics:** The normative approach to ethics, which is the largest branch, deals with how individuals can figure out the correct moral action that they should take. Philosophers such as the Greek philosopher Socrates and John Stuart Mill are included in this branch of ethics.
- **Meta ethics:** The meta ethics branch seeks to understand the nature of ethical properties and judgments such as if truth

values can be found and the theory behind moral principles.

- **Applied ethics:** Applied ethics is the study of applying theories from philosophers regarding ethics in everyday life. For example, this area of ethics asks questions such as "Is it acceptable to have an abortion?" and "Should you turn in your friend at your workplace for taking home office supplies?"
- **Moral ethics:** The branch of moral ethics questions how individuals develop their morality, why certain aspects of morality differ between cultures and why certain aspects of morality are generally universal.
- **Descriptive ethics:** Descriptive ethics is more scientific in its approach. It focuses on how human beings actually operate in the real world, rather than attempting to theorize about how they should operate.

IMPORTANCE OF ETHICS IN NURSING

- Ethics used to guide professional behavior of the nurses.
- It helps the teachers to know what must be taught in the education for the nurses.
- It can be used to prevent a nurse from practicing if her/his conduct is poor and clearly below the standards set by the code. **Figure 17.3** shows professional ethics.

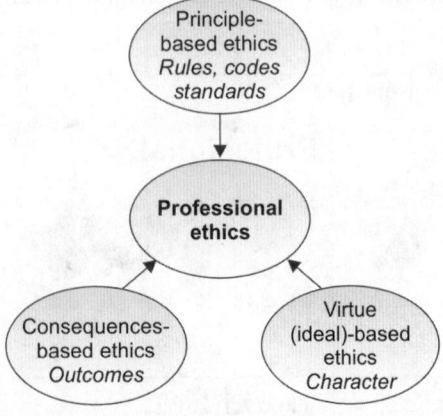

Fig. 17.3: Professional ethics.

- It can used to protect a nurse who is falsely accused of doing something wrong.
- It can also be used as a guide for direction when legal action must be taken in a lawsuit.

NIGHTINGALE PLEDGE

The pledge itself was little more than a paragraph and is reproduced below, but it must be noted that many of the ideals contained in the pledge continue to be seen in the present day code of ethics.

"I solemnly pledge myself before God and in the presence of this assembly, to pass my life in purity and to practice my profession faithfully. I will abstain from whatever is deleterious and mischievous, and will not take or knowingly administer any harmful drug. I will do all in my power to maintain and elevate the standard of my profession, and will hold in confidence all personal matters committed to my keeping and all family affairs coming to my knowledge in the practice of my calling. With loyalty will I endeavor to aid the physician, in his work, and devote myself to the welfare of those committed to my care".

This pledge was used as the basis for developing a code of ethics by the American Nurses Association (ANA) which was founded in 1896. The association presented its first draft in 1926 and a tentative code in 1940, but it was only in 1950 that a code of ethics for nurses was first established. The code was revised and amended several times afterwards as the influence of time and society changed the scope of a nurse's duties and responsibilities (Rambur, 1998). Substantial revisions took place in 1968 when the code was condensed and later in 1985 with the additional of interpretive statements. The present code as it is seen today was created in 2001 (ANA, 2001).

It must be noted that whatever shape or form the code was presented in, the basic ideas behind the code of ethics have always remained the same. As discussed by the American Nursing Association (2001), these principles are:

- Doing no harm
- Performing beneficial services
- Remaining loyal to the profession
- Honesty to oneself and the care receivers.

NURSING ETHICS

The nursing ethics provide professional standards for nursing activities which protect the nurse and the patient. In 1973, the International Council for Nurses (INC) adopted code of ethics. The fundamental responsibility of the nurse is four fold: (1) to promote health, (2) to prevent illness, (3) to restore health and (4) to alleviate suffering. The need for nursing is universal. Inherent in nursing is respect for life dignity, and rights of men. It unrestricted by considerations of nationality, race, creed, color, age, sex, politics or social status.

Nurses render health services to the individual, the family and the community and coordinate their services with those of related groups. **Box 17.1** represents ethical principles.

Nightingale pledge, 1935

I solemnly pledge myself before God and in the presence of this assembly, to pass my life in purityand to practice my profession faithfully. I will abstain from whatever is deleterious and mischievous, and will not take or knowingly administer any harmful drug. I will do all in my power to maintain and elevate the standard of my profession, and will hold in confidence all personal matters committed to my keeping, and all family affairs coming to my knowledge in the practice of my calling. With loyalty will I endeavour to aid the physician in his work, and as a 'missioner of health, I will dedicate myself to devoted service to human welfare.

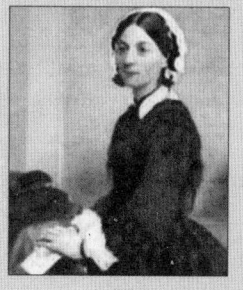

Box 17.1: Ethical principles.

Purpose
« Establish common ground among nurse, patient, family, other healthcare professional is and society for discussion of ethical questions and ethical decision making
« Permit people to take a consistent position on specific or related issues
« Provide an analytical framework by which moral problems can be evaluated

Autonomy
« Principle of respect for the person: primary moral principle
« Unconditional intrinsic value for all persons
« People are free to form their own judgments and actions as long as they do not infringe on the autonomous actions of others
« Concepts of freedom and informed consent are grounded in this principle

Beneficence
« To promote goodness, kindness, and charity
« To abstain from injuring others and to help others further their own well-being by removing harm; risks of harm must be weighed against possible benefits
« Common bioethical conflict results from an imbalance between the demands of beneficence and those of the healthcare delivery system

Nonmaleficence
« Implies a duty not to inflict harm
« To abstain from injuring others
« To help others further their own well-being by removing harm

Veracity
« Principle of truth-telling
« Belief that truth could at times could be harmful held for many years
« Consumers expect accurate and precise information revealed in an honest and respectful manner
« To develop trust between providers and patients, truthful interaction and meaningful communication must occur
« Challenge is to mesh need for truthful communication with the need to protect

Ethical Issues Involved in Nursing

Ethical issues involved in various branches in nursing. The branch/areas are:
• Nursing research
• Nursing education
• Nursing administration
• Nursing management
• Intensive care unit
• Operation theater/surgical nursing
• Medical nursing
• Community health nursing
• Child health nursing
• Mental health nursing
• Maternity nursing
• Nursing procedures

CODE OF ETHICS (FIG. 17.4)

The code of ethics will state what kind of conduct is expected from the members of a profession, what are the responsibilities of its members towards those whom they serve, their coworkers, the profession and the society as a whole. The nurse will adjust better if she understands what a wrong/right behavior in different situations is. The first such code of ethics, called the international code of nursing ethics, was adopted by the grand council of the International Council of Nurses at Sao Paulo, Brazil in 1953. It was later revised in Frankfurt, Germany in 1965 and then became known as ICN code of ethics.

The most recent revision in 1973 took place in Mexico City, Mexico and resulted in the present code for nurses, revision of the code have resulted in clearer and broader standards which can be applied in any culture.

The International Code for Nurses adopted by the International Council for Nurses (1973)

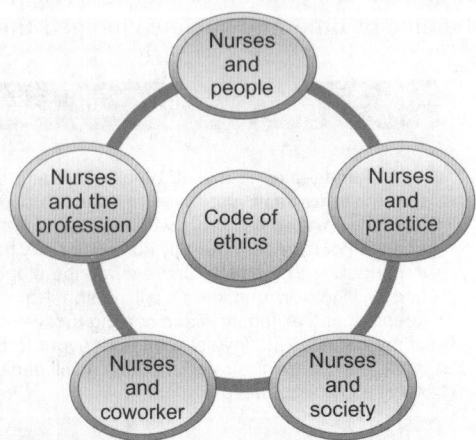

Fig. 17.4: Code of ethics.

is given in this unit. The code gives a general description of:

- What the nurse does: The four-fold responsibility of promoting health, preventing illness, restoring health and alleviating suffering.
- How nursing service should be given: Unrestricted by nationality, race, creed, color, age, sex, politics or social status; coordinated with related groups.
- To whom service is given: The individual, family and community.

The body of the code is made up of five sections.

1. **Nurses and people:** The nurse's primary responsibility is to those people who require nursing care. The nurse holds in confidence personal information's and use judgment in sharing this information.
    - The nurse's primary responsibility is to those people who require nursing care.
    - The nurse, in providing care, promotes an environment in which the values, customs and spiritual beliefs of the individual are respected.
    - The nurse holds in confidence personal information and uses judgment in sharing this information.
2. **Nurses and practice:** The nurse maintains the highest standards of nursing care possible within the reality of a specific situation. The nurse when acting in a professional capacity should at all times maintain standards of personal conduct which credit upon the profession.
    - The nurse carries personal responsibility for nursing practice and for maintaining competence by continual learning.
    - The nurse maintains the highest standards of nursing care possible within the reality of a specific situation.
    - The nurse uses judgment in relation to individual competence when accepting and delegating responsibilities.
    - The nurse, when acting in a professional capacity, should at all times maintain standards of personal conduct which reflect credit on the profession.

3. **Nurses and society:** The nurse shares with other citizens the responsibility for initiating and supporting action to meet the health and social needs of the public.
4. **Nurses and coworker:** The nurse maintains a cooperative relationship with coworkers in nursing and other fields. The nurse takes appropriate action to safeguard the individual when his care is endangered by a coworker or any other person.
    - The nurse sustains a cooperative relationship with coworkers in nursing and other fields.
    - The nurse takes appropriate action to safeguard the individual when his care is endangered by a coworker or any other person.
5. **Nurses and the profession:** The nurse acting through the professional organization participates in establishing and maintaining equitable social and economic working conditions in nursing.
    - The nurse plays a major role in determining and implementing desirable standards of nursing practices and nursing education.
    - The nurse is active in developing a core of professional knowledge.
    - The nurse, acting through the professional organization, participates in establishing and maintaining equitable, social and economic working conditions in nursing.

The international code of nursing ethics is given below:

- The fundamental responsibility of a nurse is to conserve life and to promote health. Every nurse is a teacher of health by example.
- A nurse must be adequately prepared to practice nursing and be willing to continue to learn new ideas by reading, and attending meetings.
- The nurse must learn to respect authority.
- The nurse must carry out the doctor's orders accurately and sustain confidence in the doctor, and all members of the health team.

- The nurse should report any unusual conditions or symptoms to the doctor or the in-charge nurse.

Table 17.1: Ethical values in nursing.

Themes	Sub-themes
Preserving patient dignity	• Belief in human dignity • Respect for patient privacy • Compassion for the patient • Accepting and observing the patient's rights • Fulfilling the spiritual and religious needs of the patient • Maintaining privacy for the patient's family and those present in the hospital
Practice integrity	• Careful care • Appropriate decision making • Using tact in performing obligations • Patient advocacy • Informing and training the patient
Professional commitment	• Responsibility • Having a conscience • Accountability
Forming human relationship	• Kind behavior • Trust building and gaining trust
Justice	Justice and fairness
Honesty and integrity	Honesty and integrity
Attempt to promote professional and individual competence	• Promoting personal moral traits • Professional dynamic and continuous effort • Preserving nursing reputation • Spiritual empowerment • Preserving and improving relationship with other colleagues

- The religious beliefs of a patient should be respected.
- The nurse should hold confidential all information given to her.
- When a patient requires continued nursing care, the nurse must remain with the patient until adequate relief is available.
- The nurse has the obligation to give conscientious service and, in return, is entitled to just remuneration.

- A patient should always be called by his full name.
- Punctuality is very important for every nurse.
- Obedience is very important in observing rules and regulations.
- Every nurse must have respect for authority and for rules and regulations.
- Economy is important for all nurses to practice.

ETHICAL PRINCIPLES INVOLVED IN NURSING ETHICS (FIG. 17.5)

Ethical principles actually control professionalism nursing practice much more than to ethical theories. Principles encompass basic promises from which rules are developed. Principles are the moral norms that nursing, as a profession, both demands and strives to implement to every day clinical practice. Ethical principle that the nurse should consider when making decisions are as follows:

1. **Respect for persons:** Respect for persons not only applies to clinical situations, but also to all life's situations. It directs individuals to treat themselves and others with a respect inherent to man's humanness. It requires recognition on a sense that all mankind shared a common human destiny. The respect to persons needs to be simplified as it affects nursing practice.

2. **Respect for autonomy:** Autonomy that individuals are able to act for themselves to the level of their capacity. It is the right of individual to govern their actions according to their own purpose and reason. Respect for autonomy requires that persons honor another's right to govern him or her. The legal doctrine of informed consent is the direct reflection of autonomy. So it requires that health personnel obtain a patient's informed consent for treatment and for participation in research. The followings are required for a patient to give informed consent for either:

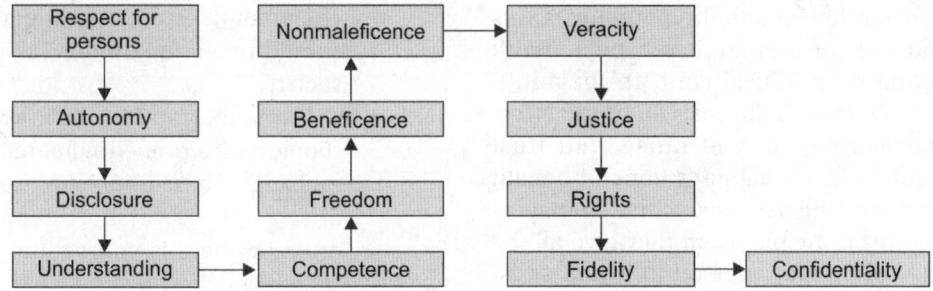

Fig. 17.5: Ethical principles involved in nursing ethics.

- **Disclosure:** Adequate presentation of relevant information about the proposed treatment or study.
- **Understanding:** Adequate comprehension of the disclosed information.
- **Voluntary agreement:** Free assent, influenced by external controlling factors.
- **Competence:** Adequate decision making capacity. There are three type of autonomy, i.e., freedom of action, freedom of choice and effective deliberation.

3. **Respect for freedom:** The principle of individual freedom decrease that patients be exempt from control by others to select and pursue personal health goals. Nurses as a group believe that patient should have greater freedom of choice within the nation's healthcare system. This principle should be observed by staff nurses when planning patient care; by nurse manager when leading subordinates.

4. **Respect for beneficence:** The beneficence principle states that the actions one takes should promote good. It dictates that a person is obliged to help others to advance their legitimate and important interests; it requires the balancing of harms and benefits. Benefits promote the client's welfare and health, whereas harms or risks detract from the client's health and welfare. In other words, providing benefits that enhance the others welfare. Whereas balancing the benefits and harms of intervention made on the others behalf.

Professional education provides awareness that most nursing interventions are capable of producing undesirable, as well as desirable, patient outcome. Therefore, the nurse is obliged to ascertain each care measure, likelihood of success, and balance the measures probable benefits and risks in order to select interventions that maximize patient's welfare.

5. **Respect for nonmaleficence:** The corollary of beneficence, the principle of nonmaleficence states that one should do no harm. The nurse should interpret the term 'harm' to mean emotional and social as well as physical injury. Harm is thwarting, defeating, or setting back one person's interest through invasive action by another. Many nurses find it difficult to follow the principle when performing treatment and procedures that bring discomfort and pain to patients. When the principle of sanctity of human life guides healthcare decisions, the principle of nonmaleficence prohibits active and passive enthusive by caregivers of terminally ill patients. As nurse manager performing performance evaluation of subordinates should emphasize their good qualities and give positive direction for growth. Destroying the employees self-esteem and self-worth would be considered doing harm their principles.

6. **Respect for veracity:** Veracity concerns truth telling an incorporates the concept that individuals should always tell the truth. It requires professional caregivers to provide with accurate, reality-based

information about their health status and care or treatment prospect. Truth telling is an ethical concern for nurse, because truth is the basis for mutual trust between patient and nurse, and trust is the basis for patient's hope of benefit from nursing services. Nurse managers use this principle when they give all the facts of a situation, truthfully and assist their employees to make decisions. However, truth telling may be difficult in a healthcare relationship. Some information that is transmitted from nurse to patient is depressing and/or frightening, e.g., bad news about personal health status.

7. **Respect for justice:** Justice concerns the issue that persons should be treated equally and fairly. This principle of justice requires treating others fairly and giving persons their due. When there are resources to distribute in healthcare, nurses should allocate them in such a way that equal shares go to equal recipients. The following problems complicate the application of justice:

   - Not everyone is equal in every way; sometimes there are situations in which it seems that one person should receive a greater or lesser share than another.

   - Resources are limited. There is not always enough for each person to receive an equal share. Questions of justice relate to the fairness with which benefits and burdens are distributed among people. Experience in turn found various principles have to be proposed to guide fair distribution of society's good are as follows:

     ◆ Each person should receive an equal share.

     ◆ The amount given to each person should be proportional to his or her need.

     ◆ The amount given to each person should be proportional to the amount of his or her work effort.

     ◆ The amount given to each person should reflect the value of his or her work product.

     ◆ The amount given to each person should reflect his to her value to society.

     ◆ The amount given to each person should be determined by free market exchange. These principles usually arise in times of short supplies or when there is competition for resources of benefits.

8. **Respect for rights:** Right is an entitlement to behave in certain way under circumstances, such as nurse's entitlement to freely express personal beliefs and preferences by voting in a political election. Another right is the prerogative to define another's behavior in selected situations, such as manager's prerogative to give assignments to subordinates. A right is also a claim to a specific good, service or prerequisite such as tea break time. Right is also used to mean agreement with justice, law and morality. So right may be mental rights or legal rights related to respective profession.

   - The patient has the right to every consideration of his privacy concerning his own medical care program.

   - The patient has the right to expect that all communications and records pertaining to his care should be treated as confidential.

   - The patient has the right to expect that within its capacity a hospital must make reasonable response to the request of a patient for services.

   - The patient has the right to obtain information as to any relationship of his hospital to other healthcare and educational institutions in so far as his care is concerned and any professional relationships among individuals, by name, who are treating him.

   - The patient has the right to be advised if the hospital proposes to engage in or perform human experimentation affecting his care or treatment and has the right to refuse to participate.

   - The patient has the right to expect reasonable continuity of care.

- The patient has the right to examine and receive an explanation of his bill regardless of source of payment.
- The patient has the right to know what hospital rules and regulations apply to his conduct as a patient.

9. **Respect for fidelity:** Fidelity is keeping one's promises or commitments. The principle of fidelity holds that a person should faithfully fulfill his duties and obligations. Fidelity is important in a nurse because a patient's hope for relief and recovery rests on evidence of caregiver's conscientiousness. Nurse Managers abide by this principle when they follow through on any promise they have previously made to employees, such as promised leave, a certain shift to be worked or a promotion to perception within the unit.

10. **Respect for confidentiality:** Confidentiality is the duty to respect privileged information. The principle of confidentiality provides that caregivers should respect a patient need for privacy and use personal information about him or her only to improve care. Nurses should practice confidentiality to decrease patient vulnerability and share from widespread knowledge of personal information divulged during care.

Table 17.2 summarizes ethics versus etiquette.

STATEMENTS OF ETHICAL RESPONSIBILITY

- Caring demands, the provision of helping services that is appropriate to the needs of the client and significant to others.
- Caring recognizes the client's membership in a family and community, and provides for the participation of significant others in his or her care.
- Caring acknowledges the reality of death in the life of every person, and demands that appropriate support provided to the dying person and family to enable that to prepare for, and to cope with death when it is inevitable.

Table 17.2: Ethics versus etiquette.

Ethics	Etiquette
Ethics refer to the moral principles that govern our behavior	Etiquette is a set of rules indicating the proper and polite way to behave
Ethics is related to principles	Etiquette is related to behavior
Ethics can mean different things to different people	Etiquette can differ according to culture, ethnicity, religion, country, etc.
Ethics is personal; the right and wrong are judged individually	Etiquette is social; it is not created by an individually

- Caring acknowledges that the human person has the capacity to fact up to health needs and problems in his or her own unique way, and directs nursing action in a manner that will assist the client to develop, maintain or gain personal autonomy, self-respect and self-determination.
- Caring, as a response to a health need, requires the consent and the participation of the person who is experiencing the need.
- Caring dictates that the client and significant others have the knowledge and information adequate for free and informed decisions concerning care requirements, alternative and preferences.
- Caring demands that the needs of the client supersede those of the nurse.
- Caring acknowledges the vulnerability of a client in certain situations and dictates restraint in actions which might compromise the client's rights and privileges.
- Caring involving a relationship which is, in itself therapeutic, demands mutual respect and trust.
- Caring acknowledges that information obtained in the course of the nursing relationship is privileged and that requires the full protection of confidentiality unless such information provides evidence of serious impending harm to the client or to a third party, or is legally required by the courts.

- Caring requires that the nurse represents the needs of the client and that the nurse takes appropriate measures when fulfillment of these needs is jeopardized by the actions of other persons.
- Caring acknowledges the dignity of all persons in the practice of educational setting.
- Caring acknowledges respects and draws upon the competencies of others.
- Caring establishes the conditions for the harmonization of efforts of different helping professionals in providing required services to clients.
- Caring seeks to establish and maintain a climate of respect for the honest dialogue needed for effective collaboration.
- Caring establishes the legitimacy of respectful challenge and or confrontation when the service required by the client is compromised by in competency, incapacity or negligence or when the competencies of the nurses are not acknowledged or appropriately utilized.
- Caring demands the provision of working conditions which enable nurses to carry out their legitimate and responsibilities.
- Caring demands resourcefulness and restraint accountability for the use of time, resources, equipment, and funds, and requires accountability to appropriate individuals and/or bodies.
- Caring requires that the nurse bring to the work situation in education, practice, administration or research, the knowledge, affective and technical skills required, and that competency in these areas be maintained and updated.
- Caring commands fidelity, oneself, and guards the right and privilege of the nurse to act in keeping with an informed moral conscience.

MEANING AND RELATIONSHIP OF PROFESSIONAL ETHICS AND ETIQUETTES

Etiquettes mean good manners. We all learn certain standards of social etiquette in daily life. It means that we know how to behave with courtesy and respect as we relate with other people. For e.g., we learn when it is correct to remain seated or to rise in different kinds of social situations. We also learn how to make another person feel welcome comfortable and at ease, much of what we learn to do in these relationships depends upon the social customs of the community in which we live.

Professional etiquette means "good manners" in professional relationship just as we learn social etiquette, we must learn that etiquette is acceptable and expected of us in our professional relationships. It is essential for successful working, relationships with those in authority nursing colleagues, members of other professions, patients and those in society.

To help us learn what professional etiquette is expected of us the following discussion is centered upon professional relationships and standards of behavior which have been developed and accepted by the nursing profession. It must be remembered that these standards will vary according to the society in which they are practiced in all situations. However professional etiquette is based upon the same characteristic that is consideration and respect for others.

Nothing is more important than practicing these two things in everyday behavior. Developing good relationships in all area of life will help you to become a better person and will lead you to develop greater cooperation and understanding in your professional relationships and activities.

Professional etiquette: Etiquette means good manner, it tells how to behave with courtesy and respect as we relate with other people. Professional etiquette means good manner in professional relationship. It is essential for successful working relationship with those in authority, nursing colleagues, and members of other profession, patients and those in society. It must be remembered that these standards will vary according to the society in which they are practiced. Professional etiquette is based upon the characteristics, which are consideration and respect for others.

Employment etiquette: Professional success and reputation depend upon practicing good professional etiquette. Advertising in nursing journals and newspaper, direct contact with institutions and professional organizations and informal contacts with experienced nursing personnel's are the best sources of information about vacant positions. Application for a position may be sent through a letter or application with or without a resume, an application form supplied by an employer or by personal interview.

Resigning from a position: Resignation letter should be submitted in good business form, well in advance, of your planned departure, depending upon the circumstances. Early notification is helpful for staffing and planning by the administration under which you presently work. A resignation should never be written unless you are sure that you are leaving. The letter of resignation should be typed or printed clearly in approved business form on plain white paper. Your reasons for leaving should be expressed in a polite, honest and objective manner. You should also express appreciation for the experience you have had and express regret for the necessity of leaving. You should hand over charge to another responsible person before you quit the hospital. Proper notification is professional and important when submitting a resignation. A notice of one month is considered courteous except in emergency cases. Professional success and reputation depend upon practicing good professional etiquette.

PROFESSIONAL ETIQUETTES FOR NURSES

Etiquette is a code of good manners that a nurse should follow. The nurse is an important member of the health team that must work in cooperation and harmony for the care of the sick. For a smooth functioning and a good interpersonal relationship, you as a nurse should follow certain essential good manners.

- The nurse should be courteous to all. Be gentle and polite in your talk.
- The nurse should greet your seniors, coworkers, your patients, etc., with appropriate words and according to the time of the day, e.g., good morning, good evening.
- The nurse should address the seniors with proper title, e.g., sir, madam, sister, mister, miss, etc.
- Stand up when people of higher rank enter your room.
- Stand up when answering questions in the classroom.
- Open the door for the senior and stand aside for them to pass.
- Excuse yourself when overtaking a senior person.
- Stand aside and give way to senior when you cross them on the ways, e.g., in the corridors, on the staircases, etc.
- Maintain silence wherever and whenever necessary, e.g., classroom, library, study room and dormitories.
- Keep your dress neat and tidy (series arranged and the hair put up).
- While on duty never use any form of jewelry that may interfere with work.
- Obey seniors without arguing.
- Help the seniors to carry a heavy load if you find them on the way.
- Say "thank you" when someone is doing a favor for you, and also when someone corrects you.
- Get prior permission from the sister in-charge before you take any article from any department.
- Do not delay the answers to the questions. Give the answer immediately and appropriately.
- Always be punctual.
- Avoid thumb sucking and nail biting.
- In an assembly, let the senior take the seat first.
- Keep eye contact and sit face to face when listing to someone.
- Say "Excuse me" even if you hurt others accidentally.
- Never let others secret go out of you.
- Always close the door after getting into a room or when you get out of the room, if so desired.

Provision 1	• Practice with compassion and respect for inherent dignity, worth and unique attributes of every person
Provision 2	• Commitment to the patient whether an individual, family, group, community or population
Provision 3	• Promote, advocates for and protects the rights, health and safety of the patient
Provision 4	• Authority, accountability, and responsibility for nursing practice makes decisions takes consistent action with the obligation to promote health and to provide optimal care
Provision 5	• Owes the same duty to self as others including the responsiblity to promote health and safety, presevere wholeness of character and integrity, maintain competence and continue personal and professional growth
Provision 6	• Through individual and collective effort, establishes, maintains and improves the ethical environment of the work setting and conditions of employment that are conducive to safe, quality health care
Provision 7	• In all roles and settings, advances the profession through research and scholarly inquiry, professional standards development and the generation of both nursing and health policy
Provision 8	• Collaborates with other health professionals and the public to protect human rights promote health diplomacy and reduce health disparities
Provision 9	• Collectively through its professional organizations, must articulate nursing values, maintain the integrity of the professional and integrate principles of social justice into nursing and health policy

Fig. 17.6: Professional etiquettes for nurses.

- Knock at the door and wait for the answer before you enter into other's room.
- Do not cover the mouth while talking to others. Cover your mouth when you cough or sneeze.
- Excuse yourself before you interfere with others engaged in talking or doing some work.

- The nurse should not give and receive any gifts or present especially from the patients and their relatives.

Ethical Dilemma (Fig. 17.7)

Ethical dilemmas are situations in which there is a difficult choice to be made between two or more options, neither of which resolves

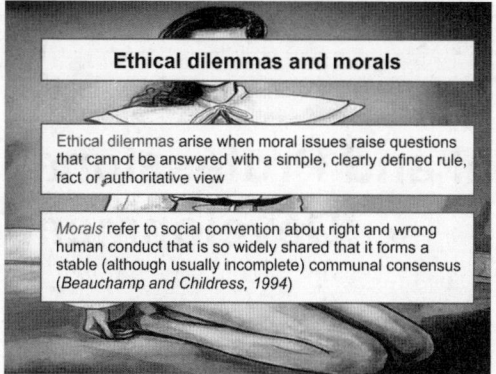

Fig. 17.7: Ethical dilemmas and morals.

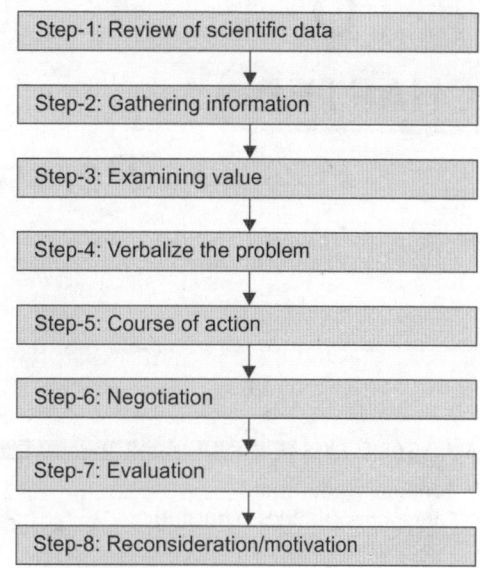

Fig. 17.8: Steps to process an ethical dilemma.

the situation in a manner that is consistent with accepted ethical guidelines. When faced with an ethical dilemma, a person is faced with having to select an option that doesn't align with an established code of ethics or societal norms, such as codes of law and religious teachings, or with their internal moral perceptions of right and wrong. Explore ethical dilemma examples to see how you might handle these difficult situations?

Nurses often face ethical dilemmas when caring for patients. Ethical dilemmas come in various forms and for several reasons. The following are five main reasons why nurses face ethical dilemmas in nursing?

1. Patients or their loved ones must make life or death decisions
2. The patient refuses treatment
3. Nursing assignments may contradict cultural or religious beliefs
4. Nursing peers demonstrate incompetence
5. Inadequate staffing

Nurses in all disciplines face ethical challenges from time to time. The best way to describe and identify an ethical dilemma in nursing is to consider how a situation makes you think and feel. Ethical dilemmas create a conflict between two courses of action that are both correct but represent different principles or values. If a situation involves doing something right and wrong at the same time and one of those actions negatively impacts the other action, this is what creates the dilemma. **Figure 17.8** shows how to process ethical dilemma.

CONCLUSION

Nursing ethics is a branch of applied ethics that concerns itself with activities in the field of nursing. Nursing ethics shares many principles with medical ethics, such as beneficence, nonmaleficence and respect for autonomy. It can be distinguished by its emphasis on relationships, human dignity and collaborative care. The need of nursing is universal. Inherent in nursing is respect for life, dignity, and rights of man; it is unrestricted by considerations of nationality, race, creed, color, age, sex, politics or social status. Nurses render health services to the individual, the family, and the community and coordinate their services with those of related groups.

18

Personal and Professional Development

- Continuing education
- Career opportunities in nursing
- In-service education

- Expanded role of the nurse
- Futuristic nursing

INTRODUCTION

Many professions require that members of their profession continue learning new and changing skills to retain their credentials or even licenses. For example, certified public accountants in most states are required to take continuing education hours every year to keep their licenses current. Continuing education is any course of study offered by an educational institution, association, professional society or organization for the purpose of providing continuing education for nursing home administrators.

Continuing education program are usually short-term and specific, a certificate may be offered for completion of a course. It is not to be confused with academic degree-granting

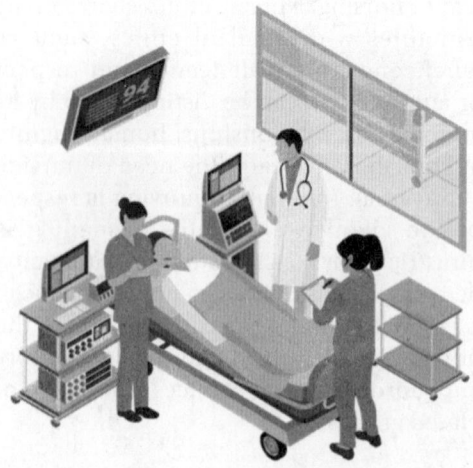

Fig. 18.1: Professional activities of a nurse in health care.

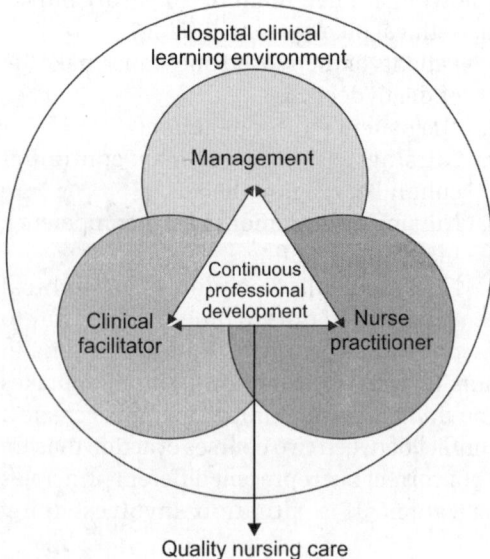

Fig. 18.2: Continuing education program for the nurse.

programs such as advanced education or post graduate education.

CONTINUING EDUCATION

Continuing education means the phenomenon of ever learning which does not stop at any particular stage. It includes all learning opportunities which would be taken up after full time education has stopped. It is the resumption of the process of studying or learning which might have interrupted

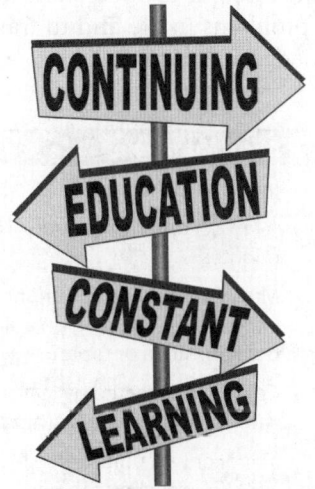

Fig. 18.3: Updating the knowledge and skill by continuing education.

because of some economic, professional and personnel compulsion of the individual.

Continuing education program provide teaching and learning strategies that are based upon the learning theory which states that adult learners should participate in the development of their learning objectives.

Definition

- The American Nurses Association (ANA) has defined continuing education as "learning activities", intended to build upon the education and experience bases of the professional nurse for the enhancement of practice education, administration, and research or theory development.
- Continuing education is a formal, organized educational programs designed to promote the knowledge, skills and professional attitudes of nurses.

Objectives of CE: Continuing education helps the employee to:
- Keep up-to-date with new concepts and development in the health field.
- To increase their basic knowledge and skills and develop positive attitudes.
- Develop an ability to analyze problems and to work with others.
- Meet the challenge of changes in technology.

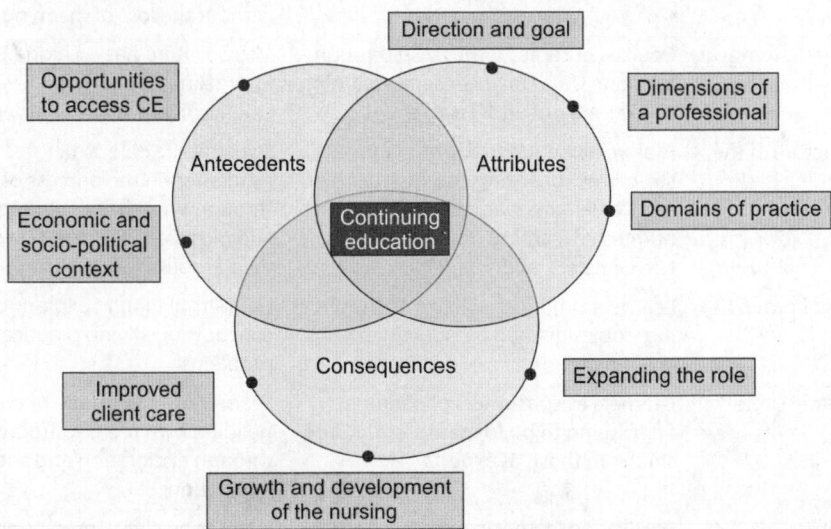

Fig. 18.4: Importance of continuing education.

- Maintain standards of health care at acceptable level.
- Help in setting standards within the health care team.
- Help in career development.
- Motivate staff for better patient care.
- Meet new needs of the community.

Purpose of CE:

- Documenting attendance at the designed seminars or course of institution. Licensing bodies in a number of fields impose continuing education requirements on members who hold licenses to practice within particular profession.

- These requirements are intended to encourage professionals to expand their knowledge base and them up-to-date on new departments.
- Depending on the field, these requirements may be satisfied through college or university course work, extension courses or conferences and seminars attendance.

Need for continuing education:

- Kothari Education Commission also suggested that education institutions should arrange ad-hoc courses which will make people to understand and solve their problems in life and to train wider knowledge and experience.

Table 18.1: Difference between micro and macro learning.

		Macro learning	Micro learning
1.	Learning context	Formal learning	Informal learning
2.	Time spent	Several hours	A few seconds up to about 15 minutes
3.	Content type	Learning modules, comprising and structuring a broader range of ideas or topics and combining learning objects	Microcontent as small chunks of information, focusing on a single definable idea or topic
4.	Content creation	Content created by subject matter experts, usually with authoring tools	Content co-created by learners with web 2.0 and rapid e-learning tools
5.	Content aggregation and fragmentation	Learning objects usually need to be combined with other learning objects to enable full understanding; content can be easily split for re-use and restructuring	Microcontent units are self-contained as they can be understood without any additional information: microcontent cannot be divided into smaller pieces without the loss of meaning
6.	Content retrieval	Courses or topics retrievable through a unique URL. However single learning objects are not addressable	Microcontent has a unique URL (permalink), which make even small chunks of information retrievable
7.	Structure of the learning cycle	Hierarchic, sequential, pre-planned structures consisting of a number of units or lessons, each combining a number of learning objects, such as texts, images, audio, video	Dynamic, flexible structures created by learners in the process of learning through syndication, aggregation and modification, based on such data as social tags and bookmarks
8.	Target group	Learners aiming at gaining an insight into topics defined by domain experts	Learners aiming at exploring concepts or solving practical problems
9.	Learner's role	Learners as consumers of content, attempting to build mental structures similar to those of experts	Learners as prosumere of content, building own mental structures through exploration and social interaction
10.	Learner participation	Focuses on learner-content interactions	Focuses on social interactions between learners

- Learning through continuing education is also essential for the rural people, who must acquire full knowledge about rapid advancement of agricultural and economic techniques just as urban people have to acquire commercial techniques.
- Indian Education Commission has rightly stated about it, "Education does not end with school, but it is a lifelong process."
- Continuing education programmed provide teaching and learning strategies that are based upon learning theory which states that adult learners should participate in the development of their learning objectives.
- Continuing education is the most essential requirement of the adult today. He can enjoy a better, healthier and more successful life only if he continues his education up to end of his life.

National policy on CE: According to NPE, adult education can be successfully implemented by involving continuing education. Hence these kinds of implemented by involving continuing education. Hence these kinds of education are to be combined. It is possible to implement adult and continuing education programs through various ways, such as:

- To setup continuing education centers in rural areas.
- To educate workers through their employers trade unions and concerned agencies of government.
- To provide post-secondary education institutions.
- To provide books, libraries and reading rooms.
- To use radio, TV and film as mass and group learning media.
- To create learners groups and organizations.
- To design programs of distance learning.
- To organize assistance in self-study.
- To organize vocational training programs based on needs and interests of learners.

Programs of action on NPE: Continuing education is any training or classes that one takes after completing formal education. Continuing education can be college classes taken after completing a formal degree program or seminars and training taken to improve one's job skills.

- **Program of action** given by the ministry of Human Resource Development, Government of India has been fully formulated. First of all it is considered that continuing education is regarded as an indispensable aspect of the strategy of human resource development and of the goal of creation of learning society.

Table 18.2: Need of continuing education.

Competency	Definition
Patient-centered care	Recognize the patient or designee as the source of control and full partner in providing compassionate and coordinated care based on respect for patient's preferences, values, and needs
Teamwork and collaboration	Function effectively within nursing and inter-professional teams, fostering open communication, mutual respect, and shared decision-making to achieve quality patient care
Evidence-based practice (EBP)	Integrate best current evidence with clinical expertise and patient/family preferences and values for delivery or optimal health care
Quality improvement (QI)	Use data to monitor the outcomes of care processes and use improvement methods to design and test changes to continuously improve the quality and safety of health care systems
Informatics	Use information and technology to communicate, manage knowledge, mitigate error, and support decision-making
Safety	Minimize risk of harm to patients and provides through both system effectiveness and individual performance

Note: Adapted from QSEN, 2009.

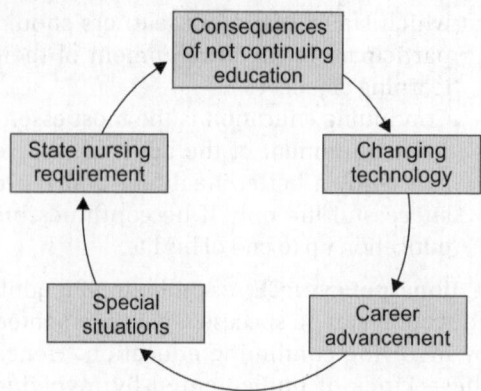

Fig. 18.5: Aims of continuing education.

- **Continuing education** aims at post literacy for neo literates and school drop outs for retention of literacy skills continuation of learning beyond elementary literacy and application of this learning to improve their living conditions. However the continuing education goes beyond post literacy and its instruments.
- **Program of book promotion** will be undertaken on the lines indicated in the policy. Libraries and reading rooms in educational institutions should be opened to the public in the evening and necessary additional grants should be provided to them for this purpose. The voluntary efforts for establishment of reading room and libraries should be encouraged. Radio, TV films should be encouraged for sub-serving the objectives of education and recreation.
- **Agencies of continuing education** are parallel system of education, ad-hoc or short-term courses, open universities, distance education scheme, libraries, special part-time courses, special institutions and mass medias.

CAREER OPPORTUNITIES IN NURSING

The goal of profession is nursing is to confirm and expand the present body of nursing knowledge, which in turn contribution to improved health care. Establishing a scientific base of nursing knowledge will provide nurses with most current principles of practice, e.g., if it could be demonstrated through research that one method of thermometer disinfections proved to be more effective than another, the better method could be adopted; a comparative study of the different methods of teaching family planning could aid in the selection of the best method for researching family planning; if a study of patient's comfort suggested that a relationship between high level of stress and visiting hours existed, visiting hours could be reduced and the effectiveness of reduced visiting hours could be further evaluated.

Nursing career: Nursing shortages are often a symptom of wider health system or Nursing shortages are not just a problem for nursing stated Christine Hancock of Nurses. They are a health system problem, which undermines health social ailments, nursing in many countries continues to be undervalued as 'Women's work', and nurses are given only limited access to resources to make them effective in their jobs and careers. Health care is labor intensive and demands more nursing service. Policy makers in many countries have already recognized this fact and making necessary changes to attract the best nursing services in numbers and quality. Increases in demand are created due to these policies.

- Be a serious student with proficiency in the health sciences.
- Assume legal, moral and ethical accountability for your actions.
- Use good judgment, and be loyal to patients and to the profession.
- Demonstrate unbiased compassion for all by respecting all people regardless of age, race, social status, sexual orientation and religious beliefs.
- Show highest degree of motivation to keep up with trends and research in the profession and to value life-long learning.
- Learn to handle catastrophe and crisis, and everyday challenges, in a confident, efficient, and caring way.
- Have good mental and physical health, plenty of stamina and endurance, a sense.

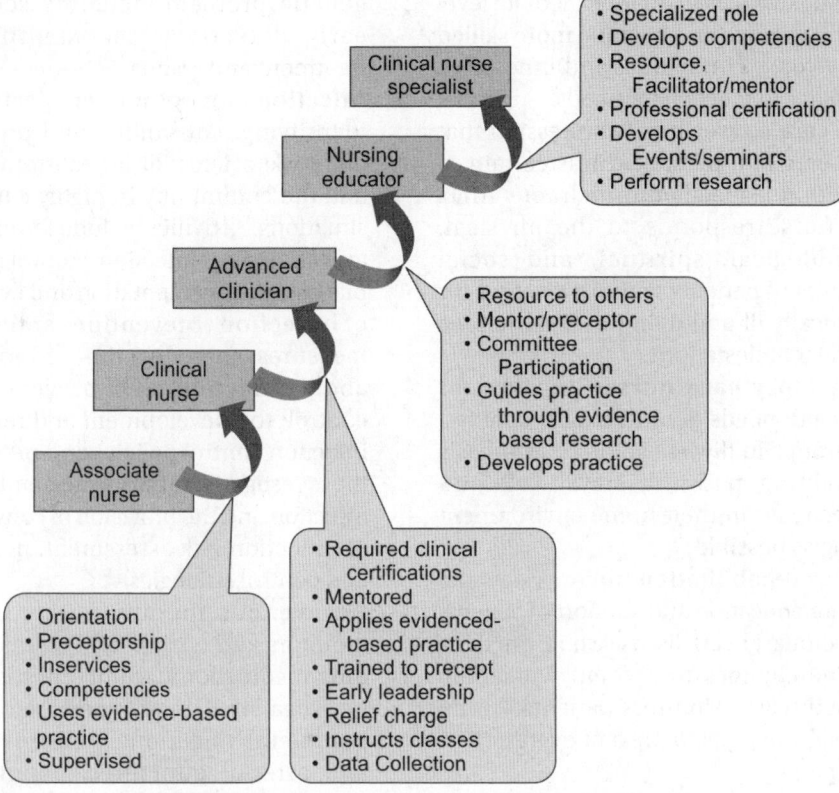

Clinical nurse
specialist

• Specialized role
• Develops competencies
• Resource,
  Facilitator/mentor
• Professional certification
• Develops
  Events/seminars
• Perform research

Nursing
educator

Advanced
clinician

• Resource to others
• Mentor/preceptor
• Committee
  Participation
• Guides practice
  through evidence
  based research
• Develops practice

Clinical
nurse

Associate
nurse

• Required clinical
  certifications
• Mentored
• Applies evidenced-
  based practice
• Trained to precept
• Early leadership
• Relief charge
• Instructs classes
• Data Collection

• Orientation
• Preceptorship
• Inservices
• Competencies
• Uses evidence-based
  practice
• Supervised

Fig. 18.6: Career path and professional development in nursing.

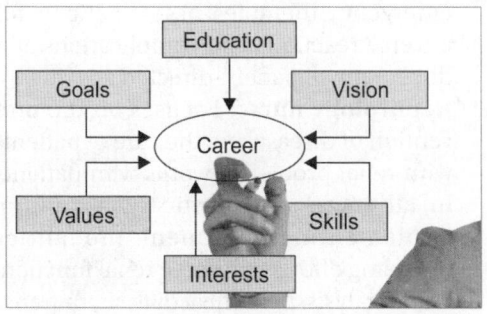

Fig. 18.7: Career opportunities in nursing.

Career opportunities in nursing:

• **Nurse anesthetist:** Provides care to patients before, during and after surgery or delivery. Specific activities include physical assessment, preoperative teaching, and preparation, administration and maintenance of anesthesia. Responsible for constantly monitoring every function of the patient's body while the patient is anesthetized. Provides care during the recovery period and as part of follow-up monitoring during the postoperative course.

• **Nurse educator:** As the name suggests, the responsibilities include a verity of roles including teaching, research, and patient care. Central to effective teaching is the solid clinical skills developed from clinical practice. Nurse educator is responsible for lesson planning, instructing, evaluating learning, counseling, and assisting with solving learning problems. Serves as a primary resource for theory and knowledge development in the discipline of nursing.

• **Staff nurse:** The entry-level nurse or nurse without any specialization is called staff nurse whose responsibilities include making nursing judgments based on scientific knowledge and relies on procedures and standardized care plans. The staff nurse has an incredibly complex job and advances to an intermediate level with experience and become more skilled in developing individual and innovative care plans to meet client needs.

- **AIDS care nurse:** This is profession that takes care of a person who is certain to die within a specified time frame. AIDS care nurse responds to the physical, psychological, spiritual, and social concerns of patients with AIDS, cares for chronically ill and dying with numerous clinical manifestations.
- **Ambulatory care nurse:** Provides for the health needs of individuals, families, and groups in diverse settings. Emphasis on helping patients stays well and independent in their home environment as long as possible.
- **Cardiac rehabilitation nurse:** Meets the need for education and support of patients with coronary heart disease who are making lifestyle changes to prevent worsening of the disease. Monitors patients during physical workouts to prevent overexertion and or injury.
- **Correction nurse:** Provides for the health care of inmates in correctional facilities such as juvenile offender homes, jails prisons and penitentiaries.
- **Endoscopy nurse:** Provides essential care of patients undergoing procedures for screening, diagnosis and or treatment of gastrointestinal disorders and may specialize in endoscopy.
- **Genetic nurse:** The genetic nurse care for people's genetic health—those with genetic problem-including screening, early detection, risk identification, treatment and testing.
- **Infection control nurse:** Specializes in identifying, controlling and preventing outbreaks of infection in healthcare settings and the community in highly contagious situations. Activities include the collection and analysis of infection-control data; the planning, implementation and evaluation of infection prevention and control measures; the education of individuals about infection risk, prevention and control; the development and revision of infection control policies and procedures; the investigation of suspected outbreaks of infection and the provision of consultation on infection risk assessment, prevention and control strategies.
- **Intravenous therapy nurse:** Initiates, monitors and terminates therapies including medications, antineoplastic agents, investigational drugs, blood products, and parenteral nutrition, performs venous and arterial punctures, maintain the intravascular side including tubing and dressings, monitor for infections, initiate emergency therapies, assess patients for adverse reactions and complications and document all patient-directed activities.
- **Nephrology nurse:** Focuses on the prevention of disease and the care of patients with renal problems; works with patients in all stages of chronic renal failure, implementing treatment modalities including efforts to reserve renal function, hemodialysis, peritoneal dialysis, or transplant.
- **Neuroscience nurse:** Care for individuals who have a dysfunction of the nervous system including alterations in consciousness and cognition, communication, mobility, rest and sleep, sensation and sexuality; plans and implements interventions to support bodily functions, promote healing, encourage adoption to persistent neurological difficulties and teaches patients and families about the illness.

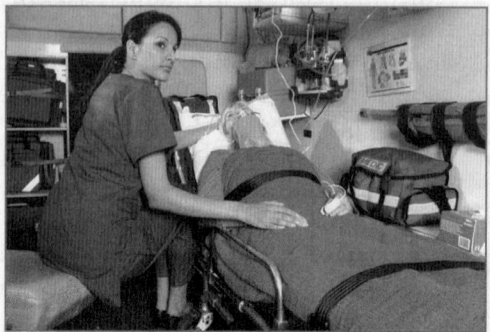

Fig. 18.8: Ambulatory care nursing.

- **Occupational health nurse:** Occupational health nursing combines concepts of public health and nursing theory in an orientation toward primary prevention or keeping healthy workers healthy and includes managing workers' compensation records and counseling employees.
- **Oncology nurse:** Cares for patients with the diagnosis of cancer in various settings; utilized an empathic and caring approach to patients whose diagnostics and treatment are often painful and life-threatening, administers chemotherapy, conducts patient teaching, and manages illness-treatment-related symptoms.
- **Ophthalmic nurse:** Provides care to persons with disorders of the eyes including blindness or visual impairment; functions range from patient teaching to assistance in surgery.
- **Perioperative nurse:** Provides for the surgical patient's needs by assessing, planning and implementing nursing care patient receive preoperatively, intraoperatively and postoperatively. Nursing activities performed by the preoperative nurse include patient assessment, creating and maintaining a sterile and safe environment.
- **Orthopedic nurse:** Cares for the actual and potential health problem related to musculoskeletal function; relies on a holistic approach in their assessment of the impact of musculoskeletal conditions on self-care, patient management of the environment, available patient resources, and support systems.
- **Prenatal nurse:** Cares for women, infants and their families from the onset of pregnancy through the first month of the newborn's life (prenatal period); monitors the pregnancy, assesses the progression of labor; monitors the status of mother and body, maintains a sense of calm and comfort during labor; fosters the new mother-infant relationship, teachers parenting skills, and assesses and supports the mother in her recovery from childbirth; evaluates the newborn's early adjustment to life.
- **Psychiatric nurse:** Should possess the art of using one's self in therapeutic ways to assist patients to affect changes in self-understanding and behavior. Views individuals from a holistic perspective, taking into account both physical and mental health needs while focusing on human behavior.
- **Plastic and reconstructive surgical nurse:** Cares for patients undergoing cosmetic and maxillofacial surgery, laser and microsurgery and nonsurgical treatments to correct esthetic problems.
- **Rehabilitation nurse:** The rehabilitation nurse cares for individuals who are experiencing temporary, progressive, or permanent illness or disabilities that are extensive enough to alter their normal functioning and interrupt their lifestyle.
- **Respiratory nurse:** Promotes pulmonary health for individuals, families, and communities, and cares for persons with pulmonary dysfunction throughout the lifespan. Respiratory nursing may be preventive, acute or critical, or rehabilitative.
- **Transplantation nurse:** Cares for recipient and living-donor patients throughout the transplantation process from and state disease to preoperative to intraoperative experience to aftercare and long-term follow-up.
- **Trauma nurse:** Trauma nursing involves responding quickly to a wide variety of single and multisystem trauma involving

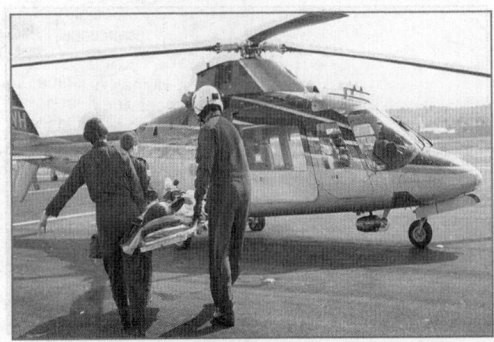

Fig. 18.9: Flight nurse.

different patient needs, ages, cultures and severity of presenting symptoms. The trauma nurse must respond with decisiveness and clarity to unexpected events by assessing, intervening, and stabilizing patients about whom there is minimal information.

- **Flight nurse:** Involves emergency and non-emergency air surface transport of ill and injured patients. This includes interfacility transport and emergency 'scene calls' for trauma and medical emergencies.
- **Forensic nurse:** Forensic nursing combines clinical nursing practice with the law enforcement arena. It involves the investigation and treatment of victims of sexual assault, elder, child and spousal abuse, unexplained or accidental death, trauma and assault as well as perpetrators of these and any criminal activity.
- **Holistic nurse:** Involves all aspects of wellness and healing of a holistic nature; holism being defined as the mind, body, spirit connection; that it, treating the whole person, not just a disease of symptom.

- **Medical editor/author:** Involves all aspects of writing, editing and proofreading technical material for use in biomedical research, education and training, sales and marketing and other communication forms.
- **Military nurse:** Provide all aspects of traditional nursing care and practice in both peace and wartime settings through various branches of the military service. Classifications include active duty, reserves, and civilian employment.

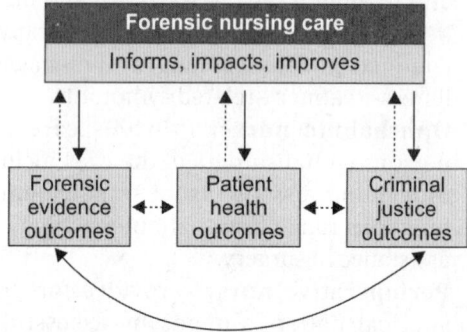

Fig. 18.11: Forensic nursing care.

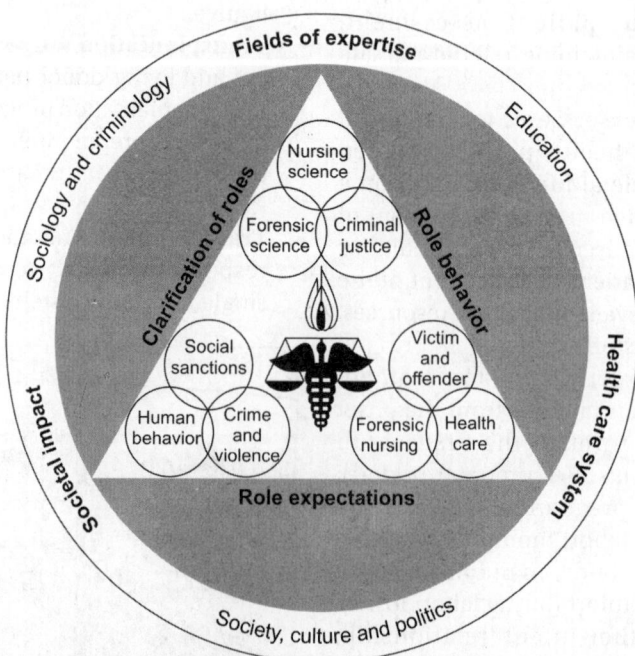

Fig. 18.10: Legal and ethical issues in nursing.

- **Pediatric nurse:** Provides comprehensive care to children, adolescents and their families in various settings. Responds to the physical and psychosocial aspects of health and illness, concern for health promotion and disease prevention, management of physical and mental disabilities, and response to acute and chronic illness.
- **Nursing informatics:** Involves all aspects of computerization as it relates to nursing and healthcare practice.
- **Nurse anesthetist:** Perianesthesia nursing provides intensive care to patients as they awaken from anesthesia. The perianesthesia nurse prepares patients for the surgical experience, monitors and supports safe transition from anesthetized state to responsiveness, and readies patients for discharge from perianesthesia care unit.
- **Career healing touch:** Nursing encompasses autonomous and collaborative care of individuals of all ages, families, groups and communities, sick or well and in all settings. Nursing includes the promotion of health, prevention of illness, and the care of ill, disabled and dying people. Advocacy,

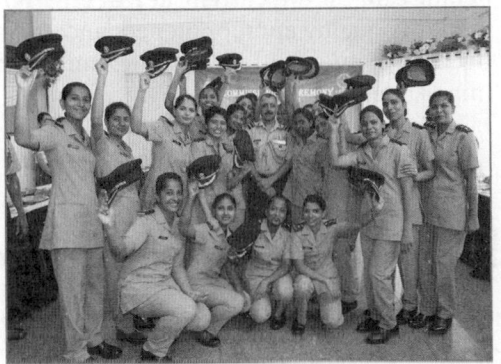

Fig. 18.12: Military nursing services.

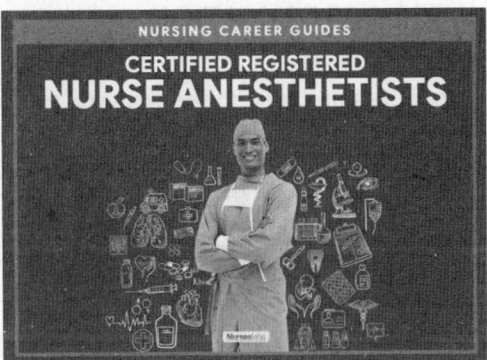

Fig. 18.14: Certified nurse anesthetists.

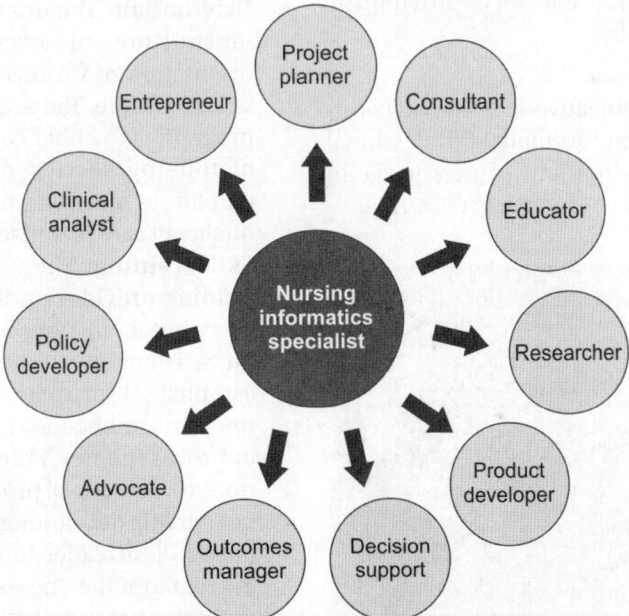

Fig. 18.13: Role of nurse in nursing informatics.

promotion of a safe environment, research participation in shaping health policy and inpatient and health system management, and education are also key nursing roles.

Nurse extends a caring hand; give a healing touch, a curing wish, and a mother's touch unconditionally to the person with a health condition of experiencing trauma. If personal and professional satisfaction and rewards are what you're looking for by caring the lives of others, nursing is for you. Nursing education makes intellectual demands on the student. Nursing career needs lot of stamina and patience.

IN-SERVICE EDUCATION

In-service education is defined as learning experiences provided in the working setting for the purpose of assisting staff in performing their assigned functions in that particular agency.

Definition: The American Nurses Association defined as "Planned education activities intended to build upon the educational and experiential bases of the professional nurse for the enhancement of practice, education, administration, and research or theory development to the end of improving the health of the public.

Aims and objectives:
- The primary objective of in-service education is the improvement of professional practice, development of person as an individual and a responsible citizen.

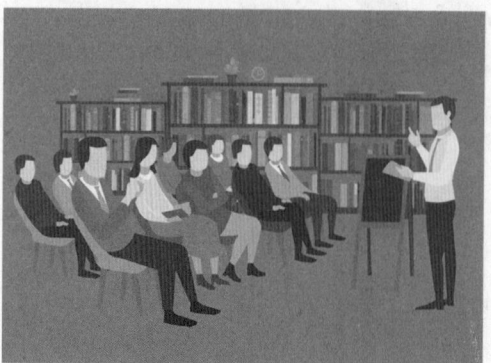

Fig. 18.15: In-service education.

- It keeps enthusiastic in their learning and makes them to seek latest knowledge.
- It enables to implement the knowledge with skill and ability.
- It improves the health care delivery to the public enhancing the quality of effective nursing practice.
- It develops interest and job satisfaction.
- By acquiring current and up to date knowledge, confidence is developed among them.

Need for in-service program: Need for in-service education for professional nurses is influenced by research and advances in health care. In the current health environment the quality appropriateness and effectiveness of interventions assume increasing importance.
- **General in-service education:** This program is short-term learning experiences related to topics required to all staff, e.g., CPR, fire safety.
- **Specific in-service education:** This type of education programs are also short-term but are designed to meet the needs of a particular group of staff in a clinical area.

Components of in-service education:
- **Orientation:** The orientation influences the structure and content of individualized orientation of various groups of nursing service people. The goal of the orientation program is to enhance the competencies of nursing service personnel so that employees may continuously improve the quality of care provided to patients.
- **Skill training:** The new employee skill training provides an idea about how to carry out the assigned function complex ones. It enables to meet the standards established for quantity and quality of the performance and job satisfaction it improves the new employees skill in the routine and special procedures.
- **Leadership development:** The staff should have skills in leadership and management in order to guide a new employee in caring outpatient care activities. At present the hospitals are recognizing the development

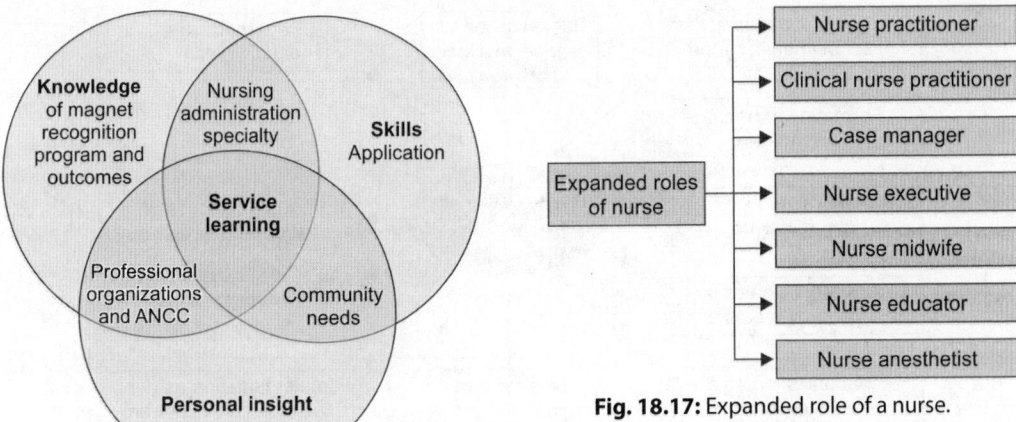

Fig. 18.16: Components of in-service education.

Fig. 18.17: Expanded role of a nurse.

of leadership and management qualities among the staff members.

- **Continuing education:** The international council of nurses emphasized the importance of continuing education for nurses in order to ensure safe and effective nursing care it consists of a large number of educational programs and activities. It is the necessary for all the level of nursing personnel to deal with the needs of nursing oneself aware of all the development in the field of the specialization.

EXPANDED ROLE OF THE NURSES

Contemporary nursing requires that the nurse possess knowledge and skills in a variety of areas. But changes in nursing have expanded the role to include increased emphasis on health promotion and illness prevention, as well as concern for the client as a whole. The contemporary nurse functions in the interrelated roles of care giver, clinical and ethical decision maker, protector and client advocate, case manager, rehabilitator, comforter, communicator, and teacher.

Care giver: As care giver, the nurse helps the client regain health through the healing process. Healing is more than just curing a specific disease, although treatment skills that promote physical healing are important to care givers. The nurse addresses the holistic health care needs of the client, including measures to restore emotional, spiritual, and social well-being. The care giver helps the client and family set goals and meet those goals with a minimal cost of time and energy.

Clinical decision maker: To provide effective care, the nurse uses critical thinking skills throughout the nursing process. Before undertaking any nursing action, whether it is assessing the client's condition, giving care, or evaluating the results of care, the nurse plans the action by deciding the best approach for each client. The nurse makes these decisions alone or in collaboration with the client and family. In each of these situations, the nurse collaborates and consults with other health care professionals.

Protector and client advocate: As protector the nurse helps maintain a safe environment for the client and takes steps to prevent injury and protect the client from possible adverse effects of diagnostic or treatment measures. Confirming that a client does not have an allergy to a medication and providing immunization against disease in a community-based practice are examples of the nurse's protective role. In the role of client advocate, the nurse protects the client's human and legal rights and provides assistance in asserting those rights if the need arises. For example, the nurse may provide additional information for a client who is trying to decide whether to accept treatment.

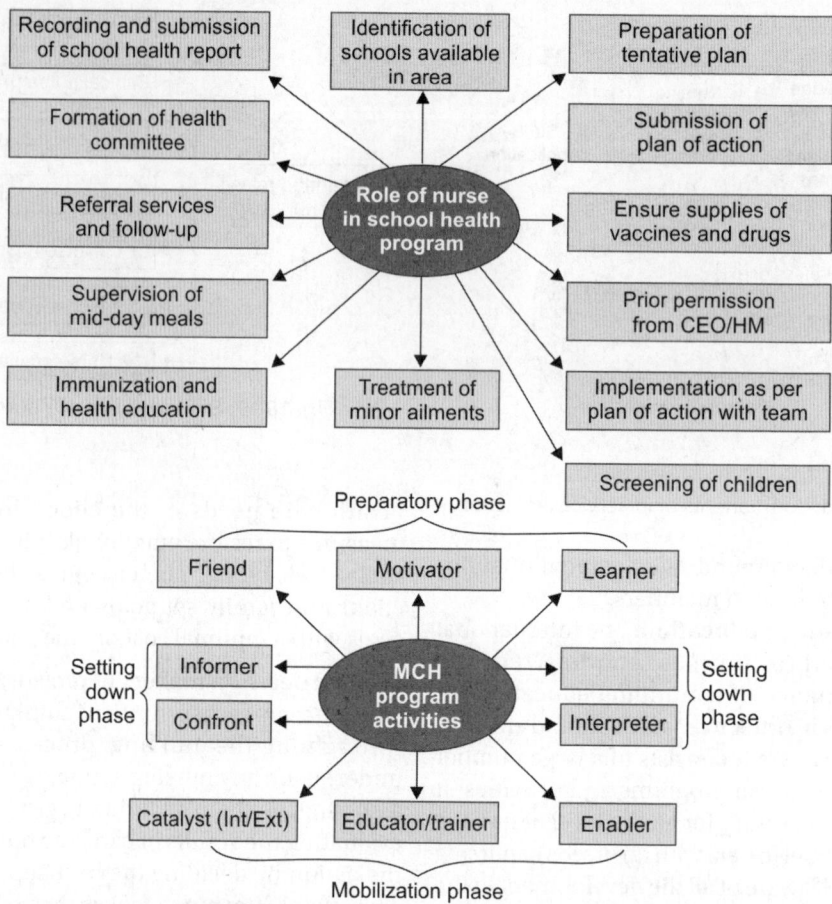

Fig. 18.18: Role of nurse in school health and MCH services.

The nurse may also defend clients' rights in a general way by speaking out against policies or actions that might endanger client's well-being or conflict with their rights.

Case manager: As case manager, the nurse coordinates the activities of other members of the health care team, such as nutritionists and physical therapists, when managing a group of clients' care. In addition, nurses must also manage the own time and the resources of the practice settings.

Rehabilitator: Rehabilitation is the process by which individual's maximal levels of functioning after illness, other disabling events. Frequently clients experience physical or emotional impairments that change their lives, and the nurse helps them adapt as fully as possible. Rehabilitative and restorative care activities range from teaching clients to walk with crutches to helping clients cope with lifestyle changes often associated with chronic illness.

Comforter: The role of comforter, caring for the client as a person, is a traditional and historical one in nursing and has continued to be important as nurses have assumed new roles. Because nursing care must be directed to the whole person rather than simply the body, comfort and emotional support often help give the client strength to recover. While carrying out nursing activities, nurses can provide comfort by demonstrating care for the client as an individual with unique feelings and needs. As comforter, nurses should help the client reach therapeutic goals rather than encourage emotional or physical dependence.

Communicator: The role of communicator is central to all oilier nursing roles. Nursing involves communication with clients and families, other nurses and health care professionals, resource persons, and the community. The quality of communication is a critical factor in meeting the needs of individuals, families, and communities.

Teacher: As teacher, the nurse explains to clients concepts and facts about health, demonstrates procedures such as self-care activities, determines that the client fully understands, reinforces learning or client behavior, anti-evaluates.

Progress in learning or client behavior, and evaluates progress in learning. Some teaching can be unplanned and informal, such as when a nurse responds to a question about a health issue in casual conversation. Other teaching activities may be planned and more formal, such as when the nurse teaches a client with diabetes to self-administer insulin injections. The nurse uses teaching methods that match the client's capabilities and needs and incorporates other resources, such as the family, in teaching plans.

Career roles: The proceeding roles and functions apply to all nurses in most practice settings. Career roles, on the other hand, are specific employment positions. Because of increasing educational opportunities for nurses, the growth of nursing as a profession, and greater concern for job enrichment, the nursing profession offers expanded roles and different kinds of career opportunities. Examples of career roles include nurse educators and advanced practice nurses, such as clinical nurse specialists, nurse practitioners, certified nurse midwives, anesthetists, administrators, and researchers. Additional no clinical roles include risk managers, quality improvement nurses, and product consultants.

Nurse educator: Nursing educators generally have a background in clinical nursing, which provides them with practical skills and theoretical knowledge. A faculty member in a school of nursing prepares students to function as nurses.

Nursing faculty members are responsible for teaching current nursing practice theory and necessary skills in laboratories or clinical settings. Nurse educators in nursing schools are usually required to have graduate degrees in nursing education. In addition, they generally have a specific clinical specialty and advanced clinical experience.

Nurse educators in staff development departments of healthcare institutions provide educational programs for nurses within their institution. These programs include orientation of new personnel, critical care nursing courses and instruction about new equipment or procedures. The primary focus of the nurse educator in an agency's department of client education is to teach or disabled clients and families to provide care in the home. In most wall health care agencies, however, time budget dues not permit a separate client education department. Therefore staff nurses usually incorporate education into a client's plan of care.

Advanced practice nurse: The advanced practice nurse (APN) has a master's degree in nursing, advanced education in pharmacology and physical assessment, and certification and expertise in a specialized area of practice (ANA, 1995). An APN usually works in primary, acute, restorative, or community health care agency. In addition, in the management of a disease such as cancer, diabetes, or cardiovascular or pulmonary disease or in a specific field such as pediatrics or gerontology.

Clinical nurse specialist: The clinical nurse specialist (CNS) has a master's degree in nursing and expertise in a specialized area of practice. A CNS may work in primary care, acute care, restorative care, and community-based settings. In addition, the CNS may specialize in specific diseases such as diabetes mellitus, cancer, or congestive heart failure or in a specific field such as pediatrics or gerontology. The CNS functions as an expert clinician, educator, case in manager, consultant, and researcher to plan or improve the quality of care provided to the client and family.

Nurse practitioner: The nurse practitioner provides health care to clients, usually in an outpatient, ambulatory care, or community-based setting and comprehensiveness of care. A significant percentage of primary care encounters extend beyond the boundaries of medicine and demand the expertise of the nurse. The nurse practitioner is able to establish a collaborative provider-client relationship. The major nurse practitioner categories are adult, family, pediatric, obstetrics-gynecology, and geriatric nurse practitioner. A nurse practitioner has the knowledge and skills necessary to detect and manage limited acute and chronic stable conditions. The nurse practitioner's educational preparation includes a practitioner program or a master's degree in nursing.

Adult nurse practitioner (ANP): ANP provides primary, ambulatory care to adults with a non-emergency acute or chronic illness, and in some settings tertiary care. ANPs are usually employed in ambulatory care centers or outpatient clinics and work in collaboration with a primary physician.

Family nurse practitioner (FNP): A family nurse practitioner (FNP) provides primary ambulatory care for families, usually in collaboration with a family care physician. The FNP meets the family's general health care needs, manages some illnesses by providing direct care, and guides or counsels the family as needed.

Pediatric nurse practitioner: A pediatric nurse practitioner (PNP) provides health-care to infants and children, an obstetrics-gynecology nurse practitioner (OBGYN) provides primary ambulatory care to women seeking obstetrical or gynecological health care. The nurse practitioner who is also a certified nurse-midwife may independently deliver infants. Geriatric nurse practitioner (GNP) provides ambulatory or inpatient care to older adults. The GNP's activities include

interventions for health maintenance, illness prevention, or health restoration.

Certified nurse midwife: A certified nurse-midwife (CNM) is an RN who is also educated in midwifery and is certified by the American College of Nurse-Midwives. The practice of nurse-midwifery involves providing independent care for women during normal pregnancy, labor, and delivery, as well as care for the newborn; it may include some gynecological services such as routine Papanicolaou (Pap) smears, family planning, and treatment for minor vaginal infections. A CNM practices with a health care agency that provides medical consultation, collaborative management and referral.

Nurse anesthetist: A nurse anesthetist is an RN who has received advanced training in an accredited program in anesthesiology. Nurse anesthetists provide surgical anesthesia under the guidance and supervision of an anesthesiologist, who is a physician with advanced knowledge of surgical anesthesia.

Nurse administrator: A nurse administrator manages client care and the delivery of specific nursing services within a health care agency. This administrator may hold a middle-management position, such as head nurse or supervisor, or an upper-level management position, such as assistant or associate director or director of nursing services. Functions of administrators include budgeting, staffing, strategic planning of programs and services, employee evaluation, and employee development. Middle-management position usually requires at least a baccalaureate degree in nursing, and upper-level positions generally require a master's degree.

Nurse researcher: The nurse researcher investigates problems to improve nursing care and to further define and expand the scope of nursing practice. The nurse researcher may be employed in an academic setting, hospital, or independent professional or community-service agency. The minimum educational requirement is now a doctoral degree, with at least a master's degree in nursing.

FUTURISTIC NURSING

Nursing continue to be challenged and rewarded by both new and changing opportunities and constraints. Professional nursing's image continues to be major challenge for all nurses individually and collectively. A number of forces that have affected the development of professional nursing still continue to affect significant issues which includes.

- Societal images and expectation of nurses
- Degree of the nursing professions control over the quantity and quality of practitioners
- Impact of technology and theory on nursing practices roles and setting
- Professional self-image of nurses
- Sources of financing for health care services.

Predicting the future is an occupation fraught with peril in a society and world that are changing rapidly. The changes that seem likely to occur in due course will be changes in the demographics, the deteriorating environment, risky life styles, and economics of health care and governmental regulation of health care. The changes will be accomplished by changes in both nursing practice and nursing education.

Nursing practice:

- **Demographical changes:** The trends important to future of nursing includes rising number of elderly people, continuing increase in poverty an increasing in cultural diversity in the population and a continued trend urbanization. Each has implication or nursing.

- Many older persons are healthy, but the likelihood of illness becomes greater as people age. It indicates clearly nurse of the future must be prepared to work affectively with rising number of elderly persons.

- The number of people living below the poverty lines increasing, particularly among children and elderly. When basic needs for food, clothing and shelter are unmet or uncertain, health care becomes a luxury.

- Immunizations, for children's parental care for pregnant woman, nutritious meals and other health maintaining factors are neglected even though some care has been taken on these issues

- Poor people tend to put off seeking care until illness advanced and thus harder to treat

- Preventable conditions are often not prevented due to lack of education lack of sanitation, crowded living conditions. Improper shelter, home-lessness, and host of other poverty related factors

- Nursing as a profession, is committed to provide care to all peoples, regardless of social and economic factors to take challenges to meet these issues

  - Cultural diversity refers to the array of people from different racial, religious, social and geographic backgrounds who make up a particular entity, cultural beliefs and practices of the citizens are

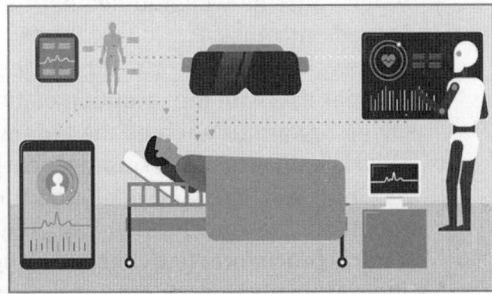

Fig. 18.19: Application of technology in nursing care.

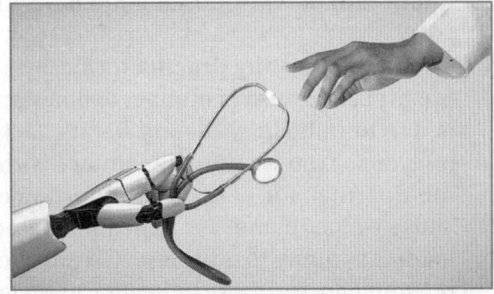

Fig. 18.20: Robotic nursing.

quite different. Each groups has its own

Health beliefs, folk remedies and conventional wisdom about health and sickness

- ♦ Nurses increasingly need to take these beliefs into considerations when planning and implementing nursing care for individuals of diverse cultural backgrounds.

- – Urbanization, that is, people moving from rural farming areas to cities has increased since the time of industrial revolution. The trend continues today and is expected to continue in the future. This will create more social problems (homelessness, drugs, gangs, mental illness, violence, crime). These spread over into suburbans and rural areas, creating further social change. Nurses of the future will be increasingly confronted with health problems created by these social phenomena.

- **Environment changes:** Major environmental tragedies such as nuclear power plant accident, burning oil wells, Tsunami, gradual decline in the qualities of the air, water, plant and animal life of the universe leads to many social and health problems. Depletion of the ozone layer, accidental lead and mercury poisonings, pesticides spilling into streams and rivers and accidental releases of radioactive steam from nuclear power plants, are all leads to health problems. The related problems of environmental deterioration and over population are health care issues that future nurses will undoubtedly have to face.

- **Changes to healthy practices:** Obesity is predisposing cause of number of illnesses is due to unhealthy dietary habits, lack of exercise, stress, having contact with multipartner for sex, AIDS. Substance abuse which in another unhealthy habit leads to many problems. Given the predominance of these unhealthy lifestyle factors, it is clear that nurses will play an increasingly important role in educating people about wellness and self-care. Nurses will also play an instrumental in educating the public about how to be involved in the development of sound public policies concerning these issues. Nursing, through its professional association, will become powerful player in the national health care politics. Nurses will form coalition with customer groups. Individual nurse become politically active as voters, campaign workers, community health activities, and political candidate. As nursing's public profits profile becomes higher, public scrutiny of the profession will increase. Consumers of nursing services will exercise their political power to pressurize nursing to provide quality health care.

- **Emerging bioethical issues:** Bioethics related to those ethical issues that are raised because of new technologies advancement in medicine and biological sciences.

- – Issues related to birth involve processes that prevent conception or terminate pregnancy prematurely as well as processes that enable conception and pregnancy to occur through technological intervention the fetal. Development sterilization, contraception and abortion on the one hand, and "test tube" conception, and artificial inseminations on the other, evoke strong feelings from various groups and individuals.

- – Each of these issues had its own ethical ramification, risks and consequences which must be weighed against the desired outcomes.

- – Issues related to life or death, which includes that with the invention of life saving apparatus such as the kidney dialysis unit, artificial respirator, heart and lung machine, and fetal monitor and with the development of new surgical procedures (e.g., fetal surgery, organ transplantation, etc.) and new technology (e.g., genetic Genetic research, fetal research), it has become necessary to redefine the terms of life and death as new technology emerges, new issues will arise, and nurses must be prepared.

Nursing education: In the future the nurses will need broad based education, assessment skills, technical competence, and the ability to deal with rapid change. The knowledge base and technology used in providing nursing care will continue to increases as well as nurses need for skill and ability in:

- Intensely acute aspects of care
- Diagnostics and decision making
- Client teaching
- Coordination of less-skilled workers
- Collaboration with client and health care professionals to improve the quality of health

In earlier days, entry level for profession was certificate level and diploma level. Now changing circumstances people are thinking that undergraduate (BSc Nursing degree) as entry level of professional nursing. Entry to nursing could conceivably occur at one of four level Diploma, (DGNM), Bachelors Degree level (UG-BSc Nursing), Masters Level (PG-MSc Nursing) or the doctoral degree (PhD Nursing).

The current pattern, entry at diploma level, with professional education at the UG Level (Bachelors degree) might be perpetuated. There are some who propose that education for entry to professional nursing be moved to the master's level rather than basic degree level. This level of education would prepare the student for combination of specialized and generalized practice appropriate for developing health care delivery system. All students would need prior general education and possible a bachelor's degrees for entry into nursing, which would strengthen the liberal arts and science base for practice. Since in India pre-degree course (PUC) included liberal arts and science concepts, human education PUC is made as entry into nursing both diploma and degree courses in nursing. So, it is better that after PUC-science, students can join BSc nursing degree courses. After

few years of experience in bedside nursing or community health nursing, they can join the master degree courses in nursing. After they can think of doing doctoral degree courses in nursing in their respective interest in the field of nursing.

As the coming decades sees nursing practice become more exciting and autonomous than ever, the need for strong, differentiated educational preparation for nurses at all levels will be crucial. More nurses will recognize the value of bachelor's degrees for beginning professional practice and masters degrees for specialty practices. More will pursue doctoral degrees to prepare for research and theory development. In response, colleges of nursing will expand flexible educational programs to improve access. They will also develop differentiated levels of nursing education that correspond to differentiated levels of practice.

The major challenge for nursing education in the future will be to produce a steady supply of well prepared nurse's graduates in the face of an aging faculty, rapidly changing technology, increasing cultural diversity of students and patients and budgetary constraints in higher education. So meeting continuing or advanced education needs is an individual responsibility of every nurses. It is the obligation of nurses who are responsible for their patients care, to maintain current and relevant knowledge and skills in their field. It is important for each nurse to realize that the attainment of a certificate or a degree is not an end itself. Rather, it is to be viewed as a beginning foundation upon which to build their nursing knowledge.

Nursing research: Today almost all nursing leaders and nursing organization offer professional nurse perhaps both the greatest demands and greatest rewards for nursing research. Research opportunities and needs await interested professionals in nursing. Professionals nurses are obligated both to ask the significant questions that need to be answered and to use research findings on the basis of nursing practice. Research in nursing generates the knowledge that is used in practice, while practice generates ideas of research. Nurses need to understand research as legitimate scientific inquiry. To fulfill the professional obligations in health care delivery system, the nurses have to keep following objectives. Nursing education will develop programs to educate practitioners skilled in scientific inquiry at all levels of practice:

- Nursing research will be an integral part of nursing education and nursing practice
- Nursing practice will establish an environment receptive to inquiry and professional practice.

Most nurses' to-day would probably agree that a practice based on research is desirable. Capitalizing on that agreement, the profession could begin to present different images to the public. To help actualize the motivation to base nursing practice on research, education programs need to prepare students in scientific inquiry whole also preparing them to apply theory in the conduct of professional roles.

CONCLUSION

Technologic advances have significantly affected the definition of nursing and the role of the nurse; the methods by which care is delivered have been reshaped significantly. The acute care hospital provides care to patients who are much more acutely ill and who are diagnosed with conditions from which they would not have survived 25 years ago. Today, recovery is anticipated after careful evaluation and treatment that can require diagnostic procedures (e.g., angiography, sonography, or tomography), delicate medical procedures, and specialized critical care nursing that requires a host of variously prepared health care providers. Critical thinking skills are essential to the successful performance of the diverse tasks expected of a nurse. Nurses in many positions have been required to assume ever-greater levels of responsibility. Only recently are nurses beginning to receive the official authority, autonomy, and recognition that should accompany those responsibilities.

19

Legislation in Nursing

LEARNING OBJECTIVES

- Common legal issues
- Legal responsibilities of a nurse
- Legal perspectives in nursing
- Legal issues related to nursing registration
- Patient's bill of rights

- Legal safeguarding of nurse
- Negligence in nursing practice
- Standards of nursing practice
- Malpractice in nursing practice

INTRODUCTION

The law constitutes body of principles recognized or enforced by public and regular tribunals have the administration of justice. The law is the body of principles recognized and applied by the state and the administrations of justice. Law is that portion of the established thought and habit which has gained district and formal recognition and the shape of uniform rules backed by the authority and power of the government. Legal framework for nursing practice is shown in **Figure 19.1**.

Definitions

- **Common law:** Common law is law that results from previous legal decisions. They are based on legal precedent.
- **Statutory law:** Statutory law is law that is passed by a legislative body such as the state's legislature or the US Congress.
- **Constitutional law:** Constitutional law is law that is included in the Constitution of the United States of America and its amendments.
- **Administrative law:** Administrative law is rules and regulations that are legally enacted to support some statutory law. For example,

nursing boards enact administrative rules and regulations relating to state enacted laws such as the state's nurse practice act and legislated continuing education requirements for the relicensure of nurses.

- **Criminal law:** Criminal law, part of public law, covers acts that are illegal and against the law. Criminal law includes felony and misdemeanor infractions of the law.
- **Civil law:** Civil law, also part of public law, covers torts and contract laws.
- **Torts:** Torts are civil laws that address the legal rights of patients and the responsibilities of the nurse in the nurse patient relationship. Some torts specific to nursing and nursing practice include things like malpractice, negligence and violations relating to patient confidentiality.
- **Unintentional torts:** Unintentional torts include things like malpractice and negligence.
- **Intentional torts:** Intentional torts include things like false imprisonment, assault, battery, breaches of privacy and patient confidentiality, slander and libel.
- **Liability:** Liability is vulnerability and legal responsibility, simply stated. For example, nurses are liable when they fail to carry out doctor's orders.

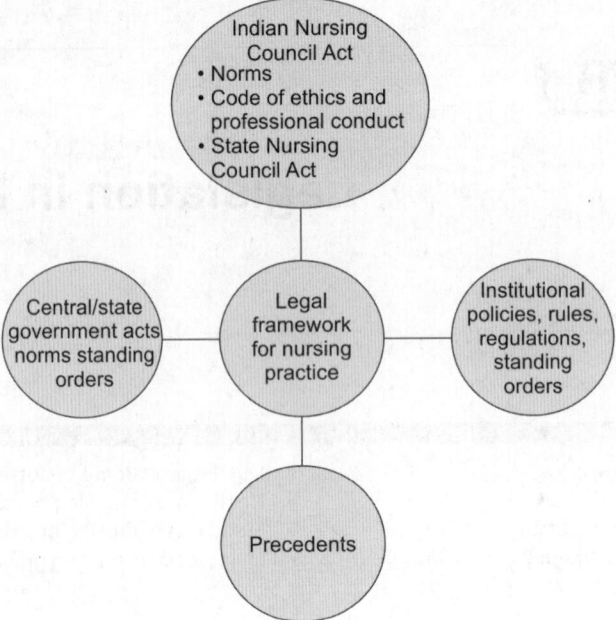

Fig. 19.1: Legal framework for nursing practice.

- **Respondeat superior:** Respondeat superior is the legal doctrine or principle that states that employers are legally responsible for the acts and behaviors of its employees. Respondeat Superior does not, however, relieve the nurse of legally responsibility and accountability for their actions. They remain liable.
- **Negligence:** Negligence is a nonintentional tort. Negligence occurs when the nurse fails to follow established policies, procedures and standards of care in the same manner that another "reasonable" nurse would do in the same situation.
- **Malpractice:** Malpractice, also a nonintentional tort, has six elements. The elements of malpractice include a duty, a breach of duty as a nurse, reasonable foreseeability that the nurse's act has a connection with the patient injury that occurred, the patient was harmed, the link that act directly led to the harm and the patient has the right to financial compensation or damages.
- **Assault:** Assault, an intentional tort, is threatening to touch a person without their consent.

- **Battery:** Battery, another intentional tort, is touching a person without their consent.
- **False imprisonment:** False imprisonment is restraining, detaining and/or restricting a person's freedom of movement. Using a restraint without an order is considered false imprisonment.
- **Defamation:** Defamation is making false statements about a person in writing or orally that leads to the destruction of a person's reputation.
- **Slander:** Slander is oral defamation of character using false statements.
- **Libel:** Libel is written defamation of character using false statements.

TYPES OF LAWS

1. **Civil law** includes rules and regulations that specify the required course of action to be followed by an individual in business and social relationships with others. It is concerned with relationships among people and the protection of a person's rights.
2. **Criminal law** defines offences that affect public welfare and security and impose

penalties. It includes rules forbidding conduct that is injurious to public order and specifying punishments to be administered to individual who exhibits injurious conduct.

COMMON LEGAL ISSUES

- Wrong medications, wrong dosage, wrong route of administration and wrong concentration.
- Mistaken identity: Prepare the wrong patient for an operation, to exchange babies in the labor room. To exchange dead bodies in the mortuary.
- Failure to communicate.
- Maintenance of record.
- Giving explanation and getting the concerned.
- Bums and false.
- Counting sponges and instruments during surgery.
- Loss or damage to patient's property and fame.

- Euthanasia or mercy killing: Taking positive step to kill a person in order to end his suffering is a murder.

Functions of Law in Nursing

The law serves a number of functions in nursing which are to:

- Provides a framework for establishing which nursing actions in the care of clients are legal.
- Differentiates the nurses' responsibilities from those of other health professionals.
- Helps establish the boundaries of independent nursing action.
- Assists in maintaining standard of nursing practice by making nurses accountable under the law.

LEGAL RESPONSIBILITIES OF A NURSE (FIG. 19.2)

- **Responsibility of appointing and assigning:** The nurse administrators have responsibility for staffing and supervising

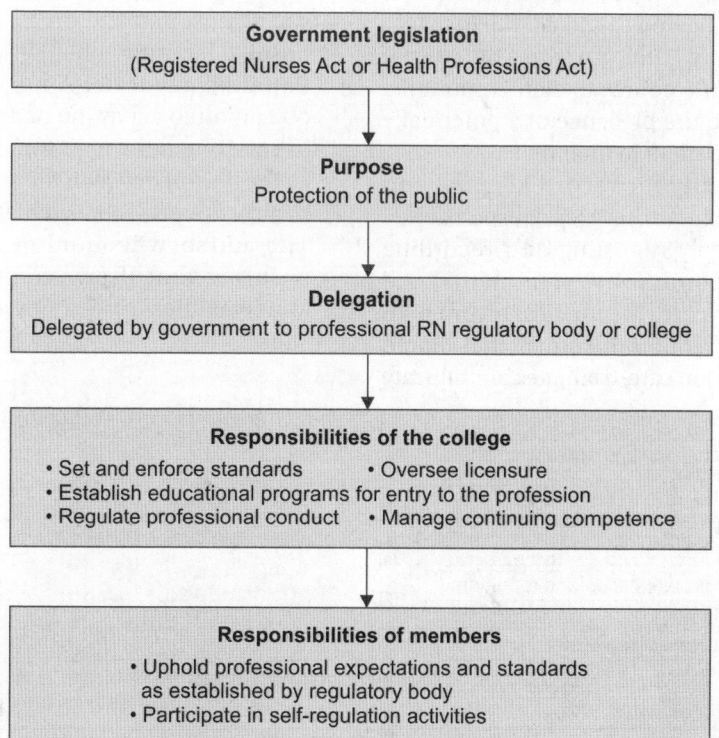

Fig. 19.2: Legal responsibilities of a nurse.

nursing units to ensure safe, effective patient care. Therefore, they have the authority to temporarily reassign a nursing employee to compensate for emergency staff shortages.

- **Responsibility in quality control:** A nurse manager's legal responsibility for quality control of nursing service imposes a duty to observe report and correct the incompetence of any patient care provider.
- **Responsibility for equipment:** To protect the patients and employees from injury, a nurse manager must ensure that all patient care equipment are fully functional and that defective equipment is promptly repaired or replaced.
- **Responsibility for observation and reporting:** Consequently nurses have a legal duty to observe patients frequently and report findings that have diagnostic or treatment value for the patient's physician and other members of the patient's treatment team.
- **Responsibility to protect public:** The nurse has a legal duty to protect the public from injury by dangerous patients. The manager must ensure that nursing personnel follow the procedures to alert community members to the presence of a potentially dangerous patient in their midst.
- **Responsibility for record keeping and reporting:** Nurses have legal responsibility for accurately reporting and recording patient's conditions, treatments and response to care. The medical record is an information source document that should be used to plan care, evaluate care, allocate costs, educate personnel, research care measure, and substantiate legal claim.
- **Responsibility for death and dying:** Nurses must be aware of legal definition of death because they must document all events that, when the patient is in their care.

LEGAL PERSPECTIVES IN NURSING (FIG. 19.4)

- **Nurse Practice Act:** Each state has what is called a Nurse Practice Act. The guidelines and laws outlined in the act pertain to all nurses who are licensed in that particular state. Nurse limitation is one of those laws. Each nurse has a limitation on what he is allowed and trained to do. He must follow the chain of command, especially with the care of a patient. If he does not have the authority or knowledge to give a prescription, analyze a laboratory report, or advise the patient on treatment, he may not legally do so. Any wrong information or practice he commits is punishable by the law and the patient or family may file a suit against him and the health agency or hospital he works for.
- **Patient's advocate:** A nurse has a legal obligation to act as the patient's advocate in case of emergency. The nurse is to act as the liaison between the patient and the healthcare provider, such as a physician. The nurse will monitor the patient, ensuring that if any complications or abnormalities arise, a physician notified

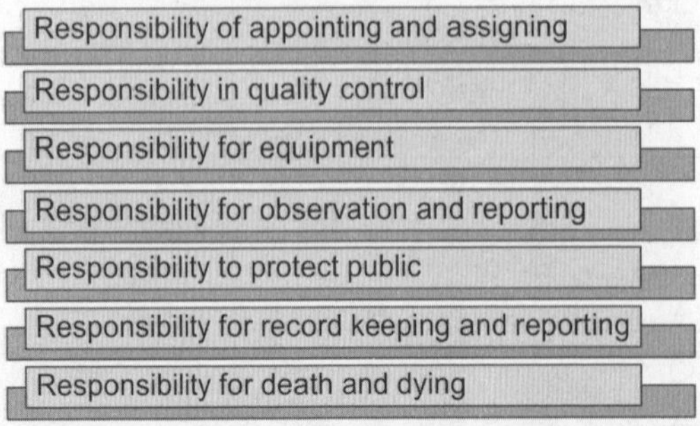

Responsibility of appointing and assigning

Responsibility in quality control

Responsibility for equipment

Responsibility for observation and reporting

Responsibility to protect public

Responsibility for record keeping and reporting

Responsibility for death and dying

Fig. 19.3: Legal responsibilities of a nurse.

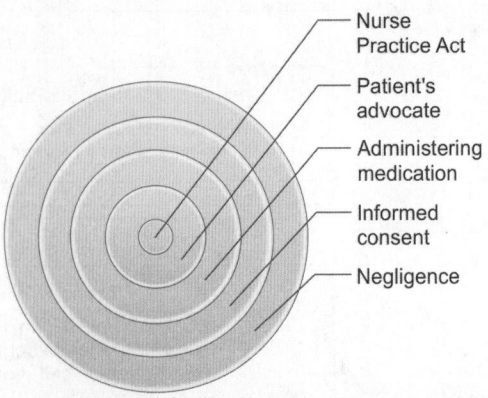

Fig. 19.4: Legal prespectives in nursing.

immediately. The nurse is legally obligated to keep the personal data and information of the patient confidential not doing so is a violation of the code of ethics for nurses.

- **Administering medication:** Nurses are responsible for administering the correct doses and medications to patients. If the nurse gives a fatal dosage amount, she may face legal malpractice suits. It is also the responsibility to research the patient's records, or ask the patient and family members if there are any allergies or complications that may pose a risk if a certain medication is administered.
- **Informed consent:** When a nurse is administering treatment, she must explain what the effects and outcomes could be, and any other important information. It is the responsibility of the nurse to confirm that the patient or family member who will sign the informed consent form is coherent, and understands all the negatives and aspects of the treatment. The nurse, patient, or patient family member will sign the informed consent form in front of a witness, a physician or another nurse. Not having this legal document signed and in front of a witness could be a legal issue for the nurse if complications arise during treatment.
- **Negligence:** It is the responsibility of the nurse to monitor the patient. If a patient calls for a nurse to come and assist him in going to the restroom, for example, the nurse is to assist, or if he/she is busy with another patient, have another nurse assist the patient. Ignoring the patient or responding after a lengthy delay could be considered negligence, and if the patient is hurt from trying to move himself, the nurse could face legal suits. Also, it could be considered negligence if a physician orders the nurse to administer a prescription, and the nurse did not do so.

LEGAL ISSUES RELATED TO NURSING REGISTRATION

A registered nurse (RN) is a nurse who has graduated from a college's nursing program or from a school of nursing and has passed a national licensing exam. A registered nurse helps individuals, families, and groups to achieve health and prevent disease. They care for the sick and injured in hospitals and other healthcare facilities, physicians' offices private homes, public health agencies, schools, camps, and industry. Some registered nurse, are employed in private practice. A registered nurses scope of practice is determined by each state's Nurse Practice Act. It outlines what is legal practice for registered nurses and what tasks they may or may not perform. Nurse Practice Acts also dictates the scope of practice for nurse practitioners (NPs). An example is prescriptive authority for NPs. In some states, NPs can practice completely autonomously and prescribe any category of medications. In other states, NPs cannot prescribe controlled substances and may only practice with the collaboration of a physician.

Civil law penalties for registered nurses: Registered nurses have penalties that are inflicted on them for transgressions such as medical malpractice and breach of confidentiality. These civil law penalties can cause them to be suspended or banned from the nursing practice.

License revocation or suspension procedure: According to Tennessee law, the reasons for a Tennessee registered nurses license being denied, suspended or revoked are: fraudulent activity with respect to certification, established' I guilt before a court of law, medical negligence or malpractice, mental dysfunction, unprofessional conduct, drug use and complicity in a crime with another.

PATIENT'S BILL OF RIGHTS

In 1973, the American Hospital Association adopted Patient's Bill of Rights as national policy statement and distributed it to its members in the healthcare organizations throughout the nation. There are twelve rights summarized below:

1. The patient has a right to a considerate and respectful care.

2. The patient has a right to obtain complete and concerned information concerning the diagnosis, treatment and prognosis from his physician for the patient's expected understanding.

3. The patient has a right to receive the necessary information from his physician regarding the treatment and the procedures involved in it.

4. The patient has a right to refuse the treatment to the extent permitted by the law and to be informed about the medical consequences of his action.

5. The patient has a right to privacy concerning his own medical care program.

6. The patient has a right to expect all communications and records pertaining to his care should be treated as confidential.

7. The patient has a right to expect within the capacity a hospital must make reasonable response to the request made by the patient for services.

8. The patient has a right to obtain information as to any relationship of his hospital to other healthcare institution a care is concerned.

9. The patient has a right to be advised if the hospital proposes to engage him in or perform human experimentation affecting his treatment.

10. The patient has a right to expect reasonable continuity of care.

11. The patient has a right to examine and receive an explanation of his hospital bills regardless of the source of payment.

12. The patient has a right to know what hospital rules and regulations apply to his conduct as a patient.

Rights of patients is discussed in **Figure 19.5**.

STANDARDS FOR BREACH SANCTIONS (FIG. 19.6)

Important practice standards for breach sanctions: The disparity in organizational response to employee malfeasance has a far-reaching impact on the healthcare industry. Consequences include the following:

• **Confusing message:** An inconsistent organizational response to a breach sends a confusing message to both staff and the public. Healthcare workers moving from one organization to another find differing tolerance levels for enforcing the same directives.

Patients have the right to:

1. Be treated for the life-threatening, chronic disease of addiction with honesty, respect and dignity

2. Know what to expect from treatment, and the likelihood of success.

3. Be treated by licensed and certified professionals

4. Evidence-based treatment

5. Be treated for co-occurring behavioral health conditions simultaneously

6. An individualized, outcomes-driven treatment plan

7. Remain in treatment as long as necessary

8. Support, education and treatment for their families and loved ones

9. A treatment setting that is safe and ethical

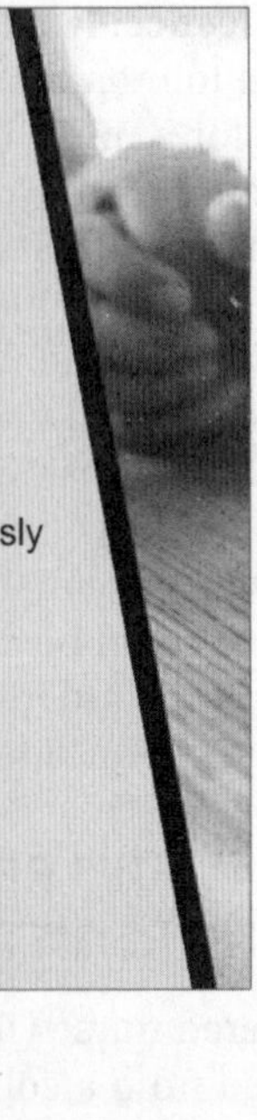

Fig. 19.5: Rights of patients.

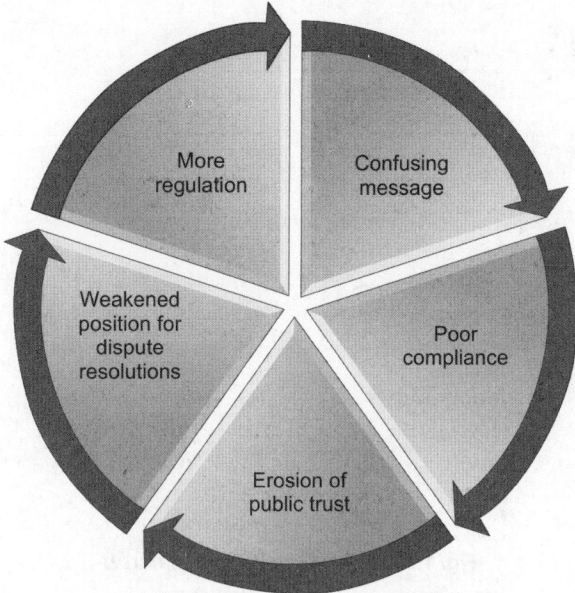

Fig. 19.6: Standards for breach sanctions.

- **Poor compliance:** Staff in organizations with less stringent enforcement may weigh the level of risk to themselves against the potential advantages. Inequity in sanction application encourages poor compliance by individuals who know they will escape any serious consequence for breaching privacy and security policies.
- **Erosion of public trust:** Public trust is eroded when significant variation is blatantly apparent in how healthcare organizations respond to a privacy or security breach both within and across entities and systems. The public must feel assured their personal health information has sufficient protections across the healthcare spectrum, particularly in this era of health information exchange.
- **Weakened position for dispute resolutions:** Inequitable application of sanctions can affect the outcome of personnel actions at arbitration and grievance proceedings. Unequal penalties for similar offenses undermine the organization's ability to prevail in dispute resolutions.
- **More regulation:** Poor and inconsistent implementation of privacy and security safeguards invites further state and federal intervention. Such laws place an additional administrative and financial burden on facilities. If the industry does not self-correct, then it leaves open the door to state and federal government intervention.
- **Questionable research:** The validity of research may be called into question when privacy or security breaches are not handled consistently and expeditiously patients.

LEGAL SAFEGUARDING OF NURSE (FIG. 19.7)

- **Licensure:** All nurses who are in nursing practice have to possess a valid licensure, issued by the respective State Nursing Council/Indian Nursing Council.
- **Good Samaritan laws:** In response to health professionals, fear of malpractice claims, most states enacted.

  Good Samaritan laws that exempt doctors and nurses from liability when they render help during emergency. These laws limit liability and offer legal immunity for people helping in an emergency.

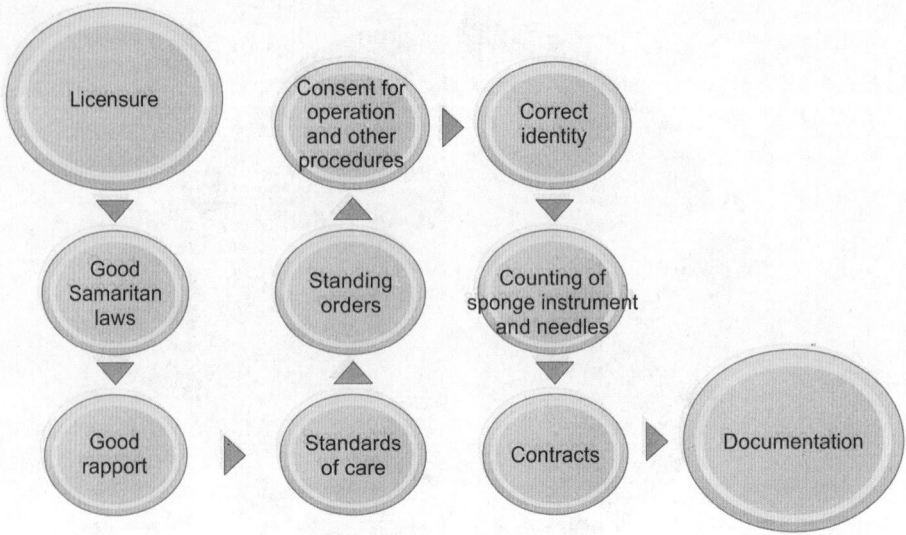

Fig. 19.7: Legal safeguarding of nurse.

- **Good rapport:** Developing good rapport with the client is very important to prevent malpractice. The ability to develop good rapport with client is dependent on the nurse having good interpersonal communication skills, e.g., listening.
- **Standards of care:** All professional practicing in the medical field are held to certain standards when administering care. It is always better to follow standards of care to avoid malpractice and do not attempt anything beyond the level of competence.
- **Standing orders:** Although a nurse may not legally diagnose illness or prescribe treatment, she or he may after assessing patients condition apply standing orders or treatment guideline that have been established by the physician or doctor as appropriate for certain problems and conditions.
- **Consent for operation and other procedures:** A patient coming into hospital still retains his rights as a citizen and his entry only denotes his willingness to undergo an investigation or a course of treatment. Any investigation or treatment of a serious nature, or an operation in which an anesthetic is used, requires the written consent of the patient.
- **Correct identity:** The nurse or the midwife has the great responsibility to make sure that all babies born in the hospital are correctly labeled at birth and to ensure that at no time they are placed in the wrong cot or given to the wrong mother.
- **Counting of sponge instrument and needles:** Nurses advocate that sponge, instrument and needle counts be performed for all surgical procedures taking place in operation theater. When an instrument left in a patient's body the nurse will probably be liable for any patient injury caused by the presence of foreign body.
- **Contracts:** A contract is a written or oral agreement between 2 people in which goods or services are exchanged.
- **Documentation:** Documentation is by far the best once a lawsuit field. The medical record is a legal document admissible in court as evidence.

AREAS OF PATIENT'S BILL OF RIGHTS (TABLE 19.1)

Table 19.1: Eight key areas of Patient's Bill of Rights.

Sl. No.	Areas	Description
1.	Information for patients	The patient has the right to accurate and easily understood information about your health plan, healthcare professionals, and healthcare facilities. If you speak another language, have a physical or mental disability, or just don't understand something, help should be given so you can make informed healthcare decisions.
2.	Choice of providers and plans	You have the right to choose healthcare providers who can give you high-quality health care when you need it.
3.	Access to emergency services	If you have severe pain, an injury, or sudden illness that makes you believes that your health is in danger, you have the right to be screened and stabilized using emergency services. You should be able to use these services whenever and wherever you need them, without needing to wait for authorization and without any financial penalty.
4.	Taking part in treatment decisions	You have the right to know your treatment options and take part in decisions about your care. Parents, guardians, family members, or others that you choose can speak for you if you cannot make your own decisions.
5.	Respect and non-discrimination	You have a right to considerate, respectful care from your doctors, healthplan representatives, and other healthcare providers that does not discriminate against you.
6.	Confidentiality (privacy) of health information	You have the right to talk privately with healthcare providers and to have your healthcare information protected. You also have the right to read and copy your own medical record. You have the right to ask that your doctor change your record if it is not correct, relevant, or complete.
7.	Complaints and appeals	You have the right to a fair, fast, and objective review of any complaint you have against your health plan, doctors, hospitals or other healthcare personnel. This includes complaints about waiting times, operating hours, the actions of healthcare personnel, and the adequacy of health care facilities.
8.	Consumer responsibilities	In a healthcare system that protects consumer or patients' rights, patients should expect to take on some responsibilities to get well and/or stay well (for instance, exercising and not using tobacco). Patients are expected to do things like treat healthcare workers and other patients with respect, try to pay their medical bills, and follow the rules and benefits of their health plan coverage. Having patients involved in their care increases the chance of the best possible outcomes and helps support a high quality, cost-conscious healthcare system.

BREACH OF DUTY (FIG. 19.8)

Examples of breach of duty, which may be considered negligent under certain circumstances, may include "doing something which a reasonably prudent person would not do, or the failure to do something which a reasonably prudent person would do, under circumstances similar to those shown by the evidence".

- **Injury:** For an injury to be considered caused by negligence, records must show that the nurse failed to perform her duties with the patient in question. In such cases, the failure of duty must then be proven as directly related to the injury of the patient. For example, if a nurse fails to give medications as directed then the patient's condition worsens or he dies, the nurse may be found negligent.

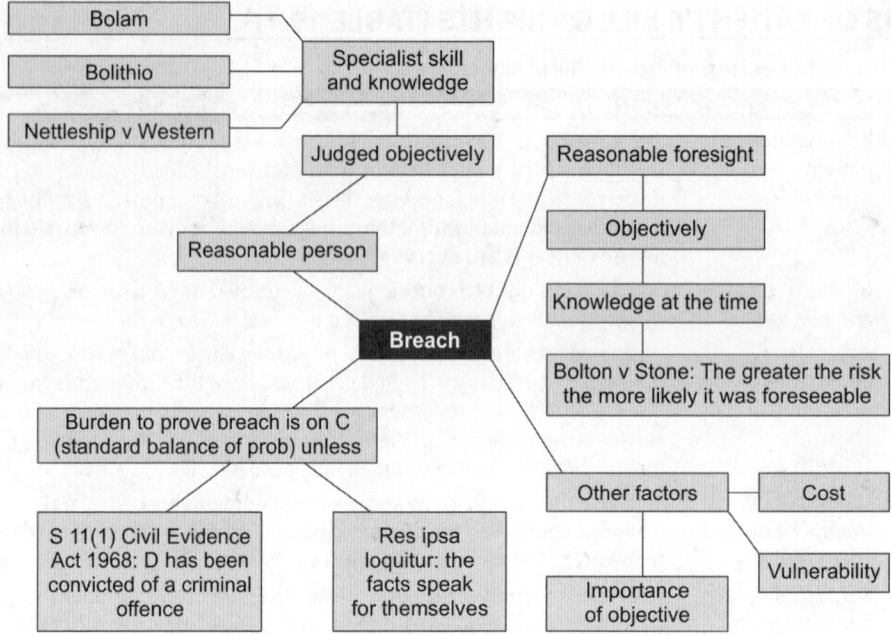

Fig. 19.8: Breach of duty.

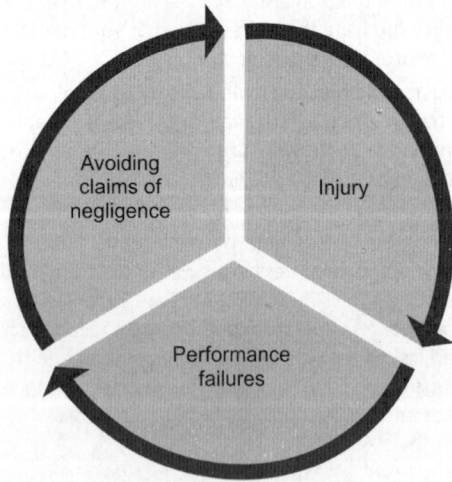

Fig. 19.9: Breach of duty.

- **Performance failures:** Inadequate nursing skills or attention to tasks may result in a suit of negligence against a nurse who chronically fails to provide approved standards of care. Such incidents include, but are not limited to, habitual medication errors, failure to follow protocol or orders and improper use of equipment.

- **Avoiding claims of negligence:** A good nurse is well-informed regarding health and safety laws, as well as board regulations and customs of nursing. She is diligent in preventing injuries and falls, knowing her duties and is familiar with medications and dosage ranges for all patients under her care. A good nurse will avoids negligence when she practices good communication with patients and physicians and works within legal guidelines.

NEGLIGENCE IN NURSING PRACTICE

Negligence occurs when a nurse performs an act that is deemed below a competence level that is expected of someone in their position. Consequences to the nurse can range from suspension or firing to malpractice suits and loss of license. Neglect can be intentional or unintentional and can occur for many different reasons:

- **Charting:** Failing to record vital information on the patient's chart can be considered negligent, especially if it results in further damage.

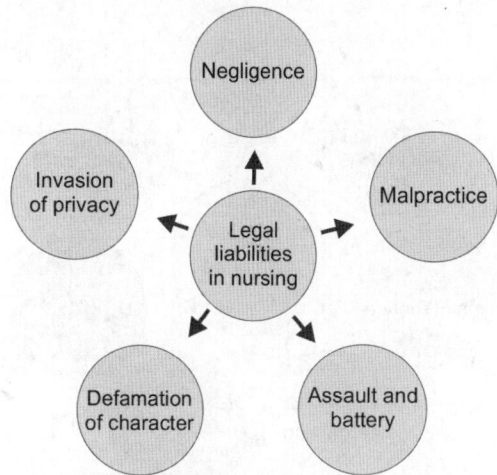

Fig. 19.10: Legal liabilities in nursing.

- **Doctor's orders:** Failing to follow a doctor's orders can be grounds for malpractice if it results in damage to the patient.
- **Confirming patient identity:** Before giving a patient medication or performing a medical procedure, the nurse must be sure that the right patient.
- **Intentional neglect:** Many cases of neglect result from poor planning and other unintentional errors in judgment, but sometimes a nurse knows she is doing something wrong and chooses to do it anyway.

Legal liabilities in nursing is shown in **Figure 19.10.**

MALPRACTICE IN NURSING PRACTICE

Malpractice is one type of negligence and includes professional misconduct, breach of a duty or standard of care, illegal or immoral conduct or failure to excise reasonable skill, all of which lead to harm. Malpractice also professional misconduct performed in professional practice, any unreasonable lack of skill in professional duties or illegal or immoral conduct that results in injury or death to the client or consumer.

Common malpractices issues are:
- Leaving foreign objects inside the client's body during surgery.

- Failure to observe and report a change in the patient's condition.
- Failure to get informed consent from the patient.
- Medication error, giving wrong medication to the patient or wrong dosage.
- Failure to follow physicians order.
- Delaying patients care or failure to monitor the patient.
- Incorrectly performing a procedure or trying to perform a procedure without training.
- Documentation error.
- Failure to provide patients education.

Avoiding nursing malpractice

Nursing is a highly respected and rewarding career, but it can also be very stressful and demanding. Even so, nurses make every effort to meet and exceed standards of care. The nurse should keep abreast of standards of care and standards of practice. Always follow facility policies and procedures to the letter. Above all, document. Be sure to note the date and time on nurses' notes, and record all patient assessments and nursing interventions.

STANDARDS OF NURSING PRACTICE

Nurses are judged against specific standards of care. Simply put, standards of care delineate what nurses should do in the performance of their role. Standards of practice are more specific and outline how the care is to be delivered. For example, a standard of practice for a critical care nurse might be: vital signs will be monitored continuously and recorded on the patient's medical record every fifteen minutes for the first 24 hours following admission. Standards of care are outlined within the state's Nursing Practice Act, facility departmental policy/procedure manuals, and within the specific area of practice.

Definition

- Standards are as broad statement of quality. It is a definite level of excellence or adequately required, aimed at possible. It agreed upon achieved level of performance, considered proper and adequate for a specific purpose against which actual performance is compared. So standard is an acknowledge measure of comparison for quantities or qualitative value, criterion, norm.

- Standard are an established rules or basis of comparison in measuring or judging capacity, quality context and value of objects in the same category. The term norm is frequently used synonymously with standard in the literature. Selected standards are reliable and relevant for the category being compared.

Purposes of Standards

- Standards give direction and provide guidelines for performance of nursing staff.
- Standards provide a baseline for evaluating quality of nursing care, ranging from excellent care to unsafe care.
- Standards help improve quality of nursing care, increases effectiveness of care and improve efficiency.
- Standards may help to improve documentation of nursing care provided, i.e., maintaining record of care.
- Standards may help to determine the degree to which standards of nursing care maintained and take necessary corrective action in time.
- Standards help supervisors to guide nursing staff to improve performance.
- Standards may help to improve basis for decision-making and devise alternative system for delivering nursing care.
- Standards may help justify demands for resources association.
- Standards may help clarify nurses area of accountability.
- Standards may help nursing to define clearly different levels of care.

Legal safeguard is shown in **Figure 19.11.**

Characteristics of Standards

- Standard statement must be broad enough to apply to a side variety of settings.
- Must be realistic, acceptable, attainable
- Nursing care must be developed by members of nursing profession, preferable

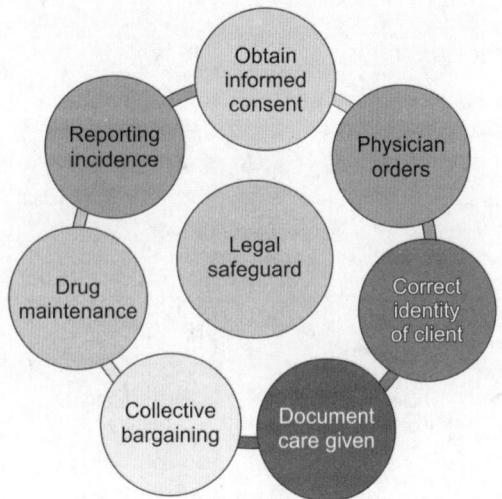

Fig. 19.11: Legal safeguard.

nurses practicing at the direct care level with consultation of experts in the domain.
- Should be phrased in positive and indicate acceptable performance.
- Nursing care must be express what desirable optional level is.
- Must be based on current knowledge and scientific practice.
- Must be reviewed and revised periodically.
- May be directed towards an ideal, i.e., optional standards or may only specify the minimal care that must be attained, i.e., minimum standard.

Sources of nursing care standards: The standards can be established developed, reviewed to enforce by variety of sources.
- Professional organization, e.g., Trained Nurses' Association of India (TNAI), Government nurses association in Karnataka
- Licensing bodies, e.g., statutory bodies Indian National Council (INC), Medical Council of India (MCI), Dental Council of India (DCI), etc.,
- Institutions/healthcare agencies, e.g., university hospitals, health centers.
- Department of institutions, e.g., Department of Nursing
- Patient care unit's, e.g., specific patient's units.
- Government units at national, State and
- Individual, e.g., Personal standards.

Box 19.1: ANA standards of nursing practice.

« **Assessment:** The registered nurse collects comprehensive data pertinent to the patient's health and/or the situation.

« **Diagnosis:** The registered nurse analyzes the assessment data to determine the diagnoses or issues.

« **Outcomes identification:** The registered nurse identifies expected outcomes for a plan individualized to the patient or the situation.

« **Planning:** The registered nurse develops a plan that prescribes strategies and alternatives to attain expected outcomes.

« **Implementation:** The registered nurse implements the identified plan.

- *Coordination of care:* The registered nurse coordinates care delivery.
- *Health teaching and health promotion:* The registered nurse uses strategies to promote health and a safe environment.
- *Consultation:* The graduate level-prepared specialty nurse or advanced practice registered nurse provides consultation to influence the identified plan, enhance the abilities of others, and effect change.
- *Prescriptive authority and treatment:* The advanced practice registered nurse uses prescriptive authority, procedures, referrals, treatment and therapies in accordance with state and federal laws and regulations.

« **Evaluation:** The registered nurse evaluates progress toward attainment of outcomes.

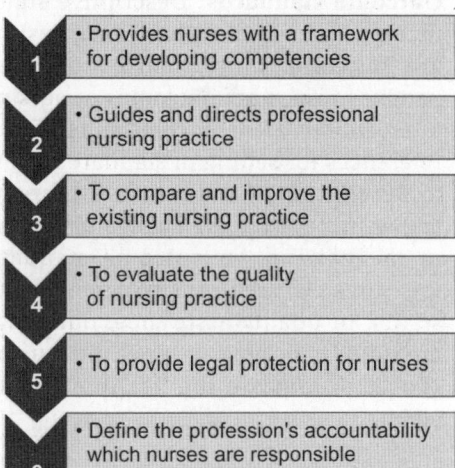

Why are standards important?

1. • Provides nurses with a framework for developing competencies

2. • Guides and directs professional nursing practice

3. • To compare and improve the existing nursing practice

4. • To evaluate the quality of nursing practice

5. • To provide legal protection for nurses

6. • Define the profession's accountability which nurses are responsible

Fig. 19.12: Importance of standards.

Standards can be classified and formulated according to frames of references relating to nursing structure, process and outcome, because standard is a descriptive statement of desired level of performance against which to evaluate the quality of service structure, process or outcomes. Importance of standards is shown in **Figure 19.12**.

- **Structure standard:** The structure is related to the framework, that is care providing system and resources that support for actual provision of care. Evaluation of care concerns nursing staff, setting and the care environment. The use of standards based on structure implies that if the structure is adequate, reliable, and desirable, standard will be met or quality care will be given.

- **Process standards:** Process standards describe the behaviors of the nurse at the desired level of the performance. The criteria that specify desired method for specific nursing intervention are process standards. A process standard involves the activities concerned with delivering patient care. In process standard there is an element of professional judgment, i.e., determining the quality of the degree of

Box 19.1 summarizes ANA standards of nursing practice.

Classification of Standards

Nursing care standards can be divided into ends and means standards. The ends standards are patient oriented, they describe the change as desired in a patient's physical status or behavior. The means standards are nursing oriented, they describe the activities and behavior designed to achieve the ends standards. Ends standards require information about the patients. A means standard calls for information about the nurse's performance. Standards are expected to understand achievable and measurable.

skill. It includes nursing care techniques, procedures, regimens, processes.

- **Outcome standards:** Descriptive statements of desired patient care results are outcome of standards, because patient's results are outcomes of nursing interventions. Here outcome as a frame of references for setting of standards refers to description of the results of nursing activity in terms of the change that occur in the patient. An outcome standard measures change in the patient's health status. In quality assurance, outcomes are stated in positive terms as the nursing goal is to improve the health status of client.

Nursing Care Standards

Helping the patient to attain and maintain health is the ultimate aim of nursing. This is also the aim of the physician, the dieticians, media, social work and other working in the hospital. Each group has a distinctive contribution to make and is independent upon others for the accomplishment of common purpose.

Nurse's observation and recording of patient's conditions and response to therapy aids the physician in carrying out his therapeutic purpose. The nurse in-charge of the community is the key person who coordinates and supports the activities of all groups. In emergencies, the physician often asks the nursing officer to carryout certain therapeutic measures for which he alone is responsible. The head nurse is the nursing officer overall in-charge, as well as the matron for efficient performance of her own duties and those of nursing personnel placed under her change.

- Deals with organization and control of the patient's environment and to secure for him maximum mental and physician comfort.
- Concerned with immediate personal care.
- She performs duties under the direction and in cooperation with the physician.
- Administrative duties of ward management.

Important Responsibilities of Nurse (Fig. 19.13)

- Maintaining general cleanliness and upkeep of the ward and its surrounding areas to provide neat and cheerful environment of the patients.
- Coming out of the instruction of the medical officers regarding treatment of patients, observing and recording the process of treatment and generally assisting the medical officer to achieve his therapeutic aim.
- Keeping the ward equipment in optimum state of readiness by prompt repairs and placement through condemnation boards.
- Supervision of care and maintenance of building furniture, fitting and arranging their reports.
- Assignment or duties for patient's care to the staff working is the ward taking into consideration the capabilities of each.
- Ensuring that all specimens are sent to the laboratory in time and results collected when due.
- Maintaining strict control over accounting and distribution of controlled and dangerous drugs.
- Requisition of diet as per instruction of the medical officer and ensuring that the diets and extras are distributed to patients as per the requisition.

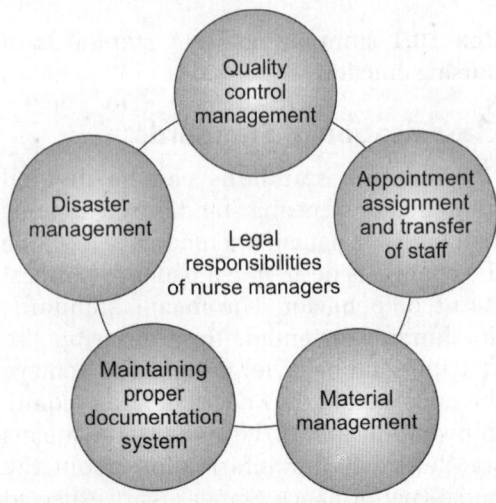

Fig. 19.13: Legal responsibilities of nurse managers.

- Maintenance of all registers and documents required in the ward.
- Overall supervision of all that happens in the ward is to ensure that the patient's treatment and recovery is as smooth and pleasant as possible.
- Training of nursing and other personnel working in the ward.

Medical Record

Certified Legal Nurse Consultant (CLNC): This is a registered nurse who uses nursing experience/medical expertise in combination with specialized legal training and comprehensive exam and certification to assist attorneys to research and develop medically related cases.

CLNC comprehensive medical record review includes:

- Thoroughly assess and organize all medical records, narrow down and identify what is irrelevant or what may be missing.
- Look for inaccuracies in documentation of condition that are inconsistent with what is regarded/believed to be accurate.
- Determine if staffing issues were a consideration (weekends, holidays).
- Address specific missing records, direct the attorney to explore more in depth request for production from the defense or plaintiff.
- Assess for evidence or signs of tampering through specialized training in detecting tampering in a medical record.
- Review and assess all relevant medical records present prior to the incident for evidence of pre-existing conditions.
- Screen cases for merit.
- Review/analyze medical records for deviations from the standards of care or institutions policies and procedures.
- Provide appropriate literature regarding treatments, standards of care, demonstrative evidence for whatever the attorney may request, and integrate them into the case analysis.
- Locating top expert witnesses in their medical fields, or the CLNC has specialized training to serve as a testifying or consulting expert to support the case
- Identify factors that caused or contributed to the injury.
- Identify and recommend potential defendants.
- Identify and review relevant medical records, hospital policies and procedures, and other essential documents and tangible items.
- Interview plaintiff and defense clients, key witnesses and experts with the attorney.
- Develop specialized written reports/chronological time lines and summaries as requested by the attorney.

Forensic Document Examiners

Especially trained legal professionals who utilize specialized equipment to detect fraud and tampering in a legal medical document. Some of the areas they may disclose include identifying different paper, different inks, indentations in the paper, and handwriting inconsistencies, to detect chronological inconsistencies and evidence of tampering in a medical record. If tampering of a medical document can be proved in a court of law, it implies dishonesty and deceit on the part of the defense, and may dramatically swing the jury's opinion in favor of the plaintiff.

Legal Consideration Involving Nursing Practice

Aside the regulation of nursing practice and standard, each hospital has their rules and codes of practice laid down to ensure safety and wellbeing of the patients. Any nurse, who do not oblige to these rules, codes of the hospital, and causes harm or injury to any patient, may be liable. Certainly, not all rules or policies covers every eventuality, hence the need for the nurse to ensure that the right patient gets the right treatment, use her professional judgment while caring for patients, do not attempt anything beyond her competence and should not exceed the limits of nursing procedures laid down. The laws governing nursing profession oblige nurses to perform their duties and responsibilities within the scope of nursing practice. Nurses have the duty to care for patients and should be cared for in the process of carrying out their lawful duties.

Common Causes of Malpractice

According to Reising and Allen, common malpractice claims arise against nurses when nurses fail to:

- Assess and monitor
- Follow standards of care
- Use equipment in a responsible manner
- Communicate
- Document.

Ways of Minimizing the Risk of Malpractice

Nurses should be cognizant of legal risks in providing care. Reising (2012) suggests that the following actions can help minimize a nurse's risk of being sued for malpractice:

- Know and follow your state's nurse practice act and your facility's policies and stay up to date in your field of practice.
- Assess your patients in accordance with policy and their physicians' orders and, more frequently, if indicated by your nursing judgment.
- Promptly report abnormal assessments, including laboratory data, and document what was reported and any follow-up.
- Follow up on assessments or care delegated to others.
- Communicate openly and factually with patients and their families and other healthcare providers.
- Document all nursing care factually and thoroughly and ensure that the documentation reflects the nursing process; never chart ahead of time.
- Promptly report and file appropriate incident reports for deviations in care.

Expectations of the nurse during ligation:

Should the unfortunate occur, and the nurse discovers herself in the midst of a legal entanglement. The first step to take is to share your observation with your immediate superior, who will in turn notify her manager or advice you on what to do immediately. It is worthy to note that you should relay information factually and accurately to your confider. It's also necessary to observed and complete all institutional procedural requirements. For instance, if your facility policy stipulated that an incident form be completed and forwarded, please endeavor to do so. Furthermore, contact your facility legal department/unit, which will assign an attorney to guide you through the case. Do not discuss the case with anyone other than your supervisor, employer, or legal representative.

Expectations of employer during ligation process involving a nurse:

The nurse is a staff of the hospital and therefore, she cannot be disclaimed according to the doctrine of respondent superior (let the master answer). The employer will notify the legal unit of the hospital for onward action. Set up an investigation panel to find out the truth. If possible, the hospital may employ the service of a lawyer to face the court, etc.

Expectations of the professional bodies during ligation of its members:

- Contact her lawyer
- Set up investigation panel
- Follow the accused to the court
- Give necessary moral and financial support to the accused provided the nurse practice within her professional boundaries.

Implication of ligation on the accused nurse:

- If a nurse was found guilty, she may lose her job or be suspended from work.
- She may be fined or be made to pay compensation.
- Her license may be revoked.
- Litigations serve as lesson to others.

If the nurse was not found guilty:

- She may be compensated adequately.
- She will be a public figure.
- The image of the nurses will improve, etc.

The nurse as a witness in the court:

A nurse may be require in the course of his professional duties to give account (evidence) of something he did or saw during his clinical duties in court as a professional witness or expert witness.

Expected Conduct of a Nurse in Court

- The nurse should be punctual to court on the day she/he was ask to appear.
- She/he should be corporately dressed.
- Her/his conduct should portray the image of nursing profession. The nurse should listen thoughtfully to all the questions put to him.
- She/he should think before he gives his answers or opinions.
- Her/his answers should be audible clear and firm and addressed to the judge and not to the counsel.
- The nurse should be courteous when answering questions.

CONCLUSION

In the nursing profession, instances of litigation can occur, despite healthcare professionals' best efforts in providing quality care. The goal of this to educate nurses regarding their responsibility and accountability to patients and the complex issues involved in basic legal situations. This course will help nurses become educated about and be alert to the legal aspects of nursing practice. Ethico-legal issues are far less common in developing countries compared with developed countries. This is partly because the populaces in developing countries are less well informed of their rights and because of fatalistic and religious beliefs in many societies in developing countries. With more awareness of the people, ethico-legal issues are likely to increase even in the developing nations.

20

CHAPTER

Profession and Related Organizations

INTRODUCTION

Organizations provide a means through which united efforts are made to elevate standards of nursing education and practice. It also offers a means of voicing and opinions, developing our abilities and keeping informed of new trends. Nursing regulatory bodies are also known as 'Professional Associations, which are responsible for the licensing of nurses within their respective province or territory. These regulatory bodies set the enforced standards of nursing practice, monitor and enforce standards for nursing education, monitor and enforce standards for nursing practice and set the requirements for registration of nursing professionals. The professional nurse must be aware of these associations so as to participate in various nursing professional activities of these organizations. To be a part of these associations, the nurse must have

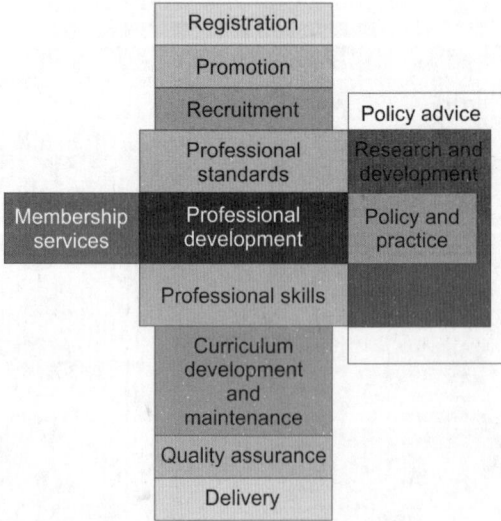

Fig. 20.1: Importance of professional membership.

life membership with these organizations through proper registration which is must.

FUNCTIONS OF PROFESSIONAL BODIES

- These associations provide a means through which the professional development of a nurse can be channeled with the authority because of its representative character.
- These associations also provide the nurses with the opportunities for expression of their viewpoints, development of their leadership qualities and abilities.
- These associations keep the nurses informed of professional news and trends throughout the country and worldwide.
- Roles of regulatory and professional bodies is shown in **Figure 20.2**.

INDIAN NURSING COUNCIL

The Indian Nursing Council (INC) is an autonomous body under the Government of India, Ministry of Health and Family Welfare was constituted by the Central Government under Section 3(1) of the Indian Nursing Council Act, 1947 of Parliament in order to establish a uniform standard of training for nurses, midwives and health visitors.

AIMS OF INC

The aim of legislation in nursing is best achieved through introduction of a 'Nurse Practice Act' having statutory regulation which makes provision for establishment of nursing council. Since health is a state subject,

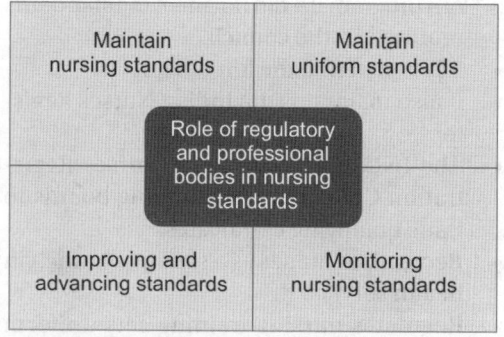

Fig. 20.2: Role of regulatory and professional bodies.

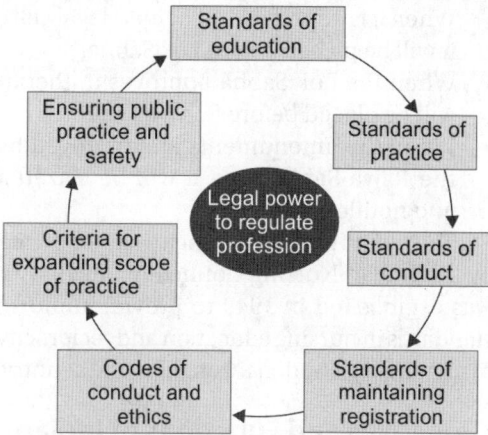

Fig. 20.3: Legal power to regulate profession.

there is nursing council at the state level which formulates their policy as per the guidelines provided by the INC. The members of the State Nursing Council is majority from the nursing profession. Nursing Council functions with enactment of an Act by the state legislature. The Act prescribes the licensures and the state council has to register the members of the profession.

The Central Government has established INC which is a central council of the country established by an Act of Parliament in 1947.

The purpose of INC is to formulate a national policy for training and practice of nursing depending mainly on the culture and philosophy of the country. Thus INC is required to prescribe the syllabus for the training of nurses of all levels, e.g., MSc BSc (N), GNM ANM, LHV, etc., and the minimum requirements for the recognition of any institution offering such a course. Nursing personnel has to be identified with an appropriate educational program for each level in the system of the country. The council has the authority to prescribe training institutions periodically to ensure its functioning abiding the standard prescribed.

INC to be made following process is needed:
- A proposal is to be sent to Govt. of India Ministry of Health and Family Welfare.
- Ministry of Health will consult Ministry of Law.
- It will go to cabinet (legal cell).

- When it is approved by cabinet (legal cell), it will be placed before Lok Sabha.
- When the Lok Sabha approves it, then it will be placed before Rajya Sabha.
- When the amendments are approved by the Rajya Sabha then it will be Gazeted and notified.

The Indian Nursing Council was authorized by the Indian Nursing Council Act of 1947. It was established in 1949 to provide uniform standards in nursing education and reciprocity in nursing registration throughout the country.

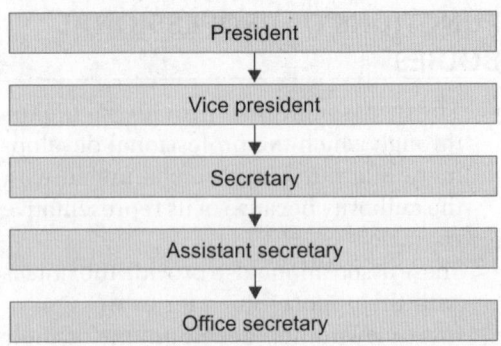

Fig. 20.4: Organization structure of Indian Nursing Council.

Objectives and Functions of Indian Nursing Council

- To establish and monitor a uniform standard of nursing education for nurses midwife, auxiliary nurse midwives (ANM) and health visitors by doing inspection of the institutions.
- To recognize the qualifications under section 1 O(2)(4) of the Indian Nursing Council Act, 1947 for the purpose of registration and employment in India and abroad.
- To give approval for registration of Indian and Foreign Nurses possessing foreign qualification under section 11(2)(a) of the Indian Nursing Council Act, 1947.
- To prescribe the syllabus and regulations for nursing programs.
- Power to withdraw the recognition of qualification under section 14 of the Act in case the institution fails to maintain its standards under Section 14 (1)(b) that an institution recognized by a State Council for the training of nurses, midwives, ANMs or health visitors does not satisfy the requirements of the council.
- To advise the State Nursing Councils, Examining Boards, State Governments and Central Government in various important items regarding nursing education in the country.

Organizational Structure of Indian Nursing Council Committee (Fig. 20.4)

- **Executive committee** of the Council is constituted to deliberate on the issues related to maintenance of standards of nursing programs.
- **The nursing education** committee is constituted to deliberate on the issues concerned mainly with nursing education and policy matters concerning the nursing education.
- **Equivalence committee** is constituted to deliberate on the issues of recognition of foreign qualifications, which is essential for the purpose of registration under section 11(2)(a) or (b) of the INC Act, 1947, as amended.

Functions of INC

- It provides uniform standards in nursing education and reciprocity in nursing registration.
- It has authority to prescribe curriculum for nursing education in all states.
- It has authority to recognize program of nursing education or to refuse recognition of a program if it did not meet the standards required by the council.
- It is registering the foreign nurses.
- It also maintains the Indian Nurses Register.
- The INC authorizes State Nurses Registration Council and examining boards to issue qualifying certificates.
- Recognizes nurses as a separate branch in health service.
- Regulates nursing training sets uniform standard types of training for nurses throughout the country.

- Construct syllabus, e.g., ANM, GNM, BSc (N), MSc (N), etc.
- Laid down requirements for admission of students.
- Set up minimum standard of a schools and colleges of Nursing.
- Certificates on completion of training.
- Recognition of qualifications (basic and higher).
- Effect of recognition any recognized qualification shall be sufficient qualification for enrolment in any state register.
- Power to enquire information as to course of study and training and examination from any state from time to times as required.
- Inspection of the schools and colleges of nursing.
- Withdrawal of recognition of nursing institutions.
- Maintenance of Indian Nurse Registers.
- Power to make regulations.
- To regulate nursing practice.
- Permits title, badges, uniforms for registered nurses.
- Uphold the standard of nursing.
- Publications.

INTERNATIONAL COUNCIL OF NURSES

The International Council of Nurses (ICN) was founded in 1899 by Mrs Bedford Fenwick. It is federation of nonpolitical and self-governing national nurses association. The ICN is the global voice of nursing. The main purpose of the ICN is to provide the means through which the national associations can share their interests in the promotion of health and care of the sick **Figure 20.5** shows logo of ICN.

It was founded by Mrs Bedford Fenwick in cooperation with nursing leaders from many countries. In 1900, the council's constitution was adopted and the first meeting was held at the World Exposition in Buffalo, New York. Their headquarter is established at Geneva in Switzerland.

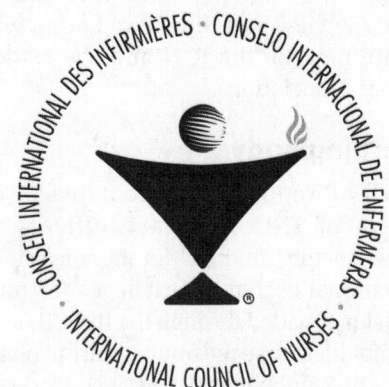

International Council of Nurses
The global voice of nursing

Fig. 20.5: Logo of International Council of Nurses (ICN).

Objectives of ICN

- To promote the development of the strong National Nurses Association.
- To assist National Nurses Association to improve the standards of nursing education and practice.
- To assist National Nurses Association to improve the status of nurses within their countries.
- To serve as the authoritative voice for nurses and nursing internationally.

Activities

- The ICN has published the Code for Nurses.
- It makes the policy statement on health and social issues.
- It also maintains and improves the status of nurses and standard of nursing around the world.
- The council works to improve the nursing education and practice by publishing the guidelines for National Nurses Association.

The governing body of the ICN is the Council of National Representatives, which is made up of the ICN honorary officers and the presidents of the national member associations.

The ICN publishes the International Nursing Review and the News Letter, which give the news of the ICN and the National Member Association.

Governing Body

Council of National Representatives which consists of INC honorary officers and president of the National Member Association. International exchange privileges for nurses have been provided through the INC. This gives the individual nurse the opportunity to observe and obtain employment in other countries and also contributes to improvement of standards.

The Activities of ICN:

- Making the code of nurses.
- The world wide accepted definition of a nurse.
- A book of ethics "The nurses Dilemma".
- Policy statement on health and social issues.
- Arrange exchange program for study and employment.
- Maintain a register on professional qualification of people.
- Conducting seminars around the world to maintain relationship.

The international relationships: The ICN has close relationship with many of the world's major international organizations such as WHO, ILO, UNESCO, UNICEF, Red cross and its allied leagues. This relationship helps ICN to have related concerns in the healthcare field and allows keeping abreast of trends affecting the future of nursing.

Functions of ICN

- The division of nursing education
- The division of nursing service
- The division of social and economic welfare.

TRAINED NURSES ASSOCIATION OF INDIA

The Trained Nurses Association of India (TNAI) is a national professional association of nurses **(Fig. 20.6)**. The present name and organization were established of nurses. The present name

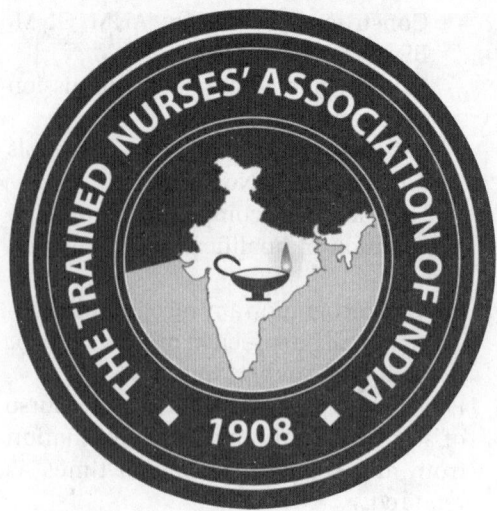

Fig. 20.6: Logo of Trained Nurses Association of India (TNAI).

and organization were established in 1922 but its history of development goes back to 1905. The TNAI had its beginning in the Association of Nursing Superintendent which was founded for all nurses to participate at same level.

The level of organization moves to the district state and national levels. Members of the TNAI are usually most active on the level of the local unit. Activities and conferences however are planned regularly by the estate branches and provide opportunities for valuable professional participation and development of the individual member.

Governing Body of TNAI

The governing body of the TNAI is the council which is assisted by standing committees for economic welfare, nursing research and finance. A fulltime salaried secretary was first appointed in 1935. A salaried assistant secretary who also serves as the advisor to the Student Nurses Association (SNA) was appointed in 1983.

Aims of TNAI

The aims of TNAI center upon needs of the individual member and problems in the nursing profession as a whole, such aims include up grading, development and standardization of nursing education,

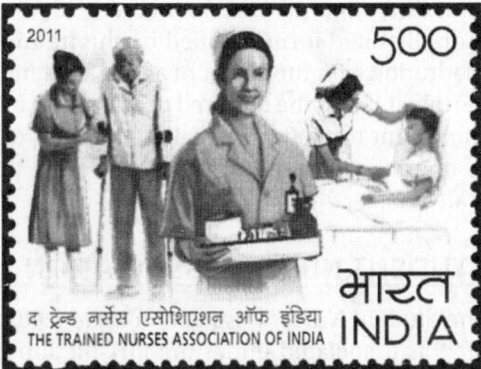

Fig. 20.7: Indian postal stamp of TNAI.

improvement of living and working conditions for nurses in India and registration for qualified nurses.

Various activities of the TNAI implement its aims. It was active in helping to formulate basic nursing curricula when it first organized. More recently, it has promoted the development of courses in higher education for nurse. It gives scholarship for nurses who wish to goon for advanced study either in India or abroad.

The TNAI also stimulates action to organize the state nurses and midwives registration councils. It also helps to remove discrimination against male nurses and initiates study and improvement of economic condition for nurses.

Membership of TNAI: The Trained Nurses Association of India membership is obtained by application and submission of a copy of your state registration certificate. Transfer membership from the Student Nurses Association by having a certificate sent from the institution in which the student studied within six months after completing the course. A reduced fee is offered to those who transfer membership directly from SNA.

Publications of TNAI

The Trained Nurses Association of India publishes. "The Nursing Journal of India", monthly. Another impressive publication is the "Indian Nursing Year book". This contains important reports, trends and statistics about nursing profession in India.

STATE NURSING COUNCIL

State Nurses Registration Council is independent and recognized as a body that can make statues and prescribe by laws for trained nurses and prospective nurses who are undergoing various nursing programs. Although, it is an independent body but it has to obtain approval from state government for all the laws passed by it and decision taking. This council helps to maintain a register of names of professional nurses. Registration is must for the diploma and degree courses in nursing. Registration system helps to maintain the high standard amongst the professional nurses. Registration serves a legal protection to the nurse and also to the public as it prevents disqualified and incompetent persons to practice nursing.

The training of nurses, midwives, health visitors and ANMs is to a large extent controlled by the Nurses Registration Councils in the states. Registration in State Nursing Council is very necessary to be registered in order to practice officially as a professional nurse. Registration councils are functional in all the states of India and they are affiliated to INC.

Each state nurse registration council maintains a register of names of professional nurses. The names of these nurses are also put into Indian Nurses Registration Council. All the diploma and degree holder nurses have to register with State Nurses Registration Council.

Functions of State Nurses Registration Council

- To accredit and inspect schools of nursing in their state.
- To conduct examinations for General Nursing and Auxiliary Nursing courses.
- To prescribe rules of conduct, take disciplinary actions.
- Registration of nurses and midwives in their state.
- Maintenance of register of nurses, midwives and others.
- To renew registration and upgrade registration.

The State Nursing Council is an autonomous statutory registration body for registering qualified nurses, midwives, ANMs, MPHWs and health visitors. A council has president/vice president, registrar and staff of the council. The functions of the council includes the registration of qualified nursing professionals, regulation of training programs by conducting inspection, checking malpractice and maintaining professional ethics, foreign verification, coordinating with the INC and with various other government departments and universities. The council conducts inspection for the institution, who are conducting the programs such as ANM, MPHW, DGNM, BSc (N), Post basic BSc (N), MSc (N) and Diploma in nursing education and administration. The council ensures that all facilities are available for conducting any of the nursing program before granting permission. It also conducts the surprise and periodical inspection to identify the deficiencies in that institution. If necessary, it also conducts reinspection to ensure that the deficiencies are rectified. It periodically sends communication to all the educational institutions to inform the issues of importance to nursing and health.

Activities

- To look after the various nursing educational programs run under its territory.
- To conduct exams of GNM and ANM in its areas.
- To issue certificates of registered nurse and registered midwife to the qualified nurses.
- Maintenance of various records such as the names and addresses of all-registered nurses, registered health visitors, registered midwives, registered nurse dais, registered trained dais in Punjab.

Renewal of Registration

The registration once done has to be renewed after a specific period of time or after attainment of higher education in nursing. It is done in respect to keep a control on registered persons practicing the profession in the state. The renewal process includes sending a dually filled form certified by the training institution with the copies of all the academic certificates and the required process fees. It is important to renew the registration in order to upgrade the status of the nurse within the state register.

STUDENT NURSES ASSOCIATION

The Student Nurses Association organized in 1929 is associated under the jurisdiction of the TNAI, in addition to providing a means of personnel and professional development for the nursing students. It serves as a source of membership for the parent organization. In addition the TNAI serves as the advisor for the SNA.

Objectives of SNA

- To help the students to uphold the dignity and ideals of the profession for which they are qualifying.
- To promote a corporate spirit among students for the common good for all.
- To furnish nurses in training with advance in their courses of study leading to professional qualifications.
- To encourage leadership ability and help students to gain a wide knowledge of nursing profession in all of its different branches and aspects.
- To increase the students social conducts and general knowledge in order to help them to take their place in the world when they have finished their training.
- To encourage both professional and recreational meeting, games and sports.
- To provide a special section in the nursing journal of India for the benefits of students.
- To encourage students to participate in the student nurses exhibition and to attend national and regional conferences.

Functions of SNA

- Project undertaking
- Sociocultural activities
- Exhibitions, public speaking and writing
- Organization of conferences

- Maintenance of SNA diary
- Propagation of profession
- Improvement of nursing education to improve health care
- Aid in the development of the nursing student
- Encourage optimal achievement in the professional role of the nurse.
- Fund raising

Organization Activity

Organization activities in the SNA are similar to that of the TNAI. The beginning level of organization is the local unit established in a teaching institution. It then moves on to the state and national level as in the TNAI. Members of the local unit are guided and assisted by the president of their unit who is a professional nurse, member of the TNAI and serves only as an advisor. The vice-president, who presides at all meeting and secretary of the unit must be students. State level advisors are active members of the TNAI elected by the state branches. There is a salaried full time secretary on the national level who is also a member of the TNAI and who is appointed by the TNAI council.

Membership: Membership fees in the SNA is minimal and easily met by the nursing student. The arrangement for transfer of membership to the TNAI has made in convenient for the new professional nurse to establish membership in the parent organization immediately.

CHRISTIAN MEDICAL ASSOCIATION OF INDIA

The Nurse's League of the Christian Medical Association of India (CMAI) was founded in 1930.

Christian Medical Association of India (CMAI) is a registered, non-profit, charitable organization. CMAI is the health arm of National Council of Churches in India (NCCI). They undertake programs in training, researcher community service, institutional consultancy, policy advocacy, interface of theology and medicine, information dissemination and others.

Objectives of CMAI

- Prevention and relief of human suffering irrespective of caste, creed, community, religion and economic status.
- Promotion of knowledge of the factors governing health.
- Coordination of activities for training doctors, nurses, allied health professionals and others involved in the ministry of healing.
- Implementation of schemes for comprehensive health care, family planning and community welfare.
- Rendering health in calamities and disasters of all kinds.

Functions of the Nursing Examination Board

- To coordinate and bring a uniform standard of nursing education, in accordance with the requirements of the Indian Nursing Council and State Nursing Council.
- To verify the eligibility requirements of the students before each examination.
- To arrange to conduct examination and issue diploma certificates to successful candidates.
- To maintain and enhance the educational standards of Schools of Nursing by arranging continuing education programs/ workshops/exhibitions.
- To prepare the calendar of events at the beginning of each academic year.
- To decide the disciplinary action against students/concerned staff in case of malpractice in examinations.
- To nominate members for the panel of examiners for Ist, IInd and IIIrd year of GNM nursing examinations.
- To appoint the examiners before annual and supplementary examination.
- To appoint an auditor to audit the board accounts.

Current Objectives

- To promote cooperation and encouragement among Christian nurses.
- To promote efficiency in nursing education and services.

- To secure the highest standard possible in Christian Nursing Education through the Christian Schools of Nursing
- To consider the special work and problems of Christian nurses working.

Nursing considered being an occupation now attains the status of profession.

MEDICAL COUNCIL OF INDIA

According to Indian Medical Council Act, 1956, the council consists the following members:

- One member from each state other than a union territory to be nominated by the Central government in consultation with the state government concerned.
- One member from each university, to be elected from amongst the members of the medical faculty of the university, by members of the senate of the university or in case of the university has no senate, by members of the court.
- One member from each state in which a state medical register is maintained to be elected from amongst themselves by persons enrolled on such register who possess the medical qualifications included in the first and second schedule.
- Seven members to be elected amongst themselves by persons who possess the medical qualifications.
- Eight members to be nominated by the Central Government. The members of the Council from amongst themselves elect the President and Vice – President of the Council.

Objectives and Functions of MCI

- Inspection or visitation with a view to maintain proper standard of medical education of India.
- Permission to start new medical colleges, new courses, including PG of higher courses, increase of seats, etc.
- Recognition of all India Medical registers of persons who hold any of the recognized Medical qualification or for the time being registered with any of the State Medical Councils or Medical Council of India.

- Maintenance of all India Medical registers of persons who hold any of the recognized Medical qualification or for the time being registered with any of the State Medical Councils or medical council of India.
- **Registrations:** Permanent registration, provisional registration and registration of additional qualifications.
- Issue of good standing certificates for doctors going abroad.

DENTAL COUNCIL OF INDIA

The Dental Council of India is a statutory body constituted by an Act of Parliament. Dentists Act, 1948 (XVI of 1948) with the main objective of regulating the dental education, dental profession, dental ethics in the country and recommend to the Government of India to accord permission to start a dental college, start higher course and increase the seats. The council celebrated the inaugural function of the golden jubilee of the Dental Council of India at Mumbai on 21st September 1998, which was inaugurated by the Honorable Minister of State for Health and Family Welfare.

Meeting of the council: During the year general body of the council meeting were held 17th and 18th April, 1998 and 21st to 23rd September 1998. Executive committee meeting was held on 16.04.98. The council received 23 applications in prescribed form/scheme from the central government for: i. establishing new dental college's, ii. Staring MDS courses, iii. increase of seats in BDS/MDS courses for evaluation and recommendation by the council in accordance with the provision of the section 10A of the Dentists Act, 1948.

Goals and Objectives of DCI

- **Decentralization of power:** It is collectively distribute the autarchy to other members in order to initiate a team approach towards the work of the council.
- **Transparency in assignments**—in order to prevent unwanted speculation on the ways the council functions. It would

be the foremost objective to ascertain transparency.

- **CDE program**—in order to keep the general practitioners abreast with the latest development in the fate of dentistry, regular CDE programs relevance to renewal of registrations is something
- **Surprise visits**—with an increase in the rise of dental colleges coming up in various part of the country it is imperative for us to keep a check on their functioning and surprise visits.

INDIAN RED CROSS

Indian Red Cross was established in 1920, and women in close co-operation with national and international agencies. At present it has 400 branches which are functioning all over the country. The Indian Red Cross is interested I providing care for war veterans, in maternity and child welfare, in emergency relief, in health education for the public and in nursing education.

Functions of Indian Red Cross

- It provides blood bank facilities.
- It offers first aid training with its branch St John Ambulance Association for men and home nursing courses to women.
- It provides relief worked at the time of disaster like earthquakes, flood or famine or war.
- It supplies milk and medical supplies like medicines, vitamins and other to hospitals, dispensaries, meet centers and render family planning services.
- It assists in the related research activities and offer scholarship to nurses to upgrade them.
- It publishes and distributes materials on child care and mother craft. Indian set up, the President of India is the President of the Association. Its affairs are managed by an executive committee, the chairman of which is nominated every year by the President. The Government of India gives a grant in aid to the Indian Red Cross Society.

UNITED NATIONS INTERNATIONAL CHILDREN'S EMERGENCY FUND (UNICEF)

UNICEF was established in 1946 as United Nations International Children's Emergency Fund. To deliver post war relief to children, later renamed as United Nations Children's Fund. It concentrates its assistance on development activities aimed at improving the quality of life for children.

The head quarters of UNICEF are at New York in USA and there are Regional Offices for South East Asia is established at New Delhi in India. UNICEF got close collaboration with WHO. UNO, UNDP, FAO and UNESCO.

Functions of UNICEF

- **UNICEF started** functioning in close collaboration with other specialized agencies of UNO and assisted in the prevention and control of communicable diseases like malaria, tuberculosis, leprosy, Yaws, trachoma, etc. Which were more prevalent in children?
- **In India UNICEF** supported the BCG immunization program from the start. It also assisted in the manufacture of DPT vaccine. Subsequently UNICEF shifted its attention to primary health care with focus on MCH services. IT laid stress on immunization, supplementary feeding of children and control of deficiency diseases by the provision of vitamin A solution, iodized salt and iron and folate tablets.
- **UNICEF took considerable** interest in the provision of piped water supply basic sanitation and formal and non-formal education. It provided substantial aid to primary health centers in India, by way of equipment, vehicles, bicycles, delivery kits, drugs, milk and other supplies.

GOBI Strategy by UNICEF

Currently UNICEF is engaged in affecting child health revolution through.

GOBI strategy promoting growth monitoring, oral rehydration, breast feeding, and immunization program and ICDS programs.

Regional organizations of UNICEF: UNICEF has a decentralized organizational structure with its headquarters in New York and separate regional offices for eastern and southern Africa, Central and West Africa, and North Africa, South Central Asia, Australia and New Zealand and Japan. UNICEF also maintains a Geneva office. The south Central Asia region includes India, Mongolia, Afghanistan, Sri Lanka, Nepal and Maldives.

UNICEF in India: UNICEF is assisting India with the collaboration to UNESCO. In the expansion of educational institutions and improvement of teaching sciences, science laboratories, equipment, working tools, libraries, audio-visual aids, helping training programs for nurses, midwives and health auxiliary personnel, etc.

In rural health aspects:
- Provided equipment and drugs to primary health centers BCG vaccination program.
- Assist in field of medical education and training.
- Assist in development of rural health services.
- Provided equipment for daily plants in various parts of India, e.g., Mumbai, Gujarat, Karnataka, Uttar Pradesh, West Bengal, Andhra Pradesh and Tamil Nadu.

UNITED NATIONS EDUCATIONAL, SCIENTIFIC AND CULTURAL ORGANIZATION (UNESCO)

- **UNESCO** is the United Nations Educational, Scientific and Cultural Organization. It contributes to peace and security by promoting close collaboration among nations through education, science and culture. It furthers universal respect for justice, rule and law, human rights and fundamental freedoms.
- **UNESCO** is sometimes believed to have originated from the International Institute of Intellectual cooperation. August 1st 1945 the Government of Britain communicated the revised draft to the Allied and Associated powers and invited them to an International Conference in London.
- **UNESCO** is an intergovernmental organization with membership of 158 countries and 2 associate members (British Virgin Islands and Netherlands Antilles) at present. The first session of the General Conference of UNESCO was first conceived as UNESCO – without the 'S'. The person who successfully promoted the "S" was the US poet Archibald MacLeish.
- **UNESCO** took possession of its new headquarters at palace de Fontenoy in Paris in September 1958. As against only 26 members in 1946, the membership at present stands at 158 nations. This has meant considerable increase in the responsibilities and resources of the organization. On November 4th 1986 UNESCO completed 40 years of its existence.

UNESCO Activities

The activities of UNESCO fall under the following broad heads education, natural sciences, social sciences, human sciences, culture, communication, co-operation with nongovernmental organizations and publications. Typical activities of UNESCO include the organization in various parts of the world of conferences and meeting of experts, coordination of international scientific efforts, standardization of documents and procedures, clearing house services, assistance to non – governmental organizations a wide range of publications and the establishment of international agreements to which states are invited to adhere or confirm.

Indian National Commission for cooperation with UNESCO: The main functions of the national commission are to serve as a link between UNESCO and institutions working in this country in the field of education, science and culture to advise the Government of India on matters relating to UNESCO and to promote understanding of the aims and policies of UNESCO among the people of India.

UNITED STATES AGENCY FOR INTERNATIONAL DEVELOPMENT (USAID)

USAISD was started in 1961. It provides grants and loans for a number of projects designed to improve the health of the people. The US Government presently extends aid to India through three agencies.

Agencies of United States

- United States agency for International Development (USAID)
- The public law -food for peace program.
- The US export – import bank.

USAID on Health in India

- Malaria eradication program
- Medical education
- Nursing education
- Health education
- Water supply and sanitation
- Control of communicable diseases
- Nutrition
- Family planning

Recent trends: The recent trends in assistance from the USA are increasingly in the support of agricultural and family planning programs.

UNITED NATIONS DEVELOPMENT PROGRAM (UNDP)

The United Nations Development Program was established in 1966 contributes towards increasing the pace of development in the third world countries. It supports all phases of socio-economic development including agriculture, industry, education, health and social welfare. It is the main source of funds for technical assistance. The basics objective of the UNDP is to help poorer nations develop their human and natural resources more fully.

THE FOOD AND AGRICULTURE ORGANIZATION (FAO)

The Food and Agriculture Organization was formed in 1945 with headquarters in Rome. It was the first United Nations Organization specialized agency created to look after several areas of world co-operation. FAO's primary aim is to increase agriculture production to keep pace with growing population in the world.

The chief aims are:
- To increase the efficiency of farming, fisheries and forestry.
- To improve the condition of rural people.
- To ensure that the food is consumed by the people who need it in sufficient quantities and in right proportions.
- To develop and maintain a better state of nutrition throughout the world.
- To help nations raise their living standards.

Objectives of FAO: The FAO has organized a World Freedom From Hunger Campaign (FFHC) in 1960. The primary objective of FAO is towards ensuring that the food is consumed by the people who need it in sufficient quantities and in right proportions to develop and maintain a better state of nutrition throughout the world.

FAO and Other Organizations

- The FAO also collaborating with other International agencies such as UNICEF, WHO in applied nutritional program.
- The joint WHO/FAO expert committee have provided the basis for many co-operative activities—nutritional surveys training courses, seminars and the coordination of research programs on brucellosis and other zoonoses.

CO-OPERATIVE FOR AMERICAN RELIEF EVERYWHERE (CARE)

CARE is a non-governmental organization which was started is 1946. It began working in India in 1950. CARE was found in North America in the wake of the Second World War in the year 1945. It is one of the world's largest independent, non-profit, non-sectarian international relief and development organization.

Objectives of CARE India: The primary objective of CARE—India was to provide food for children in the age group of 6-11 years. From mid 1980's CARE – India focused its food support in the ICDS program and in development of programs in the areas of health and income supplementation.

CARE: India and projects: CARE India is helping the following projects:
- Integrated nutrition and health project.
- Better health and nutrition project.
- Anemia control project.
- Improving women's health project.
- Improved health care for adolescent girls project.
- Child survival project.
- Improving women's reproductive health and family spacing project.
- Konkan integrated development project.
  It has been helping with the school midday meal scheme. Apart from this, it also provides help in the fields of medicine, literacy vocational training and agriculture.

CARE-India works in partnership with Government of India, state governments, nongovernmental organizations, etc.

ROCKEFELLER FOUNDATION

The Rockefeller foundation is a philanthropic organization chartered in 1913 and endowed by Mr John D Rockefeller. Its purpose is to promote the well-being on mankind throughout the world. It is a non – governmental agency that started functioning in India from 1920. The foundation contributed meaningfully to the implementation of public health programs and the advancement of social and agricultural sciences. The main area of interest has been medical education and research.

Activities of Rockefeller Foundation
- Training of competent teachers and research workers.
- Sponsoring of visits of a large number of medical specialists from the USA.
- Providing grants in aid to selected institutions.
- Development of medical college libraries.
- Population studies.
- Assistance to research projects and institutions.

FORD FOUNDATION

Ford Foundation was started as a contemporary of the Rockefeller foundation. Ford Foundation is an organization which is dedicated to the field of rural health services and family planning.

Activities of Ford Foundation
- It provides help in short-term training programs in community health.
- Pilot projects of health services.
- RCA projects and research programs in family planning.

The Ford Foundation has provided help in the water supply and drainage of sewage systems in Kolkata and the establishment of National Health and Family Welfare Institute in Delhi.

COLOMBO PLAN

Colombo Plan is a cooperative venture of a unique kind which was inaugurated in 1950 by 20 governments of common wealth countries to provide economic development in south and south east Asian countries, e.g., Australia, Canada, Japan, New Zealand, Britain, and America are its members.

Objectives
- Colombo plan is attempting to raise the living standard by cooperating and reviewing the development programe.
- Colombo plan is attempting to raise the living standard by cooperating and reviewing the development programs.
- Colombo plan aims at preparing a model of development plan together. Under the Colombo help is provided for industrial and agricultural development, but some support has also been given to health

promotion mostly through fellowship. All India Institute of Medical Science (AIIMS), New Delhi was made under the Colombo Plan with financial support from New Zealand.

WORLD BANK

World Bank is a specialized agency of the United Nations. It was established with the purpose helping less developed countries raise their living standards. The bank provides financial and technical support for projects of economic development.

Objectives: World Health Bank's primary objective is to help in raising the standards of living in comparatively poor or under-developed countries.

Functions of World Bank: World Bank collaborates with WHO in supporting public health programs on water supply, good production and population control and AIDS Control. World Bank is generally concerned with projects involving energy, transport, railways, industries, education, agriculture family planning, health and environment, etc.

CONCLUSION

Nurses are prepared to collaborate with a healthcare team to effectively perform treatments and procedures. Thus, nurses manage patient care. They ensure cohesive and coordinated care for successful patient outcomes. Healthcare should address a patient's cultural, spiritual and mental needs. They are dedicated to the advancement of the knowledge and practice of professions through developing, supporting, regulating and promoting professional standards for technical and ethical competence.

4

Nursing Administration and Ward Management

TERMINOLOGY

Management: Management is the art of securing maximum results with a maximum of effort so as to secure maximum prosperity and happiness for both, the employer and employee, and give the public the best possible services.

Manager: A person who is in-charge of running business or organization.

Administration: Administration is the organization and direction of human and material resources to achieve desired ends.

Objectives: Objectives are the purposes which the organization wishes to achieve.

Strategies: Strategies helps the organization to decide what their major roles are and policies which help them achieve the final goal.

Manual: Manual is a book of easy directions concerning the administration and procedure, e.g., nursing procedure manual.

Rule: Rule is a direction, telling what may or may not be done. It is a specific guide for action.

Project: A project is a plan or design for something that is to be done. It is an idea which is all worked out.

Budget: Budget is a plan covering all phases of operation of a business expressed in monetary units and is time-bound.

Forecasting: It is used to anticipate future problems and events. It is the prediction of the future course of action.

Manpower planning: It may be defined as a process by which an organization ensures right number of people and right kind of people at the right place, at the right time, doing things for which they are economically most suitable.

Coordination: Coordination is balancing and keeping together team by ensuring a suitable allocation tasks are preformed with due harmony among the members themselves.

Planning: Planning is the management function of anticipating the future and the conscious determination of a future course of action to achieve the desired results.

Recruitment: Recruitment has defined as the process of searching for prospective employees and stimulating them to apply for jobs in the organization.

Placement: Placement is the process of determining which of the several positions those are available

and within the competence of the candidates will be most suitable to him and assigning that job to the selected candidate.

Orientation: It is a fusion process for integrating the new employee with the organization. Orientation makes new employee feel at home and helps to adjust him to the new environment.

Performance appraisal: It is a systematic appraisal of the employee's personality triads and performance on the job and is designed to determine his contribution and relative worth to the firm.

Leadership: Leadership is interpersonal influence exercised in a situation and directing through communication process, towards the attainment of a specified goal or goals.

Authority: Authority is the right to give orders and power to exact obedience.

Models: Models are graphic or symbolic representations of phenomena that objectify and present certain perspectives or points of view about nature or function or both.

Management by objectives (MBO): Management by objectives is a process in which there is periodic agreement between a superior and subordinate, on the subordinate's objectives for a particular period and a periodic review of how well the subordinate achieved those objectives.

Supervision: Supervision is the activity of management that is concerned with the training and discipline of the workforce. It includes follow-up to assure the prompted and proper execution of order.

Motivation: Motivation refers to the way in which needs (urges, aspirations, desires) control, direct, or explain the behavior of human beings.

Communication: Communication is the passing of information and understanding from a sender to receiver. Communication is vital to the directing function of management.

Coordinating: Coordinating is the act of synchronizing people and activities so that they function smoothly in the attainment of organization objectives.

Controlling: Controlling is regulation of activities in accordance with the requirements of plans.

Decision-making: Decision making is a complex, congrutive process often defined as choosing a particular course of action. Decision making is the heart of all administrative and managerial functions. Decision-making is the process of choosing between alternatives to achieve a goal.

Staffing: Staffing is the systematic approach to the problem of selecting, training, motivating and retraining professional and non-professional personnel in any organization. It involves manpower planning to have the right person in the right place.

Human resource management: Human resource management deals with personnel of the organization. It is needed to be obtained and retain employees or to get and keep workers.

Personnel management: Personnel management is that activity in an enterprise which serves to mold human resources into an effective organization provides opportunity for maximum individual contribution, under desirable working conditions.

Carrier planning: Carrier planning is a process which optimizes in interdependence of the individuals and also their organizational relationship. Carrier planning can often be translated into programs and the organizational environment.

Supervision: Supervision is a process by which worker are helped by a designated staff member to learn according to their needs, to make the best use of their knowledge and skills and to improve their abilities so that they do their jobs more effectively and with increasing satisfaction to themselves and the agency.

Audit: Audit is a systematic and official examination of a record, process or account to evaluate performance. Audit is an independent appraisal activity within the organization for the review of accounting, financial and other operations as a basis of service to the management.

Medical audit: It is a systematic, critical analysis of the quality of medical care, including procedures for diagnosis and treatment, the use of resources and the training outcome and quality of life for the patient.

Nursing audit: Nursing audit is an evaluation of nursing service, it is related to planning, delivery and evaluation of care; it is an important component of nursing care.

Standard: Standard is a broad statement of quality. It is a definite level of excellence as adequately required, aimed at or possible. It agreed upon achievement level of performance, considered properly and adequately for a specific purpose against which actual performance is compared.

Quality assurance: Quality assurance program is an on-going, systematic process designed to evaluate and promote excellence in the health care provided to patients. Quality assurance requires evaluation of three components of care: structure, process, and outcome.

Peer review: It is a process by which employees of the same profession, rank, and setting evaluate one another job performance against accepted standards.

Hospital: Hospital is an institution for the care, cure, and treatment of the sick and wounded for the study of disease and for the training of doctors and nurses.

Nursing care: Nursing care is the person to person application of scientific principles for the sake of achieving physician's therapeutic purposes for patients, and for the sake of their health maintenance and the prevention of illness.

Case method: Case method nursing provides nurses with high autonomy and responsibility. In the case method each patient is assigned to a nurse for total patient care while that nurse is on duty.

Functional nursing: Functional method of nursing care is a technical approach to nursing care that emphasizes the dependent functions of nursing practice. The available staff on the unit, for a particular period of time, is assigned to selected functions such as vital signs, treatment, medications.

Team nursing: Team nursing is based on in which a group of professionals and nonprofessional personnel work together who identify, plan, implement and evaluate comprehensive client-centered care.

Modular or District nursing: Modular or district nursing is a modification of team and primary nursing. It decreases the sense of isolation and unrealistic expectations often associated with primary nursing.

Progressive patient care/client care: Progressive patient care is a method in which client care areas or units provide various levels of care, e.g., intensive care unit for critically ill, post-intensive care unit, regular care units, convalescing unit, and self care unit.

Primary nursing: It involves total nursing care, directed by a nurse on a 24 hours basis as long as the client is under care.

Managed care: Managed care is a unit based care system that can be used with any nursing care delivery system in any clinical setting. It uses standard critical paths with nursing care plans, analysis the positive and negative variations from critical paths, and uses them in change of shift reports.

Case management - Focuses on the entire episode of illness, including all settings in which the client receives care. it emphasizes achievement of outcomes in designed time frames with limited resources.

Collaborative practice: Collaborative practice can include inter-disciplinary teams, nurse-physician interaction in joint practice or nurse-physician collaboration in care giving. Collaboration is cooperative and assertive.

Evaluation: Evaluation is a judgmental process and it reflects the beliefs, values, and attitudes of participants of the program. It also helps in decision-making that leads to suggestions for actions to improve participant's effectiveness and program efficiency.

Philosophy: Philosophy is a system of motivating belief and principles those direct actions of a particular group during goal pursuit. The philosophy of a nursing department determines goals of the nursing workforce, which in turn influences patient care objectives established by each nurse.

Accountability: Accountability is the obligation to provide reasoning for one's actions to the persons who delegate authority for that action. The conscientious nurse exhibits accountability toward her/his employer, the patient, and government agency or insurance company that pays for the patient's health care.

Nursing care outcome: A Nursing care outcome is the end result of nursing interventions, a measurable change in the state of a patient's health that is occasioned by nursing action.

Criterion: A Criterion is the value free name of a variable that is known to be a reliable indicator of quality, e.g., it has been shown that the type and amount of a nurse's educational preparation affect the quality of her or his patient care decisions.

Norm: A Norm is current level of performance of a selected work group with reference to a given criterion. An objective is a goal towards which effort is directed. To be effective a goal should be expressed in observable, measurable terms and should include a target date for fulfillment.

Critical clinical indicator: A critical clinical indicator is a quantitative measure that can be used as a guide to monitor and evaluate the quality of important patient care activities.

Measurement: Measurement is the objective process of determining capacity, quantity or dimension of an object phenomenon, or outcome.

Quality health care: Quality health care is the appropriate application of medical science and nursing science knowledge to patient care, while balancing the hazards associated with each intervention with the benefits resulting from the intervention.

21

CHAPTER

Administration and Management

INTRODUCTION

Administration is concerned with the "what" and the "how" of government. The "what" is the subject matter, the technical knowledge of a field which enables the administrator to perform its tasks. The "how" is the technique of management, the principles according to which cooperative programs are carried to success. Each is indispensable; together they form the Synthesis called administration. Public administration consists of getting the work of Government done by coordinating efforts of people, so that they can work together to accomplish their set tasks. Administration embraces activities which may be highly technical or specialized such as public health and building of bridges. It also involves managing, directing and supervising the activities of thousands, even millions of workers so that some order and efficiency may result from their efforts.

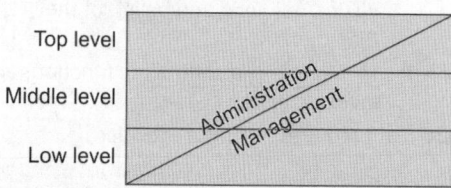

Fig. 21.1: Administration and management.

DEFINITION

- Administration is the activities of groups cooperating to accomplish common goals.
  Herbert A Simon
- Administration may be defined as the management of affairs with the use of well thought out principles and practices and rationalized techniques to achieve certain objectives. **Goel**
- Management may be defined as the art of securing maximum results with a minimum efforts so as to secure maximum prosperity and happiness for both employer and employee and give the public the best possible service. **John Mee, 1963**
- Administration is the organization and use of men and materials to accomplish purposes. It is the specialized vocation of managers who have skills of organizing and directing men and material just as definitely as an engineer has skill of building structure. **James L**

NATURE/FEATURES OF ADMINISTRATION

Administrative process is intellectual, social dynamic and creative as well as continuous.

The features or nature of administration are as follows:

- It is universal: Because irrespective of the nature and objectives of the organization, all basic elements of administration such as planning, organizing, staffing, directing, coordinating, reporting, and budgeting can apply for its effective achievement of goals.
- It is holistic: The whole process of administration embraces the organization and its function in entirely, i.e., involve total activities of the organizations.
- It is intangible; since administration is visualized as abstract. It cannot be transferable, so every organization has to develop its own administrative style within the content of functional elements of administration.
- It is a continuous and ongoing process. The cycle of administration goes on continuously.

- It is goal oriented; administration is always struggling to achieve the laid down goals and objectives of the organization.
- Administration has group of people to achieve the objective; it needs social and interpersonal contact or relationship to achieve the goal.
- It is dynamic; administration has the elements of flexibility and adaptability and adjustability rising to the needs and demands of different situations.
- It is creative or innovative; an effective administration existed administration. Provides innovation, offers and invites creative ideas to its organizational teams.

PHILOSOPHY OF ADMINISTRATION

Administration is a moral act and also a moral agent. Public administration is of pivotal importance in the developing countries, like India, which is engaged in a massive effort to

Difference between Administration and Management in Nursing

Basis of difference	Administration	Management
Nature of work	It is concerned about the determination of objectives and major policies of an organization.	It puts into action the policies and plans laid down by the administration.
Type of function	It is a determinative function.	It is an executive function.
Scope	It takes major decisions of an enterprise as a whole.	It takes decisions within the framework set by the administration.
Level of authority	It is a top-level activity.	It is a middle level activity.
Nature of status	It consists of owners who invest capital in and receive profits from an enterprise.	It is a group of managerial personnel who use their specialized knowledge to fulfil! the objectives of an enterprise.
Nature of usage	It is popular with government, military, educational, and religious organizations.	It Is used in business enterprises.
Decision making	Its decisions are influenced by public opinion, government policies, social, and religious factors.	Its decisions are influenced by the values, opinions, and beliefs of the managers.
Main functions	Planning and organizing functions are involved in it.	Motivating and controlling functions are involved in it.
Abilities	It needs administrative rather than technical abilities.	It requires technical activities.

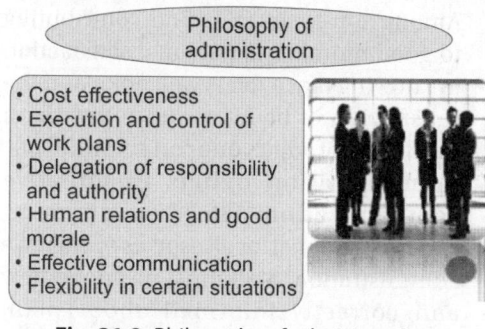

Philosophy of administration

- Cost effectiveness
- Execution and control of work plans
- Delegation of responsibility and authority
- Human relations and good morale
- Effective communication
- Flexibility in certain situations

Fig. 21.2: Philosophy of administration.

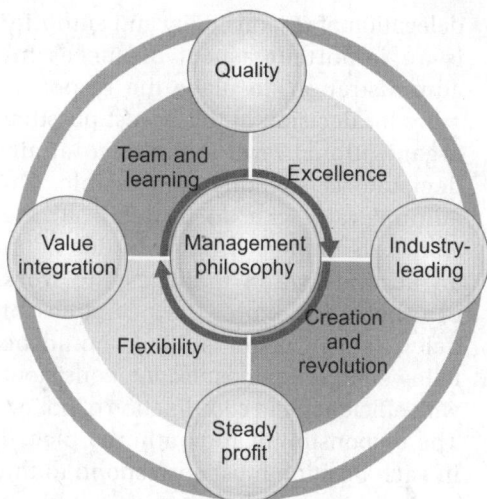

Fig. 21.3: Management philosophy.

lift themselves from a state of poverty, squalor and disease to a level of general happiness and prosperity, and which employ it as the instrument of change and development. No plan can succeed if its administrative implications are not fully realized and commensurate administrative machinery not provided.

A country's progress is, thus largely determined by the quality of its public administration. The contents of public administration today are more positive in nature for it is now engaged in looking after myriad needs of human life—health, education, recreation, sanitation, social security and others. It is therefore, a creative factor, its motto being the welfare of society.

- It must bring into sharp focus, all elements entering into administrative action should, then, be integrated and brought into a system of proper and unified relationship.
- Where possible principles are developed, bearing in mind that they are valid guidelines to future action under substantially similar conditions.
- Administration is concerned with both ends and means. A skillful fusion of the two is the test of administrative excellence.
- A good administrative system should communicate to the stakeholder's feelings of widespread satisfaction.

The philosophy underlying the whole field of administration, particularly as it applies to health work, is based on the following key points:

- **Administration believes in cost-effectiveness:** In the management or adminis-

tration of any enterprise or organization, the quality, quantity, timing, and cost of the work necessary to reach the objective of the enterprise are interrelated factors which must be given constant attention. If the resources of health work, in trained persons and in finances were unlimited, the need for constant attention to these factors would not be so great. But the limitation in the number of trained personnel and the lack of adequate financial resources are major obstacles to greatly improved health in the world today. We must monitor our resources carefully to accomplish as much as possible with what we have available.

- **Administration believes in execution and control of work plans:** One of the greatest possible contributors to wastage of our precious resources, whether at the local or national level, is the failure of those at any level of administration, and at all stages in the management of the activity, to base all decisions on verifiable facts. There should be no tolerating errors in administrative action, which occur, because someone failed to get all those facts. In the evolution, execution and control of work plans, obtaining the factual evidence should always be the first step.

- **Administration beliefs in delegation of responsibility and authority:** The delegation of responsibility and authority is an important aspect of successful administration, to place the responsibility for decision at the lowest possible organizational level in order to attain decision as speedily as possible. No administrator can do in detail all the work he is administering for; by definition an administration manages the work of others. Therefore, the principles of delegation of responsibility should be followed to the utmost extent, consistent with efficiency and coordination of policy. The responsibility and authority placed in each position must correspond to the responsibility which the position carries.

- **Administration beliefs in human relations and good morale:** Since the function of administration is to attain an established objective through the management of people, administration is deeply concerned with human relations. Find the individual worker in any enterprise, including health work, feels about a situation. One of the facts of the situation which the administrator must take into account assessing the total situation. Good morale of the staff is essential to the success of any undertaking and that morale is affected by both financial and non-financial factors. For the financial factor, the amount of remuneration is often less important to morale than the knowledge that remuneration of each individual is fair, as compared with that of other staff in the same organization or institution.

Among non-financial factors contributing to good morale is a personal satisfaction in knowing that a job is well done and the satisfaction of being associated with an institution of which one can be proud of.

- **Administration beliefs in effective communication:** Effective communication is essential for all aspects of effective administration. Staff must be adequately and correctly informed about plan, methods, schedules, problems, events and progress. It is necessary that instructions, knowledge and information be passed on for practical application to all concerned, and that they may be so clearly presented as to rule out any misinterpretation or misunderstanding. Proper and adequate communication is not just in one direction, it requires two way communications. Administrators must be certain that they know and understand the problem of workers for whom they are responsible. Communications must flow from the bottom-up, as well as from top-down.

- **Administration beliefs in flexibility in certain situation:** Administration must be completely flexible to meet the changing needs of the situation.

PRINCIPLES OF ADMINISTRATION

The science of administration attempts to discover and impart principles of administration. Principles can mean either of two things, i.e., ethical nature and generalization of behavior. The first is of an ethical nature; the administration may say we ought to do this list

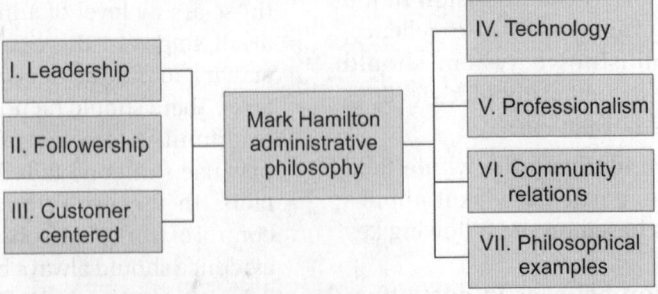

Fig. 21.4: Mark Hamilton administrative philosophy.

of things in this way. Here the ethical impulse is paramount. Thus, we ought to admit every child that is sick and brought to our door. Or, we ought not let a patient leave, until we are absolutely certain that he is capable of returning to work the next morning, at least to get as strong as he was before he was afflicted.

These are standards ambitions, expressions of what is supremely good in the conduct of the enterprise. This is the meaning of ethical nature of principle. Another meaning of the word "principle" is a generalization from behavior, a succinct statement that experience has shown that if "A" (a purpose) is to be attained, then "B" (a train of policies and activities) must be employed.

Henri Fayol Principles of Administration or Management

Since principles may be considered as widely accepted statements which are found to be true and reflective of life situations. To sum up, with fourteen principles of administration were identified by the Henry Fayol as follows:

- **Division of work** in any organization administrator or manager cannot perform all the activities to achieve its objective. So there should be division of work according to managerial and non-managerial, or according to jobs grouped according to departments, e.g., Department of Nursing, Department of Pharmacy, and Department of Medicine and so on.
- **Authority, responsibility, and accountability:** If the person has to perform job assignment effectively according to their own qualification and experience, or convention there should be delegation of authority and responsibility needed, which in turn helps to get accountability.
- **Discipline:** For smooth running of administration to achieve objectives, there should be proper observance of the rules, regulations, norms, decorum, manners, code of ethics and respect; this requires to be enforced within the organization by the managers.
- **Unity of command:** In any organization the subordinates should be supervised by

a single superior to whom he/she should be accountable.
- **Unity of direction:** In any organization, there should be one supervisor to give direction to his/her subordinates.
- **Subordination of individual interest to organizational interest:** This implies that narrow selfish interest should be overcome or should turn to common and broad interest of the organization for its welfare, e.g., collective bargaining (more salary, more production).

Fourteen management principles of Henri Fayol	
1.	Division of work or division of labor
2.	Balancing authority and responsibility
3.	Discipline
4.	Unity of command
5.	Unity of direction
6.	Subordination of individual interests to the general interest
7.	Remuneration
8.	Centralization
9.	Scalar chain
10.	Order
11.	Equity
12.	Stability of tenure of personnel
13.	Initiative
14.	Esprit de corps

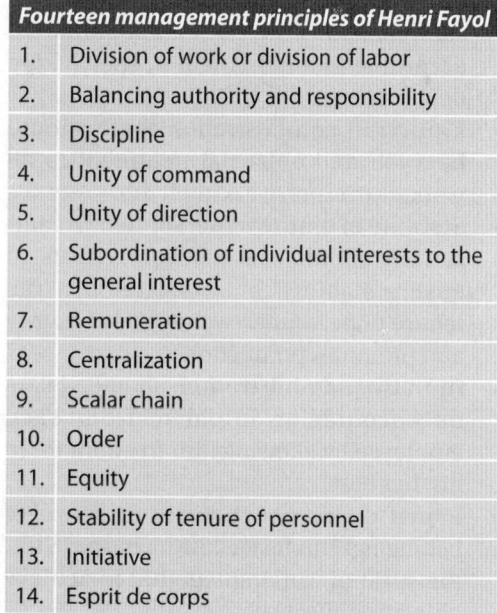

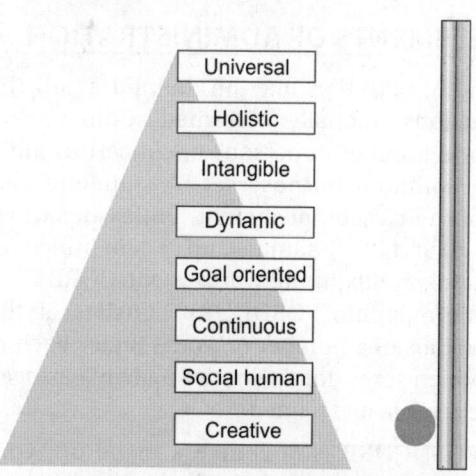

Fig. 21.5: Nature of administration.

- **Remuneration of personnel:** There should be fair policy for payment to the personnel justifying the workload, job hazards, efficiency and quality of performance.
- **Centralization:** There should be an amount of greater and larger authority resting with top level managers.
- **Scalar chain of command:** Which implies that there is chain or link of directional instructions from the top level to the lowest rank of organizational members in the hierarchy.
- **Order:** In an administration there should be proper, systematic arrangement of staff, materials, supplies and equipment according to requirement of specific job departments.
- **Equity:** In administration there should be a fair and impartial treatment to all workers irrespective of their job.
- **Stability of tenure of personnel:** Organizations should make proper efforts to ensure stability and continuity in the tenure of personnel, which gives security and promotes productions.
- **Initiative administration:** should always be encouraging initiative from each employee by allowing him freedom to do his/her best.
- **Esprit de corps:** It refers to sense of belonging. This fosters the team spirit, i.e., the spirit of working together to achieve objectives effectively.

ELEMENTS OF ADMINISTRATION

Administration may be defined as all the actions rationally performed by one person or a number of persons in concert to fulfill a common purpose set by someone else of their accomplishment. Professor Luther Gullick (1937): summed up certain principles or elements in the word "POSDCORB". The hieroglyphic POSDCORB consists of the initials of a number of words under each of which some administrative activity has been classified and named.

POSDCORB is of course a made up word designed to call attention to the various functional elements of the work of a Chief Executive because "administration" and "Management" have lost all specific content. POSDCORB is made up of initials and stands for the following activities:

'P' stands for planning: That is working out a broad outline, the things that need to be done and the methods for doing them to accomplish the purpose set for the enterprises or of the purpose in hand.

'O' stands for organizing: That is the establishment of the formal structure of authority through which work of subdivisions are arranged, defined and co-ordinate for the defined objectives. Other words building up the structure of authority through which the entire work to be done arranged into well-defined subdivisions and coordination.

'S' Stands for staffing: That is the whole personnel function of bringing in and training the staff and maintaining favorable conditions of work. In other words, staffing is appointing suitable persons to the various posts under the organization and the whole of personnel management.

'D' stands for directing: That is the continuous task of making decision and embodying them, specific and general orders and instructions

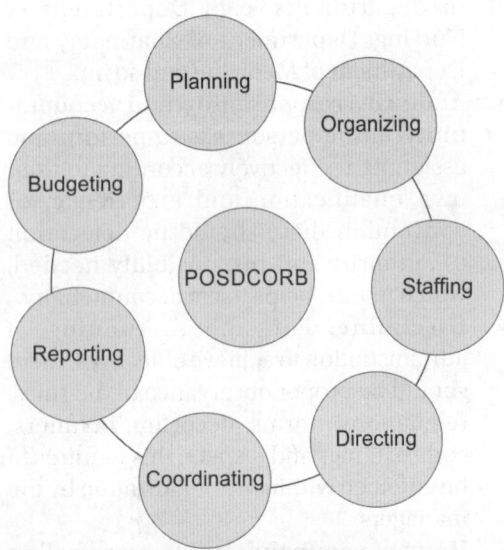

Fig. 21.6: POSDCORB.

and serving as leader of the enterprise. Making decisions and issuing orders and instructions embodying them for the guidance of the staff.

'CO' stands for Coordinating: That is the all important duty of interrelating the various parts of the work and eliminating of overlapping and conflict.

'R' stands for Reporting: That is keeping those to whom the executive is responsible informed as to what is going on, which thus includes keeping himself and his subordinates informed through records, research and inspection.

'B' stands for Budgeting with all that goes with budgeting in the form of fiscal planning, accounting and control. In American phraseology, budget stands for the whole of financial administration.

FUNCTIONS OF ADMINISTRATION

Planning

Planning means to decide in advance what is to be done. It charts a course of action for the future. It is an intellectual process and it aims to achieve a coordinated and consistent set of operations aimed at desired objectives.

Essentials of Good Planning

- Yields reasonable organizational objectives and develops alternative approaches to meet these objectives.
- Helps to eliminate or reduce the future uncertainty and chance.
- Helps to gain economical operations.
- Lays the foundation for organizing.
- Facilitates coordination.
- Helps to facilitate control.
- Dictates those activities to which employers are directed.

Organizing

- Once the objectives have been established through planning, management concern must turn to developing an organization that is capable of carrying them out. The management function of organizing can be defined as, "relating people and things

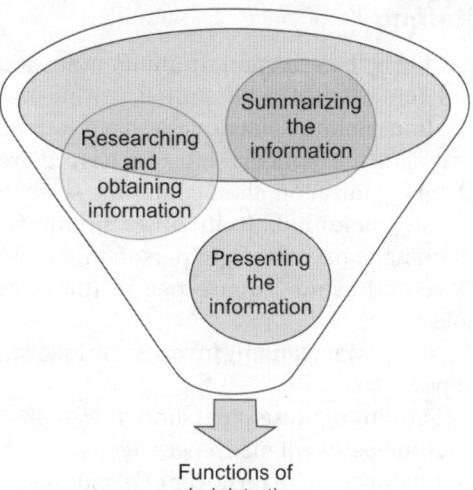

Functions of administration

Fig. 21.7: Functions of administration.

to each other in such a way that they are all combined and interrelated into a unit capable of being directed toward the organizational objectives."

- Work activities required for the organizational performance are separated through
  - **Horizontal differentiation** (i.e.. Dividing the organization into operational units for more effective and efficient performance.)
  - **Vertical differentiation** (i.e., Establishes the hierarchy and the number of levels in the organization.

The formal organization depends on two basic principles:

- **Responsibility:** Responsibility in an organization is divided among available personnel by grouping the functions that are similar in objectives and content. This should be done in a manner that avoids overlaps and gaps as much as possible. Responsibility may be continuing or it may be terminated by the accomplishment of a single action.
- **Authority:** When responsibility is given to a person, he must also be given the authority to make commitments, use resources and take the actions necessary to carry out his responsibilities.

Staffing

Staffing is the selection, training, motivating and retaining of a personnel in the organization. Before selection we have to make analysis of the particular job, which is required in the organization, then comes the selection of the personnel. It involves manpower planning to have the right person in the right place and avoid "square peg in the round hole".

Manpower planning involves the following steps.

- Scrutiny of present personnel strength.
- Anticipation of manpower needs.
- Investigation of turnover of personnel.
- Planning job requirements and job descriptions.

Directing

Directing means the issuance of orders, assignments and instructions that permit the subordinate to understand what is expected of him, and the guidance and overseeing of the subordinate so that he can contribute effectively and efficiently to the attainment of organizational objectives.

Directing includes the following activities:

- Giving orders
- Making supervision
- Leading
- Motivating
- Communicating

- **Giving orders:** The central task in directing is giving orders. The order is the technical means through which a subordinate understands what is to be done. To facilitate this there are certain characteristics of good orders which manager should be aware of:
  - The order should be clear, concise and consistent to give sufficient information to ensure understanding.
  - Order should be based on obvious demands of a particular situation, it seems logical to the subordinates and not just an arbitrary whim of the manager.

  - The tone of the order is very important. The manner in which the manager delivers the order has a great deal to do with its acceptance by the subordinate.
  - Whenever possible, the reason for the order should be given. A subordinate will accept an order more readily if he understands the need for it.
  - In some instances the manager uses delegation of authority instead of issuance of orders for avoiding too many specific orders.

- **Supervision:** Supervision is the activity of the management that is concerned with the training and discipline of the work force. It includes follow up to assure the prompt and proper execution of orders. Supervision is the art of overseeing, watching and directing with authority, the work and behavior of other.

- **Leading:** Leadership is the ability to inspire and influence others to contribute to the attainment of the objectives. Successful leadership is the result of interaction between the leader and his subordinates in a particular organizational situation. There are number of styles of leadership that have been identified such as autocratic, democratic participative leadership. The continuum of leadership styles, ranges from the completely authoritarian situation with no subordinate participation to a maximum degree of democratic leadership, enabling the subordinate to participate in all phases of the decision making process.

- **Motivating:** Motivation refers to the way in which the needs (urges, aspirations, desires) control, direct or explain the behavior of human beings. The manager must motivate, or cause, the employee to follow directives.

- **Communicating:** Communication is the passing of information and understanding from a sender to receiver. Communication is vital to the directing function of the management; one way to visualize this importance is to view the manager on one side of a barrier and the work group on the other. Communication is the means the manager has of reaching through the barrier to attain work group activity.

Coordinating

It is the act of synchronizing people and activities so that they function smoothly in the attainment of organization objectives. Coordination is more important in the health services organization, because functionally they are departmentalized. Different kinds of organization require different amount of coordination.

Basic Approaches to Coordination

- Corrective coordinations are those coordinative activities that rectify the present error or correct a dysfunction in the organization.
- Preventive coordination comprises those coordinative activities that are aimed at preventing the occurrence of anticipated problems of coordination, or at least minimizing the impact of these problems.
- Regulatory coordination comprises those coordinative activities that are aimed at the maintenance of existing structural and functional arrangements in the organizations.
- Promotive coordination has those coordinative activities that are aimed at attempting to improve the articulation of the parts of the organization, or to improve the existing organizational arrangements without regard for specific problems.

Controlling

Controlling can be defined as the regulation of activities in accordance with the requirements of plans.

Steps of control: The control function, whether it is applied to cash, medical care, employee morale or anything else, involves four steps.
- Establishments of standards.
- Measuring performance

- Comparing the actual results with the standards.
- Correcting deviations from standards.

Reporting and Recording

Reports are oral or written exchanges of information shared between caregivers or workers in a number of ways. A report summarizes the services of the person, personnel and of the agency. Reports are written usually daily, weekly, monthly or yearly.

Purposes of Reporting

- To show the kind and amount of services rendered over a specified period.
- To illustrate progress in reaching goals.
- As an aid in studying health conditions.
- As an aid in planning.
- To interpret services to the public and to the other interested agencies.

Records and reports must be functional, accurate, complete, current, organized and confidential.

Budgeting

Budgeting, though primarily recognized as a device for controlling, becomes a major part of the planning process in any organization. It is expressed in financial terms and based on expected income and expenditure. Budget is the heart of administrative management. It serves as a powerful tool of coordination and negatively an effective device of eliminating duplicating and wastage.

Features of Budget

- Should be flexible.
- Should be synthesis of past, present and future.
- Should be product of joint venture and cooperation of executives/department heads at different levels of management.
- It should be in the form of statistical standard laid down in specific numerical terms.
- It should have support of top management throughout the period of its planning and supplementation.

DIFFERENCE BETWEEN ADMINISTRATION AND MANAGEMENT

S. No.	Concept	Administration	Management
1.	Meaning	It means which determines the objective policies and directive principles of organization	It means which is related to the achievement of goals board of directors or governor.
2.	Term	Term used in civil institutions	Term used in companies, factories, firms-for work done through others.
3.	Enforcement	It enforced on rules: difficult and traditional	Enforced on results: innovative and imaginative.
4.	Results	The results cannot be measured easily	The results can be measured.
5.	Steps of process	Planning, organizing, staffing, directing, coordinating, recording, budgeting and evaluation.	Planning, organizing, directing, motivating, leading, controlling and evaluation.
6.	Coordination	Coordination of physical and human endeavor.	Coordination of individual and commodity.

NURSING ADMINISTRATION

Nursing management is performing leadership functions of governance and decision-making within organizations employing nurses. It includes processes common to all management like planning, organizing, staffing, directing and controlling. Nursing Administration is usually more of a broad scale job - like working in a hospital as the entire hospital's Patient Care Administrator (the ultimate nursing supervisor that deals with hospital-wide issues). The nurse administrator generally does not have a staff of nurses that are responsible for hiring and firing for an individual unit, but might hire nurse managers for the units, etc. The nurse administrator helps create patient care policies that affect the nursing care that is given and work with hospital-wide upper management. It is more behind the scenes work. And one 'almost' always need a master's degree.

Definition

- A nurse administrator is that person who is charged with the financial decision making, staff administration and policy making as concerns nurses

in an establishment. Such a nurse also supervises nursing staff, establishes work schedules, maintains medical supply inventories, and manages resources to ensure high-quality patient care.
- A nurse manager is an administrative position, within the medical profession and whose holder is charged with planning, organizing, staffing, directing and controlling
- Nurse administrators have a group of nurses working directly under them who, in addition to supervision, a nurse administrator also allocates resources to them accordingly. Building team efficiency and minimizing the risk of burnout are some of the responsibilities that a nurse administrator will have to take up.

Qualities of administrator: A nurse manager coordinates the work of other nurses with varying skills, education levels, and personalities while providing patients with safe and high-quality care. A few qualities of a good nurse manager are being a good leader and role model for their staff. Nurse Managers need to ensure that their unit or department is running smoothly at all times. The nursing staff looks up to their manager for clinical expertise and advice.

Communication and flexibility are also important traits that good nurse managers possess.

Responsibilities of nurse administrator: A nurse administrator will work in a variety of health care environments. They often manage a team of nurses, or a specific nursing unit or shift. They are fully trained in the implementation of nursing procedure and must hold their team of nurses accountable for their actions. Nurse administrators can interact directly with patients but often are assigned to a more managerial role. Nurse Administrator responsibilities may include:

- Overall responsibility for nursing patient care
- Establishing and documenting administrative procedure for the nursing team
- Promoting the development of nursing staff
- Budgeting and maintaining practice and standard guidelines
- Communication between practice and nursing staff
- Scheduling and supervising of nursing staff
- Analyzing nursing treatment and diagnosis decisions
- Troubleshooting and patient consultation
- Team building exercises and employee counseling.

A **Nurse Administrator** is highly trained and has knowledge of nursing procedure and protocol. They work as pivotal leaders in an organization and may aspire to chief executive positions. People drawn to this specialty want to be leaders in health care. They enjoy managing processes and people. Nurse Administrators are qualified to work in a variety of positions in the health care environment.

DIFFERENCE BETWEEN NURSE ADMINISTRATOR AND NURSE MANAGER

The terms nurse administrator and nurse manager are sometimes used interchangeably,

there is usually a difference in the overall responsibility, duties and salary for the two positions. A nurse administrator is usually responsible for a group of departments, an entire hospital or several hospitals, while a nurse manager is more likely to have the responsibility for one or more nursing units within a hospital or other healthcare organization. A nurse administrator often reports to the Chief Executive Officer in the organization or to a Vice President directly below the CEO, while nurse managers generally report directly to the nursing administrator.

- **Titles:** A nurse administrator may also be called a Director of Nurses, a Nurse Executive or a Vice President of nursing. In some organizations, the term Chief Nurse Executive is used to denote the nurse administrator. As these titles indicate, the scope of a nurse administrator's responsibilities is usually very broad. The nurse manager might have responsibilities that seem similar but on a smaller scale. Nurse Managers may also be known by the term head nurse or chief nurse.
- **Skills and responsibilities:** Both positions need basic business skills such as financial management and experience in areas such as human resources, strategic planning and systems thinking. Although both positions usually have financial and budgeting responsibilities, a nurse manager will develop and manage a budget for a nursing unit or department such as a critical care unit or emergency room. The nurse administrator, however, might need to budget for multiple nursing departments and may also be responsible for support services such as a transport department or home care.
- **Education and credentialing:** Nurse managers might have diploma or associate degrees, although many organizations prefer a bachelor's degree in nursing. A nurse administrator is nearly always have masters or doctoral level degrees in nursing or a related field such as health care administration. Certification in nursing management is available from

the American Nurses' Credentialing Center; the minimum educational level for certification is a bachelor's degree.

- **Accountability and patient care:** Both nurse administrators and nurse managers usually have 24-hour accountability for their areas of responsibility, although there might also be charge nurses or assistant nurse managers assigned to a particular shift or unit who provide management support. Nurse Managers may provide direct care to patients, depending on the size of the unit, the availability of staffing and the demands of their management duties. It is unusual for a nurse administrator to work at the bedside.

- **Wages:** Nurse Administrators tend to have higher wages than a nurse manager, although wages vary according to practice setting, locality, education and experience.

CONCLUSION

Administration is an enabling process, and in the sense in which it is usually understood, it covers the whole art of carrying into effect any policy, plan or undertaking, whether conceived by government, public or private agency. It may, however, go further than the single entire function of applying known rules to given cases, for in its widest form, it must embrace leadership, policy making and planning. Managers address complex issues by planning, budgeting, and setting target goals. They meet their goals by organizing, staffing, controlling and problem solving. The nurse manager can assist the staff to think strategically about what it is doing and what it should be doing for its clients, for example, in today's world of cost containment, examining what clients pay for the care they receive from the health care professionals

22

Management Process

LEARNING OBJECTIVES

- Planning
- Organization
- Staffing
- Directing/leading

- Control
- Budget
- Hospital

INTRODUCTION

A process is a series of steps or actions which lead to achieve a goal, and it is dynamic. Nurses are familiar with the application of nursing process, such as assessing, diagnosing, planning, implementing and evaluating the patient care in the health care management of their patients/clients in any setting. Similarly, nurse leaders must also be aware of various steps involved in the management process. Generally, the students are aware of managing their learning activities during their professional carrier, and in their work in professional practice. Some of the individuals

basically organized but some will learn through exposure to certain situations during their practice. The effective nurses are those who really understand and consciously apply the principles of management to practice.

PLANNING

Planning is important for socioeconomic development. It helps to conceive and achieve results in an atmosphere and spirit of true democratic situation, wherein different agencies at various levels are involved in the policies of the Government for welfare of its people. Planning is essentially a

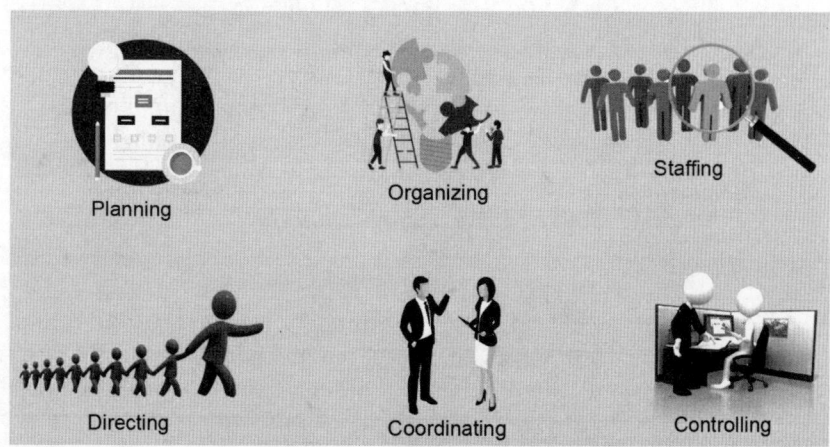

Fig. 22.1: Management process.

process of making choice between available alternatives at all levels of decision-making. It is the exercise of intelligence to deal with facts and solutions as they are find a way to solve problems. So, planning is an essence, an organized, conscious and continual attempt to select the best available alternative to achieve specific goods.

Planning is one of the major fundamental elements of administration. In planning stage, decisions are made about what needs to be done, how and when it has to be done, by whom and with what resources. Planning is an intellectual process of making decisions and it aims to achieve a co-ordinated and consistent set of operations aimed at desired objectives. For any work, planning is very essential.

Definitions of Planning

- Planning is a process of determining the objectives of administrative effort and devising the means calculated to achieve them. **—Millet**
- Planning is a process of setting formal guidelines and constraints for the behavior of the firm. **—Assoff and Brundinharg**

- Planning is a continuous process of making entrepreneurial decisions systematically and with the best possible knowledge for their future, organizing systematically the effort needed to carry out these decisions and measuring the results of the decisions against expectations through systematic feedback. **—Drucker**

Principles of Planning

- Planning must focus on purposes. It should always be based on a clearly defined objective.
- Planning is a continuous and iterative process which includes series of steps, so continuity and flexibility should be maintained in planning cycle.
- Planning should be simple and there should be provision for proper analysis and classification of actions.
- In planning, there should be a good harmony with organization and environment-political as well as economical etc.
- Planning is hierarchical in nature and must have an organizational identification.

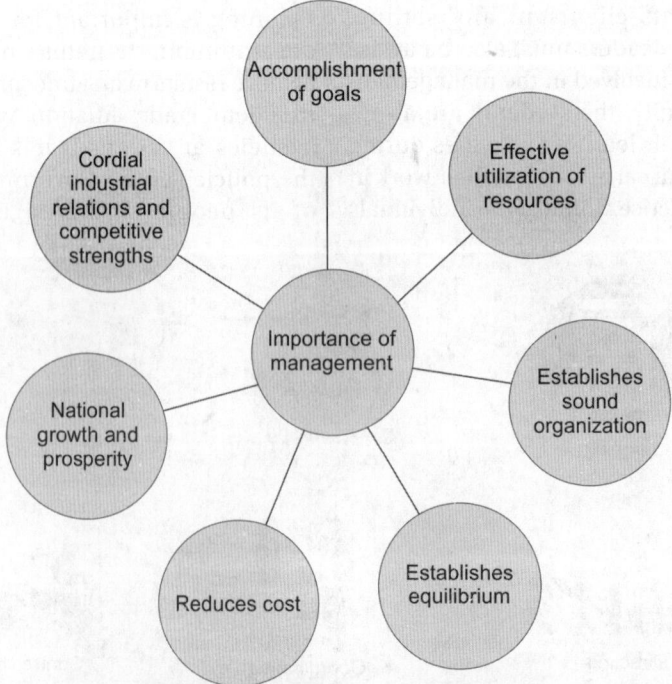

Fig. 22.2: Importance of management.

- Planning should be pervasive activity covering the entire organization with all its departments, sectors, and different levels of administration, and it should be balanced.
- Planning must be precise in its objective, scope and nature. It should be realistic in its scope and pinpoint the expected results.
- In planning, the provision should be made to use all available resources.
- Planning should always be documented so that the entire concerned are fully committed to the implementation of the program.

Importance of Planning

- It attempts to offset uncertainty by foreseeing the future and bringing about preparedness for the happing in the future.
- It focuses attention on the objectives or goals of the organization and their achievement.
- It leads to economy in operation through the selection of the best possible course of action.
- It helps in controlling the activities by providing measures against which performance can be evaluated.
- It helps in coordinating the operations of organizations since a well-considered

plan embraces and unifies all the divisions in an organization.

Characteristics of Planning

Planning has number of characteristics as given below:

- **Primacy:** Planning is an important element in the administration that usually precedes other elements or functions of administration. Obviously without setting the goals to be reached and lines of action to be followed, there is nothing to organize, to direct, or to control in the enterprises.
- **Continuity:** Planning is a continuous and never-ending activity of an administrator or manager to keep the enterprise as a going concern. One plan begets another plan to be followed by a series of other plans in quick succession. Actually, a hierarchy of plans operates in the enterprise at anytime. Planning gets used up where tomorrow becomes today and calls for further planning day-in and day-out. Again, incessant changes make replanning a continuous necessity.
- **Flexibility:** Planning leads to the adoption of a specific course of action and the rejection of other possibilities. This confinement to one course takes away flexibility. But if future assumptions upon which planning are based prove wrong, the course of action has to be adapted to altered situations for avoiding any deadlock. Accordingly, when the future cannot be molded to conform to the course of action, flexibility is to be in grained in planning for adapting the course of action to demands of current situation.

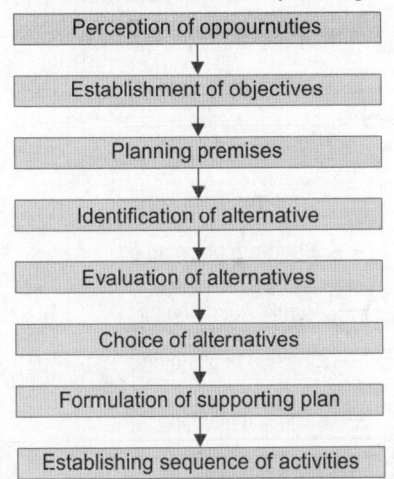

Flowchart 22.1: Need for planning.

Perception of oppournuties

Establishment of objectives

Planning premises

Identification of alternative

Evaluation of alternatives

Choice of alternatives

Formulation of supporting plan

Establishing sequence of activities

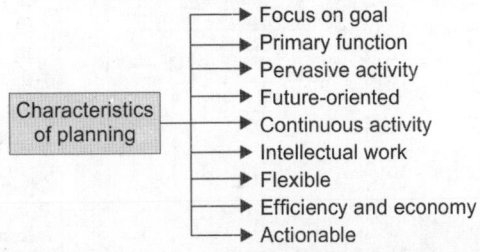

Flowchart 22.2: Characteristics of planning.

Characteristics of planning
- Focus on goal
- Primary function
- Pervasive activity
- Future-oriented
- Continuous activity
- Intellectual work
- Flexible
- Efficiency and economy
- Actionable

Compartment of Planning

- **Objectives:** Objectives are basic plans which determine goals or end results of the projected action of an enterprise. By setting goals, objectives provide the foundation upon which structure of plan can be built.
- **Policies:** Policies are written statements or oral understanding. In some, they are general terms for governing actions in repetitive situations. Realization of objectives is made easy with the help of policies, as policies provide standing solutions to problem.
- **Procedures:** Procedures indicate the specific manner in which a certain activity is to be performed. They are more definite and specific guides to action, but only for fulfillment of objectives.
- **Program:** Program welds together different plans for implementing them into completely and orderly course of action. Programs are necessary for both repetitive (routine planning) and non-repetitive (creative planning) course of action.
- **Budget:** Budgets are plans continuing statements of expected results in numerical terms; i.e. rupees, man-hours, product units and so forth.

Types of Planning

Planning must be done at several levels and each has its own particular problems and configuration of the planners and methods. Planning may be classified as directional planning, administrative planning, and operational planning.

- **Directional planning:** It is often called policy planning, and is concerned with the broad general direction of the program, i.e. setting the framework of intent and philosophy within which the program will proceed, and with relating the program to the broad planning of the community in which the program will function. For example, State level planning at Directorate or Secretariat of States or Union (Center).
- **Administrative planning:** It is concerned with the overall implementation of the policies developed and with the mobilization and co-ordination of the personnel and material available in the administrative unit for the effectuation of the service. For example, Medical

Flowchart 22.3: Types of planning.

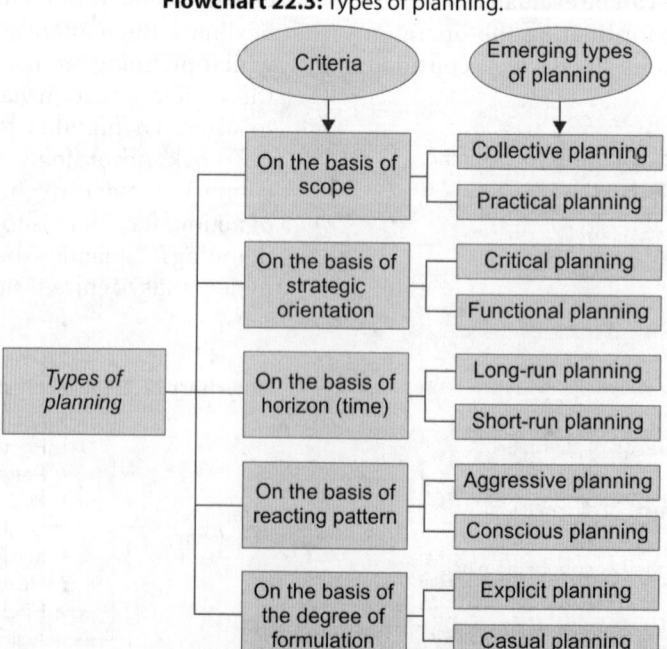

Superintendent of major hospitals or district Surgeon of district hospitals or Medical Suptd. of Primary health centre are responsible for administrative planning.

- **Operational Planning:** It is concerned with the actual delivery of the service to the community. For example, nursing personnel of all level are planning to deliver proper service to the community either in hospital or community. Planning may be classified as long-range and short-range and also strategic and operational. There are similar activities involved and long-range and short-range planning and also strategic and operation planning.
  - **Strategic planning,** usually, the strategic and long-range planning is undertaken by the top level which involves following activities:
    - ◆ Detail analysis of strength, weakness, opportunities, and threats (SWOT) of organization both internal and external environment.
    - ◆ Developing philosophy and formulation of policies and objectives on the basis of analysis of the organization.
    - ◆ Allocation of resources on the basis of priority.
    - ◆ Evaluation of activities to increase efficiency.

- ◆ Providing proper direction to avoid duplication of services.
- **Operational planning,** usually, this operational and short-range planning is undertaken by middle or supervisory level personnel. This involves:
  - ◆ Planning for a few months to a financial year.
  - ◆ Planning for details budgeting, provision for short-range goods and it should be achieved within given period.
  - ◆ Extensional aspect of long range plan.

Sometime, it can applied our nursing situation. Budgeting time and related budgetary other provision for providing nursing care in according to events and situation arises.

Methods of Planning

Planning is a process of analyzing and understanding a system, formulating its goals and objectives, assessing its capabilities, designing alternative courses of action or plans for the purposes of achieving these goals and objectives, evaluating the effectiveness of these plans, choosing the preferred plan, initiating the necessary action for its implementation and monitoring the system to ensure the implementation of the plan and its desired effect on the system. Health planning is an orderly process of defining community health problems, identifying correct needs and surveying the resources to meet them, establishing priority goals that are realistic and feasible and projecting administrative action to accomplish the purpose of the proposed program.

The above statement of planning process gives us series of steps in planning which include:

- Analysis of the health situation,
- Establishment of objectives and goals,
- Assessment of resources,
- Fixing priorities,
- Write-up the formulated plan,
- Programming and implementation, and
- Evaluation.

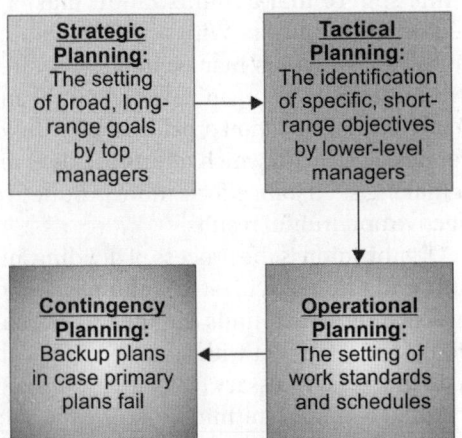

Fig. 22.3: Methods of planning.

ORGANIZATION

Definitions of Organization

- Organization is the form of every human association for the attainment of common purpose the process of relating specific duties or function in a whole.

  —J D Mooney

- Organization is the process of combining the work in which individuals and groups have to perform with the faculties necessary for its execution. So that the units so formed provide the best channels for efficient, systematic, positive and co-coordinated application of the available.

  —Olive Sheldon

- Organization is a system of co-operative activities of two or more persons.

  —Chester Bernard

- Organization consists of the relationship of individual to individuals and groups to groups which are related as to bring about an orderly division of labour **—Pfiffiner**

- An organization is a combination of necessary human beings, equipment, facilities and appurtenances, materials and tools assembled in some synthetic and effective co-ordination in order to accomplish some desired and designed objective. But when one speaks of the organization, reference is usually to the body of persons who have been brought together to carry on the enterprises and who are being taught up as an entity.

  —O. Tead

- Organization is the arrangement of personnel for facilitating the accomplishment of some agreed purpose through allocation of functions and responsibilities. **—L. White**

Aims of Organization

- To increase managerial efficiency in a number of ways.
- To ensure an optimum use of human efforts through specialization.
- To make use of all resources.
- To place a proportionate and balanced emphasis on various activities.
- To facilitate co-ordination in the enterprises.
- To provide training and developing managers.
- To encourage individuals growth development according to individual potentials through job enrichment, training and participation.
- To invite creative and innovative ideas to working through adopting human relations approach.
- To prevent overlapping.

Nature of Organization

The policy of plan having been decided, the near step is organization, and it is perhaps in this sphere that administration makes it greatest contribution. With a view to getting things done by others, management is required to pay attention on organizing personnel and their work. Organization provides the means of avenues along with which efforts are directed for making such joint efforts more productive, effective and fruitful results.

Organization is the process of dividing and combining the activities. It is the process of organization which finds the means, human and material to meet with situation foreseen. To do this, it is necessary to:

- Make careful determination of what jobs are to be done and what workers are required to do them.

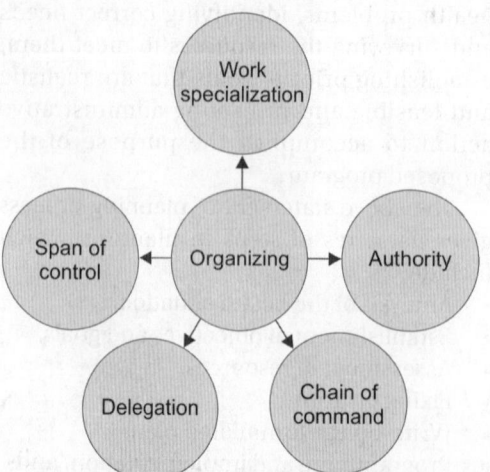

Fig. 22.4: Aims of organization.

- Assess the amount of materials, tools, and equipment needed for the accomplishment of the work.

Administration which carries the responsibility of accomplishing results through the effort of other people is concerned not only with the direction, but also with the development of people. The organization of work is very much a human affair, in which results, through visibly depending on materials and equipment, cannot be accomplished except by human effort. The purpose of organization is to unify that effort and a clear understanding of human relationship is necessary if the desired result is to be obtained.

Importance of Organization

- Organization increases managerial efficiency in a number of ways. It provides the structure, within which the functions of administration are performed.
  - It avoids delay, duplication or confusion in performance and remove, friction or rivalry among personnel.

- Analysis of objectives of institution provides all pertinent activities.
- Activities in turn are allocated to particular individuals.
- Assignment of fixed duties helps to add certainty and promptness in their work.
- Organization ensures an optimum use of human efforts through specialization and also makes use of all resources, determines needs for innovative and new technologies in terms of cost effectiveness and accomplish objectives. Details job specification helps for right persons are placed in the right position on the basis of their knowledge, skill, and experience.
- Organization places a proportionate and balanced emphasis on various activities. Money and efforts can be spent proportionately with the importance of activities.
- Organization facilitates co-ordination in the enterprises.

Different departments and section, positions and jobs functions welded

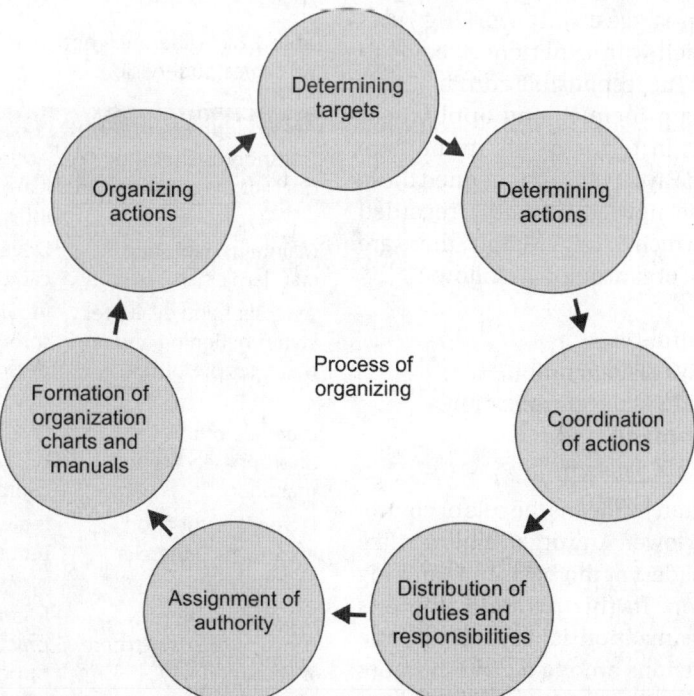

Fig. 22.5: Process of organization.

together by structural relationship of the organization.

- Organization provides scope for training and developing managers. Encourages individual's growth and development of personnel according to individual potentials through job enrichment, training and participation.
- Organization helps to consolidate growth and expansion of the enterprise/institution. It helps in growth and development of the establishment, in planning for need based change through appropriate division and allotment of works.
- Organization invites creative and innovative ideas to working through adopting human relations approach.
- Organization prevents the growth of laggards, wirepuller, intriguers, or other forms of corrupters.
- Unsound organization becomes the breeding ground of corruption, dishonesty and such odd things.

Principles of Organization

In the words of White (1955), the principles of organization suggest only working rules of conduct which with experience seems to have validated. The responsible administrator must know the principles and apply them with judgment in terms of his immediate situation. Henri Fayol (1947) has defined these principles as "acknowledged truths, regarded as preview on which to rely". Mainly, there are six principles of organization as follows:

- Hierarchy,
- Span of control,
- Integration vs disintegration,
- Centralization vs decentralization,
- Unity of command, and
- Delegation.

Hierarchy: Hierarchy means the rule or control of the higher to lower. Any organization is like a pyramid, broadest at the base and tapering towards the top. In this pyramid, there is hierarchy. Organization is, essentially, the division of functions among a given number of persons. The distribution of functions and responsibilities is both horizontal and

vertical. An organization structure grows both horizontally and vertically. When additional levels are added in an organization structure, it is called vertical growth. But when more functions or more positions are added without increasing the number of level, it is called horizontal growth. Vertical distribution creates levels like top management, middle management, supervision and the level of specific performance. Strictly speaking, these levels cannot inherent superiority and inferiority. However, due to the difference in nature of responsibility of various levels, the difference in the salary scales as between different levels and difference in the qualifications and qualities of the personnel manning various levels, superior, subordinate relationship does emerge in the organization.

Span of control: Span of control means the number of subordinates an officer can effectively supervise. It is simply the number of subordinates or the units of work that an administrator can personally direct. In other words, the number of subordinates that a supervisor can personally direct or supervise is known as "span of control". There is no

Table 22.1: Difference between line management and clinical supervision.

Line Management	Clinical Supervision
Is responsible for the goals of the organization	Addresses the learning needs of the individual practitioner
Maintains minimum standards	Develop excellence in clinical practice
Assessees and evaluates staff functioning and manages performance	Provides relationship through which personal/ professional development occurs
Is carried out by an appropriately trained manager	Is conducted by a properly trained clinical supervisor
Is a normal function about which there is no choice	Is always and of its nature voluntary
Is a management function to ensure there is accountability	Is individual practitioners opportunity for learning and Development

agreement as to the exact number, but there exist a general agreement that the shorter the span, the greater will be contact and consequently more effective control. That there is a limit to the span of controls of every person or officer is readily admitted. The 'span of control' is related to psychological problem of 'span of attention'. None of us can attend to more than a certain number of things at the same time. The number to which one can do attend is ones 'span of attention'. 'Span of control' is nothing but the span of attention applied to these works of supervision and control of subordinates. But the span of control is greatly determined by the type of activity and by the supervisor's capability.

Integration vs Disintegration: Integration means unification in administrative language, integration means connecting one or more of hitherto independent organization with the rest of the organizational structure of the country by placing them under the Chief Executive directly or through some department. It involves the abolition of the independent status of agencies, e.g. independent regulatory commissioners. An integrated administrative system, therefore, is one, all the parts of which are connected together through common ultimate subordinates to the Chief Executive of the country. In such system, the line of authority runs unbroken from the Chief Executive, through various levels to all the parts of the system, so that there are no loose ends anywhere. A disintegrated system, on the other hand, has got a number of loose ends in the shape of independent establishments and directly elective persons at which or whom the line of authority from the Chief Executives stops short and it is broken.

Centralization vs decentralization: Centralization stands for concentration of authority at or near the top. An organization is said to be centralized if most of the power of decision is vested in the top level so that the lower ones have to refer most problems to the head of the organization or his immediate subordinates for decision.

Decentralisation means that the Central Authority gives certain power to the local authorities. A decentralized organization is one in which the lower levels are allowed the discretion to decide most of the matters which come up, reserving comparatively a few bigger and more important problems only for those higher up. Decentralization has five aspects, two of which are administrative, one political, one geographical, and one functional.

These are as follows:
- Delegation of authority in such a way that large areas of discretion are entrusted to subordinate officers and comparatively few questions are referred to Chief at the apex.
- Broad grant of power to individual component parts of the organization and retention of only certain essential powers of control in the head office.
- Much power in the hands of elective bodies and consider popular participation in administration.
- Freedom to field units or agencies away from headquarters and near to people. Functional autonomy to the various departments in respect of their several functions. Whereas centralization is the opposite of above five aspects of arrangements.

Neither centralization nor decentralization can be accepted in an absolute principle of good organization under these circumstances; experts or administrators either plead for

Table 22.2: Difference between integration and disintegration.

	Integration	Disintegration
Individual	• Duty and/or privilege of certain newcomers • 'Assimilation' • Participation	• 'Hostile environment' • Exclusion (from services etc.) • 'Organized disintegration' towards asylum-seekers
Collective	• Social/ community cohesion • Inclusive societies and/ or institutions	• Social conflict • Fragmentation • Lack of trust • Institutional racism • 'Soziale Desintegration'

Table 22.3: Comparison chart.

Basis for Comparison	Centralization	Decentralization
Meaning	The retention of powers and authority with respect to planning and decisions, with the top management, is known as Centralization	The dissemination of authority, responsibility, and accountability to the various management levels, is known as Decentralization
Involves	Systematic and consistent reservation of authority	Systematic dispersal of authority
Communication Flow-	Vertical	Open and Free
Decision Making	Slow	Comparatively faster
Advantage	Proper coordination and leadership	Sharing of burden and responsibility
Power of decision making	Lies with the top management	Multiple persons have the power of decision making
Reasons	Inadequate control over the organization	Considerable control over the organization
Best suited for	Small sized organization	Large sized organization

Flowchart 22.4: Unity of command advantages.

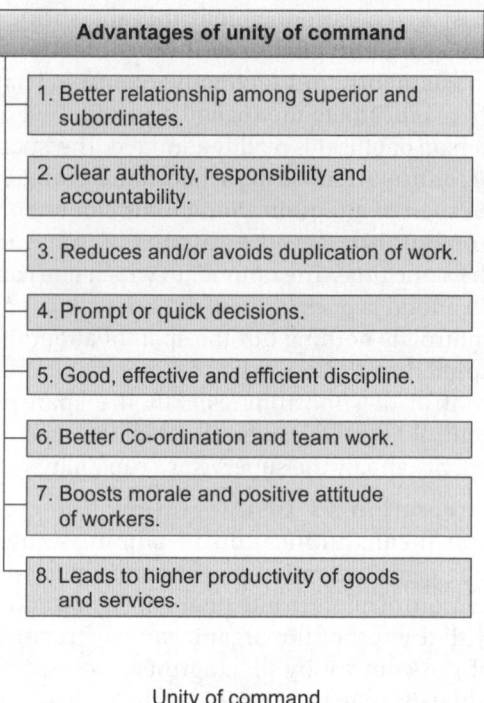

Advantages of unity of command

1. Better relationship among superior and subordinates.
2. Clear authority, responsibility and accountability.
3. Reduces and/or avoids duplication of work.
4. Prompt or quick decisions.
5. Good, effective and efficient discipline.
6. Better Co-ordination and team work.
7. Boosts morale and positive attitude of workers.
8. Leads to higher productivity of goods and services.

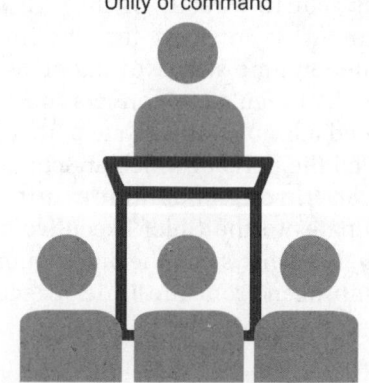

Unity of command

Fig. 22.6: Unity of command hierarchy.

compromise between the two principles, or else maintain that each case for the application

Unity of command: Unity of command means that no individual employee should be subjected to the orders of more than one immediate superior. The concept of unity of command requires that every member of an organization should report to one and only one leader. Henri Fayol is a great advocate of this principle, meant that an employee should receive orders from one superior only. When it is jeopardy, order disturbed and stability threatened, diversity of command may also result in the subordinates playing off one superior against another or other. All this may cause confusion and blurring of responsibility.

It is true that command, orders or guiding should always come from one delegating supervisor; otherwise there are chances of shortage of duties, of abusing authority and of evading accountability. Theoretically, the principle of unity of command appears to be unassailable; in practice has some important exceptions to it. For example, an individual employee is frequent subjected to a dual control, i.e., one administrative and the other technical or professional. The head of the professional colleges of the Government has academic control by it. Universities and has administrative control by the respected Government.

Unity of command helps increasing co-ordination in the organization. Co-ordination me negatively the removal of conflicts, working at cross-purposes, and overlapping from administration; positively co-ordination's aim is to secure co-operation and team work among the numerous employees engaged in the work of the organization.

Delegation: In an organization, usually, all authority legally belongs to the head of the organization, but in practice no head can

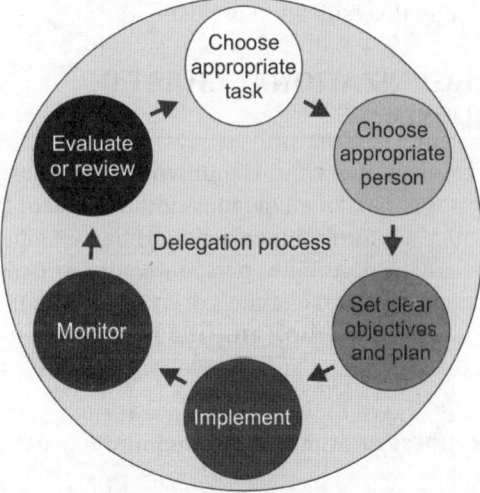

Fig. 22.7: Delegation process.

actually exercise all the powers legally vested in him, he would be overwhelming with detail; so there is a need that sufficient authority has to be given to every employee to enable him to do his job. The device of distributing his authority is 'delegation. Delegation means conferring of specified authority by a higher authority. It is devolution authority by a person to his agent or subordinate, subject to his right of supervision control. As an integral part of the organizing process, delegation has three essential aspects or dimensions:

1. *Assignment duty:* As one person cannot perform all the tasks, he must allocate a part of his work to subordinates for the purposes of accomplishment by them.

2. *Grant of authority:* If the delegated duty is to be discharged by subordinates, they must be entrusted with requisite authority for enabling them to make such work performance. While granting authority to subordinates, the executive, some reserve authority should be retained with him for his own performance.

3. *Creation of accountability:* Delegation of duties implies accountability from the side of subordinates. With the allocation of powers and duties, there must be logically the obligation on the part of subordinates to render an account of their performance. Because of this accountability, the manager must keep for himself some

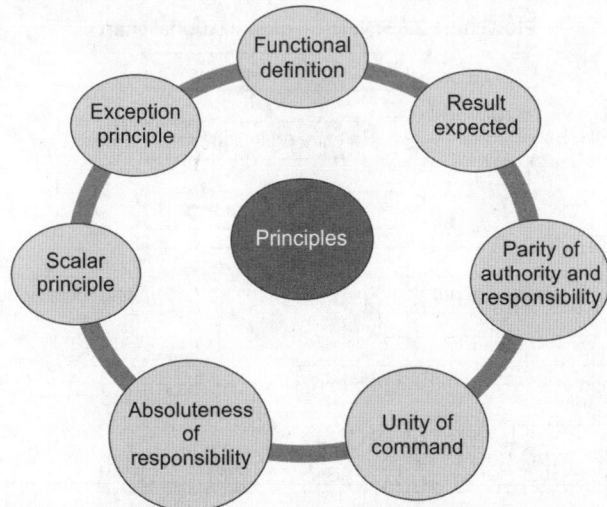

Fig. 22.8: Principles of delegation.

reserved authority and duties for directing, regulating and controlling the course of work undertaken by his subordinates.

Principles of Delegation

There are four fundamental principles which serve as guides for effective delegation.

1. Assignment of duties in terms of expected results.
2. Parity of authority and responsibility. While assigning duties to subordinates, there should be equality of authority and responsibility.
3. **Clarification of limits of authority:** It is the clear limit of authority that permits subordinates to exercise initiative to develop their personal capacity through freedom of action and to know their area of operation.
4. **Unity of command:** As employee should receive orders from one superior only. So subordinates should always be placed under the guidance, control and supervision of one supervisor/superior who will set up work priorities and will arrange for co-operation.

Advantages of Delegation

- Delegation serves as a vehicle of co-ordination. The various levels of the organization are used more appropriately.
- A sound system of delegation tends to develop an increased sense of responsibility and enhanced potential work capacity of individual employees.
- It reduces the executive burden—it relieves the superior of time-consuming, minor duties and allows him to concentrate more effectively on major responsibilities of his own position.
- Delegation minimizes delay when decisions have no longer to be referred up the line.
- Proper delegation of authority is conductive to an effective control over operation.
- As delegation provides the means of multiplying the limited personal capacity of the superior it is instrumental for encouraging and diversification of business.

ORGANIZATIONAL CHART IN NURSING

Organizational chart is a drawing that shows how the parts of an organization are linked. It depicts the formal organizational relationships, areas of responsibility, persons to whom one is accountable and channels of communication. It is a diagram shows the different positions and departments, and the relationships among them.

Purposes of organizational chart: It is used to show:

- The formal organizational relationships.
- Areas of responsibility.

Flowchart 22.5: Vertical organizational chart.

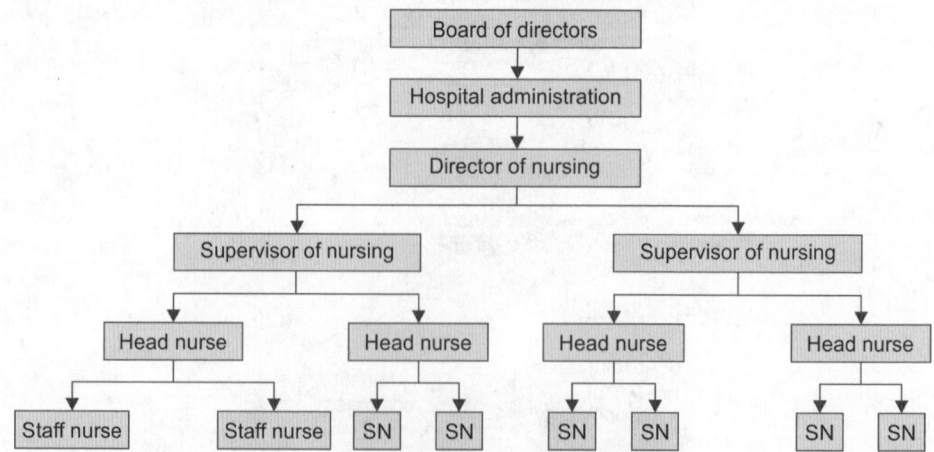

Vertical organizational chart

- Persons to whom one is accountable.
- Channels of communication.

Characteristics of an Effective Organizational Chart

- Be accurate, clear, simple, and updated.
- Shows the chain of command, lines of authority, responsibility, and relationships.
- All members of the department should be notified when any change occurs.

Principles of Organizational Chart

- The chart should have a clear title.
- It should be dated.
- The higher management should be shown at the top, while most junior position at the end of the chart.
- Positions of equal seniority should be shown at the same level.
- For clarity, details should be well spaced.
- Solid lines must be used to indicate flow of authority; staff relationships can be shown by a dotted line.
- Colors may be used to distinguish between departments.

Types of organizational chart: There are three types of organizational charts: Vertical, horizontal and circular charts.

- **Vertical charts:** It shows high-level management at the top with formal lines of authority down the hierarchy, are most common.
- **A left-to-right (horizontal) charts:** It shows the high-level management at the left with lower positions to the right. It shows relative length of formal lines of authority, helps simplify understanding the lines of authority and responsibility.
- **Circular charts:** It shows the high-level management in the center with successive positions in circles. It shows the outward flow of formal authority from the high-level management. It reduces status implications.

Organizational Chart Helps in Nursing

- To plan, provide and evaluate nursing care for patient and families.

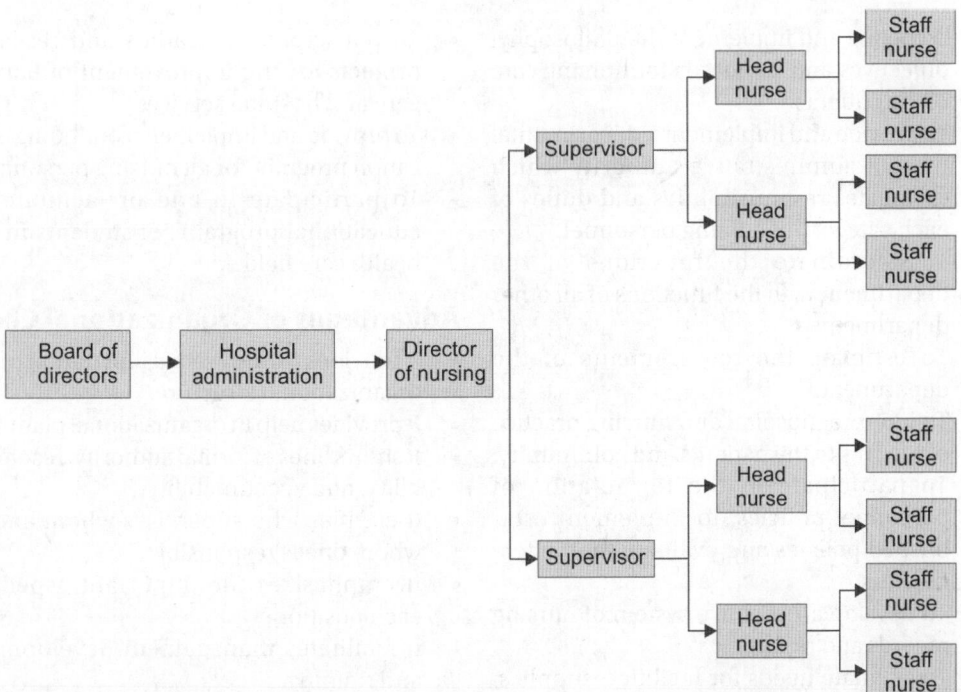

Fig. 22.9: Left-to-right (horizontal) organizational chart.

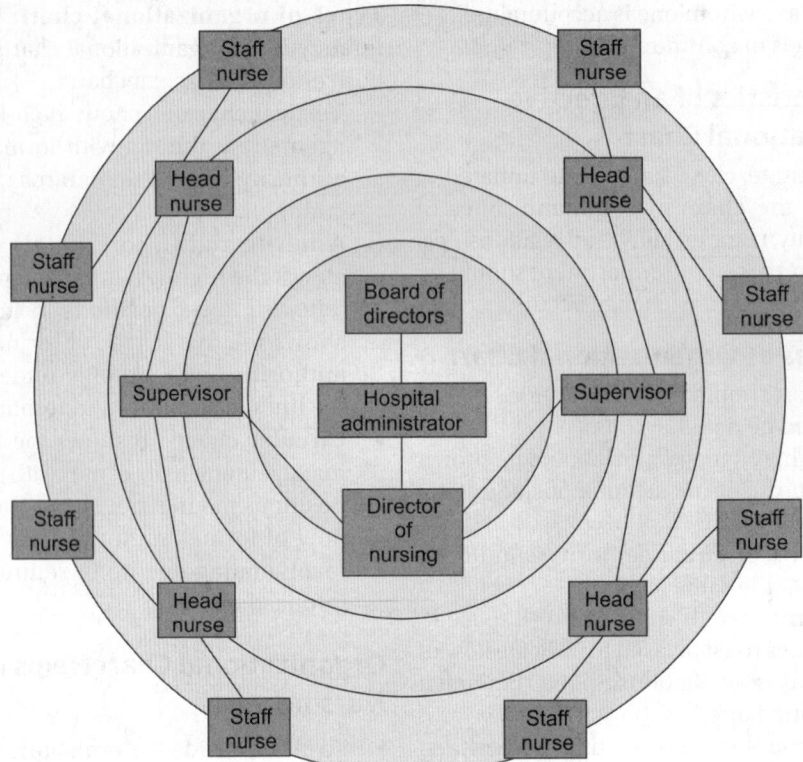

Fig. 22.10: Circular organizational chart.

- To define and implement the philosophy, objectives and standards for nursing care of the patients.
- To provide and implement a departmental plan of administrative authority which delineates responsibilities and duties of each category of nursing personnel.
- To coordinate the functions of the department with the functions of all other departments.
- To estimate the requirements of the department.
- To interpret hospital and nursing practice objectives to the patients and community.
- To participate in the formulation of personnel policies, to implement established policies and evaluate their effectiveness.
- To develop an effective system of nursing records and reports.
- To estimate needs for facilities, supplies, and equipment.
- To participate in financial planning.

- To participate in studies and research projects for the improvement of patient care and hospital services.
- To provide and implement continuing education program for all nursing personnel.
- To participate in and or facilitate all educational programs of students in the health care field.

Advantages of Organizational Chart

- It provides a quick visual illustration of the organizational structure.
- It provides help in organizational planning.
- It shows lines of formal authority, responsibility, and accountability.
- It clarifies who supervises whom and to whom one is responsible.
- It emphasizes the important aspect of each position.
- It facilitates management development and training.
- It is used to evaluate strengths and weakness of current structure.

- It provides starting points for planning organizational changes.
- It describes channels of communication.

Disadvantages of Organizational Chart

- Charts become outdated quickly.
- Does not show informal relationship.
- Does not show duties and responsibilities.
- Poorly prepared charts might create misleading effects.

STAFFING

Staffing refers to the continuous process of finding, selecting evaluating and developing a working relationship with current or future employees. The main goal of staffing is to fill the various roles within the organization with suitable candidates. Staffing is the process of hiring eligible candidates in the organization or company for specific positions. It also improves the quality and quantity of work done by the company because they have staffed the optimum people. Job satisfaction rates are likely to increase because everyone is well-suited for their position and is happy to be doing their specialty of work. Higher rates of productive performance from the company are also common, as they have staffed the right people to do their jobs. It provides employees the opportunity for further growth and development.

Definitions of Staffing

- Staffing involves choosing competent and suitable personnel for different positions in the organization.
- Staffing may be defined as the management function of employing and developing human resources for carrying out various managerial and non-managerial activities of the organization.
- Staffing basically involves matching jobs and individuals.
- Staffing involves making people suitable to jobs, while organizing is concerned with creation of jobs.

Objectives of staffing: The staffing function of management is the most important and significant on account of the following:

- Without people, human resources, organizations become empty entities and cannot achieve the objectives for which they have been established.
- All other managerial functions: planning, organizing, direction, and control become non-starters without the required personnel for carrying out these functions.
- Performance of an organization depends to a large extent on the efficiency and effectiveness of the other managerial functions which depend on the efficiency with which staffing function is done.
- Staffing is responsible for retaining and developing there right people both in terms of quality and in number and placing them to right jobs to take full advantage of human resources efficiently.
- Staffing function makes an organization strong and capable of meeting the changing situations as it is rightly responsible for developing abilities, skills and efforts

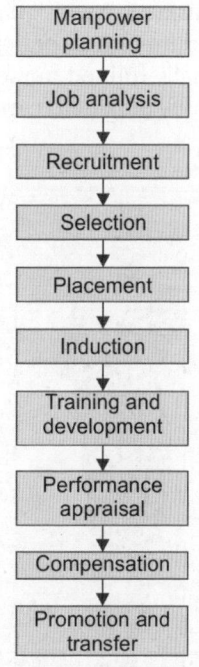

Flowchart 22.6: Process of staffing.

of it personnel through training and development programmes.

- Physical, financial and other resources of the organization are efficiently allocated and utilized, only through the function of staffing since it is the people who have to use all other resources.

Mission and Philosophy of Staffing

Mission of Staffing

- To ensure maximum utilization of human resources.
- To discover and obtain competent personal for various job.
- Adequate staffing ensures continuous survival and growth of enterprise.
- To improve job satisfaction, morale of employees through objective assessment.
- To meet the crisis at the time of emergency.
- To deliver good quality of care and attain job satisfaction and patient satisfaction.

Philosophy of Staffing

- The nurse administrator believes that it is possible to match (nurse) staff's or Employees knowledge and skill to the patient care, therefore it save way to attain the job satisfaction with quality of care.
- Nurse administrator believes that only professionally trained nurses can provide a high quality of patient care.

- Nurse administrator believes that only professionally skillful nurses can handle critically ill patients by providing technical and humanistic care.
- Nurse administrator believes that a professional nurse can treat chronically ill patient, provide health education, and provide rehabilitative care which is more complex.
- Nurse administrator believes that by determining patient needs and doing patient assignment only job quantification and job analysis can be done.
- Nurse administrator believes that all sortz of nursing related plans for example., master rotation plan, duty roster should be done only by nursing heads.
- Nurse administrator believes that staffing plan to be delegated to each unit level head nurse so that each ward activities, details of each shift are planned well.

Importance of Staffing

The staffing function is the life blood of an organization, even with increased use of computer technology, the importance of human resource cannot be over emphasized. As has been stated by TB Greenfield, a thinker on educational administration "organization do not think, act, achieve goals (or) make decisions. The staffing function

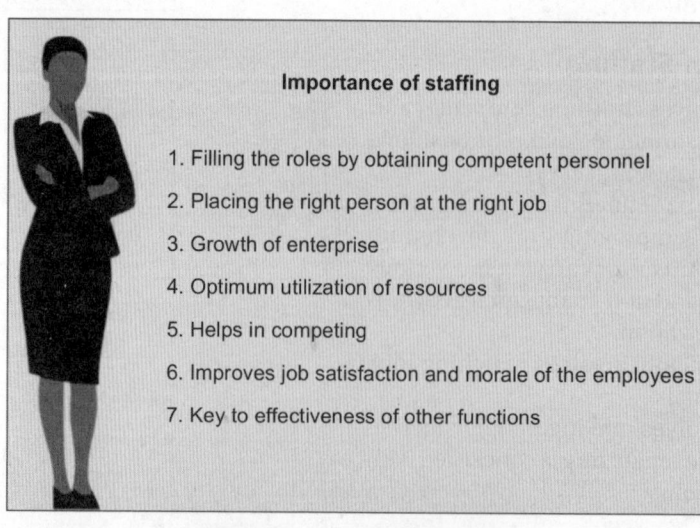

Importance of staffing

1. Filling the roles by obtaining competent personnel
2. Placing the right person at the right job
3. Growth of enterprise
4. Optimum utilization of resources
5. Helps in competing
6. Improves job satisfaction and morale of the employees
7. Key to effectiveness of other functions

Fig. 22.11: Importance of staffing.

of management is the most important and significant on account of the following:

- Without people, human resources, organizations become empty entities and cannot achieve the objectives for which they have been established.
- All other managerial functions-planning, organizing, direction and control become non-starters without the required personnel for carrying out these functions.
- Performance of an organization depends to a large extent on the efficiency and effectiveness of the other managerial functions which depend on the efficiency with which staffing function is done.
- Staffing is responsible for retaining and developing there right people both in terms of quality and in number and placing them to right jobs to take full advantage of human resources efficiently.
- Staffing function makes an organization strong and capable of meeting the changing situations as it is rightly responsible for developing abilities, skills and efforts of it personnel through training and development programs.
- Physical, financial, and other resources of the organization are efficiently allocated and utilized, only through the function of staffing, since it is the people who have to use all other resources. To carry out effective nursing care is also dependent on many factors. They are as follows:
  - **Type of service:** Each type of service, such as medicine, surgery, obstetrics, pediatrics, etc. differs in the nursing hours required. For example, more nurses are needed for children than for adults, and isolated patients need more nursing.
  - **Acuteness of illness:** The degree of illness affects the amount of nursing care needed. In some studies, acutely ill and therefore completely dependent patients have been known to require 430 minutes in the first (morning), 186 in the second (afternoon), and 124 during the night shift.
  - **Experience of nurses:** Graduate nurses are usually more mature in judgment,

more skilled and able to work more rapidly (efficiently). Student nurses in upper classes are more experienced and skilled than younger students.
- **Amount and quality of supervision:** Nurses who are well-supervised learn to use their time more efficiently.
- **Availability of nursing aides:** Nursing aides (variously called nursing assistants, nursing orderlies, etc.) can play an important role in saving time of nurses if properly trained. Nursing assistants/medical assistants, who are nursing aides, take on many nursing tasks in military hospitals, thereby significantly reducing the nurse to patient ratio in military hospitals.
- **Teaching function:** Inexperienced medical students often need assistance and supervision from nurses. There are more treatments and tests performed on patients in a teaching hospital. More nursing staff is needed to meet these demands in teaching hospitals.
- **Plan of nursing units (wards):** In an open type of ward, the patients are in full view of nurse, and it is easier to see what is happening. Therefore, supervision of the patients is easier. In wards where patients are housed in small units (Rig's pattern), more number of nursing staff are required.
- **Physical facilities:** Good functional planning of physical facilities minimizes avoidable walking and waste of time of nurses.
- **Location of equipment and supplies:** Time-saving equipments and their availability at nursing units save nurses' time. A central supply department and flash sterilizers are two examples.
- **Working hours and shifts:** When the staff is able to work only certain fixed hours and days, the result is inflexibility, and more nurses are needed to adequately cover all parts of the day.
- **Hospital routine:** Although reports and record keeping are essential, more complex the system of record keeping and reporting, the more nursing time is

consumed in clerical work. Availability of a less technical person to handle telephone communications, direct visitors, assemble charts and papers, and check supplies, etc. enhances nurses' time available for nursing.

- **Assignment method:** Other things apart, the functional method of assignment of work is more efficient than case or team method. The team method where the assignment of duties is based upon analysis of functions to be performed, competencies available and supervision required is a popular method and is quite effective if properly organized and supervised.

Steps of Staffing

- Planning for staffing vis-à-vis size, composition, nature and time frame.
- Recruitment and selection.
- Placement of staff an orientation to members of staff.
- Training and development of all categories of staff.
- Formulation of policies for promotion and transfer to prevent stagnation and frustration.
- Formulation of policies for rewarding performance and punishing non-performance.
- Development of potentials through job enrichment, value generation and self-development.

Functions of Staffing

- The first and foremost function of staffing is to obtain qualified personnel for different jobs position in the organization.
- In staffing, the right person is recruited for the right jobs; therefore it leads to maximum productivity and higher performance.
- It helps in promoting the optimum utilization of human resource through various aspects.
- Job satisfaction and morale of the workers increases through the recruitment of the right person.

- Staffing helps to ensure better utilization of human resources.
- It ensures the continuity and growth of the organization, through development managers.

Recruitment

Recruitment refers to the discovery and developments of the sources of require personnel so that sufficient number of candidates will always be available for employment in the organization. It involves identifying an attracting job candidate who has the required abilities, attitudes and motivation so as to meet the manpower requirements of the enterprise.

Definition: Recruitment has been defined as "the process of searching of prospective employees and stimulating them to apply for jobs in the organizations".

Methods of Recruitment

- **Transfer:** A transfer refers to the shifting of an employee from one job to another without a drastic change in the responsibilities and status of the employee.
- **Promotion:** It involves shifting an employee to a higher position carrying higher responsibilities, higher status and more pay.
- **Advertisements:** Advertising in newspaper or trade and professional journals is a very popular source of recruitment.
- **Employment agencies:** The government of India has set up a network of employment exchanges throughout the country. These exchanges maintain detailed records of job seeker and refer appropriate candidates to the employers.
- **Educational institutions:** Colleges and institutes of management and technology have become a popular source of recruitment for technical professional and managerial jobs.
- **Recommendations:** Applicants introduced by present employees, for their friends and relatives may prove to be a good source of recruitment.
- **Casual callers:** Many well reputed business organizations draw a steady stream of unsolicited applicants in their offices. Such

Table 22.4: Advantages and disadvantages of recruitment methods.

Methods	Advantages	Disadvantages
Placement of announcements in newspapers	• Low costs targeting • Accessibility for all potential applicants	A large number of competing advertisements
Placement of announcements on TV, radio	Possible colorful advertisement serving	Relative expensiveness Low targeting
Direct recruitment of graduates	"Cheapness" of graduates the enthusiasm of "young blood" current knowledge	Lack of work experience of applicants
Internet recruiting	• Low costs • Easy selection • A large number of applicants	Underdevelopment of Internet culture among the older population
Contacting recruiting agencies	• Short time costs • Professional selection	High costs Incompetence of recruiters in the required professional sphere
Headhunters	Recruitment hard-to-find specialist	High costs • Slowness in carrying out the order • The possibility of disclosure of confidential information • Incompetence of recruitment in the required professional sphere

Flowchart 22.7: External recruitment methods.

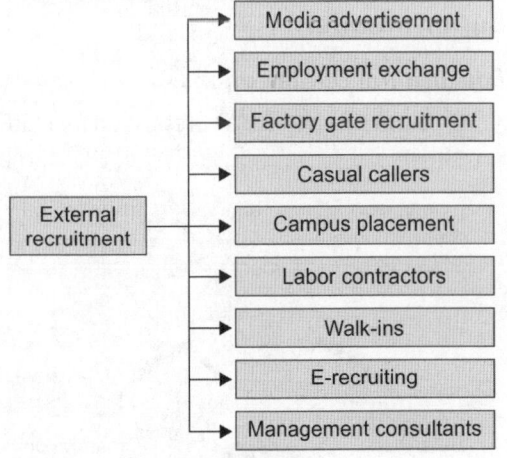

Selection

After recruitment, selection procedure has to be implemented. Selection process relates to the securing of relevant information about an applicant. This information can be obtained in different ways. Selection is actually matching people with the job. It is only the quality of human force that matters much in the organizations. It is essential; therefore, to select quality men for placing them in right positions render quality services. Selection of men is a critical activity. It is a process of choosing from among the candidates from outside, the most suitable persons for the current position or for future positions.

Placement

Placement may be defined as "the determination of the job to which an accepted candidate is to be assigned," and his assignment to that job. It is a matching of what the supervisor has reason to think he can do with the job demands (job requirements): it is a matching of what he imposes (in strain, working conditions), and what he offers in the form of payroll, companionship with others,

job seekers can be a valuable source of manpower.

- **Direct recruitment:** Under this source of recruitment a notice is placed on the notice board of the enterprise specifying the details of the jobs available.
- **Labor contracts:** Labour contracts maintain close contacts with laborers and they can provide the required number of workers at short notice.

promotional possibilities, etc. A proper placement of worker reduces employee turnover, absenteeism and accident rates, and improves morale.

Training

Training is an activity, which involves the development of hidden talent of an individual and uses it for the benefit of the organization. It is directed towards maintaining and improving current jobs and developing skills in employees for future jobs too. After the candidates are selected for various jobs, there is a need for management, to provide for their 'Training' and 'Development.' The efficiency of our organization depends very much on training and development. New employees have to learn new skills, and since their motivation is likely to be high, they can be acquainted relatively easily with the skills and behavior expected in their new position. But training of existing employees is a tough job. They may refuse to take training, as they have to change their established ways of doing their jobs. Whether the employees are new or existing, there is need for the management to provide for their training. This is because the efficiency of any organization depends very much on the training and development of personnel.

Retaining

Employee retention involves taking measures to encourage employees to remain in the organization for the maximum period of time. Organization is facing a lot of problems in employees retaining these days. Employees stay and leave organizations for some reasons. The reason may be personal or professional. These reasons should be understood by the employer and should be taken care of. The organizations are becoming aware of these reasons and adopting many strategies for employee retention.

Promotion

Promotion is a term which includes a change and calls for greater responsibilities and usually involves higher pay and better terms and conditions of service and, therefore, a higher status or rank. Promotion is an upward movement or advancement of an employee in the organization to another job which commands better pay, prestige or status and higher challenges, responsibilities, opportunities, better working environment and hours of work facilities.

JOB DESCRIPTION

A job description is a list of duties and activities a person is to perform and is based on the level of preparation and training of a person. A job description will include his obligations and the person or persons to whom he is responsible. Very often the job descriptions are prepared by top level administrative staff and in charge nurse has participation in preparing them. Sometimes, she has to put into practice the hospital general job descriptions to hospital ward situation. When there are clear job descriptions, the assignment of duties is much easier.

Job Description of Nursing Superintendent

Educational Qualifications

- **General Education:** As prescribed for staff nurse.

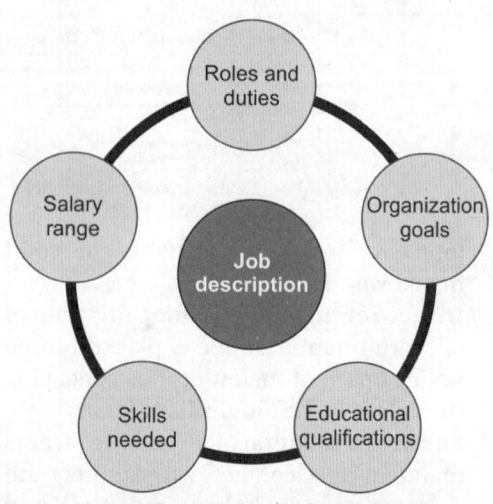

Fig. 22.12: Job description.

- **Professional Education:** As prescribed for staff nurse.
- **Registration:** As prescribed for staff nurse, Registered with Karnataka Nursing Council.
- **Experience:** Should have experience as senior staff nurse.

Standard Norms

Since, it is the second level nursing supervisory role, it needs at least the Nursing Superintendent Gr II for three senior staff nurses (1:3).

Job Summary

She/he is responsible for developing and supervising nursing services of a department or a floor consisting of two or more wards or units managed by the senior staff nurses. These units may be inpatient wards, outpatient department clinics, operation theatres, obstetric units, central supply department, etc. She/he is responsible to the Nursing Superintendent Gr I.

Patient Care and Ward/Unit Management

- Organizes and plans nursing care activities of the department of floor according to the hospital policies and service needs.
- Plans staffing pattern and the other necessary requirements of her/his department.
- Complies and submits nursing statistics to the concerned authorities.
- Conducts and attends to the departmental and interdepartmental meetings/conferences from time-to-time.
- Makes regular rounds of her/his department.
- Ensures to the safety and general dealings of the department.
- Looks into general comforts of the patient and his/her relatives.
- Receives report from the Night Supervisor of her/his departments.
- Evaluates nature and quantum of care required in each unit/ward.
- Makes rotation plan for the nursing staff and domestic staff under her/his jurisdiction.

- Plans ward management with the each ward/unit.
- Reinforces the principles of good ward management in ward.
- Helps ward/unit supervisors to procure their ward/unit.
- Supervises the proper use and care of the equipment and supplies in the department.
- Acts as the public relation officer of the unit and deals with the problems faced by the ward supervisor if any, especially with Group "D" employees, patient attenders.
- Keeps the nursing superintendent Gr I and office informed of the needs of the nursing units/wards under her/his charge and of any special problem/problems.
- Officiates in the absence of Nursing Superintendent Gr I.

Educational Function

- Arranges classes and clinical teaching of nursing students in the department, related to the specialty experience.
- Implements the ward teaching programme and clinical experience of the students with the help of doctors and nurses.
- Does counseling and guidance of staff and students.
- Arranges and conducts staff development programs of her/his department.
- Assists in planning for and participation in the training of auxiliary personnel.

Responsibilities of Head Nurse

The head nurse is the nursing officer overall in charge of a ward unit. She is responsible to the medical officer in charge as well as the matron for efficient performance of her own duties and those of nursing personal placed under her charge. This dual authority over her activities sometimes leads to conflict and clash of personalities. The functional authority of the physician requires the nursing officer to carry out his instructions for treatment of the patients whereas he has no authority to relieve her of the patients whereas he has no authority to relieve her of her duties or change her if she does not perform her functions adequately. That is the responsibility of the matron or the CO.

Similarly, in ward management, there might be orders and counter orders originating from two sources of authority over her knowledge and a thorough understanding of each others responsibilities to manage a ward efficiently. Some of the important duties of a head nurse are given below:

- Carrying out the instructions of the medical officers regarding treatment of patients, observing and recording the progress of treatment and generally assisting the medical officer to achieve his therapeutic aim.
- General cleanliness and upkeep of the ward and its surrounding areas to provide neat and clearful environments for the patients.
- Supervision of care and maintenance of buildings, furniture, fittings and arranging their reports through the CM.
- Keeping the ward equipment in optimum state of readiness by prompt repairs and replacement through condemnation boards.
- Assignment or duties for patients care to the staff working is the ward taking into consideration the capabilities of each.
- Indenting the collection of various items of medical and QM and other stores.
- Ensuring that all specimens are sent to the laboratory in time and results collected when due.
- Maintaining strict control over accounting and distribution of controlled and dangerous drugs.
- Requisition of diet as per instructions of the medical officer and ensuring that the diets and extras are distributed to patients as per the requisition.
- Ensuring that sufficient linen is available in the ward.
- Maintenance of all the registers and documents required in the ward.
- Overall supervision of all that happens in the ward is to ensure that the patient's treatment and recovery is as smooth and pleasant as possible.
- Training of nursing and other personnel working in the ward.

Job Description of Staff Nurse

Educational Qualifications

- **General:** Pre-University course/10+2 or equivalent exam.
- **Professional:** 3 years General Nursing/9 months/6 months Midwifery/Psychiatric Nursing Diploma certificate, recognized by Indian Nursing Council.

Or

Revised General Nursing and Midwifery/Psychiatric nursing Diploma/Certificate Recognized by Indian Nursing Council.

Or

Basic BSc Nursing from a Recognized University according to Indian Nursing Council norms.

- **Registration:** Registered with the Karnataka State Nursing Council/Indian Nursing Council (INC).

Standard Norms and INC (Nurse: Patient Ratio)

- General Wards
  - 1:3 (Hospital attached with school or college of nursing).
  - 1:5 (Hospital not attached with school or college of nursing)
- ICU, ICCU and other specialty 1:1 for 24 hours.
- Labour room 4 in each shift.
- Operation theatre 3 for 24 hours per table.
- Out-patient department 1 in each clinic room of the OPD.
- Casualty and emergency 1:1 in each shift
- Paediatric unit 1:2 beds
- And 30 per cent leave reserve post of staff nurses should be maintained.

Job summary: Staff nurse is a first level professional nurse who provides direct patient care to one patient or group of patients assigned to her/him during duty shift and assist in management of wards/units/special departments. She/he is directly responsible to

Senior Staff Nurse or ward in charge Nurse/ Nursing Superintendent Gr II.

Duties and Responsibilities

Direct Patient Care

- Carry out the procedures of admission and discharge of the patient.
- Makes beds of serious patients and helps or guides students or Group "D" employees to make beds, by supplying linen.
- Maintains personal hygiene and comforts of the patient.
- Attends to the nutritional needs of the patient and feeds the helpless patients.
- Maintains clean and safe environment for the patient.
- Implements and maintains ward policies and routines.
- Co-ordinates patient care with other team members.
- Take rounds with the doctors when called to list new orders and see that they are carried out.
- Performs various technical tasks related to nursing care.
  - Administration of medication, i.e., tablets, injections, infusions and transfusion on prescription, or according to standing instructions.
  - Assisting doctors in various medical and surgical diagnostic procedures by preparing patients and getting ready with required things.
  - Performing simple diagnostic procedures viz, urinalysis hemoglobin %, etc.
  - Collecting and sending of specimens for laboratory diagnostic procedures.
  - Recording of vital signs, i.e. temperature, pulse, respiration and blood pressure.
  - Performing gastric lavage, giving enema, etc.
  - Prepares patients for operations and see that he/she is sent to operation theatre with all necessary papers and medications.
  - Takes care of eyes, ears, back, bowel, bladder, perineum, and breast, etc. whenever needed.
  - Observes all patient conditions and take suitable action accordingly and/ or reports changes to ward in charge and/or the doctor.
  - Give expert bed-side nursing to all patients.
  - Attends last offices in case of a patient dying during shifts and arrange to preserve dead body in mortuary, or hand over the body with respect to concerned family members/relatives/authorities.

Ward/Unit Management

- Helps the ward in charge to carry out her/ his work or act as ward in charge during their absence.
- Maintains general cleanliness of the ward and the sanitary annexure.
- Supervises the duties of Group "D" employees and guides them and reports accordingly.
- Writes the diet register and supervises the distribution of diet and report if any, necessary.
- Maintains scheduled poisonous drug registers.
- Supervises nursing care and other tasks carried out by the students.
- Maintains duty room trays, sterilizes instruments and see that procedural trays are in readiness.
- Take over from duty nurse of the previous, new and serious patients, instruments, supplies, drugs, etc., and handover the same accordingly.
- Maintains all the records pertaining to ward/unit.
  - Maintains case papers, investigation reports, etc.
  - Maintains vital signs charts, intakeoutput charts and other special charts if necessary.

- Takes special care of medico legal case papers and records.
- Writes day and night orders and maintains ward statistics.

STAFF DEVELOPMENT

Staff development is the process directed towards the personal and professional growth of nurses and other personnel, while they are employed by a health care agency. Staff development refers to all training and education provided by an employee to improve the occupational and personal knowledge, skills and attitudes of vested employees. Staff development activities consist of the training and education provided by an employer to improve employee's occupational knowledge, skills and attitudes and to provide the employee with the opportunity to grow professionally.

Meaning of staff development: Staff development refers to the continuing improvement of the nursing personnel. It also includes setting standards for jobs, providing on-the-job growth experiences, considering potential growth opportunities in all assignment planning, supervising and appraising performance proficiencies and assuming responsibility for reparative or corrective training measures. Staff development program are designed to motivate learner in the way of the train and education to improve their knowledge, skills, and attitudes.

Importance of Staff Development

- Focuses on developing nursing skills and knowledge.
- Introduces the employees to new situations and orientated to philosophy, soils, politics, and physical sanities.
- It provides job-related counseling, which involves promoting the professional growth of employees.
- It provides learning experiences in the work setting for the purpose of refining and developing new skills and knowledge related to job performance.
- It is planned and organized around learning experiences in variety of setting.
- To reduce staff turnover and absenteeism.

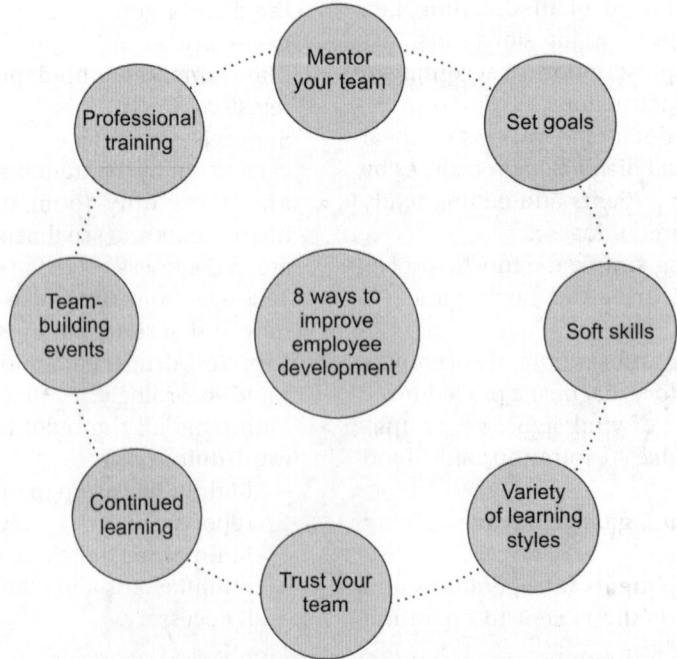

Fig. 22.13: 8 ways to improve employee development.

Objectives of Staff Development

- To assist each employee to improve performance in present position.
- To keep pace with medical sciences.
- New development in medical science and technology.
- New diagnostic and treatment techniques.
- To motivate each staff member and create a sense of security and loyalty.
- To improve work productivity and for promotion.
- To reduce staff turnover, absenteeism and tardiness.
- To acquire personal and professional abilities that maximizes the possibility of career advancement.

Role of Head Nurse in Staff Development

- Involves staff members in developing high standards of patient care and in establishing objectives and criteria for their attainment.
- Discover leadership's skills and creative abilities among staff and arrange for their development.
- Encourage staff to participate in planning for the improvement of nursing care and to apply findings of nursing practice research.
- Provide learning opportunities for professional advancement of staff in order to develop to their highest potential.
- Share in planning and participate in staff educational programs of professional and non-professional personnel.
- Allot time for discussions, observations, and questions.
- Set a good example in everyday practice.

STAFF WELFARE

The institution should serve various facilities for the staff members to enable them to function effectively at their work. The institution expects from its staff a commitment to serve, in the spirit of god, the patients and others who come in search of the services. Some of the provisions provided are unique

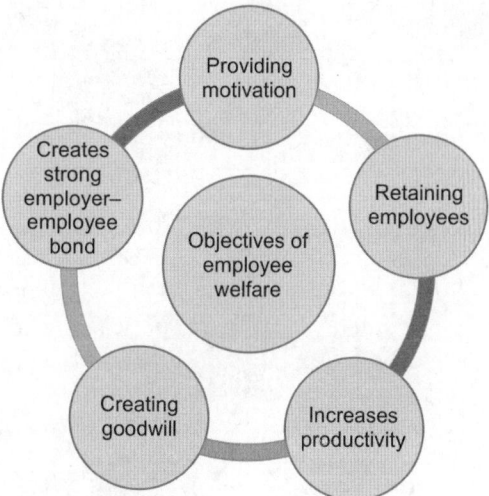

Fig. 22.14: Objectives of employee welfare.

to the institution and we believe will faster a fellowship and friendship amongst the staff to develop a team spirit which is critical for successful medical services.

Purposes of Staff Welfare

- It motivates the staff to work effectively.
- It improves interest to serve to the particular institution.
- It facilitates the staff member to participate with full involvement.
- It improves the team work in the institution.

Faculty Improvement Techniques

- Encourage and stimulate faculty.
- Take positive attitude towards problems of teachers.
- Provide resources and facilities for the implementation of instructions.
- Give recognition to abilities.
- Create a climate which stimulates creative participation by faculty members.
- While making changes in the curriculum, invite suggestions from the faculty.
- Given opportunity to plan, experiment, and explore.
- Assist in developing teaching techniques.
- Maintain good relation with faculty members.

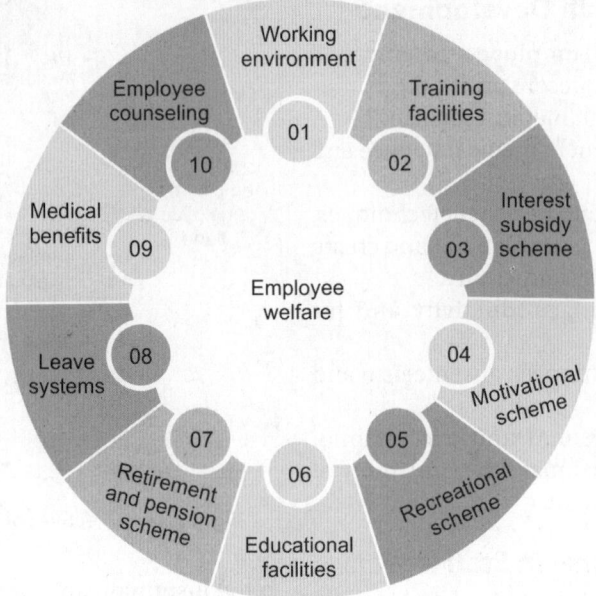

Fig. 22.15: Employee welfare.

Staff welfare activities: The conditions under which the teaching staff have an effect on the implementation of the program besides contributing towards the stability of the staff. Frustrations, conflicts, resignations, and frequent requests for transfer can often be reduced when there are clearly defined policies related to hours of work, teaching load, welfare of the staff and other matters. The policies should be written down known to everyone.

Some of them are:
- Employees provident fund,
- Gratuity benefit,
- Maternity benefit,
- Risk allowances,
- Compensations for work injuries,
- Family pension schemes,
- Employee state insurance.

Types of faculty welfare include:
- Opportunity for leave on the basis of leave rules by the institution policies
- These leave rules incorporate existing annual leave, maternity leave, sabbatical leave, study leave, leave on loss of pay, official leave.

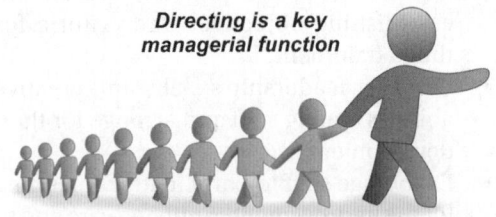

Fig. 22.16: Directing the employees.

- Gratuity-cum-retirement benefit scheme
- Hospital concessions.
- Staff special superannuation benefit scheme for long-term service.
- Provident fund.
- Death benefit schemes.
- Providing opportunity to develop cognitive skills by staff development programs, in-service program and continuing education programs.

DIRECTING/LEADING

Direction means giving the order to start the operation for the implementations of a policy or plan. It is the managerial effort that is applied for guiding and inspiring the working team to make better accomplishments in the organization, so it includes the necessary guidance and instructions for carrying out the order given, and the removal of any doubts or difficulties which may arise in the course of execution or implementation.

Definitions of Direction

- According to Koontz and O'Donnell, "Direction is a complex function that includes all those activities which are designed to encourage subordinates to work effectively and efficiently in both the short- and long-run.
- According to Ernest Dale, direction is telling people what to do and seeing that they do it to the best of their ability.
- According to Haimann, direction consists of the process and techniques utilized in issuing instructions and making certain that operations are carried on as originally planned.

Characteristics of Direction

The nature and characteristics of direction can be summed up as follows:
- Direction is an important function of management and it is also considered as the essence of management.
- It is concerned with the direction of human efforts towards enterprise objectives. Hence, direction deals exclusively with people.
- It helps in achieving coordination among the various operations of the enterprise. Coordination is a necessary by-product of good directing.
- The purpose of planning, organizing, and staffing is achieved only after the performance of directing function.
- It exists at every level, location and operation throughout the enterprise. It must be performed by every manager at different levels of the enterprise. Hence, direction is a pervasive function of management.
- Direction is a continuing activity. A manager never ceases to direct his subordinates and he must continuously

Box 22.1: Features or characteristics of directing.
- It is concerned with issuing of orders and instructions to the subordinates.
- It is guiding and counseling the subordinates in their work with a view to improving their performance.
- It is supervision of the work of subordinates to ensure that it conforms to plans.
- Directing is pervasive, because it is performed at all levels of management.
- It is a continuous process, because it deals with the continuous guidance to be provided by the superiors to their subordinates.
- It always follows a top down approach.
- It provides linkage between other managerial functions, such as planning, organising, and staffing.

supervise the execution of his orders or instructions by the subordinates.
- Direction stimulates the organization and its staff to execute the plans for achieving the desired actions and results. Hence, it is called management-in-action. Earnest Dale has stated that direction constitutes the life spark of the enterprise which like electric power sets it into motion.
- It motivates commands, communicates, supervises the staff and controls the organization.
- It also provides the necessary leadership in the business.
- It facilitates in securing cooperation of the employees for attaining the objective of the organization.

Principles of Direction

Direction is a complex function as it deals with human behavior. Effective direction is an art which a manager can learn through experience.

However, the following principles are helpful in achieving effective direction:
- **Harmony of objectives:** Direction become effective when the goals of members of the organization are in complete harmony with and complementary to the goals of the organization. A manager should direct

Flowchart 22.8: Principles of directing.

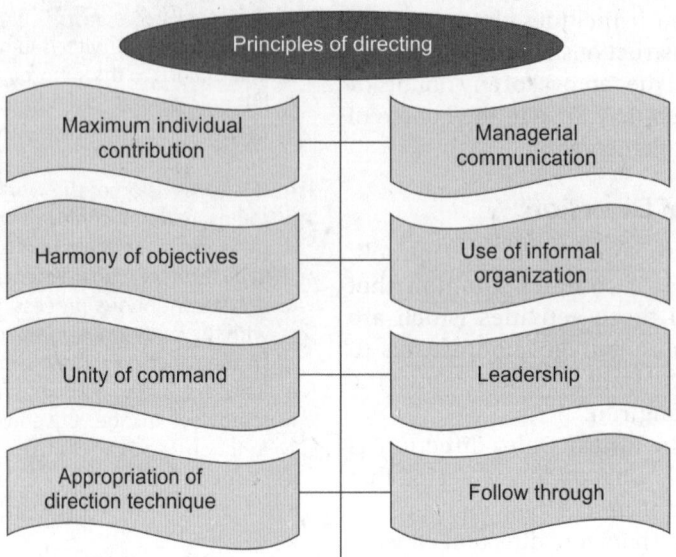

the subordinates in such a way that they perceive the enterprise objectives to be in their personal interest.

- **Unity of command:** A subordinate should at a time receive orders and instructions from one superior only. This is necessary to avoid conflicting orders, problem of priorities, and division of loyalty, indiscipline and irresponsibility.

- **Direct supervision:** Every superior must maintain face-to-face or direct contact with his subordinates. Direct supervision improves the motivation and morale of employees, increases their loyalty and provides the immediate feedback.

- **Managerial communication:** Communication is an important instrument of direction. Efficient communication is a two way process. Two way communications gives the subordinate a chance to express their feeling and the boss to know the feelings of subordinate. The manager should explain the policies and practices to subordinate and the results expected of them.

- **Individual contribution:** Efficient direction leads to the attainment of objectives at minimum cost. Performance becomes effective when every individual in the organization makes a distinct and maximum possible contribution to the organizational objectives.

- **Strategic use of informal organization:** Managers should understand, accept and use the informal groups to supplement and support the formal organization. They can increase the effectiveness of direction by securing the cooperation of informal leaders.

- **Effective leadership:** Dynamic leadership is essential to effective direction. A manager must possess the qualities of a good leader. He should guide and counsel his subordinates not only on work problems but on their personal problems too.

- **Appropriate techniques:** The techniques used for direction should be appropriate to the people, task, and situation. Standard operating procedures are not always helpful in direction.

- **Efficient motivation:** Cooperation of subordinates can be secured if they are ready to act for the organization voluntarily. People will volunteer themselves for the accomplishment of goals, if they are properly induced and motivated.

- **Follow-through**: Direction is a continuous process. Mere issuing of orders and instructions is not enough and it is essential to ensure that the work is done in the desired manner.

Techniques of Direction

The directing function of management consists of the following elements:
- Issuing orders and instructions.
- Supervising people to ensure that subordinates performance conforms to the plan.
- Motivating subordinates to strive whole-heartedly subordinates in the best way of accomplishing their jobs.
- Providing leadership to guide and counsel subordinates in the best way of accomplishing their jobs.
- Communicating with subordinates to create mutual understanding and teamwork.
- Maintaining discipline and rewarding effective people.

Issuing Orders in Direction

The issuing orders and instructions are essential steps in the process of directing subordinates. An order or instruction initiates, modifies, guides, and terminates activities in the organization. The terms order, instructions, directive, and command are used interchangeably in management literature.

According to Koontz and O' Donnell, order is defined as directional techniques, an instruction is understood to be a charge (command) by the superior requesting a subordinate to act or reflect from acting in a given circumstances.

Characteristics of Good Orders

- The order should be clear and complete so that it easily understood by the subordinates.
- The order should be reasonable and attainable, i.e., within the authority of subordinates.
- The order must be complete with the objectives of the organization and with the interests of subordinates.

- The order should be appropriately worded so that it does not appear offensive.
- The orders should specify the time within which it should be carried out and completed.
- All orders should follow the chain of command.
- Face-to-face suggestions are preferable to long distance orders.
- Attitudes and habit patterns necessary for the caring out of an order should be created in advance.
- An order should be depersonalized and made an integral part of a given situation.
- The order should be constantly followed up and should incorporate the suggestions made by the subordinates when it is issued.

Elements of Direction

The directing functions of the manager include the following:

Delegation: Delegation is the process by which the manager assigns specific tasks/ duties to worker with commensurate authority to perform the job. Delegation is an important methods of organizing and also a skill required to a manager. A manager by dividing his work and shared his responsibilities with others, he can smoothly and effectively with delegation. By delegating well defines tasks and responsibilities, the nurse manager can be freed of voluble time that can well be spent on planning and evaluating nursing programs and activities.

Supervision: Supervision is working together to achieve the organizational goals. Supervision can be defined as a process by which the subordinates are according to their needs by their immediate superiors to make the best use of their abilities so as to do their jobs efficiently and affectively and with increasing satisfaction to themselves and to the organization in which they function.

Leadership: Leadership is the lifting of man's visions to higher sights, the raising of man's performance to a higher standard, the building of man's personality beyond its normal limitations. Leadership is the process of influencing the thoughts and actions of other people (a person or a group) to attain the desired objectives.

Motivation: Motivation is the process of channeling a person's inner drives so that he wants to accomplish the goals of the organization. Motivation is a behavioral concept by which we try to understand why people behave as they do. It concerns those dynamic processes which produce a goal-directed behavior. A goal-directed behavior always begins with the individual feeling certain needs (also referred to as drives or motives). These needs give an energizing thrust to the individual toward certain goals or incentives which he perceives (rightly or wrongly) as possible satisfier of his needs.

Communication: Communication is the basic element of human interactions. It is one of the most vital components of all nursing practice. A great deal of nursing practice involves interpersonal communication skills. For example, communication between the nurse and other members of health team, personnel in other health care agencies or the public. Communication is also a component of therapy, nurses who communicate effectively are able to initiate change that promotes health, establish a trusting relationship with patients and with others, and prevent legal problems associated with nursing practice.

Coordination: Coordination is the orderly synchronization or fitting together of the interdependent efforts of individuals, in order to attain a common goal. For example, in a hospital, the activities of doctors, nurses, ward attendants, and lab technicians must be properly synchronized if the patient is to receive good care. Similarly, in a modern enterprise, which consists of a number of departments, such as production, purchase, sales, finance, personnel, etc. there is need for all of them to properly time their interdependent activities and to efficiently reunite the sub-divided work.

CONTROL

Control is one of the important functions of management. It is closely related to other functions of management, such as planning, organizing, staffing, and directing. It is said that planning is the basis, action is the essence, delegation is the key and information is the guide for control. It is the process through which managers assure that actual activities confirm to the planned activities. Therefore, control functions consist in verifying whether everything occurs in conformity with the plan adopted, the instructions issued and principles established.

Definitions

- **According to EFL Brech,** "Control is checking current performance against predetermined standards contained in the plans with a view to ensuring adequate progress and satisfactory performance."
- **According to Billy E Goetz,** "Management control seeks to compel events to conform to plans."
- **According to George R Terry,** "Controlling is determining what is being accomplished, that is, evaluating the performance and, if necessary, applying corrective so that the performance takes place according to plans."

Characteristics of Managerial Control

The main characteristics of managerial control are given below:

- **Control is a continuous process:** As long as an organization exists some sort of

Flowchart 22.9: Characteristics of controlling.

control is required. Just as the navigator continually takes reading to ascertain whether he is relative to a planned course, so should the business manager continually take reading to assure himself that his enterprise or department is on course. Control is dynamic not static.

- **Control is forward looking:** Control aims at future because one can control future events and not the past. However, control is in the nature of follow-up to other functions of management. It involves review of past performance and one cannot measure the outcome of an event which has not taken place. But the corrective action decided on the basis of past experience is taken for future.

- **Control process is universal:** Control process consists of the same elements irrespective of the type of organization or function to be controlled. It is the responsibility of every manager to regulate on-going activity and to keep the operations focused towards goal attainment.

- **Control involves measurement:** To control means to check or monitor actual performance, to keep a watch on activities. It requires measuring results against pre-established targets and review of the outcome of activities. But control not only involves checking current performance. It also suggests guidelines for future course of action. It helps to steer events towards targets so as to make things happen. Evaluation and measurement is the heart of control process.

- **Control is an influence process:** Control seeks to structure events and to condition behavior. It is designed to curb undesirable trends and to shape the pattern of future events. It induces people conform to certain norms and standards.

Steps in Control Process

- Establishing standards.
- Measuring and comparing actual results against standards.
- Taking corrective action.

I nursing service, standards may be set up on the basis of structure, process, and outcome.

The structure standards include physical facilities, organizational characteristics, financial resources, staffing, equipment and supplies, etc.

The process standards are nursing techniques, procedures and other activities, quantity and quality of care, adequacy and appropriateness of care, etc. The outcome

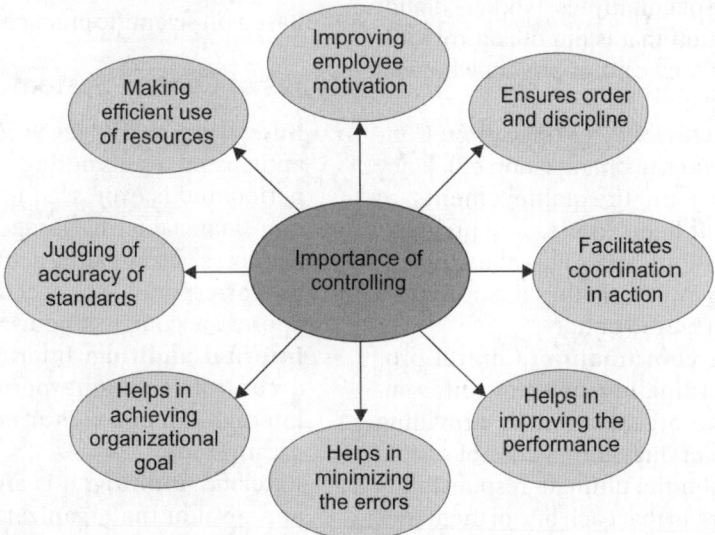

Fig. 22.17: Importance of controlling.

standards are patient satisfaction of personnel engaged in patient care, low accident rates, very few complication, promptness in the performance of task of meeting the policies of the hospital, etc.

Importance of Controlling

- **Facilitates decision-making:** The process of control involves correct actions to bring actual performance and standards together. Corrective measures involve right decisions as to what and how deviations to be rectified. Executive decisions are primarily control decisions.
- **Facilitates decentralization:** Executives like to delegate and decentralize authority, when there is an effective system of control. They can ensure through control that the decisions taken by subordinates are consistent with policies of the organization and whether the delegated authority is being properly used.
- **Stimulates action:** Control provides the basis for further action by spotting and correcting mistakes. It prevents recurrence of mistakes. By pointing out shortcomings in planning and other functions, control helps to ensure that the plans are properly implemented.
- **Enhances employee morale:** A good control system is vital to the motivation and morale of employees. Workers do not like a situation that is out of control for it means that they cannot predict what will happen to them.
- **Promotes efficiency of operation:** Control contributes to organization efficiency by focusing on the achievements of objectives. It helps to measure progress, detect deviations, and adjust operations. It tells management whether the objectives are being achieved or not.
- **Promotive coordination:** Control promotes coordination between different units of the organization by providing them unity of direction. A control system stresses upon the ultimate responsibility of managers so that each one of them tries to work in harmony with the others.

- **Psychological pressure:** The existence of a control system has a positive impact on the behavioral of employees. They become cautious while performing their duties because they know that they are being observed and their performance will be evaluated against the standards.

Essentials of Good Control System

- Suitability and appropriateness to the needs of the organizational functioning.
- Timely and forward looking. It should report deviations promptly. This would help the managers to take immediate corrective actions before the problems develop.
- **Objective:** Objective controls specify the expected results in clear and definite terms.
- **Flexible:** It should be adjusted to the changing needs of the organization.
- **Economical:** The benefit derived from the control system should be more than the cost involved.
- Simple and acceptable to the personnel in the organization.
- **Motivating:** It should motivate the people for a high level of performance.
- It should detect deviations from the standards and should provide for solutions to the problems that cause deviations.
- Based on scientific practice.

Types of Control System

- **Budgeting:** A budget is a statement of anticipated results during a designed with period and is expressed in financial and non-financial terms. Budgetary control is a process of comparing actual results with the corresponding budget data in order to approve accomplishments.
- **Internal auditing:** Internal auditing is a control technique performed by an internal auditor who is an employee of the organization.
- **External auditing:** It is an independent appraisal of the organization's financial amounts and statements. The external

auditor is a qualified person who has to certain the annual profit and loss account and prepares a balance sheet after careful examination of the relevant books of account and documents.

- **Reports:** A major parts of control consists of preparing reports to provide informations to the management for the purpose of control and planning.
- **Standing order and limitations:** These are also considered as control technique used by management.
- **Job description:** Job description can be considered as a standard set to provide excellent service in view of the objectives of the organization.
- **Personal observation/supervision:** A manager can also exercise fruitful control over his subordinates by observing them while they are engaged in work.
- **Program evaluation and review technique (PERT):** PERT is primarily oriented towards achieving better managerial control of time spent in completing a project.
- **Human resources accounting:** The concept of human resources accounting is of recent origin. They maintain accounts in the human resource department.

Advantages of Control

- It prevents faulty operations and creates a good base for future faultless operations and help in taking sound decisions.
- Control systems help taking corrective measures in case the plan activity is deviated from original designs and also assist in adopting follow-up actions.
- Control systems provide a good opportunity for decentralization of authority.
- Control brings about co-ordination in planned activity.
- Workforce in the organization will be disciplined by adopting good control system and brings about operational efficiency.

BUDGET

Budgeting, though primarily recognized as a device for controlling, becomes a major part of the planning process in any organization. Literally, the word "budget" means a Leather bag or sachet to carry official papers in. From that association, it came to mean those papers themselves, more particularly the papers containing the financial proposals for the year. The word "budget" derived from the old English word "budgettee" means a sack or pouch which the Chancellor of the Exchequer used to take out his papers for laying before the Parliament, the Government, and financial scheme for the ensuing year. Now the term budget refers to the financial papers, certainly not to the sack.

Definition: "Budget" is a concrete precise picture of the total operation of an enterprise in monetary.   **—HM Donovan**

Purposes of budget: Budget supplies the mechanism for translating fiscal objective into projected monthly spending pattern.
- Budget enhances fiscal planning and decision-making.

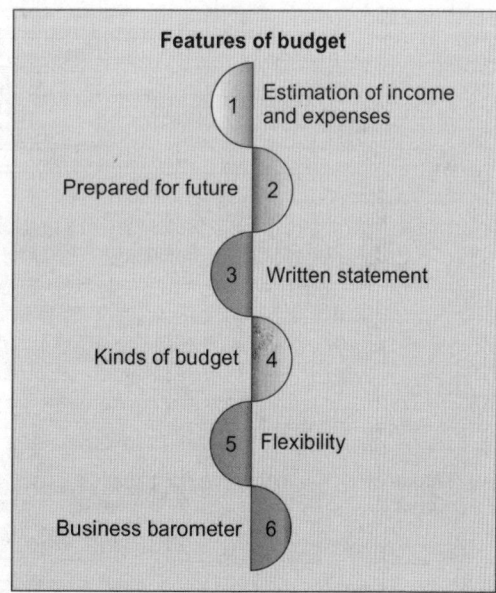

Fig. 22.18: Features of budget.

- Budget clearly recognizes controllable and uncontrollable cost areas.
- Budget offers a useful format for communicating fiscal objectives.
- Budget allows feedback of utilization of budget.
- Budget helps to identify problem areas and facilitates effective solution.
- Budget provides means for measuring and recording financial success with the objectives of the organizations.

Features of Budget

- It should be flexible.
- It should be synthesis of past, present, and future.
- It should be product of joint venture + co-operation of executives/department heads at different levels of management.
- It should be in the form of statistical standard laid down in specific numerical terms.
- It should have support of top management throughout the period of its planning and supplementation.

Importance of budget: Budget is a numerical description of expected income and planned expenditure for an organization for a specified period of time. It is a concrete, precise, picture of the total operation of an enterprise/organization/institution in monetary term, i.e. finance.

The following point serves the importance of budget:

- Budget is needed for planning for future course of action and to have a control over all activities in the organization.
- Budget facilitates co-coordinating operation of various departments and sections for realizing organizational objectives.
- Budget serves as a guide for action in the organization.
- Budget helps one to weigh the values and to make decision when necessary on whether one is of a greater value in the program than the other.

Principles of budget: Budget is an operational plan for a definite period, usually a year, expressed in financial terms and based on expected income and expenditure.

Flowchart 22.10: Classifications/types of budget.

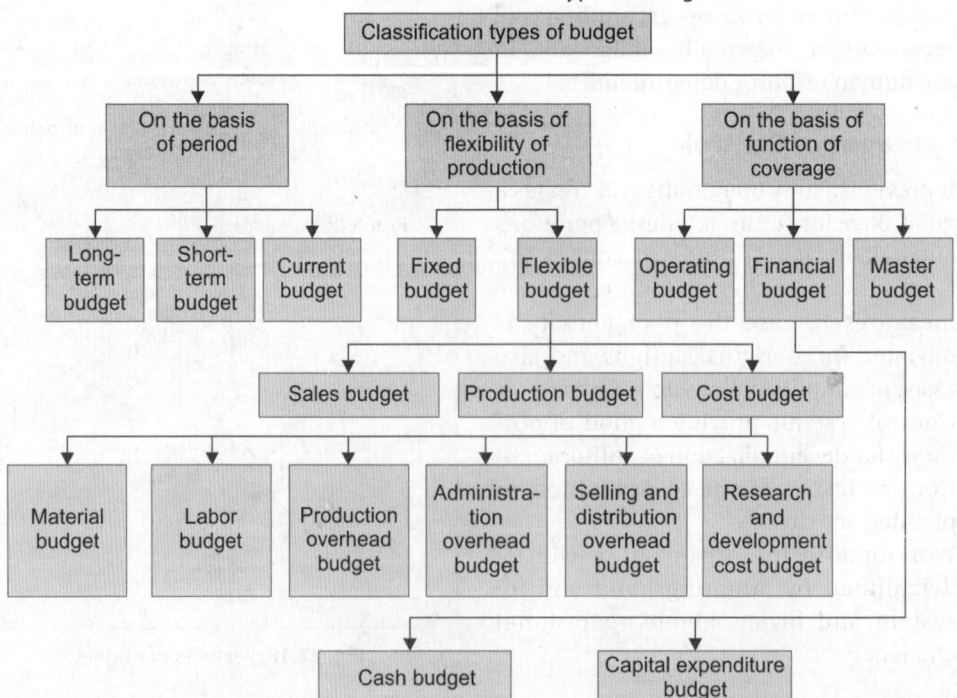

Budget needs certain principles as given below:

- Budget should provide sound financial management by focusing on requirement of the organization.
- Budget should focus on objectives and policies of the organization. It must flow from objectives and give realistic expression to the way of realizing such objectives.
- Budget should ensure the most effective use of scarce financial and non-financial resources.
- Budget requires that program activities planned in advance.
- Budgetary process requires consistent delegation for which fixed duties and responsibilities are required to be allocated to managers at different level for framing and executing budget.
- Budgeting should include co-coordinating efforts of various departments establishing a frame of reference for managerial decisions, and providing a criterion for evaluating managerial performance.
- Setting budget target requires an adequate checks and balance against the adoption of too high or too low estimate. Utmost care is a must for fixing targets.
- Budget period must be appropriate to the nature of business or service and to the type of budget.
- Budget is prepared under the direction and supervision of the administrator or financial officer.
- Budgets are to be prepared and interpreted consistently throughout the organization in the communication of planning process.
- Budget necessitates a review of the performance of the previous year and an evaluation of its adequacy both in quantity and quality.
- While developing a budget, the provision should be made for its flexibility.

Classifications of budget: Budget consists mainly three sections, i.e., manpower budget, capital expenditure budget, and operating budget. The manpower budget includes wages and other benefits provide for regular and temporary workers. The capital expenditure budget includes purchases land, buildings, and major equipment of considerable expense and long life. The operational budget includes the cost of supplies, minor equipment, repairs and overhead expenses. There are several types of budget as follows:

- Incremental budget is one based on estimated changes in present operation, plus percentage increase for inflation, all of which is added to previous year budget.
- Open ended budget is a financial plan in which each operating manager presents a single cost estimate for what is considered optimal activity level for each program in the unit, without indicating how the budget should be scaled down if less funding is available.
- Fixed-ceiling budget is a financial plan in which the uppermost spending limit is set by the top executive before the unit and divisional managers develop budget proposals for their areas of responsibility.
- Flexible budget consists of several financial plans, each for a different level of program activity. It is based on the fact, that operating conditions rarely conform to expectations.
- Rollover budget is one that forecasts program, revenues and expenses for a period greater than a year, to accommodate program that are larger than annual budget cycle.
- Performance budget is based on functions, which allocate functions, not divisions, e.g. direct nursing care, in service education, quality improvement, and nursing research. Program budget is one where costs are computed for a total program, i.e., group total costs for each service program, e.g., MCH, FP, UIP, etc.
- Zero base budgets require the nurse manager to examine, justify each cost of every program both old and new, in every annual budget preparation.
- Sunset budget is designed to "self destruct" within a prescribed time period to ensure the cessation of spend in by a predetermined date.

- Sales budget is the starting point in a budgetary program, since sales are basic activities which give shape to all other activities. Sale budgets are compiled in terms of quantity as well as of value.
- Production budget is the budget that aims at securing the economical manufacture of products and maximizing the utilization of production facilities.
- Revenue and expense budget is expressed in financial terms and takes the nature of a proforma income statement for the future. It may be prepared in a detailed form or in an abstract statement showing the items of profit and loss under classified headings.
- Capital expenditure budget is prepared for assuring planned timely capital investment in the business to ensure the availability of capital at the right time over longer period.
- Cash budget is prepared by way of projecting the possible cash receipts and payments over the budget period.

An essential requisition for budget preparation will includes:
- **Forecasting:** Sound forecasting may be related to making decisions on purchases, expansion, advertising, services, working capital needs, etc.
- **Accounting:** Well-conceived accounting system must be needed to compare the budget information with actual accomplishment. The cost information tells as to how much it will cost to produce or give service.
- **Lines of authority:** Budget preparation, operation, and supervision need/require clearly defined lines of authority.
- **Budget committee:** Budget needs budget committee in an organization (i) to receive and approve all forecasts, departmental budgets, periodic reports showing comparison of actual and budgeted income and expenditure, and (ii) to request for special studies of deviations from the budget and consider revision of budget to meet changed conditions.

- **Business policies:** Clearly defined business policies serve as basis for budget preparations.
- **Statistical information:** In the form of figures, i.e. estimates regarding the budget terms are essential for budget.
- **Support:** Top level management support is essential to ensure successful installation of the budget program.
- **Period of budget:** Length of budget period (usually a year) should be specified.

Steps in Budgeting: While designing and implementing a planning program, the nurse administrator/manager should follow steps as given below:
- Review the goals of the agency or hospital to identify activities of highest priority, because these are most likely to receive funding.
- Review the objectives of the existing programs and written for proposed programs to ensure that achievement of these objectives will support agency.
- Existing programs are revised and proposed programs designed to maximum goal accomplishment.
- Manpower, capital, and operating expenses are computed for each program, old and new.
- Alternative methods are identified for realizing designated objectives and price of each alternative is determined.
- Comparisons are made to determine which alternative is most cost-effective.
- A budget request is developed which details a fiscal plan for the preferred program indicates alterative methods for meeting the same objective, and explains why the recommended program is preferred.

For Nursing in Hospital

- Request the assistant nursing officers and supervisors to present their needs for the coming year by a specified date, and confer with those who have presented such need.
- Review the budget appropriation and actual expenditure for the current year

in conjunction with statistical data as to the numbers and distribution of patient, nursing hours, per patient by services, operations and others.

- Ascertain whether any changes are contemplated, such as opening new facilities for patients or changes in other departments, which affect the nursing services required.
- Prepare the program which the new budget is to cover in terms of the nursing hours to be given to patients, the distribution of the hours among the various groups of personnel, the ratio of supervisors and head nurses to patients' care and the provision for the administration of nursing unit.
- Determine the percentage of salaries of personnel who have both educational and nursing service function to be allocated to each function on the basis of time devoted to each.
- Estimate the requirement for the coming year from the information supplied as the expenditure for supplies, equipment, and repairs to date.
- Prepare a summary of new needs, both personnel and material with data to support the request.

The budget report submitted to the head of the nursing department after carefully reviewed by her/his associates.

HOSPITAL

The English word 'hospital' originates from the latin word "HOSPILE" and also some are of the view that it comes from the French word 'hospitale' as do the words 'hostel' and 'hotel'. The three words hospital, hostel, hotel, all are derived from same source, are used in different sense, but basically the meaning of the word will be the same. For example, in hotel, hotel authorities take care of the clients, who wish to stay there and client will receive the hospitality according to their ability. In hostel also, the hostel authorities are expected to treat their clients by providing basic amenities and other facilities as needed by their clients.

In the same hospital authorities also receive their clients as their guests and are expected to show hospitality than those of hotel or hostel. Likewise all these three institutions are meant or treating their clients, but style of treatment will be different. Now the term 'hospital' means an establishment temporary space occupied by the sick or injured. In other words, the hospital is an institution in which sick or injured persons are treated.

Definitions of Hospital

- According to WHO, "The hospital is an integral part of a social and medical organizations, the function of which is to provide for the population complete health care, both 'curative' and 'preventive' and whose outpatient services reach out to the family and it's environment; the hospital is also a center for the training of health workers and biosocial research.
- According to Steadman's Medical Dictionary, Hospital is an institution for the care, cure and treatment of the sick and wounded, for the study of diseases and for the training of doctors and nurses.
- According to Blakiston's New Could Medical Dictionary, "Hospital is an institution for medical facility primarily intended, appropriately staffed, and equipped to provide diagnostic and therapeutic service in general medicine and surgery (or) in circumscribed.

Objectives of the hospital: As stated in the definition and philosophy of the hospital, its main objective is to:

- Provide optimum health services to all people irrespective of race, color, caste, and creed and regardless of socio-economical status.
- Provide care, cure, and preventive service to all people irrespective of race, color, caste, creed and economic and social status.
- Protect the human rights of clients while taking care in its jurisdiction/in all areas of its services.
- Provide training for professionals, i.e., doctors, nurses, pharmacists, dentists,

---

Box 22.2: Objectives of the hospital.

« **Improved patient care:**
- By making information belonging to patients seen at other hospitals available at the hospital, where the patient is currently being treated. This is particularly important in light of referral system for patients from district to regional and central hospitals in the province.
- By improving the accessibility of patient related information to health care professionals during the treatment process, through improved medical records handling and shorter turnaround time for the release of diagnostic information, such as laboratory and special investigation results.
- By improving patient administration procedures resulting in shorter waiting times and better service to patients.

« **To form an integral part of a larger quality improvement program in the department through:**
- The re-engineering and standardization of patient administration and management procedures across hospitals.
- Provision of information to do performance evaluation and health care audit.

« **To improve the management efficiency of hospitals through:**
- The facilitation of decentralized financial management capacity at hospital level.
- Improved revenue collection.
- Improved management decision-making through the availability of integrated management information.
- Cost savings through the identification of primary cost-drivers at hospital level and the monitoring of mechanisms introduced to lower costs.

---

and others technical personnel who are involving in health care services.

- Provide in-service/continuing education in all discipline professional/technical personnel involving health care. For updating their knowledge, skills, etc.
- Participate/conduct research (and investigations in basic and applied bio-medical, social and technological sciences) that will benefit patient care, improve the community health status, the management of hospital services and the education of individual who perform the required service.
- Define its leadership role in the community and possibly the region depending upon its size, type and facilities in relation to regional area planning of hospital.

Scope of hospital: As stated in the objectives of the hospital, an optimum health care service have the basis of scientific method, and should be applied in a personalized manner with full recognition and attention to personal dimensions in client needs and are carried out within a framework of social responsibility. It should be available and accessible to everyone who needs it through his own community. The optimum health services consist of following elements.

- **Team approach:** The care of the needy person will be taken by the team of professional members (Doctors, Nurses, etc.) arid paraprofessionals, technicians under the leadership of medically qualified persons with integration and co-ordination.
- **Contents of service:** A spectrum of services that includes diagnosis, specific treatment, rehabilitation, education, and prevention.
- **Co-ordination:** Clients' care will cover the co-ordinated efforts of all agencies, which have the required facilities at all levels.
- **Continuity of care:** Continuity of client care will be available and rendered by the particular agency with specific services whenever needed.
- **Integration:** Organization of the hospital care of both ambulatory and non-ambulatory patients into a continuum with common integrated services.
- **Evaluation and research:** Periodic evaluation programs and provision of conducting research included in the optimum health services for adequacy in meeting needs of the patients and the community.

Flowchart 22.11:: Types of hospital system.

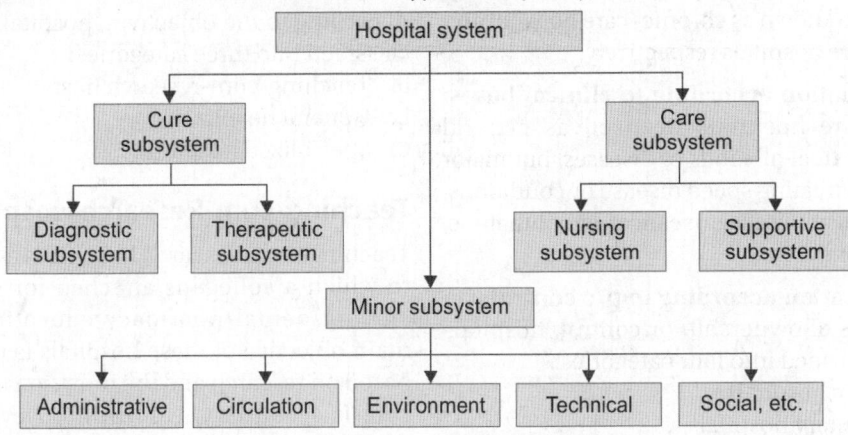

Functions of the Hospital

- Patient Care of the sick and injured and restoration of the health of a diseased person without any discrimination.
- **Diagnosis and treatment of disease:** There are diagnosis and treatment services to in-patients. Within this broad function there are many subdivisions of medical, surgical, obstetrical, gynec, pediatric, psychiatric and other forms of care and rehabilitation. Involved in the entire inpatient services are various modalities, including nursing, dietics, pharmaceutical skills, laboratory, and X-ray services and varying refinement of diagnosis and therapy.
- **Out-patient services:** There are services to out-patients with an equally wide range of specialties and technical modalities.
- **Medical education and training:** Hospital provides professional and technical education for many classes of health personnel. They must work in hospital to receive proper training of their choice, i.e. medical, nursing, pharmacy, dental, lab technicians, X-ray technicians, etc.
- **Medical and nursing research:** Since accumulation of different types of patients, the hospital provides the basis for scientific investigation into causes, diagnosis, treatment and nursing management of diseases, and hospital administration, ward/unit administration in hospitals.
- **Prevention of disease and promotion of health:** Hospital provides services

to surrounding populations that may be preventive care and promoting their health. There are many ways that hospitals, as centers for technical skills, can offer services to people before they are sick or can protect patients from the hazards of disease beyond that for which they have come to the hospital.

Classifications of Hospitals

Hospitals have been classified in many ways. Each hospital is distinct in its characteristic as it differs in structure, functions, performance, and the community it serves. However, we can classify the hospitals into different types depending upon different criteria. The most commonly accepted criteria for classification of the modern hospital are according to:

- Length of stay of patient (long-term and short-term),
- Clinical basis,
- Ownership/Control basis,
- Objectives,
- Size,
- Management,
- System of medicine.

Classification according to length of stay of patient: A patient stays for a short-term in a hospital for treatment of disease that is acute in nature, such as pneumonia, peptic ulcer, gastroenteritis, etc. A patient may stay for a long-term in a hospital for treatment of diseases that are chronic in nature, such as tuberculosis, leprosy, cancer and psychosis.

The hospital according to long-term and short-term also known as chronic- care hospital and acute care hospitals respectively.

Classification according to clinical bases: These are hospitals licensed as general hospital; treat all kinds of diseases, but major focus on treating speed disease or conditions, such as heart disease, or cancer, or ophthalmic, or maternity, etc.

Classification according to p/c control: On the basis of ownership or control, hospitals can be divided into four categories:
a. Public hospitals,
b. Voluntary hospitals,
c. Private/charitable/nursing homes,
d. Corporate hospitals.

Public hospitals: Public hospitals are those run by the central or state governments or local bodies on non-commercial lines. These may be general hospital or specialized hospitals or both.

Voluntary hospitals: Voluntary hospitals are those which are established and incorporated under the Societies Registration Act. 1860; or Public Trust Act, 1882 or any other appropriate act of central or state governments. They are run with public or private funds on a non-commercial basis.

Private nursing hospitals/nursing homes: Private nursing hospitals/nursing homes are generally owned by an individual doctor or a group of doctors. They run the hospital or nursing home on commercial basis. They accept patient suffering from infirmity, advanced age, illness, injury, chronic, disability, etc. But, do not admit patient suffering from communicable disease, alcoholism, drug addiction, or mental illness. Usually, they prefer patient from wealthy families.

Corporate hospitals: Corporate hospitals are hospitals which are public limited companies formed under the Companies Act. They are normally run on commercial lines. They can be either general or specialized or both (e.g., Hinduja hospital, Mallya hospital, Apollo Group of Hospitals, etc.).

Classification according to the objectives: According to the objectives, hospitals can be classified into three categories:
a. Teaching-cum-research hospitals,
b. General hospitals,
c. Specialized hospitals.

Teaching-cum-Research Hospital

Teaching/cum/research hospital is a hospital to which a college is attached for medical cursing/dental/pharmacy education. The main objective of these hospitals is teaching based on research and the provision of health care is secondary, e.g. AIIMS, New Delhi, PGMERI, Chandigarh, JIPMER, Pondicherry, K R Hospital, Mysore, Victoria hospital, Bangalore belong to this type.

General hospitals: General hospitals are those which provide treatment for common diseases and conditions. All establishments permanently staffed by at least two or more doctors, which can offer inpatient accommodation and provide active medical and nursing care for more than one category of medical discipline, such as general medicine, general surgery, obstetrics and gynecology, pediatrics, etc. The main objective of these hospitals is to provide medical care to the people. While teaching and research is secondary and incidental, e.g. all district and taluk or PHC or rural hospitals belong to this type.

Specialized hospitals: Specialized hospitals are hospitals providing medical and nursing care primarily for only one discipline or a specific disease or condition of one system. In other words, these hospitals concentrate on a particular aspect or organ of the body and provide medical and nursing care in that field, e.g. tuberculosis, ENT, ophthalmology, leprosy, orthopedics, pediatrics, cardiology, mental health/psychiatric, oncology, STDs, maternal, etc. The specialized department, administration attached to a general hospital will not be considered as specialized hospital.

Isolation hospitals: Isolation hospital is a hospital in which the persons are suffering from infections/communicable diseases requiring isolation of the patients, e.g., Epidemic Diseases Hospital, Bengaluru.

Classification According to Size

On the basis of health committee report, it is recommended that the following pattern of development of hospitals to be adopted according to size, i.e. bed strength.

- Teaching hospital 500 (bed to be increased according to the number of students),
- District hospital 200 (may be raised up to 300 beds depending upon population),
- Taluk hospital 50 (may be raised depending upon population to be served),
- Primary health centers 6 (may be increased up to 10 depending upon needs).

Classification According to Management

- **Union government/government of India:** All hospitals administered by the Government of India, e.g. hospital run by the railways, military/defence, or public sector undertakings of the Central Government.
- **State governments:** All hospitals administered by the state/union territory. Government authorities and public sector undertaking operated by the state/union territories, including the police, prison, irrigation department, etc.
- **Local bodies:** All hospitals administered by local bodies, i.e. municipal corporation, municipality, zila parishad, panchayat, e.g. corporation maternity homes.
- **Autonomous bodies:** All hospitals established under special act of parliament or state legislation and founded by the central/state government/union territory, e.g. AIIMS, New Delhi, PGI, Chandigarh, NIMHANS, Bengaluru, KMIO, Bengaluru.
- **Private:** All private hospitals owned by an individual or by a private organization, e.g., MAHE, Manipal, Manipal Hospital, Bengaluru, Hinduja Hospital, Mumbai, etc.
- **Voluntary agencies:** All hospitals operated by a voluntary body/a trust/charitable society registered or recognized by the appropriate authority under Central/State Government laws. This includes hospitals run by missionary bodies and co-operatives.

Classification According to System

According to the system of medicine, we can classify the hospital as follows:

- Allopathic hospitals,
- Ayurvedic hospitals,
- Homeopathic hospitals,
- Unani hospitals,
- Hospitals of other systems of medicine.

POLICIES AND PROCEDURES FOLLOWED IN THE ORGANIZATION

Policies provide the framework within which the decision-makers are expected to operate while making decisions relating to the organization. They are a guide to the thinking and action of subordinates for the purpose of achieving the objectives of the business successfully. According to George R. Terry, "Policy is a verbal, written or implied overall guide setting up boundaries that supply the general limits and directions in which managerial action will take place." Thus, the policies are a guide to thinking and action of those who have to make decisions. Policies; A policy is general guideline for decision making.

It sets up boundaries around decisions, including those that can be made and shutting out those that cannot. In so doing, it channelizes the thinking of the organization members so that it is consistent with the organizational objectives.

Advantages of Policies

The advantages of policies are as follows:

- Policies ensure uniformity of action in respect of various matters at various organizational points. This makes actions more predictable.
- Policies speed up decisions at lower levels because subordinates need not consult their superiors frequently.

- Policies make it easier for the superior to delegate more authority to his subordinates without being unduly concerned because he knows that whatever decision the subordinates make will be within the boundaries of the policies.
- Policies give a practical shape to the objectives by elaborating and directing the way in which the predetermined objectives are to be attained.

Types of Policies

Policies may be variously classified on the basis of sources, functions, or organizational level.

- **Classification on the basis of sources:** On this basis, policies may be divided into originated, appealed, implied, and externally imposed policies.
  - **Originated policies:** These are policies which are usually established formally and deliberately by top managers for the purpose of guiding the actions of their subordinates and also their own. These policies are generally set down in print and embodied in a manual.
  - **Appealed policies:** Appealed policies are those which arise from the appeal made by a subordinate to his superior regarding the manner of handling a given situation. When decisions are made by the superior on appeals made by the subordinates, they become precedents for future action. For example, let us assume that a company allows a discount of 2 per cent to its buyers. If any customer states that he is willing to purchase in large quantities and is prepared to pay part of the price in advance, provided he is allowed 2½ per cent discount, then the sales manager not knowing what to do may approach the general manager for his advice. If the general manager accepts the proposal for 2½ per cent discount, the decision of the general manager could become a guideline for the sales manager in the future. This policy is appealed policy because it comes into existence from the appeal made by the subordinate to the superior.
  - **Implied policies:** There are also policies which are stated neither in writing nor verbally. Such policies are called implied policies. Only by watching the actual behavior of the various superiors in specific situations can the presence of the implied policy be ascertained. For example, if office space is repeatedly assigned to individuals on the basis of seniority, this may become an implied policy of the organization.

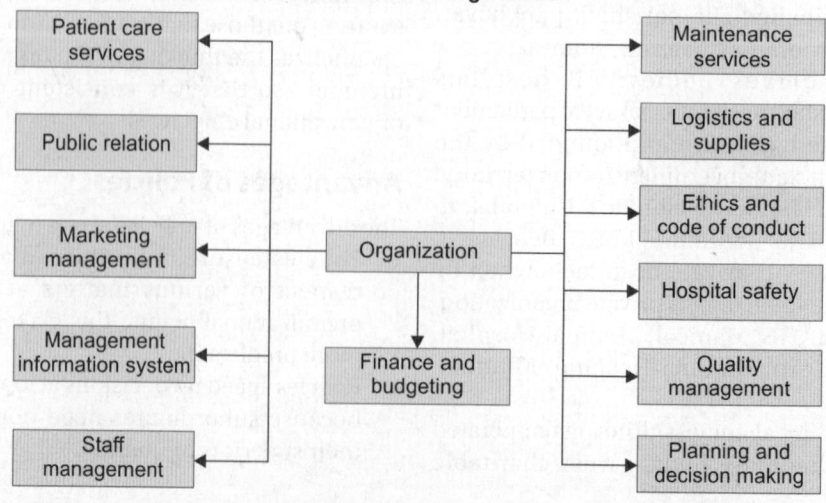

Flowchart 22.12: Role of organization in patient care services.

- **Externally imposed policies:** Policies are sometimes imposed on the business by external agencies, such as government, trade associations, and trade unions. For example, a policy might have been dictated by a government law regulating prices or by a decision of a mill owners' association limiting production or by a decision of the trade union to fill up higher posts only by promoting existing employees.
- **Classification on the basis of functions:** On the basis of business functions, policies may be classified into production, sales, finance, personnel policies, etc. Every one of these functions will have a number of policies. For example, the sales functions may have policies relating to market, price, packaging, distribution channel, commission to middlemen, etc.; the production function may have policies relating to the method of production, output, inventory, research, etc.; the financial function may have policies relating to capital structure, working capital, internal financing, dividend payment, etc.; the personnel function may have policies relating to recruitment, training, working conditions, welfare activities, etc.

Characteristics of a good policy: The characteristics of a good policy are as follows:
- Policy should help in achieving the enterprise's objectives.
- It should provide only a broad outline and leave scope to subordinates for interpretation so that their initiative is not hampered.
- Policies should not be mutually contradictory and there should not be inconsistency between any two policies which may result in confusion and delay in action.
- They should be sound, logical, and flexible and should provide a guide for thinking in future planning and action. Further, they should provide limits within which decisions have to be made.
- Policies should reflect the internal and external business environment.
- Policies should be in writing and the language of the policies should be intel-

ligible to the persons who are supposed to implement them and to those who are to be affected by them.

Guidelines for effective policy-making: Guidelines for making effective policies are as follows:
- Policies as far as possible should be in writing.
- They should be clearly understood by those who are supposed to implement them.
- They should reflect the objectives of the organization.
- To ensure successful implementation of policies, the top managers and the subordinates who are supposed to implement them must participate in their formulation.
- Conditions change and policies must also change accordingly. Hence, a policy must strike reasonable balance between stability and flexibility.
- Different policies in the organization should not pull in different directions and should support one another.
- Policies should not be detrimental to the interests of society.
- Policies should be periodically reviewed in order to see whether they are to be modified, changed or completely abandoned.

VARIOUS DEPARTMENTS OF HOSPITAL

There are many hospital departments, staffed by a wide variety of healthcare professionals, with some crossover between departments. For example, physiotherapists often work in different departments and doctors often do the same, working on a general medical ward as well as an intensive or coronary care unit. Below is a list of the main departments you will come across when you visit a hospital. Some of these units work very closely together, and may even be combined into one larger department. Each department tends to be overseen by consultants in that specialty with a team of junior medical staff under them who are also interested in that specialty.

Hospitals may have acute services, such as an emergency department or specialist trauma centre, burn unit, surgery, or urgent care. These may then be backed up by more specialist units, such as cardiology or coronary care unit, intensive care unit, neurology, cancer center, and obstetrics and gynecology. Some hospitals will also have outpatient departments and whilst others may have chronic treatment units, such as behavioral health services, dentistry, dermatology, psychiatric ward, rehabilitation services (Rehab), and physical therapy. Common hospital support units include a dispensary or pharmacy, pathology, and radiology, and on the non-medical side, there often are medical records departments and/or a release of information department.

Medical Surgical Departments in the Hospital

1. **Accident and emergency (A and E):** This department (sometimes called casualty) is where the patients are likely to be taken if you've called an ambulance in an emergency. It's also where you should come if you've had an accident, but can make own way to hospital. These departments operate 24 hours a day, every day and are staffed and equipped to deal with all emergencies. Patients are assessed and seen in order of need, usually with a separate minor injuries area supported by nurses.
2. **An-esthetics:** Doctors in this department give anesthetic for operations and procedures. An anesthetic is a drug or agent that produces a complete or partial loss of feeling. There are three kinds of anesthetic: general, regional, and local. Doctors in this department give anesthetic for operations. They are responsible for the provision of:
   - Acute pain services (pain relief after an operation),
   - Chronic pain services (pain relief in long-term conditions, such as arthritis),
   - Critical care services (pain relief for those who have had a serious accident or trauma), and
   - Obstetric anesthesia and analgesia (epidurals in childbirth and anesthetic for Caesarean section).

3. **Cardiology:** This department provides medical care to patients who have problems with their heart or circulation. It treats people on an inpatient and outpatient basis. Typical procedures performed include:
   - Electrocardiogram (ECG) and exercise tests to measure heart function,
   - Echocardiograms (ultrasound scan of the heart),
   - Scans of the carotid artery in your neck to determine stroke risk,
   - 24-hour blood pressure test,
   - Insertion of pacemakers,
   - Cardiac catheterization (coronary angiography) to see if there are any blocks in your arteries.
4. **Critical care unit:** Sometimes called intensive care, this unit is for the most seriously ill patients. It has a relatively small number of beds and is manned by specialist doctors and nurses, as well as by consultant anesthetists, physiotherapists and dietitians. Patients requiring intensive care are often transferred from other hospitals or from other departments in the same hospital.
5. **Diagnostic imaging:** Formerly known as X-ray, this department provides a full range of diagnostic imaging services including:
   - General radiography (X-ray scans),
   - Scans for A and E,
   - Mammography (breast scans),
   - Ultrasound scans,
   - Angiography (X-ray of blood vessels)
   - Interventional radiology (minimally invasive procedures, e.g to treat narrowed arteries),
   - CT scanning (scans that show cross sections of the body),
   - MRI scanning (3D scans using magnetic and radio waves).
6. **Discharge lounge:** Many hospitals now have discharge lounges to help your final day in hospital go smoothly. Patients who don't need to stay on the ward are transferred to the lounge on the day of discharge. Staff will inform the pharmacy, transport and relatives of your transfer. To help pass the

time, there are usually facilities, such as a TV, radio, magazines, puzzles, books, and newspapers. If someone feels unwell while waiting, nurses contact a doctor to come and see you before discharge.

7. **Ear nose and throat (ENT):** The ENT department provides care for patients with a variety of problems, including:
   - General ear, nose and throat diseases,
   - Neck lumps,
   - Cancers of the head and neck area,
   - Tear duct problems,
   - Facial skin lesions,
   - Balance and hearing disorders,
   - Snoring and sleep apnoea,
   - ENT allergy problems,
   - Salivary gland diseases,
   - Voice disorders.

8. **Elderly services department:** Consultant physicians specializing in geriatric medicine, this department looks after a wide range of problems associated with the elderly. This includes:
   - Stroke medicine,
   - Gastroenterology,
   - Diabetes,
   - Locomotor (movement) problems,
   - Continence problems,
   - Syncope (fainting),
   - Bone disease.

   It provides a range of services, such as home visits, day hospital and outpatient clinics. The department often has close links with other community services for the elderly.

9. **Gastroentrology:** Endoscopy involves a small thin tube with a camera on the end. This is guided down the throat to investigate problems in your esophagus and digestive system. Small surgical instruments can be guided down in the same way, meaning it can be used for diagnosis and treatment. Run by consultants specializing in bowel-related medicine, this department investigates and treats upper and lower gastrointestinal disease, as well as diseases of the pancreas and bile duct system. This includes endoscopy and nutritional services. Sub-specialties include colorectal surgery, inflammatory bowel disease, and swallowing problems. There are often endoscopy, nurse specialists linked to a gastroenterology unit who are able to perform a wide range of bowel investigations.

10. **General surgery:** The general surgery ward covers a wide range of surgery and includes:
    - Day surgery,
    - Thyroid surgery,
    - Kidney transplants,
    - Colon surgery,
    - Laparoscopic cholecystectomy (gallbladder removal),
    - Endoscopy,
    - Breast surgery.

    Day surgery units have a high turnover of patients who attend for minor surgical procedures, such as hernia repairs.

11. **Gynecology:** Reproductive organs, such as endometritis, infertility, and incontinence. They also provide a range of care for cervical smear screening and postmenopausal bleeding checks. They usually have:
    - A specialist ward,
    - Day surgery unit,
    - Emergency gynecology assessment unit,
    - Outpatient clinics.

12. **Hematology:** Hematology services work closely with the hospital laboratory. These doctors treat blood diseases and malignancies linked to the blood, with both new referrals and emergency admissions being seen.

13. **Maternity department:** Women now have a choice of who leads their maternity care and where they give birth. Care can be led by a consultant, a GP or a midwife. Maternity wards provide antenatal care, care during childbirth, and postnatal support. Antenatal clinics provide monitoring for both routine, and complicated pregnancies. High-dependency units can offer one-to-one care for women who need close monitoring, when there are complications in pregnancy or childbirth.

14. **Mircobiology:** The microbiology department looks at all aspects of microbiology, such as bacterial and viral infections. They have become increasingly high profile following the rise of hospital-acquired infections, such as MRSA and C. difficult. A head microbiology consultant and team of microbiologists test patient samples sent to them by medical staff from the hospital and from doctors' surgeries.

15. **Neonatal unit:** Neonatal units have a number of cots that are used for intensive, high-dependency and special care for newborn babies. It always maintains close links with the hospital maternity department, in the interest of babies and their families. Neonatal units have the philosophy that, whenever possible, mother and baby should be together.

16. **Nephrology unit:** This department monitors and assessees patients with kidney (renal) problems. Nephrologists (kidney specialists) will liaise with the transplant team in cases of kidney transplants. They also supervise the dialysis day unit for people who are waiting for a kidney transplant or who are unable to have a transplant for any reason.

17. **Neurology unit:** This unit deals with disorders of the nervous system, including the brain, and spinal cord. It's run by doctors who specialize in this area (neurologists) and their staff. There are also pediatric neurologists who treat children. Neurologists may also be involved in clinical research and clinical trials. Specialist nurses (epilepsy, multiple sclerosis) liaise with patients, consultants and GPs to help with any problems that may occur between outpatient appointments.

19. **Obstetrics and gynecology unit:** These units provide maternity services, such as:
    - Antenatal and postnatal care,
    - Prenatal diagnosis unit,
    - Maternal and fetal surveillance.

    Overseen by consultant obstetricians and gynecologists, there is a wide range of attached staff linked to them, including specialist nurses, midwives, and imaging technicians.

    Care can include:
    - General inpatient and outpatient treatment,
    - Colposcopy, laser therapy or hysteroscopy for abnormal cervical cells,
    - Psychosexual counseling,
    - Recurrent miscarriage unit,
    - Early pregnancy unit.

20. **Oncology:** This department provides radiotherapy and a full range of chemotherapy treatments for cancerous tumors and blood disorders. Staffed by specialist doctors and nurses trained in oncology (cancer care), it has close links with surgical and medical teams in other departments.

21. **Ophthalmology:** Eye departments provide a range of ophthalmic services for adults and children, including:
    - General eye clinic appointments,
    - Laser treatments,
    - Optometry (sight testing),
    - Orthoptics (non-surgical treatments, eg for squints),
    - Prosthetic eye services,
    - Ophthalmic imaging (eye scans).

22. **Orthopedics:** Orthopedic departments treat problems that affect your musculoskeletal system—your muscles, joints, bones, ligaments, tendons and nerves. The doctors and nurses who run this department deal with everything from setting bone fractures to carrying out surgery to correct problems, such as torn ligaments, and hip replacements. Orthopedic trauma includes fractures and dislocations as well as musculoskeletal injuries to soft tissues.

23. **Pain management clinic:** Usually run by consultant anesthetists, these clinics aim to help treat patients with severe long-term pain that appears resistant to normal treatments. Depending on the hospital, a wide range of options are available, such as acupuncture, nerve blocks, and drug treatment.

24. **Radiology:** The branch or specialty of medicine that deals with the study and

application of imaging technology like X-ray and radiation to diagnosing and treating disease. The Department of Radiology is a highly specialized, full-service department which strives to meet all patient and clinician needs in diagnostic imaging and image guided therapies.

25. **Radiotherapy:** Run by a combination of consultant doctors and specially trained radiotherapists, this department provides radiotherapy (X-ray) treatment for conditions, such as malignant tumors, and cancer.

26. **Renal unit:** Closely linked with nephrology teams at hospitals, these units provide hemodialysis treatment for patients with kidney failure. Many of these patients are on waiting lists for a kidney transplant. They also provide facilities for peritoneal dialysis and help facilitate home hemodialysis.

27. **Rheumatology:** Specialist doctors called rheumatologists run the unit and are experts in the field of musculoskeletal disorders (bones, joints, ligaments, tendons, muscles, and nerves). Their role is to diagnose conditions and recommend appropriate treatment, if necessary from the orthopedic department. The rheumatologist may need to review you regularly, either in person or via one of the rheumatology team. Alternatively, your condition may be one your GP can manage in the community. Many conditions are managed jointly between the GP and the hospital care team.

28. **Sexual health (genitourinary medicine):** This department provides a free and confidential service offering:
    - Advice, testing and treatment for all sexually transmitted infections (STIs),
    - Family planning care (including emergency contraception and free condoms),
    - Pregnancy testing and advice. It also provides care and support for other sexual and genital problems. Patients are, usually, able to phone the department directly for an appoint-

ment and don't need a referral letter from their GP.

29. **Urology department:** The urology department is run by consultant urology surgeons and their surgical teams. It investigates all areas linked to kidney and bladder-based problems. The department performs:
    - Flexible cystoscopy bladder checks,
    - Urodynamic studies (e.g., for incontinence),
    - Prostate assessments and biopsies,
    - Shockwave lithotripsy to break up kidney stones.

Nursing Service Department

Nursing services are considered one of the most important aspects in the process of distinguished medical care. Nursing division provides nursing to patients at all general and specialized clinics in addition to specialized care services to inpatients at all units.

Paramedical Departments

1. **Nutrition and dietetics:** Trained dieticians and nutritionists provide specialist advice on diet for hospital wards and outpatient clinics, forming part of a multidisciplinary team. The department works across a wide range of specialties, such as:
   - Diabetes,
   - Cancer,
   - Kidney problems,
   - Pediatrics,
   - Elderly care,
   - Surgery and critical care,
   - Gastroenterology.

   They also provide group education to patients with diabetes, heart disease and osteoarthritis, and work closely with weight management groups.

2. **Pharmacy:** The hospital pharmacy is run by pharmacists, pharmacy technicians, and attached staff. It is responsible for drug based services in the hospital, including:
   - The purchasing, supply and distribution of medication and pharmaceuticals,

- Inpatient and outpatient dispensing,
- Clinical and ward pharmacy,
- The use of drugs.

A pharmacy will provide a drug formulary for hospital doctors to use as a guide. It will also help supervise any clinical trial management and ward drug-use review.

3. **Physiotherapy:** Physiotherapists promote body healing, for example, after surgery, through therapies, such as exercise, and manipulation. This means they assess, treat and advise patients with a wide range of medical conditions. They also provide health education to patients and staff on how to do things more easily. Their services are provided to patients in the physiotherapy department itself and in rehabilitation units. Physiotherapists often work closely with orthopedic teams.

4. **Occupational therapy:** This profession helps people who are physically or mentally impaired, including temporary disability after medical treatment. It practices in the fields of both healthcare and social care. The aim of occupational therapy is to restore physical and mental functioning to help people participate in life to the fullest. Occupational therapy assessments often guide hospital discharge planning, with the majority of patients given a home assessment to understand their support needs. Staff also arranges provision of essential equipment and adaptations that are essential for discharge from hospital.

Supportive Services

1. **Public relations:** Any department in this hospital shall have two interests. One of them is internal and the other is external. Information department of the hospital will be concerned with patients as an internal public in addition to its activities and relations with parties outside the scope of the hospital. For achieving its objectives and performance of its mission. Public relations resort to the ideal use of all available media. In this regard, it participates in organizing scientific courses and media coverage of the activities of forums and conferences and scientific meetings and the visits made to the hospital for making known the activities of the hospital that are worth media coverage, and preparing materials of booklets, leaflets, and posters with the aim of education in various occasions as well as participation in expositions and health education weeks, and issuance of "health education" and performing procedures of researches and questionnaires to know the patients' feedback on services rendered by the hospital.

2. **Chaplainary:** Chaplains promote the spiritual and pastoral well-being of patients, relatives and staff. They are available to all members of staff for confidential counsel and support irrespective of religion or race. A hospital chapel is also usually available.

3. **Health and safety:** The role of the occupational health and safety department is to promote and maintain the highest possible degree of health and safety for all employees, physicians, volunteers, students and contractors, and actively participates in quality, safety and risk initiatives. Numerous health and safety issues associated with healthcare facilities include blood borne pathogens and biological hazards, potential chemical and drug exposures, waste anesthetic gas exposures, respiratory hazards, ergonomic hazards from lifting and repetitive tasks, laser hazards, hazards associated with laboratories, and radioactive material and X-ray hazards. In addition to the medical staff, large healthcare facilities employ a wide variety of trades that have health and safety hazards associated with them. These include mechanical maintenance, medical equipment maintenance, housekeeping, food service, building and grounds maintenance, laundry, and administrative staff.

4. **Social work:** Clinical social workers help patients and their families deal with the broad range of psychosocial issues and stresses related to coping with illness

and maintaining health. Social workers, resource specialists and advocates form a network that addresses the challenges families face, increases accessibility to health care and other human services, and serves as a bridge between the hospital setting and a patient's family life.

Central Sterile Supply Department

In spite of our knowledge of microbiology, availability of different methods of sterilization, use of antiseptics and also other efforts to prevent infections, hospital acquired infection continues to affect many patients. In earlier years, sterilization of instruments, dressing material, injection syringes, needles, etc. was carried out in different regions, usually near or in the user department.

Decentralization of this service has shown following disadvantages:
- Duplication of sterilization equipment
- Necessity of having additional staff in these sections
- Supervision and standardization are difficult
- Wastage of nurse's time
- Chances of negligent behavior causing false sense of security.
- Chances of accidents if safety precautions are not observed.
- Reluctance on part of other staff to handle additional work load, in case sterilization equipment of a particular section is not functioning.
- Higher expenses to the hospital due to a) Duplication of equipments, b) Recruitment of additional staff, c) Hidden cost of improper sterilization: i) Higher risk of hospital acquired infection, ii) Longer stay in hospital, iii) Higher risk of morbidity, iv) Higher risk of mortality v) expenditure on costly antibiotics.
- In case the hospital has outreach services like attached urban or rural health centers supervision is more difficult and this additional work load is resented by the hospital staff. In most of the hospitals centralization of this service has obviated

the need for having this facility scattered at different places. Establishment of central sterile supply department has resulted in many advantages to administration, clinical staff and patients.

Advantages

I. **Administration:**
- Reduction in expenditure,
- Reduction in recruitment,
- Better control and supervision,
- Improved quality and efficiency of performance, and
- Improved hospital image.

II. **Clinical staff:**
- Uninterrupted supply of sterilized items round the clock,
- Reliability,
- Less complications related to sepsis.

III. **Patients:**
- Safety,
- Avoidance of complications like wound infection, fever, HIV, or hepatitis B infection, and
- Less expenditure on antibiotics.

CSSD services cater to the needs of different sections of the hospital, namely
- Operation theatre,
- Intensive care areas,
- Emergency and casualty areas,
- Wards,
- Recovery room,
- Laboratories,
- Pharmacy, and
- OPD. services including injection section, dressing department, minor surgery theatres, etc.

C.S.S.D. does not completely eliminate other regional facilities for routine sterilization, e.g. routine instruments like tongue depressor, ENT instruments for OPD, etc. are sterilized in the respective sections.

Activities of CSSD: Sterilization of different items is performed by the trained staff using appropriate sterilization methods. Efficient functioning of CSSD also reduces the need for purchasing certain expensive disposable items.

Activities of this department are as follows:

- Receive soiled and unsterile material from different departments of the hospital.
- Sorting out these items, and a) whether the items need to be discarded b) whether the item is reusable, e.g. if torn gloves, broken syringe, cracked catheter are received they are discarded.
- Preliminary cleaning with water and disinfectant to clean out contamination.

During last few years, due to increase in incidence of infection like HIV, many hospitals have appointed hospital infection control committee. This committee ensures implementation of safety practices. Used and/or soiled linen is first rinsed in water by the user department and dipped in a plastic drum containing 2% sodium hypochlorite solution for disinfection. If user departments follow this practice work of CSSD becomes easier because if blood, pus or any other biological fluid dries up, it is difficult to remove the stains.

- If any item requires specialized method of cleaning then the same is carried out.
- Instruments, parts of equipment, tubing linen, etc. are thoroughly checked to decide whether any repair is required. If so necessary actions are taken.
- Dressing packs, linen packs, trays for specific procedures, instruments are assembled and arranged.
- Sterilization is carried out after packing the assembled items in suitable packages
- After putting labels and making entry in the supply register sterilized material is sent to the respective areas.

23

Administration of Hospital/Department/Unit/Ward

LEARNING OBJECTIVES

- Physical environment
- Therapeutic environment
- Prevention of accidents and infections in hospital
- Patient safety in the hospital
- Leadership styles
- Problem solving
- Records and reports

INTRODUCTION

The physical aspects of environment are contributing factors to client's recovery. Provision of a safe and comfortable environment for the clients and the personnel is the responsibility of the head nurse. It includes regulation of atmospheric temperature, humidity and ventilation, adequate lighting, prevention of noise, elimination of unpleasant odors, dust control, safe disposal of excreta and wastes, safe water supply, freeform vermin's, insects and animal pests, fire prevention, protection from radiation and electrocution, provision of adequate privacy, prevention of cross infection, control of visitors, cleanliness and orderliness and esthetic factors.

PHYSICAL ENVIRONMENT

Optimum environment for the patient: There are few factors which are considered as essentials to well-being, they are:

- Adequate lighting during the day and night
- Provision of an atmospheric temperature and humidity that promotes normal body functions.

- Sufficient air movement to evaporate sweats and favors vascular changes within the skin.
- Atmospheric pressure within man's tolerance.
- Provision for disposal of refuse on excreta
- Removal of dust. Injurious chemicals and pathogenic bacteria from the atmospheric air
- Reasonable cleanliness of all surface and furnishing that the individual is likely to handle.
- A dwelling place frees from insects, animal pests, fire hazards, mechanical injuries, electric shocks, radiation and poisons.
- Freedom from disagreeable odors and noises, harmony of town and design in the immediate surroundings.

Basic components of environment: The nursing unit environment is made up of two basic components.

1. **The physical component;** furniture, furnishing, lighting, etc.
2. **Psychosocial component;** created by the customs, cultural values, norms and interpersonal relationships existing in the nursing unit. It influences the patient's reaction to illness, and can play a role in

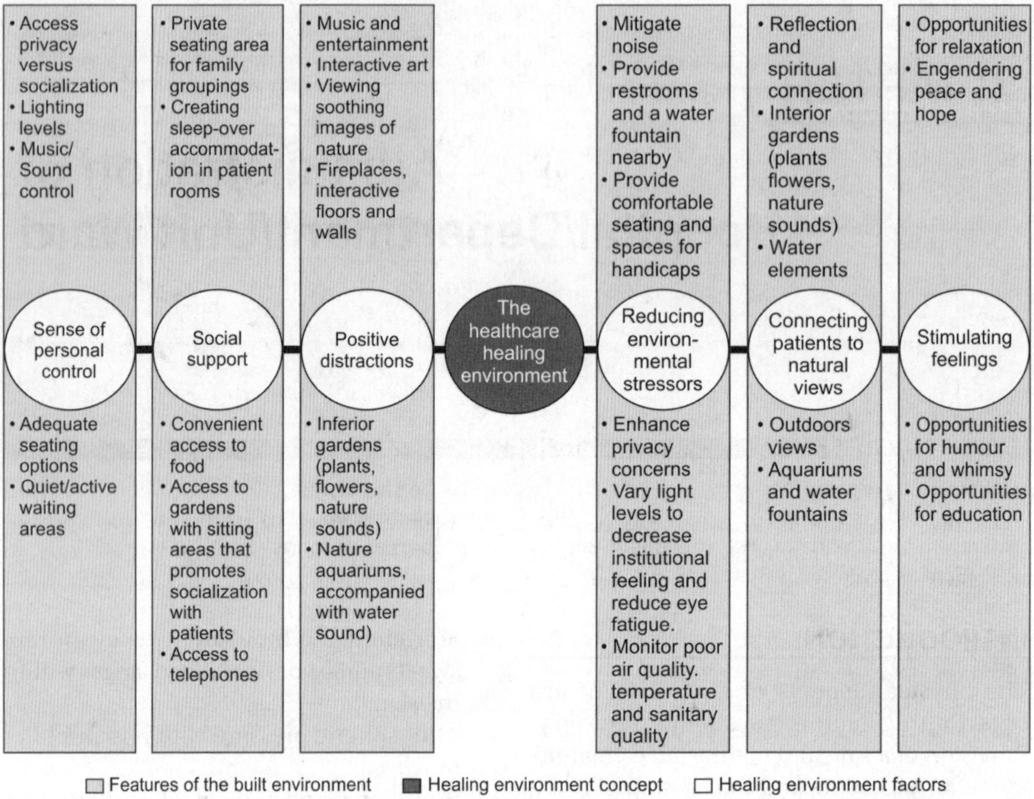

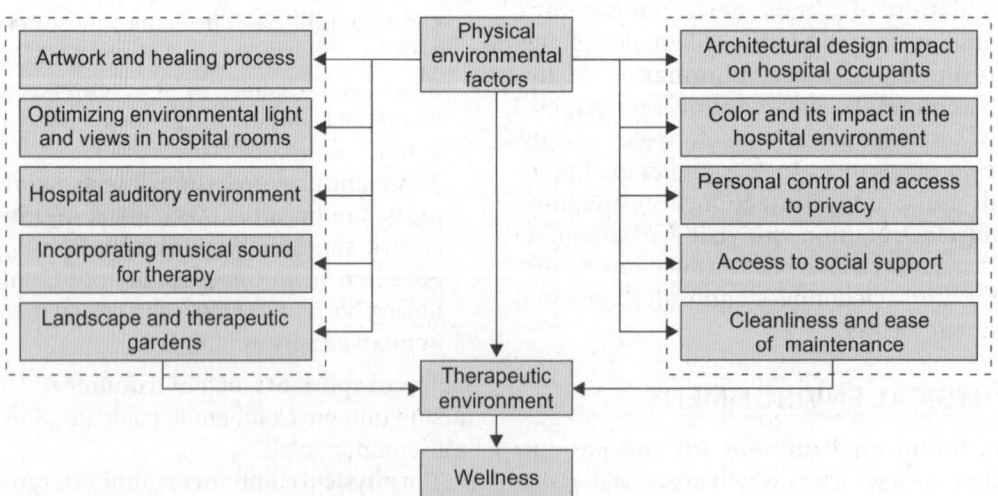

| Features of the built environment | ■ Healing environment concept | Healing environment factors |

Fig. 23.1: Health care healing environment.

Fig. 23.2: Factors influencing wellness.

his/her recovery and well-being. Therefore, the provision of a safe, comfortable and pleasant unit environment should be the aim of unit personnel and every member of the health team.

THERAPEUTIC ENVIRONMENT

Patients seek admission in the hospital because of some physical or mental illness. They have their own personality traits and social positions. They have a right to receive nursing care as well as the treatment and supportive care that will help them to get cured at the earliest moment. The speed of recovery depends upon the nursing care they receive. A nurse must remember that body mind and spirit have close relationship. And influence each other in every individual and disturbance of function of any will disturb the function of the other. Nursing care involves attention to the body, mind and spirit as well. The basic needs for love, the maintenance of dignity and social relationships need to be met. The nursing care is directed to maintain all physical and mental functions of the individual and to restore the lost functions.

Environment: Among the factors contributing to the patients speedy recovery are those from the environment. The nurse is very important part of the environment. The attitude of the head nurse towards her patients is of paramount importance.

Cleanliness, peace orderliness, neatness, ventilation and lighting are important aspects of physical environment. The nursing staff has to assume the responsibility to control these factors though some of them are belonging to the housekeeping department or technicians.

Because the effect of environment on patient care is great, the nurse has major responsibility to provide conducive environment which will contribute to peace and recovery. The modern hospital provides more privacy for the patients than was provided in olden days. Small units for two, three or four patients provide more quietness and rest than was possible in the open wards. Attention is given to pleasing effects of color of walls, floorings furnishings and linen. The arrangement of beds and furniture has gained lots of importance. More attention is nowadays paid to provide hospital environment safe, comfortable and convenient for its workers too so that it promotes their efficiency and promptness in patient. A clean environment provides clean equipment, clean linen, clean floors and walls which are relatively free from pathogenic organisms. Through unclean

contaminated equipment, it is possible to transmit infection from one patient to another.

PREVENTION OF ACCIDENTS AND INFECTIONS IN HOSPITAL

It is very important to know safety measures while working in hospital. Hospital is a place where the patient comes to get well. Ills out duty to ensure safety and protection of patients. These are:
- Physical environment
- Prevention of accident injuries and infection
- Biomedical waste management.

I. **Physical environment:** Nursing care in relation to the immediate physical environment has four major goals.
   1. To prompt safety
   2. To control communicable disease.
   3. Maintenance of physical environment in patient care unit.
   4. Guidance for cleanliness of the wards as a unit of the patient is the ultimate legal responsibility of staff for safe and effective performance.

II. **Prevention of accidents and injuries:** The nurses constantly observe the environment for hazards such as malfunctioning electrical equipment cards or tiles on the floor, inadequate lighting or improperly labeled medications one of the biggest health related concerns for nurses in environmental safety, prevention of injuries and accidents are classified according their source include mechanical, thermal, electrical and radiation chemical.
   - **Freedom from mechanical injury:** Mechanical injury can be prevented by using rails or guards on beds and windows by keeping floors dry to prevent slipping by holding the stretchers and shell chairs securely while transferring patients.
   - **Freedom from thermal injury:** Burns may occur from the application of heat. Some possible causes of fire in a hospital are smoking in bed defective

wiring explosion of gases and use of heaters and hot plates.

- **Freedom from chemical injury:** Chemical injury involves the use of too strong chemicals kept within the reach of the patient. Chemical injury can be prevented by keeping the chemicals in separate cupboards under lock and key and by using them with care.
- **Freedom from radiation:** Radiation injury occurs from, over exposure to rays of X-ray radium infrared and U-V rays. These injuries can be prevented by having trained operators and having enough protection from exposure to these rays. Freedom from bacteriological injury—bacteriologic safety has to do with the elimination of disease bearing organisms and dirt that harbors them.
- **Freedom from allergens:** Injury from allergens may results from insect bites, from materials in the environment such as feather mattresses, food, cosmetic lotions, powders, medications, etc. Prevention of allergy may be accomplished by having covers for mattresses and pillows adopting dusting without raising the dust and by testing for allergies before an agent is applied on the body.
- **Freedom from vermin insects and animal pest:** All buildings should be rat proof. Flies will find a breeding place where the dirt accumulated. Therefore the whole hospital and its surroundings should be kept clean to prevent breeding of flies, prevent the breeding of mosquitoes by removing the stagnant water and by using mosquito repellants such as DDT spray, etc.

PATIENT SAFETY IN THE HOSPITAL

Medical errors may occur in different health care settings, and those that happen in hospitals can have serious consequences. The agency for healthcare research and quality, which has sponsored hundreds of patient safety research and implementation projects,

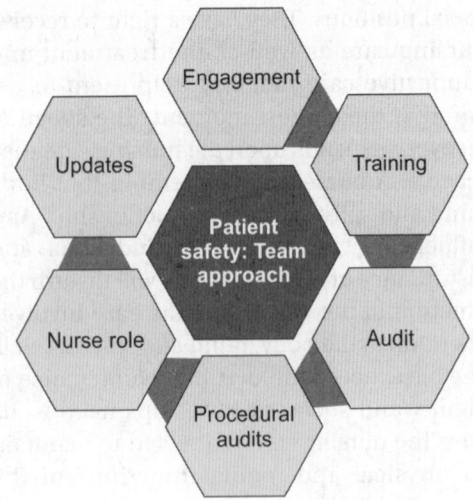

Fig. 23.3: Patient safety: Team approach

offers these 10 evidence-based tips to prevent adverse events from occurring in the hospital.

Prevent central line-associated blood stream infections: Be vigilant preventing central line-associated blood stream infections by taking five steps every time a central venous catheter is inserted—wash your hands, use full-barrier precautions, clean the skin with chlorhexidine, avoid femoral lines, and remove unnecessary lines. Taking these steps consistently reduced this type of deadly health care-associated infection to zero in a study at more than 100 large and small hospitals.

Re-engineer hospital discharges: Reduce potentially preventable readmissions by assigning a staff member to work closely with patients and other staff to reconcile medications and schedule necessary follow-up medical appointments. Create a simple, easy-to-understand discharge plan for each patient that contains a medication schedule, a record of all upcoming medical appointments, and names and phone numbers of whom to call if a problem arises.

Prevent venous thromboembolism: Eliminate hospital-acquired venous thrombo-embolism (VTE), the most common cause of preventable hospital deaths, by using an evidence-based guide to create a VTE protocol. This free guide explains how to take essential first steps, lay out the evidence and identify best practices, analyze care delivery, track performance with metrics, layer interventions, and continue to improve.

Educate patients about using blood thinners safety: Patients who have had surgery often leave the hospital with a new prescription for a blood thinner, such as Warfarin brand name: Coumadin®, to keep them from developing dangerous blood clots. However, if used incorrectly, blood thinners can cause uncontrollable bleeding and are among the top causes of adverse drug events. A free 10-minute patient education video and companion 24-page booklet, both in English and Spanish, help patients understand what to expect when taking these medicines.

Limit shift durations for medical residents and other hospital staff if possible: Evidence shows that acute and chronically fatigued medical residents are more likely to make mistakes. Ensure that residents get ample sleep and adhere to 80-hour work week limits. Residents who work 30-hour shifts should only treat patients for up to 16 hours and

should have a 5-hour protected sleep period between 10 pm and 8 am.

Consider working with a patient safety organization: Report and share patient safety information with patient safety organizations (PSOs) to help others avoid preventable errors. By providing both privilege and confidentiality, PSOs create a secure environment where clinicians and health care organizations can use common formats to collect, aggregate, and analyze data that can improve quality by identifying and reducing the risks and hazards associated with patient care.

Use good hospital design principles: Follow evidence-based principles for hospital design to improve patient safety and quality. Prevent patient falls by providing well-designed patient rooms and bathrooms and creating decentralized nurses' stations that allow easy access to patients. Reduce infections by offering single bed rooms, improving air filtration systems, and providing multiple convenient locations for hand washing. Prevent medication errors by offering

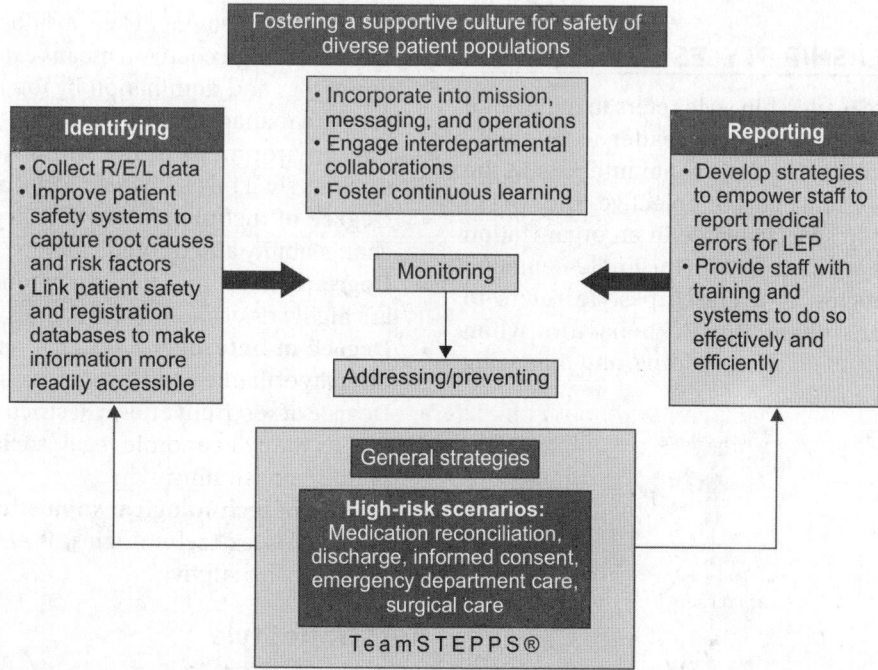

Key: R/E/L = race, ethnicity, language.

Fig. 23.4: Key recommendations to improve patient safety for LEP patient.

(R/E/L: race, ethnicity, language)

pharmacists well-lit, quiet, private spaces so they can fill prescriptions without distractions.

Measure hospital's patient safety culture: Survey hospital staff to assess your facility's patient safety culture. The Agency for Healthcare Research and Quality's (AHRQ's) free *hospital survey on patient safety culture* and related materials are designed to provide tools for improving the patient safety culture, evaluating the impact of interventions, and tracking changes over time. If the health system includes nursing homes or ambulatory care medical groups, share culture surveys customized for those settings.

Build better teams and rapid response systems: Train hospital staff to communicate effectively as a team. A free, customizable toolkit called Team STEPPS™, which stands for team strategies and tools to enhance performance and patient safety, provides evidence-based techniques for promoting effective communication and other teamwork skills among staff in various units or as part of rapid response teams. Materials can be tailored to any health care setting, from emergency departments to ambulatory clinics.

LEADERSHIP STYLES

The term leadership style refers to behavioral pattern employed by a leader to integrate organizational and personal interests in the pursuit of some goal or objective. The type of leadership style available in an organization has a great deal to do with the implementation of strategies. A leadership style refers to a leader's characteristic behaviors when directing, motivating, guiding, and managing

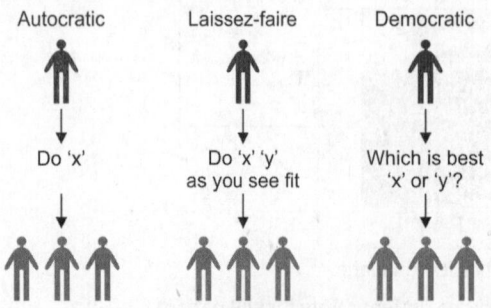

Fig. 23.5: Leadership styles.

groups of people. Great leaders can inspire political movements and social change. They can also motivate others to perform, create, and innovate.

Definition

The leadership styles are the behavioral patterns that a leader adopt to influence the behavior of his followers, i.e. the way he gives directions to his subordinates and motivates them to accomplish the given objectives.

Characteristics of Leadership Styles

- **Risk Taking**: Willingness to make high-risk, high-return decisions.
- **Technology**: Degree of commitment to planning, employment of technically qualified persons, and practice of management science techniques.
- **Organicity**: Degree of loose and flexible organizational structuring; low organicity is mechanistic in tightly structured organizations.
- **Participation**: High participation implies extensive participation of those other than the top management in key positions.
- **Coercion**: High coercion means extensive use of fear and domination by top managers as a management technique.

The environment along the following dimensions shall be characterized as follows:

- **Degree of turbulence of volatility:** Fast changeability and unpredictability.
- **Degree of hostility:** Hostile environments are highly risky and overwhelming.
- **Degree of heterogeneity:** This refers to diversity of markets and types of consumers.
- **Degree of restrictiveness:** Restrictiveness means many economic legal, social and political constraints.
- **Degree of technological sophistication:** With complex technologies, R and D is necessary for survival.

Autocratic Style

Autocratic leadership is a management style wherein one person controls all the decisions and takes very little inputs from other group

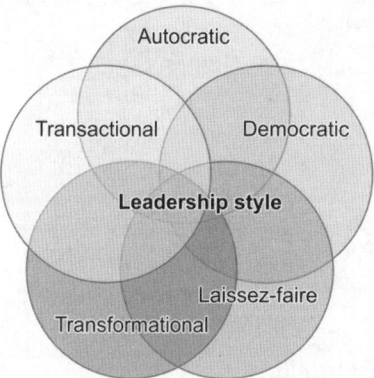

Fig. 23.6: Leadership style.

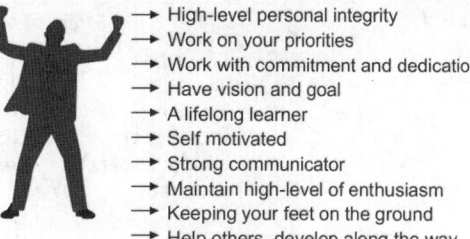

→ High-level personal integrity
→ Work on your priorities
→ Work with commitment and dedication
→ Have vision and goal
→ A lifelong learner
→ Self motivated
→ Strong communicator
→ Maintain high-level of enthusiasm
→ Keeping your feet on the ground
→ Help others, develop along the way

Fig. 23.7: 10 characteristics of a leader.

members. Autocratic leaders make choices or decisions based on their own beliefs and do not involve others for their suggestion or advice.

- In such a style of working, the superiors do not take into consideration the ideas and suggestions of the subordinates.
- The managers, leaders and superiors have the sole responsibility of taking decisions without bothering much about the subordinates.
- The employees are totally dependent on their bosses and do not have the liberty to take decisions on their own.
- The subordinates in such a style of working simply adhere to the guidelines and policies formulated by their bosses. They do not have a say in management's decisions.
- Whatever the superiors feel is right for the organization eventually becomes the company's policies.
- Employees lack motivation in autocratic style of working.

Characteristics of autocratic leadership include:

- Clear separation of leader and subordinate roles
- Focus on tasks and goals
- Clearly defined performance expectations for all team members
- Consequences for failure to comply with expectations
- A structured work environment

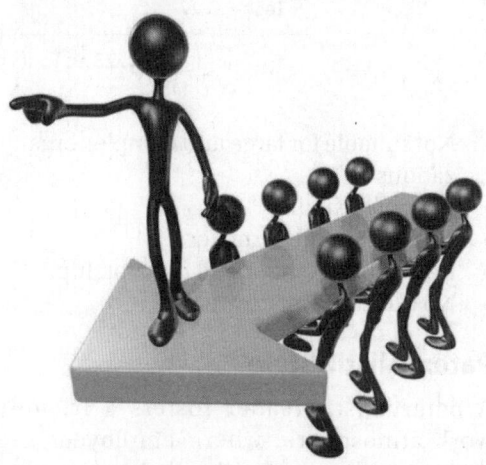

Fig. 23.8: Autocratic leadership.

- Specific processes for performing workplace tasks
- Strict adherence to established rules and policies
- The leader is the sole decision-maker

Benefits or Advantages

The main advantages of autocratic leadership can be pointed out as follows:

- Allows quick decision making
- High level of secrecy
- Simple and easy style
- Better discipline
- Increased productivity
- Suitability
- Clear chain of command
- Useful for new and incompetent employees

Drawbacks or Disadvantages

The main disadvantages of autocratic leadership can be pointed out as follows:

- Workload to the superiors
- Negative motivation

Traits of a good leadership		
• Self-motivated	• Integrity	• Innovative
• Humility	• Ability to delegate	• Honesty
• Care for others	• Communication	• Active listening
• Self-awareness	• Gratitude	• Self-confidence
• Emotional intelligence	• Learning agility	• Vision
• Self-discipline	• Influence	• Delegation
• Passion	• Empathy	• Decision-making
• Resilience	• Courage	• Problem-solving
• Accountable	• Respect	• Fair attitude
• Supportive		• Inquisitiveness
• Tech-savvy		• Empower others

Fig. 23.9: Traits of a good leadership.

- Not suitable for large and complex organizations
- Lack of flexibility
- High employee turnover
- Micromanagement and dictatorship
- No utilization of creativity.

Paternalistic Style

A paternalistic leader fosters a friendly work atmosphere, where employees see their coworkers as family. The paternalistic leadership style lays huge importance on the needs of employees and the organization.

- In paternalistic style of working, the leaders decide what is best for the employees as well as the organization.
- Policies are devised to benefit the employees and the organization.
- The suggestions and feedback of the subordinates are taken into consideration before deciding something.
- In such a style of working, employees feel attached and loyal towards their organization.
- Employees stay motivated and enjoy their work rather than treating it as a burden.

Advantages of Paternalistic Leadership

- High employee loyalty due to employees feeling like they are being heard and their needs are met.
- Good behavior is rewarded by the person at the top, often with goods and food.

- Absenteeism rates and staff turnover will decrease as emphasis is placed on the employee's needs.
- Most decisions will be made with the employees' best interests taken into consideration.
- Feedback is invited and encouraged, which improves morale and makes employees feel important.
- There is an open line of communication between the managers and the employees which will keep employees feeling important and satisfied.
- There is an understanding that the manager wants everyone to succeed, which can result in a lower amount of competition among employees.
- The manager is given the power to rule from the idea that they are the most capable in making the best decisions for the team, which fosters trust and loyalty with employees.
- Managers are very involved in the employee's personal lives, which makes the employee feel more connected at work.

Disadvantages of Paternalistic Leadership

- Just like a parent, managers will sometimes have to discipline the employee in non-traditional ways.
- Bad decisions from above cause major employee dissatisfaction.

Advantages and disadvantages

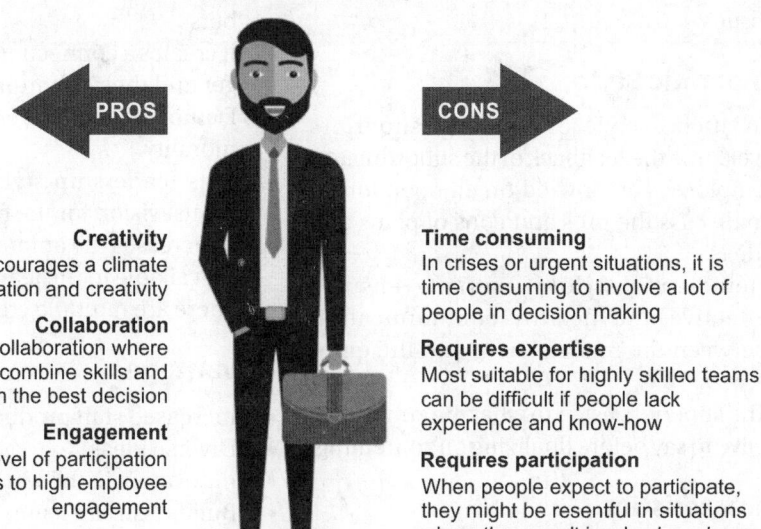

PROS

CONS

Creativity
Provides and encourages a climate of innovation and creativity

Collaboration
Facilitates collaboration where multiple people combine skills and experience to reach the best decision

Engagement
The high level of participation generally leads to high employee engagement

Time consuming
In crises or urgent situations, it is time consuming to involve a lot of people in decision making

Requires expertise
Most suitable for highly skilled teams can be difficult if people lack experience and know-how

Requires participation
When people expect to participate, they might be resentful in situations where they aren't involved or when a decision goes against them

Fig. 23.10: Democratic leadership.

Democratic leadership
Characteristics of a democratic leader

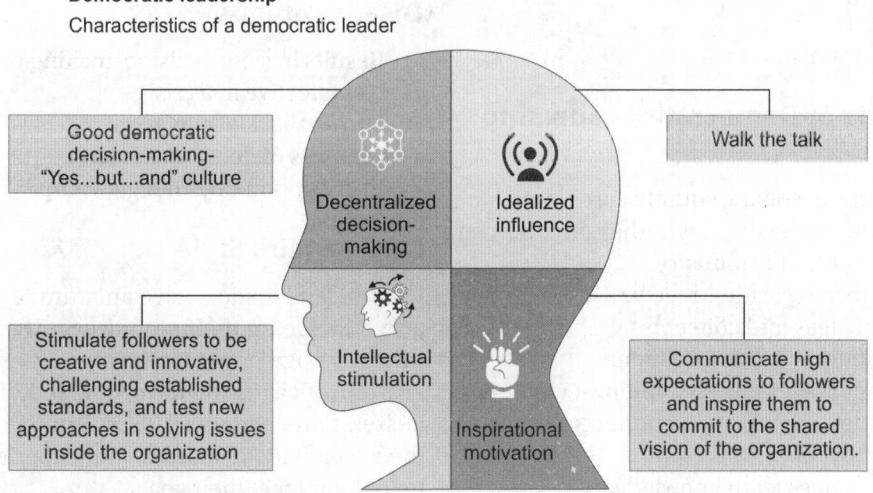

Good democratic decision-making- "Yes...but...and" culture

Decentralized decision-making

Idealized influence

Walk the talk

Stimulate followers to be creative and innovative, challenging established standards, and test new approaches in solving issues inside the organization

Intellectual stimulation

Inspirational motivation

Communicate high expectations to followers and inspire them to commit to the shared vision of the organization.

Fig. 23.11: Democratic leadership.

- The employees will become more and more dependent on the employer, which can cause an increase in necessary supervision in order to get things done in a timely and appropriate manner.
- If loyalty to the manager is not established quickly then there can be poor staff motivation.
- Issues can be caused and exacerbated with employee legislation and rights.

- Employees rely on the leader more than they would in a typical work setting. Because of this, the team can become highly competitive as they all vie for attention and affection.
- Managers can become blind with their power and make decisions that only benefit themselves.
- If roles are not well defined and employees do not know what is needed from them

there can be power struggles and internal issues.

Democratic Style

- In such a style of working, superiors welcome the feedback of the subordinates.
- Employees are invited on an open forum to discuss the pros and cons of plans and ideas.
- Democratic style of working ensures effective and healthy communication between the management and the employees.
- The superiors listen to what the employees have to say before finalizing on something.

Characteristics

- Team-focused
- Flexible
- Adaptable to change
- Engaged listeners
- Honest
- Communicative

Benefits of Democratic Leadership Style

- It helps in solving complex problems.
- It is a leadership style that anyone can practice in any industry.
- Democratic leaders receive a more diverse set of ideas and concepts.
- It enhances job satisfaction.
- It encourages honesty amongst workers.
- This leadership style connects people to their work.
- It enhances team knowledge.
- It encourages more substantial commitment levels.
- This style promotes the free flow of ideas.
- A leader who uses this style is considered more competent.
- This leadership style encourages trust and respect throughout the team.
- It takes an open and honest mind to be a using democratic leader.
- This leadership style allows a team to develop more strength. In addition, this style results in increased productivity.

- Robust connectivity between team members.
- It creates a connection between the manager and their subordinates.
- Democratic leaders emphasize values and morality.
- This leadership style can also create a robust vision for the future.
- It increases the amount of knowledge that is available to the team.
- There are multiple creative solutions.

Advantages

- Increased staff productivity
- Diverse ideas
- Innovation in the workplace and creativity
- Builds a strong team
- Increased job satisfaction
- Best for any organization
- Improved awareness about company values

Disadvantages

- Results in slow decision-making process
- Not effective in a crisis
- Shows a lack of expertise
- Chances of dealing with rejection
- Every option does not get valued

Laissez-faire Style

Laissez-faire leaders have an attitude of trust and reliance on their employees. They don't micromanage or get too involved; they don't give too much instruction or guidance. Instead laissez-faire leaders let their employees use their creativity, resources, and experience to help them meet their goals.

- In such a style of working, managers are employed just for the sake of it and do not contribute much to the organization.
- The employees take decisions and manage work on their own.
- Individuals who have the dream of making it big in the organization and desire to do something innovative every time outshine others who attend office for fun.
- Employees are not dependent on the managers and know what is right or wrong for them.

Characteristics of Laissez-faire Leaders

- Little guidance from leaders
- Employees have the ability to make decisions
- People are expected to solve their own problems
- Access to many resources and tools
- Constructive criticism from leaders
- Leaders take charge when necessary
- Leaders take responsibility for overall actions and decisions.

Advantages of Laissez-faire Leadership

- It allows team members to maximize their own leadership skills.
- It provides the people with the most experience to shine.
- It creates an environment of independence.
- It encourages team members to explore new ideas.
- It allows individual teams to create their own environment.
- It generates more individual satisfaction for the work being done.
- It provides the leader to be strategic with their skills.

Disadvantages

- It downplays the role of the leader on the team.

Laissez-faire leadership, also called delegative leadership or hands-off leadership, is the most laid-back leadership style there is. The team members are essentially given free rein to complete tasks in whatever way they please.

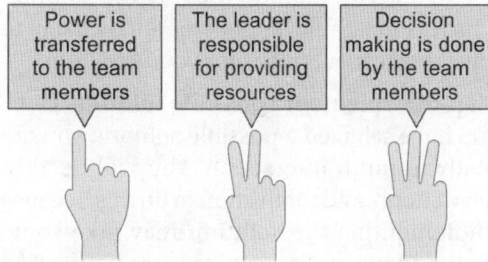

Fig. 23.12: Characteristics of laissez-faire leadership.

- It reduces the cohesiveness of the group.
- It changes how accountability is assigned within the group.
- It allows leaders to avoid leadership.
- It is a leadership style which employees can abuse.
- It can be difficult to adapt to changing situations.
- It creates opportunities for employee litigation.

PROBLEM SOLVING

Problem solving is the act of defining a problem; determining the cause of the problem; identifying, prioritizing, and selecting alternatives for a solution; and implementing a solution. The problem-solving process. Problem solving as a manager is important because it helps a company and its employees succeed. Managers who can overcome obstacles efficiently can increase their own productivity, improve job satisfaction of their team and encourage creativity within their department.

Important to Solve Problems as a Manager

- **Better team cohesion:** A manager skilled at problem solving may be a better leader for their team.
- **Workflow improvement:** When managers can efficiently remove challenges, their team can concentrate on other tasks.
- **Client and customer happiness:** Clients and customers appreciate getting accurate or well-made services or products on time.
- **Exceeding work expectations:** Managers who are skilled at problem-solving can exceed expectations and complete more work.
- **Timely project completion:** Solving problems allows employees to complete and deliver projects on time.
- **Welcoming work environment:** A manager who solves problems with their team can make their employees feel comfortable asking questions.

Skills of Problem Solving

- **Incubation:** The period between stopping conscious work on a problem and the time when we become aware of a solution or part solution. People struggling with problems often suddenly become aware of a solution after a period of incubation, during which the mind is occupied by other things.
- **Invention:** The creation of new, meaningful ideas or concepts.
- **Innovation:** Putting new ideas or concepts to a practical use, as in the development of a new product or service.

Problem Solving Cycle

A seven-step problem solving cycle: There are many different ways to solve a problem, however all ways involve a series of steps. The following is a seven-step problem solving model:

Step-1: Identify the problem: Firstly you need to identify and name the problem so that you can find an appropriate solution. You may not be clear of what the problem is or feel anxious/confused about what is getting in the way of your goals. Try talking to others, as this may help you identify the problem.

Step-2: Explore the problem: When you are clear about what the problem is you need to think about from different angles. You can ask yourself questions such as:

- How is this problem affecting me?
- How is it affecting others?
- Who else experiences this problem?
- What do they do about it?

Seeing the problem in different ways is likely to help you find an effective solution.

Step-3: Set goals: Once you have thought about the problem from different angles you can identify your goals. What is it that you want to achieve? Sometimes you may become frustrated by a problem and forget to think about what you want to achieve. For example, you might become ill, struggle to complete a number of assignments on time and feel so unmotivated that you let due dates pass.

- Improve your health?
- Increase your time management skills?
- Complete the assignments to the best of your ability?
- Finish the assignments as soon as possible?

If you decide your goal is to improve your health that will lead to different solutions to those linked with the goal of completing your assignments as soon as possible. One goal may lead you to a doctor and another may lead you to apply for extensions for your assignments. So working out your goals is a vital part of the problem solving process.

Step-4: Look at alternatives: When you have decided what your goal/s is you need to look for possible solutions. The more possible solutions you find the more likely it is that you will be able to discover an effective solution. You can brainstorm for ideas. The purpose of brain-storming is to collect together a long list of possibilities. It does not matter whether the ideas are useful or practical or manageable—just write down the ideas as they come into your head. Some of the best solutions arise from creative thinking during brain-storming. You can also seek ideas about possible solutions by talking to others. The aim is to collect as many alternative solutions as possible.

Step-5: Select a possible solution: From the list of possible solutions you can sort out which are most relevant to your situation and which are realistic and manageable. You can do this by predicting the outcomes for possible solutions and also checking with other people what they think the outcomes may be. When you have explored the consequences, you can use this information to identify the solution which is most relevant to you and is likely to have the best outcomes for your situation.

Step-6: Implement a possible solution: Once you have selected a possible solution you are ready to put it into action. You will need to have energy and motivation to do this because implementing the solution may take some time and effort. You can prepare yourself to implement the solution by planning when and how you will do it, whether you talk with others about it, and what rewards you will give yourself when you have done it.

Step-7: Evaluate: Just because you have implemented the best possible solution, you may not have automatically solved your problem, so evaluating the effectiveness of your solution is very important. You can ask yourself (and others:

- How effective was that solution?
- Did it achieve what I wanted?
- What consequences did it have on my situation?

If the solution was successful in helping you solve your problem and reach your goal, then you know that you have effectively solved your problem. If you feel dissatisfied with the result, then you can begin the steps again.

Scientific method of problem solving:

- Problem awareness
- Problem understanding
- Collection of relevant information
- Formulation of hypotheses or hunch for possible solution
- Selection of a proper solution
- Verification of the concluded solution or hypothesis

- **Problem Awareness:** The first step in problem-solving behavior of an individual concerns his awareness of the difficulty or problem that needs a solution.
- **Problem Understanding:** The difficulty or problem experienced by the individual should be properly identified by a careful analysis. He should be clear about his problem. The problem then should be pinpointed in terms of the specific goals and objectives. Thus all the difficulties and obstacles in the path of the solution must be properly named and identified and what is to be got through the problem-solving efforts should then be properly analyzed.
- **Collection of Relevant Information:** In this step, the individual is required to collect all the relevant information about the problem through all possible sources. He may consult experienced persons, read the available literature, revive his old experiences, think of possible solutions and put in all relevant efforts for widening the scope of his knowledge concerning the problem in hand.

- **Formulation of hypothesis or hunch for possible solutions:** In the light of the collected relevant information and nature of his problem, one may then engage in some serious cognitive activities to think of the various possibilities for the solution of one's problem. As a result, he may start with a few possible solutions for his problem.
- **Selection of a proper solution:** In this step, all the possible solutions, thought of in the previous step, are closely analyzed and evaluated. Gates and others (1946) have suggested the following activities in the evaluation of the assumed hypothesis or solution:
  - One should determine the conclusion that completely satisfies the demands of the problem
  - One should find out whether the solution is consistent with other facts and principles which have been well established
  - One should make a deliberate search for negative instances which might cast doubts on the conclusion.

Problem solving strategy: Problem-solving strategies are the steps that one would use to find the problem(s) that are in the way to getting to one's own goal. Some would refer to this as the 'problem-solving cycle' (Bransford & Stein, 1993). In this cycle one will recognize the problem, define the problem, develop a strategy to fix the problem, organize the knowledge of the problem, figure-out the resources at the user's disposal, monitor one's progress, and evaluate the solution for accuracy. Although called a cycle, one does not have to do each step in order to fix the problem; in fact those who don't are usually better at problem solving. The reason it is called a cycle is that once one is completed with a problem another usually will pop up. Blanchard-Fields (2007) looks at problem solving from one of two facets. The first looking at those problems that only have one solution (like math problems, or fact based questions) which are grounded in psychometric intelligence. The other that is socioemotional in nature and are unpredictable with answers that are constantly changing

The following techniques are usually called problem-solving strategies:

- **Abstraction:** Solving the problem in a model of the system before applying it to the real system
- **Analogy:** Using a solution that solves an analogous problem
- **Brain storming:** (Especially among groups of people) suggesting a large number of solutions or ideas and combining and developing them until an optimum solution is found
- **Divide and conquer:** Breaking down a large, complex problem into smaller, solvable problems
- **Hypothesis testing:** Assuming a possible explanation to the problem and trying to prove (or, in some contexts, disprove) the assumption
- **Lateral thinking:** Approaching solutions indirectly and creatively
- **Means-end analysis:** Choosing an action at each step to move closer to the goal
- **Method of focal objects:** Synthesizing seemingly non-matching characteristics of different objects into something new
- **Morphological analysis:** Assessing the output and interactions of an entire system
- **Proof:** Try to prove that the problem cannot be solved. The point where the proof fails will be the starting point for solving it
- **Reduction:** Transforming the problem into another problem for which solutions exist
- **Research:** Employing existing ideas or adapting existing solutions to similar problems
- **Root-cause analysis:** Identifying the cause of a problem
- **Trial and error:** Testing possible solutions until the right one is found.

RECORDS AND REPORTS

All professional persons need to be accountable for the performance of their duties to the public. Since nursing has been considered as profession, nurses need to record their work on completion. A record is a permanent written communication that documents information's relevant to a client's health care management. A record is a clinical, scientific, administrative and legal document relating to the nursing care given to individual family or community. The records are a practical and indispensable aid to the doctor, nurse and paramedical personnel in giving the best possible service to their clients. Recorded facts have a value and scientific accuracy for more than mere impression of memory and there are guidelines for better administration of health services. Records are the means of communications between health workers and their clients.

Purposes

- Records provide data for programme planning and evaluation.
- Records are the tools of communication between the health workers, the family and other development personnel.
- Records indicate plans for the future.
- Records provide baseline data to estimate the long-term changes related to the services.
- Records provide an opportunity for evaluating the services.
- Records help in the research for improvement of nursing care.

Every institution keeps some kinds of records. The hospital is no exception. The patients clinical record is a brief account of the personal and medical history of the patient, results of diagnostic tests, findings of medical examination, treatment and nursing care daily progress notes and advice on discharge.

Importance of Records

- Record provides an accurate and detailed account of treatments and care given to the patient. Therefore it serves as a guide for follow-up of the course of disease and future care.

- The record provides accurate information of the results of medication and treatments given to the patient. So, through the records the physician gets accurate information about the patient's conditions from day to day.
- Records are of great value in the diagnosis, treatments and nursing care.
- A record of illness and treatment saves duplication of work in the future care especially when the patient is transferred from one department to another or from one institution to another or when an attending physician is transferred and other person takes charge. In such situations it helps the patient to get prompt treatment.
- A well-written record has legal value. The records safeguard the patients, nurses, doctors and the hospital. It serves as evidence that the patient care is intelligently managed.
- Records are tools of communication among the members of the health team. It is of great value for the doctors and nurses at the shifting of duty hours.
- Records help the medical and nursing students in the clinical experience and provide data for care studies.
- Records serve as a reference material for research work.
- The patients record, registers and reports furnish the vital statistics and give information needed to evaluate the service rendered by hospital to the community.

Principles

Data taken from the patient's record points out the health problems of the country and it also provides a base line in which local, state, national and international health services are planned.

Principles of Record Writing

- Since the clinical record is a legal document, it is essential that they should

be written clearly, accurately, appropriately and legibly.
- The individual who writes them should sign all entries.
- Care to be taken not to make any error on the records. If anything is crossed out, it should be dated and initialed.
- All records should be written with black ink or typed for better legibility.
- Records should be written in chronological order as to date and time. When recording medications and treatments, note exact time and date on which they are carried out
- Records are written continuously with no blank spaces. If any space is left out, I should be crossed out, dated and signed.
- Lengthy corrections of records are written as amendments.
- Each page of the record should be properly identified with the name, age, IP no. OP. no. Date, etc.
- Use only standard abbreviations.
- Records should be truthful, brief and complete. It should include all the services given to the patients, the observations made on the patient from day to day and the results of treatments, etc.

Types of Records

- Outpatient and in-patient records
- Nurse's recording
- Doctor's order sheet
- Graphic charts of TPR
- Reports of laboratory examinations
- Diet sheets
- Consent form for operations and anesthesia
- Intake and output chart
- Reports of anesthesia, physiotherapy and other special treatment
- Registers.

General Rules for Recording

- Keep separate records or charts for each individual patient.
- It is a legal document; write it, in English, clearly, accurately, appropriately and legibly.

- Name, age, ward, date and in-patient number should be written on each page.
- All entries should be signed by the individual who makes the entry.
- All entries should be written in blue or black ink.
- Chart nursing-care and medications and other treatments only after giving them.
- It should be reliable and accurate.
- Information about patients and their care must be factual.
- Correct spelling is also important for accurate recording.
- Nurses should not allow others to record for her.
- Use only standard abbreviations.
- Do not use ditto marks or chemical formula in charting.
- Each patient should have a daily note, written by nurses on all shifts.
- The information within a record should be complete.
- Concise data are easy to understand.
- Lengthy notes are difficult to read.
- Record immediately after performing nursing activities. It should have currentness.
- It should be organized in a logical format or order.
- Nurses should maintain confidentiality of patents' record.
- Do not use blank space in the record. Keep it crossed.

NURSES' RESPONSIBILITY

Generally, nurses' notes contain the following information:
- Treatment and nursing care given by various members of the health team.
- Doctor's orders carried out by nurses.
- Nursing needs met by nurses as per doctor's order.
- Observations, e.g., vital signs, physical signs and behavioral patterns of patient.
- Response of patient to treatment and nursing care.
- Health advice given by nurses and other staff.
- Independent nursing functions are also recorded.

REPORT

Reports are oral or written exchanges of information shared between caregivers or workers in a number of ways. A report summarizes the services of the person or personnel and of the agency. Reports are usually written daily, weekly, monthly or yearly.

Purposes

- To show the kind and amount of services rendered over a specified period
- To illustrate progress in reaching goals
- As an aid in studying health conditions
- As an aid in planning
- To interpret the services to the public and to the other interested agencies.

Probably no other single factor is more vital for good administration than prompt and complete reports. They save duplication of efforts and eliminate the need for investigation to learn the facts in situation.

Types: Reports may be classified as oral and written.

Oral report: Oral reports are given when the information is for immediate use and not for permanency. For example, oral report is made by the nurse who is assigned to patient care, to another nurse who is planning to relieve her, and some of the oral reports may be made to charge nurses and nurse supervisors and also doctors. Reports are to be written when the information is to be used by several personnel, which is more or less of permanent value, for example, day and night reports, census, interdepartmental reports and other special reports, needed according to situation, events and conditions. The reports used in hospital setting usually are change-of-shift reports, transfer reports, incident reports, day, evening and night reports, legal reports.

Change-of-shift reports: These may be given orally in person by audio-taping, recording, or during rounds at the clients' bedside some of the points to be kept in mind while giving such reports are as follows:
- Provide only essential background information about client (name, sex, age,

diagnosis and medical history) but do not review all routine care procedures or tasks.

- Identify clients' nursing diagnosis or health care problems and other related causes but do not review all biographical information on case sheets.
- Describe objective measurements or observations about clients 'condition and response to health problem, Stress recent change, but do not use critical comment about clients' behavior.
- Share significant information about family members, as it relates to clients' problems do not make any assumptions about relationship between family members.
- Continuously review ongoing discharge plan. Don't engage in idle gossip.
- Relay to staff significant changes in the way therapies are given. Do not describe basic steps of a procedure.
- Describe instruction given in teaching plan and clients' response. Do not explain detailed content unless staff members ask for clarification.
- Evaluate results of nursing or medical care measures. Do not simply describe results as good or poor. Be specific.
- Be clear on priorities to which oncoming staff must attend. Do not force oncoming staff to guess what to do first.

Transfer-reports: Patients will frequently be transferred from one unit to another to receive different levels of care. A transfer report involves communications of information about clients from the nurse on sending unit to the nurse on the receiving unit. When giving transfer request, nurse should include the following information.

- Client's name, age, primary doctor, and medical diagnosis
- Summary of medical progress up to the time of transfer
- Current health status: Physical and psychosocial
- Current nursing diagnosis or problems and care plan
- Any critical assessment or interventions to be completed shortly
- Needs for any special equipment, etc.

Incident reports: Nurses usually become involved in client-related incidents as some point in their careers. They must understand the purpose of incident reports and the correct way to report information. While incident reporting, the following points are to be kept in mind:

- The nurse who witnessed the incident or who found the client at the time of incident should file the report.
- The nurse describes in concise what happened specifically objective terms, etc.
- The nurse does not interpret or attempt to explain the cause of the incident.
- The nurse describes objectively the clients, conditions when the incident was discovered.
- Any measures taken by the nurse, other nurses, or doctors at the time of the incident are reported.
- No nurse is blamed in an incident report.
- The report is submitted as soon as possible to the appropriate authority.
- The nurse should never make photocopy of the incident report.

Legal reports: Incident reports and reports on accidents, mistakes and complaints are legal in nature. There are times when a hospital is criticized for what is claimed to be negligence or poor care because of a condition that resulted in discomfort and perhaps serious harm to a patient or client. In such reports, the content is stated briefly and objectively giving all pertinent information. Accuracy, timeliness, completeness and relevancy to the problems are maintained promptly while making such reports.

Nurses Responsibility for Record Keeping and Reporting

Nurses have legal responsibility for accurately reporting and recording patient's conditions, treatments and responses to care. The medical record is a written or computerized account of a patient's illness and treatment that includes information submitted by all members of the patient health care team. The medical record is an information source document that should be used to plan care, evaluate care,

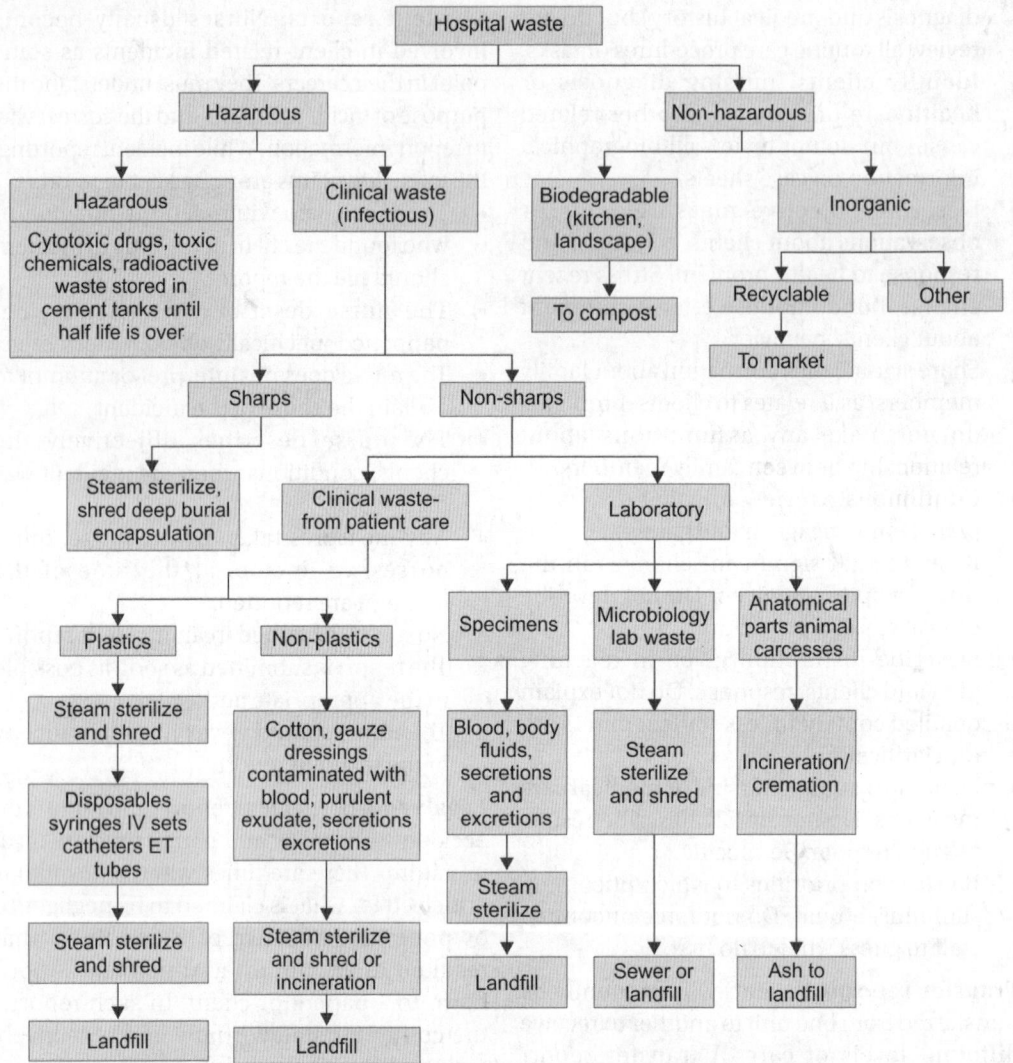

Fig. 23.13: Classification of hospital and waste and methods of treatment.

allocate costs, educate personnel, research care measure and substantiate legal claims.

Court decisions have stated that the patient's medical record is essential to proper care and the medical record is the property of the health agency. However, the patient has a property right to information contained in the report, the patient has a right to inspect and copy the record after being discharged. However, it is unadvisable to allow a patient to review his or her medical record without medical supervision and explanation because a patient is likely to misunderstand certain record notations. Failure to record significant patient information on the medical record makes a nurse guilty of negligence when the patient is injured because of a doctor's ignorance of significant information about medical history, signs and symptoms.

The medical record must be accurate to provide a sound basis for care planning. Therefore, errors in nurses charting must be corrected promptly in a manner that leaves no doubt about the facts. Every health agency should have a policy and protocol that directs that an erroneous chart entry be crossed through labeled as erroneous signed by the employee who corrects the error, and retained in the patient's record. Correct information should then be documented to replace the erroneous and corrected entries should never be destroyed. Nurses who conspire with doctors and others to falsify a patient's record for purposes of concealing a criminal violation may be found criminally liable.

Generally, the person who makes reports required by statute is immune from suit under the doctrine of the public's right to know. In many countries there are statutes that require health personnel to report instances of child abuse, ophthalmic neonatorum, communicable diseases, and births out of wedlock, gunshot wounds, suicide, rape, and use of unperceived narcotics. In reporting information about criminal acts obtained during patient care, the nurse must reveal such information only to the police, because it is considered a privileged communication. Several aspects of statutory, case, and administrative law control nursing practice and nursing management. Records and reports must be functional, accurate, complete, current organized and confidential.

- **Fact:** Information about clients and their care must be functional. A record should contain descriptive, objective information about what a nurse sees, hears, feels and smells. In the same way, any thing happens during the managing the affairs in the institutions/hospital, manager should document inferences or construction with functional information to avoid misleading, misinterpretation and any error in administration.

- **Accuracy:** A client record must be reliable. In other words, information must be accurate so that health team members have confidence in it. The use of correct measurements ensures that a record is accurate.

- **Completeness:** The information within a recorded entry or a report should be complete, containing concise and thorough information's about a client care or any event or happening taking place in the jurisdiction of manager.

- **Currentness:** Delays in recording or reporting can result in serious omissions and untimely delays for medical care or action legally, a late entry in a chart may be interpreted on negligence.

- **Organization:** The nurse or nurse manager communicates information in a logical format or order. Health team members understand information better when it is given in the order in which it occurred.

- **Confidentiality:** Nurses are legally and ethically obligated to keen information about client's illnesses and treatments confidential. In the same way certain information in management also should be kept confidential.

Any information about clients care or event taking place in the health care agencies should be communication with careful thought. All members of health team depend on recorded and reported information. Accurate information ensures continuity and quality of care, and also smooth running of administration.

24

Management of Equipments and Supplies

INTRODUCTION

Material management is concerned with providing the drugs, supplies and equipment needed by health personnel to deliver health services. The right drugs, supplies and equipment must be at the right place, at the right time and in the right quantity in order that health personnel deliver health services. Without proper material, health personnel cannot work effectively, they feel frustrated and the community lacks confidence in the health services and unless appropriate materials are provided in proper time and are required quantity, productivity of personnel will not be up to expectation.

DEFINITION

- Material management could be regarded as the function responsible for the coordination of planning, sourcing, purchasing, moving, storing and controlling materials in an optimum manner so to provide a pre-decided to the consumer at a minimum cost.
- Material management is defined as that aspect of management functions which is primarily concerned with the acquisition, control and use of material needed and flow of good and services connected with production process having some predetermined objectives in view.

BASIC PRINCIPLES OF MATERIAL MANAGEMENT

- Effective management and supervision: It deals on material function of–planning, organizing, staffing, controlling, report and budgeting.
- Sound purchasing method.
- Skillful and hard poised negotiation.
- Effective purchase system.
- Should be simple.
- Simple inventory control program.

PURPOSES OF MATERIAL MANAGEMENT

Purpose of material management is to bring about control over the acquisition, storage, retrievability, distribution, use and disposal of supplies and equipment in order to the primary responsibilities of the organization in an efficient, effective and economical manner. Material management entails two basic functions: Purchasing and storage/supply. These two functions may be carried out independently through separate stores and purchase departments, or they may be integrated into a single stores-purchase department.

- To gain economy in purchasing.
- To satisfy demand during period of replenishment.
- To carry reserve stock to avoid stock out.
- To stabilize fluctuations in consumption.
- To provide reasonable level of client services.
- Increase efficiency of healthcare systems.
- Develop knowledge and skills of health care.
- Provide materials in required quantity as and when required.

PROCESS OF MATERIAL MANAGEMENT

The process of material management involves planning, review and control of:
- Budgeting and material planning
- Demand forecasting
- Procurement
- Receipt, inspection and payment
- Storage
- Inventory control
- Issues and distribution
- Usage
- Maintenance
- Disposal
- Pilferage.

TYPES OF MATERIAL

The various types of materials used in a hospital are directly or indirectly related to the various activities that are undertaken in a hospital to achieve its objectives.

- **Drug and medicines:** Used for prevention and treatment of various types of ailments, including anesthetic agents, vaccines and such drugs required for specific purposes.
- **Supplies:** They are the materials required in the hospital for diagnosing and treating of ailments of activities related, such as

cotton, bandages, gauze or other dressing materials, syringes, needles, forceps, splints, plasters, trays, bottles, linens, utensils, which are related directly or indirectly to the treatment. Supplies may also include items of linen like draw sheet, bed cover, mattresses, pillows, masks, etc. A comprehensive list of supplies of hospital requirement has to be prepared and will need updating and modification from time to time depending upon the type of expertise, personnel or levels of technology available in the hospital.

- **Equipments and instruments:** These include various types of furniture and others instruments and equipments required are sterilizers, X-ray machines, other diagnostic equipments like auto analyzers, cell counters, Eliza readers, arterial blood gas analyzers. Oxygen and nitrous oxide gas cylinders cooking. LP gas cylinders and mechanical laundry, washing machines, incinerators for bio-waste management may also be used as tools. Ambulances and vehicles are also a part of supplies.
- **Facilities include:** Normally, the non-movable materials used for a long-term compared to equipments, which have limited life span. These include buildings, toilets, lifts, water tanks and pumps, wells, kitchen and cooking facilities, telephones and public address systems.

MATERIAL MANAGEMENT PROCEDURES

Materials are an essential resource to achieve the objectives of a healthcare organization. While about 60% of the funds of health sector are consumed to provide manpower, health care being a labor intensive activity, almost 40% of the funds are used up for providing materials. In the absence of materials required for health care activities, the manpower deployed is rendered non-functional. Therefore, it is of great importance that materials of right quality are supplied to the consumers in high quantity at right time and at right place of use. All activities involved in the achievement of above stated objectives, i.e., planning for materials, their demand, estimation, procurement, stocking and use come under the purview of term "materials planning and management".

- Taking inventory regularly and systematically
- Requisitioning at indenting according to actual needs
- Receiving and inspecting incoming items
- Storing and protecting items
- Issuing items for use
- Proper use of items.

ELEMENTS OF MATERIAL MANAGEMENT SYSTEM

Material planning and management (MP and M) is a system having numerous elements. Proper functioning of each of the elements (subsystems) coupled with inter-dependence of all the sub-systems to achieve the primary objectives are the classical characteristics of the MP and M system. The major sub-systems of MP and M system are:

- Demand estimation
- Procurement
- Receipt and inspection
- Storage
- Issue and use
- Maintenance and repair
- Disposal
- Accounting and information system

SUPPLIES AND EQUIPMENT

There must be well functioning equipment and adequate supplies to provide optimum nursing care. Insufficient and ill functioning equipment results in increased work and waste of time by the staff and may even prove danger to patient's life. Each hospital should set up a method that a sister (head nurse) or charge nurse can put a requisition for necessary equipment repairs and maintenance. All equipment should be so kept that it is easily available and as near as possible to the place where it will be required for use. Constantly

moving the place for keeping articles causes confusion and waste of time. The keys must be always carefully kept at a fixed place as certain things have to be kept in locked cupboards or store rooms. The keys must be in the ward all the time and all staff members should know where and with whom they are available. If this practice is not followed there will be difficulties and time wasted at the time of emergencies.

Some hospitals maintain a central supply of equipment and supplies. This helps to reduce the total amount needed in the hospital. However, there should be good system for the wards to avail of them and return them. The charge nurse is responsible to keep an adequate amount of equipment and supplies the ward, to see it in good conditions, repair and conveniently located.

All the personnel in the ward should clearly know who may use the articles or equipment and who assumes responsibility for it. The head nurse must watch for, and prevent waste or misuse by educating the staff in economical and appropriate use of all equipment and materials. She may sometimes arrange a ward class to enable the staff to know the cost of the equipment. There are three steps to be taken to ensure an adequate stock of available supplies the ward or unit.

1. Set a standard for the quantity of each item to be maintained on the ward all the time.
2. Have a satisfactory system for replacement of broken or worn out equipment.
3. Make regular inventories of all the items. She should draw a regular program for inventories.

PROBLEMS IN MANAGEMENT OF SUPPLY AND EQUIPMENT

- **Inadequate supply of material:** Patient's welfare and comfort is greatly affected by inadequate supply and equipment, e.g., if number of pillows is less, patient cannot be positioned properly. Lack of oxygen supply endangers the life of critically ill patient. Inadequate and insufficient equipment leads to wastage of time, increases risk of infection and complications for the patient.

- **Condition of equipment:** Pre-checking of equipment is must otherwise it will cause embarrassment to the person doing procedure.
- **Inaccessible supply and equipment:** Some articles are kept under lock and key to prevent misuse and theft which may cause delay in performing the procedure when person carrying the key is not accessible.
- **Inconveniently located equipment:** May lead to wastage of time and energy and delay in carrying out procedures. How to maintain adequate supply and equipment is the concern. The following measures should be observed: 1. Set a standard for quantity of each item kept in the ward. 2. Satisfactory system for replacing broken or worn out equipment. 3. Inventories of all items to be regularly taken.

STORE KEEPING

Functions of Storekeeping

- **Receipt of materials into storage:** Raw materials, supplies and purchased parts are usually received at a designated receiving stock, unloaded, inspected and then moved into stores keeping.
- **Record store keeping of materials in storage:** It is important to locate incoming and outgoing materials quickly and accurately, to provide the necessary information whereabout of the materials and cost keeping departments with correct and timely data.
- **Storage of materials:** The proper storage and protection of material is until they are required by authorized requisitions.
- **Maintaining stores:** Proper store maintenance measures may range from special covering or periodic lubrication to controlled atmospheric conditions.
- **Issuing stores:** This function should be performed most efficiently, promptly and accurately and a proper record should be kept of all the instance of store.

- **Coordinating storekeeping with materials control:** Duly authorized storage requisition must originate at the proper source and records of storage changes must be maintained for using the materials and cost control centers.

Protection of Stores

- **Protect goods from fire:** Store them in fire proof building and bins., with adequate automatic sprinkle provision. Adequate firefighting equipment, such as high pressure water lines, modern sprinkler systems, suitable chemical extinguishers, and, ladder should be provided.
- **To protect goods from damage** by dust Storage should be in boxes in closed cabinets. In city areas, where there are considerable dust in the atmosphere, air conditioned storage areas may prove advisable for such materials.
- **Protection against weather conditions:** Materials stored out of doors can be protected by open sheds or plastic coverings.
- **Protection against deterioration:** Some materials deteriorate with age. Such materials should not be overstocked and a first in first out storage system should be adopted.
- **Protection against theft:** Protection against theft can be insured by locking the storeroom and excluding all person not directly concerned with the receipt and issue stores. Stores should be under one authority.

INVENTORY CONTROL

Inventory control means stocking adequate number and kind of stores so that the materials are available whenever and whatever is required. Scientific inventory control results in optimal balance. Inventory control is an important aspect of material management. If the level of inventories goes up the carrying charges also increase but the procurement cost decreases. On the other hand, if we have a similar inventory, turn-over is greater requiring lesser carrying charges but more

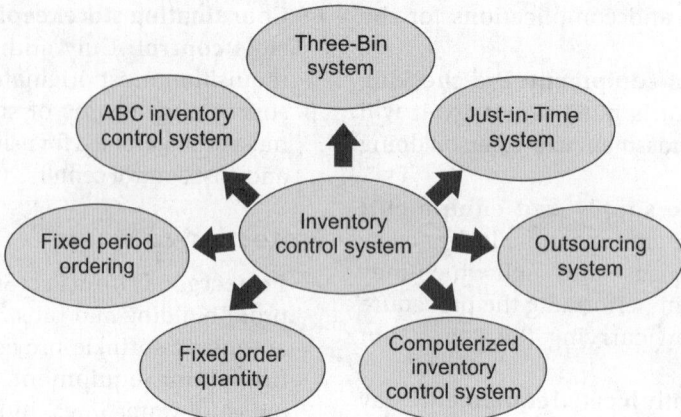

Fig. 24.1: Inventory control system.

of procurement costs, as orders have to be repeated more often.

Meaning of Inventory Control

- In healthcare system, material management is concerned with providing the drugs, supplies and equipment needed by health personnel to deliver health services.
- The right drugs, supplies and equipment must be at the right place, at the right time, and in the right quantity in order that health personnel deliver health services.
- Inventory control is an important aspect of material management.
- Inventory control is a scientific system which indicates as what to order, when to order, and how much to order, and how much to stock so that purchasing costs and storing costs are kept as low as possible.

Definition

- Inventory control is the process of maintaining the optimum needed quantity that is sufficient for smooth operation of the organization.
- Inventory management can be viewed as the process of maintaining a just adequate supply of something so that the demand pattern can be satisfied without hiccups.

Objectives of Inventory

- To reduce financial investment.
- To facilitate smooth production operation.

- If an offer of discount comes for a bulk purchase, to decide whether to go for bulk purchase or not.
- To avoid carrying cost.
- To improve quality of care with lesser inventory.
- To avoid obsolescence of inventor.

Steps in Inventory Control

- Fixing minimum quantities or ordering points and maximum quantities, or amounts to order on all materials.
- Arranging a method for allocation of material and orders which are in process.
- Creating stores accounts, which will control the store room.

Functions of Inventory Control

- To provide maximum supply service, consistent with maximum efficiency and optimum investment.
- To provide cushion between forecasted and actual demand for a material.

Principles of Inventory Management

- Determination of order quantity.
- Determination of reorder point of record level.

Advantages of Inventory Management

- Delivery in time.
- Possibility of discount for bulk purchase.

- Unforeseen circumstances can be handled to some extent.
- Workers and machinery need not idle.

Disadvantages of Inventory Management

- Working capital is tied up.
- More space required.
- Increases insurance charges.
- Increased overhead expenses.
- Charges of damage, pilferage replacement, etc. is more.
- Increase charge for obsolescence.

TECHNIQUES IN INVENTORY CONTROL

- ABC analysis (Always Better Control)
- VED analysis (Vital, Essential, Desirable)
- HML analysis (High, Medium, Low)
- FSN analysis (Fast, Slow moving and Non-moving)
- SDE analysis (Scarce, Difficult, Easy)

- **ABC analysis (Always Better Control):** It is the process of classifying items by using values as measures. ABC analysis helps us in segregating the items from one another and tells us how much valued the items is and controlling it to what extent is in the best interest of the organization. The main objective of ABC analysis is to frame policy guidelines regarding control of items.
  - ABC analysis is the analysis of the store items cost criteria.
  - It is a simple approach, which avoids being money wise.
  - The cost of each item is multiplied by the number used in a given period and then these items are tabulated in descending numerical value order.
  - It will be seen that first 10% of items approximately account for 70% value, the next 20% for 20% of value and the last 70% account for 10% of value.
  - It has been seen that a large number of items consume only a small percentage of resources and vice-versa.

- A items represent the high cost center, B items represent the immediate cost centers, and C items represent low cost centers.
- A very close control is exercised over A items while less stringent control is adequate for those in the category B, and less attention for category C.

- **VED analysis (Vital, Essential and Desirable):** The vital items are stocked in abundance, essential items, safety, stocks and very strict control. Essential items are moderate controls, purchase based on rigid requirements and reasonably strict watch. Desirable items are ordinary control, safety stocks it high, purchase based on usage estimate. The stores when subjected to analysis based on their criticality can be classified into vital, essential and desirable stores. This analysis is termed as VED analysis.
  - **Vital:** Items without which treatment comes to standstill, i.e., nonavailability cannot be tolerated.
  - **Essential:** Items whose nonavailability can be tolerated for 2-3 days, because similar or alternative items are available.
  - **Desirable:** Items whose non- availability can be tolerated for a long period. Although the proportion of vital, essential and desirable items varies from hospital to hospital depending on the type and quantity of workload, on an average vital items are 10%, essential items are 40% and desirable items make 50% of total items available. Although not included in scientific VED analysis, in some public organizations which are static or inefficiently managed, there is a peculiar category of 'U' items which can be grouped as unnecessary. These unnecessary items get purchased due to the following reasons.
    - Thoughtless continuation of previous purchase.
    - Indifferent attitude towards hospital formulary.

- ◆ Fear of change.
- ◆ Poor supervision and control.
- ◆ Unfair practice due to vested interest. The vital items are stocked in abundance; essential items are stocked in medium amounts, and desirable items we stocked in small amounts. By stocking the items in order of priority, vital and essential items are always in stock which means a minimum disruption in the services offered to the people.
- **HML analysis (High, Medium, Low):** As the name materials are classified to their unit value as high, medium and low.
- **XYZ analysis:** X items are those whose stock value are high, while Z items are those values are low. Understandably Y items fall between the two categories.
- **FSN analysis:** Movement analysis forms the basis for this classification. The items are classified as fast moving, slow moving and non-moving based on their consumption pattern.
  - It is based on rate of consumption.
  - The items can be classified into: a. Fast moving. b. Slow moving. c. Non-moving. Obsolete an understanding of the movement of items helps to keep proper levels of inventories by deciding

a rational policy or reordering. This method is based on the fact that some stock items have a much higher annual usage value than others.

- **SDE analysis:** Classification methods on source of supply, SDE classification is a system where materials are sorted out as scare to obtain, difficult to obtain and easy to obtain. SDE analysis: 1. Unit value is the basis of this analysis and not the annual consumption value. 2. Unit value > 1000 (Sanctioned by higher officials). 3. Unit value 100 to 1000. 4. Unit value < 100.
- **GOLF analysis:** In the GOLF system, classification is based on the availability and nature of supplies. Government suppliers, ordinary suppliers, local suppliers and foreign suppliers.
- **SOS analysis:** Raw material can be classified into seasonal or off season items.

CONCLUSION

A thorough understanding and use of the techniques of materials management would help in ordering the supplies when needed, controlling their use, keeping them safely and in working order. This also prevents chances of equipments and drugs as being out of stock of these reduces the usefulness of the hospital system.

25

Cost and Financing of Health Care

INTRODUCTION

Along with behavior aspect of human beings in the society, it is necessary to acquire the knowledge on the economy of human society. By economy we mean organizational and institutional structure confined to man's economic behavior. The individual economy and national economy are two different aspects of the economy of the human society. Learning about cost and financing of health care, we will get acquainted with economical aspects of individuals. In primary or primitive society, the economy is carried on a small scale, enough to satisfy the people. This can be termed as micro economy. But in a secondary society, like a nation or a country, economy is on a large scale, meant for a large group of people. This is known as macro economy. Since the economy is the management of wealth either by an individual or nation, economics is the subject which studies these activities.

DEFINITIONS

In order to study the subject of Economics, it is necessary to study the subject matter of economics, and get acquainted with basic economic terms.

- **Microeconomics:** It is that part of economics which studies and theories about the specific economic units or parts of an economic system. It studies individual behavior of the consumer, the producer in particular.
- **Macro economics:** It studies aggregate economic behavior of the entities of economic system as a whole. Economics studies four factors: 1. Land 2. Labor 3. Capital and 4. Enterprises which deliver service for, a. Production, b. Distribution of Products. These four factors are called factors of production. 1. Utility: Ability or power of a good to satisfy wants. 2. Economic goods: Such things which are scarce and carry some price called economic goods.
- **Consumption:** It is the power to consume the goods or consumer capacity to make use of the utility of commodity for the satisfaction of his wants.
- **Land:** It is the power to consume the goods or consumers capacity to make use of the utility of commodity for the satisfaction of his wants.
- **Labor:** Its source is human. It means mental and physical efforts of man used in the process of production.

- **Capital:** It includes the means of production. Machinery, factory plant, tools, equipments, raw materials, etc. are the physical capital assets. Money invested in business is called money or financial capital. Joint stock companies raise financial capital by issuing shares, debentures, etc.
- **Shares:** One of the equal parts of the capital of a joint stock company. Holding of a share gives the owner the right of part ownership of the company and the right to share the individual profit called dividend.
- **Debentures:** It means one of the equal parts of the loan capital of a company giving the holder the right fixed interest.
- **Depreciation:** The decrease in value of an asset through wear and tear, obsolescence, or any other factor that decreases its usefulness.
- **Inflation:** A persistently rising price level of all goods and services over a period of time. It is equivalent to a persistent decline in the purchasing power of money.
- **Standard of living:** Normal consumption pattern of necessities, comforts and luxuries to which an average family is normally accustomed.
- **Cost of living:** Expenditure required for maintaining a given standard of living. When prices rise, cost of living increases and the standard of living falls.
- **Rent:** It is the reward of land for its contribution to the productive activity.
- **Wage:** It is the reward of labor for its contribution to the productive activity.
- **Interest:** It is the reward of capital for its contribution to the productive activity.
- **Profit:** It is the reward of enterprise for its contribution to the productive activity.
- **Money:** It means anything which is generally acceptable as a means of payment. Currency notes, coins and chequeable demand deposits with banks are the common forms of money in a modern economy.
- **Open economy:** It means that economy which engages in foreign trade and has economic relations with the rest of the world.
- **Closed economy:** It is an economy in which there are no foreign trades and has economic relations with the rest of the world. As economy studies the wealth getting and spending activities of man, it is necessary to know the resources of the society, with which lives are maintained.
- **Choice:** It is the act of choosing among alternative goods, on the basis of criteria, such as preference of cost.
- **Morbidity:** Illness.
- **Scarcity:** Limited availability of goods in comparison to demand.
- **Tertiary level:** A higher or more advanced level. Lower levels are primary and secondary.
- **Dependent and independent variable:** If we say X causes Y or Y is explained by X, then X is the independent variable and Y is the dependent variable.
- **Investment good:** A good which is not directly used for consumption purposes but to produce consumption goods, which will, in turn be directly used.
- **Equilibrium:** A state of rest with no motivation on the part of anyone to bring about a change in existing situation.
- **Disutility:** If a thing gives disutility, it means the more you consume of that thing, the less utility you get.

MEANING OF ECONOMICS

Economics is the study of how people choose to use their limited resources, i.e., land, labor, and capital goods, to produce exchange and consumer goods and services. This can be again explained in following terms: Resources mentioned include land, labor, and capital. Here land referred as resources is permanently fixed in supply. Labor refers to human strength and talent in production, which is also known Man Power in Economics. Capital refers to a class of resources that are produced by economy system by means of machinery, buildings etc.

- **Scarcity** means inability of economy to meet the unlimited wants of the society or individual.
- **Choice:** Since resources are limited to human wants, so individual and society

has to adjust their wants to availability of resources.

- **Production** means any economic activity which is directed to the satisfaction of wants of the people. It may be goods or services, but it should satisfy the wants of consumer.
- **Exchange**: Here the goods and services are exchanged or bartered to satisfy the wants of individual, society or country.

COST OF HEALTH CARE

Cost and revenue are the two major factors that a profit maximizing firm needs to monitor continuously. It is the level of cost relative to revenue that determines the firm's overall profitability. In order to maximize profits, a firm tries to increase its revenue and lower its cost. While the market factors determine the level of revenue to a great extent the cost can be brought down by producing the optimum level of output using the least cost combination of inputs.

The price of the goods and services are determined by the interaction of demand and supply. The basic factor underlying the ability and willingness of firms to supply a product in the market is the cost of production. The cost of production provides the floor to pricing decisions. It is the cost that forms the basis for many managerial decisions like, which price to quote, whether to accept a particular order or not, whether to abandon or add a product to the existing product line, whether or not to increase the volume of output, whether to use idle capacity or rent out the facilities, etc.

Meaning of cost: When an Entrepreneur undertakes production of a commodity or service he has to pay prices for the factors when he employs for production. He thus pays wages to the laborers employed, prices for the raw materials, fuel and power used, rent for the building he hires for the production work and the rate of interest on the money borrowed for doing such business. All these are included in his cost of production. In simple language the term Cost refers to the expenses incurred by the producer to produce goods

and services. In Economics it is stated as the value of the inputs used in production is the cost of the output achieved. The value of the input is concerned not only with the physical quantities of the factors of production used, but with a monetary measure that permits to add up such unlike units as man-hours of labor, tons of raw materials and machineries to compare them in the aggregate with the value of the output produced. An entrepreneur of a Nursing Home can tell his team of doctors and supporting staff to treat 100 patients by using 75 man-hours of labor, one ton of cotton, 20 hours of ICU and supervisory services. But this does not tell the task manager whether the operation is profitable or not unless he can assign monetary values to the physical quantities of outputs and inputs involved.

The study of cost is very essential to the business manager or any entrepreneur. Normally, the management uses the concept of cost for following objectives:

- To know whether a commodity or service is worth producing at a given cost or not.
- To ascertain the money value for a product.
- To forecast whether a particular investment should or should not be made.
- To predict the profit of the business concern.
- To see that whether it is possible to produce with the existing resources.

Factors Influencing Cost of Production

The cost of production is influenced by many of its determinants. The main factors are:

- The size of the plant, i.e. Business concern, for example, A Pharmacy.
- The size of operation: Large scale or small scale.
- Managerial and labor efficiency and so on.

Types of costs: There are various types of costs which a business concern has to consider relevant for decision-making during different situations. The manner in which costs are classified or defined depends on the purpose for which the cost data are being outlined. Following are few cost concepts which are applicable in common areas of economic activities.

- **Accounting cost:** Accounting, costs are the monetary value of expenditures for supplies, services, labor, products, equipment and other items purchased for use by a business (or) other accounting entity. It is the amount denoted on invoices as the price and recorded in bookkeeping records as an expense (or) asset cost basis. The total amount of money (or) goods expended in an endeavor. It is money paid out at some time is past of recorded in journal entries and ledgers.
- **Opportunity cost,** also referred to as economic cost is the value of the best alternative that was not chosen in order to pursue the current endeavor, i.e., what could have been accomplished with resources expended in the undertaking. It represents opportunities forgone. In theoretical economics, cost used without qualification often means opportunity cost.
- **Private costs** are the costs that the buyer of a good (or) service pays the seller. This can also be described as the costs internal to the firm's production function.
- **External costs** (also called externalities), in contrast, are the costs that people other than the buyer are forced to pay as a result of the transaction. The bearers of such costs can be particular individuals (or) society at large. Note that external costs are often both non-monetary and problematic to quantify for comparison with monetary values. They include things like pollution, things that society will likely have to pay for in some way or at some time in the figure. But that are not included in transaction prices.
- **Social costs** are the sum of private costs external costs.
- **A psychic cost** is a subset of social costs that specifically represent the costs of added stress (or) losses to quality of life.
- **Path cost:** Also seen as a term in networking to define the worthiness of a path.
- **Biological cost:** In biology the biological cost (or) metabolic price is a measure of the increased energy metabolism that is required to achieve a function. Drug resistance in microbiology, for instance, has a very high metabolic price, especially for antibiotic resistance.
- **In economics**, **average cost** is equal to total cost divided by the number of goods produced (the output quantity, Q). It is also equal to the sum of average variable costs (total variable costs divided by Q) plus average fixed costs (total fixed costs divided by Q). Average cost may be dependent on the time period considered (increasing production may be expensive or impossible in the short term). Average costs affect the supply curve and are a fundamental component of supply and demand.
- **In economics, fixed costs** are business expenses that are not dependent on the level of production (or) sales. They are costs that do not change, no matter how much of a good is produced. They tend to be time-related, such as salaries (or) rents being paid per month. This is in contrast to variable costs, which are volume-related (and are paid per quantity).
- In management accounting, fixed costs are defined as expenses that do not change in proportion to the activity of a business, within the relevant period (or) scale of production. For example, a retailer must pay rent and utility bills irrespective of sales. Along with variable costs, fixed costs make up one of the two components of total cost. In the most simple production function, total cost is equal to fixed costs plus variable costs.
- **In accounting, historical cost** is the original monetary value of an economic item. In some circumstances, assets are liabilities may be shown at their historical costs, as if there had been no change in value since the date of acquisition. The balance sheet value of the item may therefore differ from the "true" value. While historical cost is criticized for its inaccuracy (deviation from "true" value), it remains in use in most accounting systems due to its simplicity, ease of use and verifiability. Various corrections to historical cost are used, many of which require the use of management judgment

and may be difficult to implement or verify. The trend in most accounting standards is a move to more accurate reflection of the fair or market value, although the historical cost principle remains in use, particularly for assets of little importance.

- **In economics and finance**, marginal cost is the change in total cost that arises when the quantity produced changes by one unit. It is the most of producing one more unit of a good. Mathematically, the marginal cost (MC) function is expressed as the first derivative of the total cost (TC) function with respect to quantity (Q). Note that the marginal cost may change with volume, and so at each level of production, the marginal cost is the cost of the next unit produced. In general terms, marginal cost at each level of production includes any additional costs required to produce the next unit. If producing additional vehicles requires, for example, building a new factory, the marginal cost of those extra vehicles includes the cost of the new factory. In practice, the analysis is segregated into short and long-run cases, and over the longest run, all costs are marginal. The factors affecting the marginal cost one negative (or) positive externalities, transaction costs, price discrimination and others.

- **Repugnancy costs** are costs borne by an individual (or) entity as a result of a stimulus that goes against that individual (or) entity's cultural mores. The cost could be emotional, physical, mental or figurative. The stimulus could be anything from food to people to an idea. These costs are perspective-dependent and individual. These costs may be different for different groups of people; countries, states, ethnicities, etc. The term allows for a clear and understandable way of representing the concept of contextual stigma in a literal and applicable sense.

- **Semi-variable cost** is an expense which contains both a fixed cost component and a variable cost component. The fixed cost element shall be a part of the cost that needs to be paid irrespective of the level of activity achieved by the entity. On the other hand, the variable component of the cost is payable proportionate to the level of activity. It shows similarities to telephone bills. One must pay line rental and on top of that a price that depends on how heavy one is using the service. So it changes with output. Another example is satellite television. A price for the box must be paid monthly and to get additional movies, more money has to be given.

- **In economics social cost** is defined as the sum of private and external costs. Economic theorists ascribe individual decision-making to a calculation costs and benefits. Rational choice theory assumes that individuals only consider their own private costs when making decisions, not the costs that may be borne by others.

- **In economics and business decision-making,** sunk costs are costs that cannot be recovered once they have been incurred. Sunk costs are sometimes contrasted with variable costs, which are the costs that will change due to the proposed course of action, and prospective costs which are costs that will be incurred if an action is taken. In microeconomic theory, only variable costs are relevant to a decision. Economics proposes that a rational actor does not let sunk costs influence one's decisions, because doing so would not be assessing a decision exclusively on its own merits. The decision-maker may make rational decisions according to their own incentives; these incentives may dictate different decisions that would be dictated by efficiency or profitability, and this is considered an incentive problem and distinct from a sunk cost problem.

DEMAND AND SUPPLY IN HEALTH CARE

Demand means desire to buy or consume something. In Economics Demand refers not only to desire but also ability and willingness to buy goods or services. It means a consumer should have desire, ability to pay for a product or service and willingness to pay for it. In microeconomic theory, demand is defined as the willingness and ability of a consumer to purchase a given product in a given frame of time. Demand depends upon the size of the total market (or) industry demand for the commodity which in turn is the sum of the demands for the commodity of the individual consumers in the market. The term demand implies a 'desire' backed by ability and willingness to pay. There term 'demand' for a commodity has always a reference to 'a price', 'a period of time' and 'a place'. Any statement regarding the demand for a commodity without reference to its price, time of purchase and place is meaningless and is of practical use.

Concepts of Demand

- **The law of demand:** The law can be explained in the following manner: "Other things being equal, a fall in price leads to expansion in demand and a rise in price leads to contraction in demand."
  Demand is a decreasing function of a price. The law of demand can be expressed in mathematical terms. i.e., $D = f(p)$ where, D represent Demand, P stands for Price and F denotes the functional relationships.
- **Demand schedule:** It refers to a statement in which we can see the different quantities demanded at various levels of price. It gives us information about quantities demanded by the consumer at different levels of price.

Important Features of the Law of Demand

- **Inverse relation:** There is an inverse relationship between price and demand.
- **Price is an independent variable** and demand is a dependent variable.
- **Qualitative statement:** It tells us only the direction of change in price and demand. But it does not indicate the quantitative changes in both price and demand.
- **Qualifying phrase:** The operation of the law is conditioned by the phrase "Other things being equal". It indicates that the law does

not have universal applicability. It indicates only the general tendency of buyers.
- **Negative slope of the curve:** Generally, the demand curve slopes downwards from left to right.

Factors Affecting Demand

The quantity of commodity purchased is dependent upon its price in the case of price demand. A careful study of the following factors is at most important to an organization/institution/firm because it enables to forecast demand (or) its sales.
- **Changing trends:** Changes in the mode of dress, beverages, any matter means a change in the demand for that commodity.
- **Change in population:** The change in the size of consuming population and in the composition of population and needs of the population fluctuates the demand of particular commodity.
- **Price:** The exact price of a commodity directly affects demand, e.g., Gold rates. As the hike in gold rate dropped the demand in public.
- **Price of the complementariness and substitute:** Complementary goods are those where one commodity possesses utility and is demanded only when the second related commodity is also available. Change in the price of one affects the demand for the other, e.g., A change in the prices of mobile batteries, and mobile charges affects the demand for mobile phones.
- **Future trend of price:** Fix trend of prices also affect demand. If it is expected that in future the prices of a commodity go up, the demand for that specific commodity
- **Climate (or) weather changes:** It is known as the demand changes according to season. In summer, (or) our specific occasions there is great demand for fruits.
- **Changes in general price level:** Sometimes it happens to rise of prices in some goods according to their need. Where people have to readjust their expenditure.
- **Changes in income:** The amount of money which a man may earn and buy

with the amount of money completely depends upon the person's income.

- **Level of income:** The demand of a commodity, others things being equal depends upon the level of income of a consumer. Level of income and demand may have relations.
- **Change in savings:** Demand of a commodity depends upon the saving rate of the society. Large saving means less money available for the purchase of goods, the demand will, therefore, decrease.
- **Goods with interconnected demand:** In the case of joining supply like wheat, the increased demand for one will lead to the cheapening of the other may stimulate its demand too, after some time.
- **Product improvement:** An improvement in the quality of goods is associated with an expansion of demand.
- **Awareness:** Improvement in the awareness of people always brings about an increase in demand.

Factors influencing demand: There are few factors influencing the demand:
- Patient factors.
- Physician factors.

Patient factors are the health status of the persons, demographic characteristics, and economic status of the persons.

Physician factors: Physician is the main factor who influences the demand of medical care among patients. Physician prescribes the drugs, admit patients into hospitals, and order the tests their influences on demand stems from the physician's dual role as advisor to the patient and provider of services.

Health care demand: The demand for health care is a derived demand from the demand for health. Health care is demanded as a means for consumers to achieve a larger stock of "health capital." The demand for health is unlike most other goods because, individuals allocate resources in order to consume and produce health.

Michael Grossman's 1972 model of health production has been extremely influential in this field of study and has several unique elements that make it notable. Grossman's model views each individual as both a producer and a consumer of health. Health is treated as a stock which degrades over time in the absence of "investments" in health, so that health is viewed as a sort of capital. The model acknowledges that health care is both a consumption good that yields direct satisfaction and utility, and an investment good, which yields satisfaction to consumers indirectly through increased productivity, fewer sick days, and higher wages. Investment in health is costly as consumers must trade off time and resources devoted to health, such as exercising at a local gym, against other goals. These factors are used to determine the optimal level of health that an individual will demand. The model makes predictions over the effects of changes in prices of health care and other goods, labor market outcomes such as employment and wages, and technological changes. These predictions and other predictions from models extending Grossman's 1972 paper form the basis of much of the econometric research conducted by health economists.

In Grossman's model, the optimal level of investment in health occurs where the marginal cost of health capital is equal to the marginal benefit. With the passing of time, health depreciates at some rate. The interest rate faced by the consumer is denoted by r. The marginal cost of health capital can be found by adding these variables: The marginal benefit of health capital is the rate of return from this capital in both market and non-market sectors. In this model, the optimal health stock can be impacted by factors like age, wages and education. As an example, increases with age, so it becomes more and more costly to attain the same level of health.

The Supply of Health Care Microeconomic and Evaluation at Treatment Level

A large focus of health economics, particularly in the UK, is the microeconomic evaluation of individual treatments. In the UK, the National Institute for Health and Clinical

Excellence (NIHCE) appraises certain new and existing pharmaceuticals and devices using economic evaluation. Economic evaluation is the comparison of two or more alternative courses of action in terms of both their costs and consequences. Economists usually distinguish several types of economic evaluation, differing in how consequences are measured:

- Cost minimization analysis
- Cost benefit analysis
- Cost-effectiveness analysis
- Cost-utility analysis.

In cost minimization analysis (CMA), the effectiveness of the comparators in question must be proven to be equivalent. The 'cost-effective' comparator is simply the one which costs less (as it achieves the same outcome). In cost-benefit analysis (CBA), costs and benefits are both valued in cash terms. Cost effectiveness analysis (CEA) measures outcomes in 'natural units', such as mmHg, symptom free days, life years gained. Finally cost-utility analysis (CUA) measures outcomes in a composite metric of both length and quality of life, the Quality Adjusted Life Year (QALY) (Note there is some international variations in the precise definitions of each type of analysis).

A final approach which is sometimes classed an economic evaluation is a cost of illness study. This is not a true economic evaluation as it does not compare the costs and outcomes of alternative courses of action. Instead, it attempts to measure all the costs associated with a particular disease or condition. These will include direct costs (where money actually changes hands, e.g., health service use, patient co-payments and out of pocket expenses), indirect costs (the value of lost productivity from time off work due to illness), and intangible costs (the 'disvalue' to an individual of pain and suffering) (Note specific definitions in health economics may vary slightly from other branches of economics).

After a careful study of Health Industry, we can conclude that the supply of health care facilities depends on internal and external factors. The internal factors are availability of funds, Government subsidy and encouragement, existence of medical personnel and drugs, etc. The external factor demand for health care, existence of Pharmaceutical companies, Laboratories, Blood Bank, etc. As the demand for health care services is inelastic, the supply of health care services is also inelastic.

Market equilibrium: Market is an economic activity of purchase and sale of goods and services at a particular level of price; it includes two market forces viz., Demand and Supply. The market equilibrium is generally achieved when aggregate demand is equal to aggregate supply.

Health Care Markets

The five health markets typically analyzed are:
- Health care financing market
- Physician and nurse's services market
- Institutional services market
- Input factors market
- Professional education market.

Although assumptions of textbook models of economic markets apply reasonably well to health care markets, there are important deviations. Insurance markets rely on risk pools, in which relatively healthy enrollees subsidize the care of the rest. Insurers must cope with adverse selection which occurs when they are unable to fully predict the medical expenses of enrollees; adverse selection can destroy the risk pool. Features of insurance markets, such as group purchases and preexisting condition exclusions are meant to cope with adverse selection.

Insured patients are naturally less concerned about health care costs than they would if they paid the full price of care. The resulting moral hazard drives up costs, as shown by the famous RAND Health Insurance Experiment. Insurers use several techniques to limit the costs of moral hazard, including imposing co-payments on patients and limiting physician incentives to provide costly care. Insurers often compete by their choice of service offerings, cost sharing requirements, and limitations on physicians.

Consumers in health care markets often suffer from a lack of adequate information about what services they need to buy and which providers offer the best value proposition. Health economists have documented a problem with "supplier induced demand", whereby providers base treatment recommendations on economic, rather than medical criteria. Researchers have also documented substantial "practice variations", whereby the treatment a patient receives depends as much on which doctor they visit as it does on their condition. Both private insurers and government payers use a variety of controls on service availability to rein in inducement and practice variations.

The US health care market has relied extensively on competition to control costs and improve quality. Critics question whether problems with adverse selection, moral hazard, information asymmetries demand inducement, and practice variations can bE addressed by private markets. Competition has fostered reduction in prices, but consolidation by providers and, to lesser extent insurers, has tempered this effect.

Competitive equilibrium in the five health markets: While the nature of health care as a private good is preserved is the last three markets, market failures occur in the financing and delivery markets due to two reasons:
- Perfect information about price products is not a viable assumption,
- Various barriers of entry exist in the financing markets (i.e., monopoly formations in the insurance industry).

The health care debate in public policy is often informed by ideology and not sound economic theory. Often, politicians subscribe to moral order system or belief about the role of governments in public life that guides biases towards provision of health care as well.

The ideological spectrum spans: Individual savings accounts and catastrophic coverage, tax credit or voucher programs combine with group purchasing arrangements, and expansions of public sector health insurance. These approaches are advocated by health care conservatives, moderates and liberals, respectively.

Medical economics: Often used synonymously with health economics. Medical economics, according to Culyer, is the branch of economic concerned with the application of economic theory to phenomena and problems associated typically with the second and third health market. Typically, however, it pertains to cost-benefit analysis of pharmaceutical products and cost-effectiveness of various medical treatments. Medical economics often uses mathematical models to synthesize data from biostatistics and epidemiology for support of medical decision making, both for individuals and for wider health policy.

Behavioral economics: Peter Orszag has suggested that behavioral economics is an important factor for improving the health care system, but that relatively little progress has been made when compared to retirement policy.

Production: It refers to creation or addition of utility. In other words, any product or service becomes useful if it is given a shape with the help of labor and capital. Production of goods and services requires the use of various inputs or factors of production which are also called as agents of production. The goods or services which are used for the production of finished goods are called inputs and what they produce in the form of final products is called output.

Factors of Production

The Classical School of Economists has classified the factors of production into four categories, viz. Land, Labor, Capital and Organization or Entrepreneurship.
- **Land** refers to surface of the earth. But in economics, land does not mean only soil. Land is synonymous with all natural resources available from air, water, from above the land surface and beneath it which can be used for production. The land is fixed in size and it has diminishing returns to scale. All those natural resources beneath the earth is also covered under the meaning of Land. The reward for Land

is rent. There are two types of rent viz., Economic Rent and Quasi Rent. Economic rent arises due to differences in fertility of land and Quasi Rent arises in short period due to scarcity of certain man made things.

- **Labor** is nothing but exertion of physical or mental work from human beings. All types of work physical or mental, done by man for a monetary reward called wages. Here, labor is human, the work done by animals is not considered as labor in economics. Wages are paid as reward for the services of labor. There are two types of Wages viz., Nominal Wages and Real Wages. Nominal wages expressed in terms of money and real wages are expressed in terms of goods and services.
- **Capital** is anything used again and again in the process of production. In other words, capital is the whole of the stock of wealth consisting of machines, tools, implements, raw materials, etc., which is used for the production of further goods. There are two types of capital viz., Money capital and Real capital. Money, capital is in terms of Money, i.e., loans, grants, etc. Recapitalize refers to all those fixed capital assets like buildings, roads, railway tracks, airports, machines, etc. Interest is a reward paid for the use of capital.
- **Organization**

  Entrepreneurship is an important factor of production which undertakes production process by allocating other factors of production. It brings together Land, Labor and capital and assign them work and bear the risk and uncertainty of production. The Entrepreneur is a real promoter of production as he initiates and directs production and bears the risk and uncertainty. The reward for the Entrepreneur is Profit. Profit can be classified as Gross Profit and Net Profit.

Production function: Production function is a functional relationship between factors of production and the goods and services produced. In other words, it refers to a technical relationship between physical inputs and physical output. Inputs are factors of production and output is the final goods and services produced. The output is a function of factors which are also called inputs. Symbolically, production function can be expressed as follows:

$Q = f (L,K,R)$ where Q is output and L,K and R are inputs which stand Labor, Capital and Raw materials, respectively.

Characteristics of Health Care Services in Market:

- **The health care market has inelastic demand.** That means the demand for health care does not change according to change in prices of services. The prices may fall or rise, but the demand remains same.
- **Supply of health care services** is independent of demand. In other words, the supply of health care facilities does not vary according to changes in demand. The nature of supply is relatively inelastic.
- **Imperfect competition,** the market is either monopolistic or oligopoly or duopoly. The level of competition is very low when compared to perfect market in case of other services or products. Generally we can see the competition between private sector and public sector health care centers. In some areas, Government enjoys monopoly market, i.e., the market without competition. Sometimes, we can observe competition among the private nursing homes but they have their own customers as they provide differentiated services.
- **Negligible selling costs:** The selling costs are the expenses incurred by the producer on promotion of sales. In product market, every producer goes for massive marketing strategies in different media of advertisements. But, in health care market less importance is given for market promotion and more is given for quality of service at hospitals and dispensaries.
- **Demand is more than supply:** The demand for health care services is more than its supply particularly in public sector health care market. Even few private hospitals and medical colleges are facing pressure from demand side.

- **No perfect knowledge:** There is no perfect knowledge about the health services market among the service providers and beneficiaries. The service providers may not be knowing the number of patients expected both in short or long period of time. The beneficiaries also may be in dark about the treatment and services available in the market.
- **Intervention of Government:** The market is controlled by the Government. The Ministry of Health controls the various public and private sector health care markets. The private sector is controlled through legislations passed by the parliament of India. Every treatment should be given after a proper diagnosis and if not they are punishable under Criminal Procedure Code and under Consumer Protection Act, 1986.
- **Profit is the secondary objective of the health care market:** Generally the public health care market does not have the motive of profit earning. But private sector health care service providers have profit making as one of the objectives of their firm.

Demand and Supply Sides of Health Care Market

The demand side of health care market is always perfectly inelastic and relatively inelastic. There will be a constant demand for health care services. The leading pharmaceutical companies are always advised to go for intensive research and development on new drugs required to meet present demand for the same. In India, the population is increasing very rapidly; the increase in population is accompanied by increase in health problems. Hence, the demand for health services never comes down. Even till today, many of the diseases are unknown and medicines are yet to be invented. The supply side of health care services market needs to be adjusted with the existing demand for the same. There is shortage of hospitals and dispensaries at rural areas. In India, about 74% of population is living in rural areas. Sometimes the hospitals are flooded with patients without proper personnel and facilities. As the private sector concentrates on profit, poor patients cannot avail the facilities from private nursing homes or clinics as the same is costly for them. Hence, it is the responsibility of the Government to provide primary health care units to all the villages throughout the country. The supply of health care services is in short of demand for health care and there is more concentration of hospitals and dispensaries in cities rather than villages.

Input-output Model: The input-output model of economics uses a matrix representation of a nation's economy, to predict the effect of changes in one industry on others and by consumers, government, and foreign suppliers on the economy. Loentief won the Nobel memorial prize in Economic sciences for his development of this model. Input-output depicts inter-industry relations of an economy. It shows how the output of one industry is an input to each other industry. Leontief put forward the display of this information in the form of a matrix. Inputs typically are enumerated in the column of an industry.

Production function: In economics, a production function is a function that specifies the output of a firm, an industry, (or) an entire economy for all combinations of inputs. In microeconomics, a production function asserts that the maximum output of a techno logically-determined production process is a mathematical production of input factors of production. Production function can be defined as the specification of the minimum input requirements needed to produce designated quantities of output, given available technology. By assuming that the maximum output technologically possible from a given set of inputs is achieved, economists using a production function in analysis are abstracting away from the engineering and managerial problems inherently associated with a particular production process.

The engineering and managerial problems of technical efficiency are assumed to be solved, so that analysis can focus on the problems of allocative efficiency. The firm is assumed to be making allocative choices concerning how much of each input factor to use, given the price of the factor and the technological determinants represented by the production function. A decision frame, in which one or more inputs are held constant, may be used; for example, capital may be assumed to be fixed or constant in the short run, and only labor variable, while in the long run, both capital and labor factors are variable, but the production function itself remains fixed, while in the very long run, the firm may face even a choice of technologies, represented by various, possible production functions.

The relationship of output to inputs is non-monetary, that is, a production function relates physical inputs to physical outputs and prices and costs are not considered. But, the production function is not a full model of the production process. It deliberately abstracts away from essential and inherent aspects of physical production processes, including error, entropy or waste. Moreover, production functions do not ordinarily model the business processes, either, ignoring the role and the relation of fixed overhead to variable costs.

INCOME

Income is the outcome of productive activity. When we work, we receive wages or payment in return for the work done. Thus, income may mean the payment or compensation received by a factor of production for its productive use. Income such as rent, wages, interest and profits are the factor incomes received in turn for services of land, labor, capital and enterprise respectively. The income can be divided into two types: National income and Personal income. An aggregate income of all the people in a community or country is known as National income, and income of an individual is known as Personal income.

National Income

- National Income is the total annual value of all goods and services produced by a country, measured in terms of money. Thus, national income data provides a summary statement of a country's aggregate economic activity. In an economy, over a given period of time, everybody works and produces something.
- A large number of goods and services are produced and exchanged during the year in the form of money.
- In real terms, it is difficult to calculate the amount in total. So their values are termed or measured in money. Thus, in turn, is termed as National Income.
  Therefore, National Income is defined as, "A national income estimate measures the volume of commodities and services turned out during a given period, counted without duplication."
- The modern economists explain the functioning of economy in generating the flow of national income, through a model of circular flow of economic activity.
- The circular economic activity exists between economic entities like households, firms and government in the functioning of an economic system. Households are the consuming units.
- Households comprise of a group of persons who spend their income on goods and services for consumption aspects of economic activity. Firms are the producing units.
- They comprise of a group of individuals and bodies, who undertake the organization of productive activity to produce goods and services. Hence, firms correspond to the production aspects of economic activity.
- As the firms sector undertakes producing activities they employ factors of production in process. These factors of production are land, labor, capital and enterprise.
- These are supplied by the households, who in turn receive the income over the services of these factors.
- The income so earned by the households is, in turn, spent for buying various goods, services from the farms producing consumable goods. In turn, firms receive income for the service rendered in terms of goods to the households. Thus household

income becomes firm's income. In this way circular flow of income takes place.

- It represents the money value of the physical exchanges involved, while real goods move from firms to households, money moves from households to firms.
- In the same way when money flows from firms to households, in return of services, in the form of land, labor, capital and enterprises, it becomes national income. This whole thing can be explained in terms of National Product=National Expenditure.

The Gross National Product (GNP) is the monetary measure of the current total output in the economy. It includes the value of only the final goods, value of all intermediate goods is excluded in the calculation of GNP, which helps to prevent double counting.

Net National Product (NNP) refers to the net output produced by a country in a year. Thus, Net National Product is derived from Gross National Product, the value of depreciation (D) or replacement allowances if capital assets. Net National Product = Gross National Product-Depreciation

This is known as Net National Product (NNP) at Current Market Price since Gross National Product also is measured in current market price. The term Gross Domestic Product (GDP) refers to the monetary value of the gross output produced by the domestic economy of a country.

METHODS OF MEASURING NATIONAL INCOME

National income can be viewed in terms of a triple identity between output, income and expenditure that is National Product = National Income (Dividend) - National Expenditure. Hence, three methods are adopted to measure the national income. 1. Output method, 2. Income method, 3. Expenditure method.

1. **The output method:** This method of measuring National Income is also known as the product method or inventory method. (A) In this method, by undertaking a census of production, the sum total of the gross value of the final goods and services in different sectors of the economy, like agriculture, industry, etc., is obtained for the current year. The value so obtained gives the Gross Domestic Product (GDP) at market prices in a closed economy. (B) In this method we add the value of export surplus, value of exports, less value of import to get the Gross Domestic Product (GDP) at market prices for the open economy. (C) From this figure we get Gross National Product (GNP) at market prices (for the open economy) by adding the net income from abroad (income received from abroad due to less payments made to the foreigners). (D) If we subtract the value of depreciation from this, we get Net National Product (NNP) at market prices. (E) To get NNP at factor price or National Income (NI), we add the value of subsidies and deduct the value of indirect (commodity) taxes. While using this method, utmost care must be taken to avoid double counting, that is, counting the same item of output more than once.

2. **The income method:** In this method of measuring National Income, all factors of payments like rent, wages, interest and profits are totaled up. Their figures are obtainable from the sources like Income Tax returns, books of accounts, reports, etc. This method is also known as factor-cost method. It gives the value of net domestic products at factor cost and to this, net incomes from abroad are added.

3. **The expenditure method:** In this method, all expenditures incurred by the households, firms and governments are added up. To the value so obtained, values of export surplus and net income from abroad are added to obtain the national income. In this method of expenditure, on current consumption, expenditure plus current investment expenditure is taken into account. Expenditure on old goods or financial investment is not to be considered.

METHOD OF ESTIMATING NATIONAL INCOME IN INDIA

In India, the Central Statistical Organization (CSO) is entrusted with the work of preparing national income estimates for the country. Since 40% of the income originates from non-industrial sector, it has been observed that unlike the developed country, where industry is the main source of income, the single method like income alone, cannot be depended upon to give a reliable estimation. Therefore, CSO adopts the combination method of income and output methods for measuring India's National Income. The output method is adopted for measuring the contribution of agricultural and manufacturing sectors. The income method is adopted for measuring the contribution of tertiary or service sector which includes small enterprises, banking and insurance, commerce and transport, professions, liberal arts, domestic service, government services, etc. By totaling up the contribution of all sectors, the value of net domestic product at factor cost is calculated. To this, indirect taxes that is sales tax, revenue tax, wealth tax, etc., are added to measure the net domestic product at market prices. To this, net income from abroad or foreign sector is added by obtaining it from the balance of payments account. This gives the national income at market prices or current prices.

ECONOMIC PLANNING

The principle of planning should be applied only as far as it is necessary. In small dose it may be useful, like a medicine, but in large doses it may kill the patient. It is very difficult to give a precise definition of Economic Planning. According to Planning Commission of India, Economic Planning is a well thought out process initiated by the Central authority (Government) to fulfill certain objectives and targets through optimum utilization of natural and human resources within a specified period of time. According to Prof. Gunnar Myrdal (a Nobel laureate), "Economic Planning is a program for the strategy of a national government in applying a system of state interference with the play of market forces, thereby conditioning them in such a way as to give an upward push to the social process."

The first to advocate the idea of planning for India was Sir M Visvesvarayya, who published in 1934 the first book on planning entitled "Planned Economy for India". In 1937, the Indian National Congress set up the National Planning Committee. It was suspended by the British Government from 1942 to 1946. The Committee was able to submit its plan only in 1949. In addition to these, several other plans were initiated, some of them are: Bombay Plan, People's Plan, Gandhian Plan, Colombo Plan, and so on.

Machinery for economic planning in India: The Planning Commission of India, as National Planning Authority has been constituted in the year 1950 under the chairmanship of the former Prime Minister of India Jawaharlal Nehru. It consists of Prime Minister as Chairman (Dr Manmohan Singh), Deputy Chairman and members include Finance Minister, Railway Minister, and Minister for Human Resource Development, and others.

The main function of Planning Commission of India is to estimate the national resources and to prepare plans for wise allocation of those resources to achieve, targeted growth in the economy within a specified period of time. It also provides suggestions and solutions to State Planning Boards for their internal economic planning. India is following Russia's Planning methodology. Accordingly, first five year plan was started in 1951.

FINANCING OF HEALTH CARE IN INDIA

Sources of Health Finance

Commercial Banks: A bank is a financial institution which accepts deposits from public and lends loans to public. Commercial banks are those banks which provide short-term loans to businessmen or industrialists. According to RBI Act of 1934, commercial banks are classified into two. They are: Scheduled commercial banks and Nonscheduled commercial banks. Scheduled bank are those commercial banks which are included in the second schedule of RBI. These banks have the combined paid up capital and reserve together up to Rs. 5 lakhs and above. These banks fulfill the conditions and obligations put in by RBI. All types of commercial banks (Indian and foreign, state co-operative banks) comes under this category. There are 286 scheduled commercial banks as on 31st March 2004. There are 196 Regional Rural banks (RRBs) and 223 public sector banks in the 286 scheduled banks.

Non-scheduled commercial banks: Those commercial banks having paid up capital and reserve up together is less than ₹ 5 lakhs. These banks are included in the second schedule of RBI Act of 1934. Till June 2004, there were only two non-scheduled banks.

Public Sector Banks: There are 19 nationalized banks under public sector banks in India along with SBI and RRBs. The SBI has 13,533 branches in India as on 30th June 2004. There are 33,211 branches of other nationalized banks and all public sector banks have 61,251 branches put together. The public sector banks are as follows:

State Bank of India: It was started by British Government in the name of Imperial Bank of India in 1923 and now it is under Government of India, performing functions next to RBI. This bank was nationalized on 1st July 1955.

The following 14 banks were nationalized on 19th July 1969. They are:

- Central Bank of India.
- Bank of India.
- Punjab National Bank.
- Bank of Baroda.
- United Commercial Bank.
- Canara Bank.
- United Bank of India.
- Dena Bank.
- Syndicate Bank.
- Union Bank of India.
- Allahabad Bank.
- Indian Bank.
- Bank of Maharashtra.
- Indian Overseas Bank.

Vijaya Bank, Andhra Bank, Corporation Bank, Punjab and Sindh Bank and Oriental Bank of Commerce were nationalized on 15th April 1980.

Private Banks: Private banks are those banks which are doing the business of banking and are not nationalized so far. There are so many Indian scheduled banks. Before the new economic policy, these banks had narrow area of operation. There was a big growth during the implementation of the new economic policy. Today, there are 32 private banks having over 5,790 branches. As usual, the performance of private banks is better than public sector banks. Put together there are 22 old banks and 10 new banks in these sectors.

Private Foreign Banks: Foreign banks are those banks based on foreign countries and are operating in India, also known as foreign exchange banks. They are incorporated in foreign countries and have its branches in India. There are 40 foreign banks in India with 218 branches. These banks provide same service like any other banks but have different focus and approach.

Growth of Commercial Banking in India: The British established Agency houses in India way back in 17th century and that was the beginning of Commercial banking in the country. "The Bank of Hindustan" was the first bank established in 1770. The Presidency bank was established in early part of 19th century for commercial purpose. The banking companies' Act of 1860 encouraged the growth of joint stock banks in India. The first Indian bank being "Oudh Commercial Bank" was established in 1881. In 1920 three Presidency banks were merged and later it was nationalized in 1955 that led to the creation of SBI (State Bank of India). There were 648 banks with 4819 branches at the time of independence. The growth of commercial banks took place at various stages. They are as follows:

- **Foundation stage or initial stage:** Legislative frame work for providing re-organization and consolidation of banking system was undertaken during this stage (1951-65).

- **Expansion stage or growth stage**: During 1960s there was lot of development and establishment of commercial banks. In this period 14 commercial banks were nationalized in the year 1969. The services of banking were expanded in full swing during this period (1965-85).
- **Consolidation stage or improvisation stage**: During this period there was lot of improvement in the performance and increase in the efficiency of service. The customer service, profitability and productivity of banks increased (1985-90).
- **Reform stage or rehabilitation stage:** There was lot of reforms in banking sector. There were lot of changes and improvement in banking. Income recognition, capital adequacy was given much importance (1991 onwards).
- **New trends were as follows:**
  - **There was lot of expansion of branches:** The number of branches, coverage of all areas (both Rural and Urban) and removal of regional imbalance were given much importance There were 67,283 branches at the end of June 2004. There was an increase in number of branches by 8 times in the last three and a half decade. The average population served per bank was around 65,000 in 1969 and now it is 15,000 populations for every branch office. There was increase in number of branches in rural areas. Public sector banks had 31,062 branches in 2004. In states like Assam, MP, Tamil Nadu, Gujarat, etc., there were expansion of branches and were nationalized. This reduced regional imbalances.
  - **Deposit mobilization:** There was reasonable growth and rise in the deposits of commercial banks. By 2004, there was a deposit of ₹ 16, 22,579 crores. There was 15% increase in total deposits in rural deposits. Rapid branch expansion, increase in growth of banking activities, lower cash reserve ratio, ideal business condition, high rate of interest on deposits are some of the reasons for deposit mobilization.
  - **Priority sector banking:** There was a remarkable progress in lending to priority sectors like Agriculture, Industry, etc. after 1969, agriculture and small scale industries were given much importance. More funds were provided for priority sector. The total credit facilities given up to year 2003 was Rs. 2,00,169 crores.

Reforms of Banking Sector: The banking sector reforms were influenced by the two reports submitted by M Narasimham Committee in 1991 and 1998. The efficiency and profitability of banking sector has increased drastically after the reforms. There is healthier competition among banks. The nine member committee was headed by M Narasimham was appointed to work on financial systems. It submitted two reports in 1991 and 1998.

Recommendations of Narasimham Committee: The main recommendation of Narasimham Committee was as follows:
- To ensure better flexibility in operations.
- To have managerial autonomy while making decisions.
- To have more and healthy competitions among banks in its activities.
- To be more professional in all the activities.

These recommendations were mainly based on assumptions that general public provides all the resources and fund of the bank. Therefore, the recommendations were to provide maximum and all types of benefits to be given to depositors and to use funds in the most rational and ideal manner. The important recommendations relating to operations of banks were as follows:
- **Statutory liquidity requirements (SLR):** The Government was recommended to reduce the SLR rate. It suggested reducing SLR rate from 38.5 to 25% over the next 5 years. It recommended that SLR to be implemented with regarding it as prudential requirement. It is not to be used by public sector as major instrument for financing.

- **Cash reserve ratio (CRR):** Committee suggested reducing CRR gradually from 15 to 5%. It recommended RBI to use more of open market operations.
- **Directed credit programs:** It recommended implementation of the concept of priority sector to be defined again and to include only marginal farmers, rural artisans, cottage industries, etc. 10% of the aggregate bank credit to be given as credit to this sector. To remove direct credit programs.
- **Structure of interest rates:** It recommended that demand force must be used to decide the level and structure of interest rate. All regulations, controls on it must be removed. To withdraw concessional rate of interest charged for priority sector and to remove subsidy on IRDP loans.
- **Structural reorganization of the banking sector:** It suggested having more efficiency and transparency in the operations and management of banking service. To reduce the number of public sector banks. It suggested having four-tier hierarchy to be established for banking structure. Banking structure consists of 3 or 4 large banks of international character which includes SBI, 8 to 10 national banks and local banks. SBI to be at the top and become international, while national banks to have network all over the country and rural banks to finance agriculture and other agricultural activities.
- **Nationalization of banks:** It recommended govt. to make declaration that no more banks will be nationalized.
- **Starting up new banks.** Committee recommended RBI to give permit to public and private sector banks to set up new branches. These banks must have the required capital to start new branches and also to follow other requirements set in by RBI. It suggested RBI not to treat Public and private banks separately.
- **Foreign banks:** It suggested RBI to allow foreign banks to be allowed to operate all over India. To give permission to set up joint venture relating to merchant and investment operations of the bank.

- **Bad and doubtful debts:** It recommended to set up ARF (Asse Reconstruction Fund) to take over part of bad and doubtful debts at discount from financial institutions and nationalize banks.
- **Wipe of dual control:** The double control of banking system done by both RBI and division of banking from Ministry of Finance to be removed.
- **Total autonomy to banks:** Full autonomy to be given to public sector banks. These banks must be given free hand to implement latest technology and introduce new work culture as per the requirement.
- **Total disinvestment:** It recommended certain percentage of shares of public sector banks to be allowed for disinvestment.
- **Subsidies to rural banking:** Public sector banks to have more rural banking subsidies and to take over rural branches. These must be on par to regional rural banks.
- **Staff recruitment:** Political favors to be avoided relating to the appointment of persons at the key positions. Staff recruitment to be main part of reforms in the banking sector. Independent panel of experts must be responsible to appoint chief executive of the bank.
- **Updating of services of banking:** Committee recommended computerizing all the activities of banking and to increase the efficiency of activities of banks.

Cooperative sector: It is one of the form of organization where persons join voluntarily on the basis of equality and to promote economic interest of all persons. In this form people join or come together in a systematic manner to protect themselves from exploitations from economically rich class, and to protect mutual interest. "One for all and all for each" is the motive of any cooperative sector.

Cooperative Movement in India: Cooperative movement started at the end of 19th century in India. In states like Punjab and Uttar Pradesh several credit societies were established. In 19th century, Sir Frederic

Nicholson was sent by Government of Madras to study cooperative movement in Germany. In 1895, he submitted the report and suggested to establish Raiffeisen model type of societies in India. In 1901, "famine commission" recommended for the establishment of Cooperative societies. In 1904, Government of India passed act called as "Cooperative Societies Act", which became the main basis for cooperative movement in India. This act gave lot of opportunities for establishment of societies following Raiffeisen model. These societies had few limitations like no differences between societies in rural places and in cities. There was not much chance for credit societies.

"New Cooperative Society's Act" was in 1912 to overcome these limitations.

Every state established cooperative societies, which was due to the implementation of cooperative act in 1912. There was lot of societies coming up during Second World War. Post independence cooperative movement was in full swing. It was implemented as per five years plan. Karnataka, Tamil Nadu, Haryana were few among many states where there was drastic development of cooperative societies. Cottage, small scale and rural industries were ideal to have cooperative societies.

Progress after l950-India had the largest cooperative sector in this period. There were 1.05 lakhs agricultural cooperative societies, having 44 lakhs members. It had 37.25 crores as working capital with advances up to 37 crores. There were around 91,000 agricultural cooperative societies, 7,460 Primary agricultural cooperative societies and around 2,900 primary cooperative societies in 1998. The total credit provided in this period was around Rs. 4,700 crores with total working capital of Rs. 10,718 crores.

HEALTH PLANS IN INDIA

A conscious and well designed schemes and programs for better health for the entire population are called Health Plans. In India, though the proportion of amount spent or health care services are less, the Government with the help of NGOs is striving very hard to take the primary health care facilities to every citizen of the country. Now, we shall discuss briefly the objectives, outlays and achievements of each plan with reference to health services.

- **First Five Year Plan (1951-1956).** The first five year plan gave top priority to Agriculture and Community Development. About Rs. 291 crores was kept for this. It aimed at correcting disequilibrium in the economy caused by the war (1948 with Pakistan) and the Partition of the country. Rs. 553 crores was spent on social services, i.e., on health und other services. The total outlay for the plan was fixed at, Rs. 2,378 crores. For health and family planning about Rs. 140 crores was allocated. During the first five year plan, the GDP (Gross Domestic Product) increased by 17.5% per annum. In respect of social services, there was an increase of about 33% in the number of children attending the primary schools. As regards health programs, while the increase in the number of hospitals and dispensaries was moderate, a large scale program of control of malaria and filarial was executed. The first five year plan was an instrumental in bringing about a marked improvement in the level of production, both in agriculture and Industry.

- **Second Five Year Plan (1956-61):** The second plan aimed at rapid industrialization with a particular emphasis on the development of basic and heavy industries. It also aimed at creating health care infrastructure under social services to mankind. The total plan outlay was Rs. 4,800 crores. Out of which, Rs. 890 crores was reserved for Industrial development and mining. The social services got 19.7% share in the outlay. The social services include health, education, creation of employment opportunities, etc. Rs. 225 crores was fixed for Health and sanitation. The achievements of the second plan were more than expectations. The growth of National Income was 18% and the target was 12%. A significant development was achieved in Industrial Progress. India is now producing progressively increasing quantities of machines and transport equipment for use in agriculture and transport and for such industries as chemicals and pharmaceuticals, textiles, cement, paper, etc. There was a considerable expansion of health services. A large number of hospitals, dispensaries, health units and maternity and child health welfare centers were opened and special programs for water supply and sanitation, control of contagious diseases and expansion of training facilities were undertaken by the Government.

- **Third Five Year Plan (1961-66):** The main objectives of the third plan were to secure an increase in national income of over 5%; to achieve self-sufficiency in food grains; to expand basic industries like steel, chemical industries, fuel and power; and so on. The total outlay was fixed at Rs. 11,600 crores of which Rs. 855 crores was allocated to social services including health services. The top priority was given to Transport and Communication. The provision of Rs. 342 crores was made in the third plan for health and family planning programs as against Rs. 140 crores and Rs. 225 crores during first and second five year plans respectively. The number of hospitals and dispensaries were increased to 14,600 from 12,600 by the end of the plan period, doctors from 70,000 to 81,000, nurses from 27,000 to 45,000, primary health units from 2,800 to 5,000, medical colleges from 57 to 75, annual admissions to these colleges from 5,800 to 8,000 and maternity and child welfare centers from 4,500 to 10,000.

- **Annual Plans (1966-69):** The fourth five year plan could not be launched because of many reasons. Firstly, country had to face attacks from China and Pakistan. Secondly, inflationary situation, i.e., a continuous rise in prices leading to plan-cost escalation and lastly, non-availability of foreign capital.

During annual plans overall development of the country's economy was targeted. Importance was given to agriculture and rural development, economic growth with social justice. The plan outlay for the first annual plan (1966-67) was Rs. 2,081 crores out of which Rs. 300.88 crores was allotted for social services, for second annual plan (1967-68) the outlay was Rs. 2, 246 crores out of which about 10% of funds were allocated to social services and during third annual plan (1968-69) it was Rs. 2,337 crores of which about Rs. 22.98 crores was allocated for health and family planning. In aggregate Rs. 140 crores was kept exclusively for health care.

- **Fourth Five Year Plan (1969-1974):** The main objective of this plan was economic growth with stability and social justice Stabilizing price or controlling inflation was a major target of fourth plan. Raising GDP over 5.5% per annum with a marginal increase in agricultural production was one of the main aims of this plan. The total outlay was fixed at Rs. 24,398 crores of which Rs.435 crores was allotted for Health, Rs.315 crores for family planning and Rs.406 was allocated for Water Supply and sanitation. Efforts were made to strengthen the primary Health services particularly in the rural areas for undertaking preventive and curative measures. The total planned outlay was Rs.435 crores while actual outlay was Rs.335 crores. About 331 new primary health care centers, 10,200 sub-centers and 26,000 hospital beds were made available. But the Mudaliar Committee's recommendation of one bed for 1,000 people and one doctor for 3,000-3,500 persons had not yet been realized. The main features of progress in health care were–increasing rate of the rural health services, popularity of mass vasectomy camps, in-depth evaluation studies of various organizations, passing of Medical Termination of Pregnancy Act, an experimental population project to study alternative approach to family planning efforts, popularity of Nirodh, success of Post partum scheme, initiative of population education, etc.

- **Fifth Five Year Plan (1974-79):** Though this plan was for full five years, it was abruptly ended by 1978 itself because of change of Government at the center. The plan aimed at 5.5% growth in National Income, extended programs of social welfare, a national program of minimum needs, agricultural and rural development, etc. The plan outlay was fixed at Rs. 39,322 crores out of which Rs. 682 crores was fixed for health care; Rs. 497 crores for family planning; and Rs. 971 crores for water supply and sanitation were allocated. Under Minimum needs program, Rs. 291.47 crores was allocated for rural health. The objectives were an integrated approach to the three services for the vulnerable group, increasing the accessibility of the services to the rural areas, further development of referral services, intensified campaign against communicable diseases, improvement of education and training under Minimum Needs Program. The Primary Health Center Complex—one for each block— were the nucleus of health services. The delivery of the integrated health service was to be through multipurpose health auxiliaries—a new category of para-medical personnel to be specially trained. The strategy in respect of nutrition was to attach the problem at its root level i.e., the pregnant women, lactating mothers and pre-school children of weaker sections. Feeding programs were to be integrated with health and welfare which included minimum health care, immunization and environmental sanitation.
- **Sixth Five Year Plan (1980-85):** The sixth plan could not be started immediately after Fifth Five year plan because, there was acute inflationary pressure during 1979-80 and a setback in the functioning of critical sectors like power, coal, railways and steel and a steep rise in price of petroleum products. This plan was formulated for taking into the achievements and shortcomings of the past three decades of planning, recent economic development vision of future. There was also a change of Government at the center. The Congress Government was replaced by Janatha Government. The rolling planning concept (Prof. Gunnar Myrdal's concept of Economic Planning) was introduced during 1979-1980 (Annual Plans). The plan mainly aimed to launch a direct attack on the problems of unemployment, under-employment and massive low-end poverty, keeping in view the need to achieve higher rate of growth or sustained growth towards self reliance. The Congress Government started the plan with a new strategy of Mahalanobis which gave importance to rapid economic growth via heavy industries. The original total outlay for the sixth plan was kept at Rs. 97,500 crores and the revised was Rs. 1,09,292 crores of which Rs. 15,917 crores was spent on social services including health services.

The progress of social sector during this sector was 6.6% against the target of 5.5%. The objective of Minimum Needs Program which aimed at improving the living conditions of the poor and also promoting their education and health were almost fulfilled. During the plan period, provision of primary and subsidiary health centers, family planning measures, etc. were largely fulfilled. Under family planning services, the percentage of eligible couples effectively protected increased from 22.5% in 1979-80 to 32% in 1984-85. The rural areas were improved by assured water supply to 1, 92,000 out of the 2,3 1,000 villages.

- **Seventh Five Year Plan (1985-90):** The basic objectives of this plan were growth, modernization, self-reliance and social justice. It targeted to reduce poverty and to create employment opportunities. It also aimed to extend Green revolution (a spectacular increase in the agricultural production due to application of scientific methods of cultivation) benefits to entire part of India.

The total outlay was fixed at Rs. 1, 80,000 crores of which Rs. 31,545 crores was allotted to social services. The medical and public health was allocated with Rs. 3, 689 crores and family welfare got Rs. 3,121 crores. The rate of growth of GDP was 5.6% per annum. The agricultural sector grew by 4.1% and industries by 8.5%. Many chemical industries were encouraged with latest lab equipment. Maximum importance was given to rural health and family planning measures. Many programs like universal immunization, pulse polio program were launched. Under universal immunization program to improve the health of children, vaccines were provided to control six diseases like TB, Diphtheria, Pertussis, Tetanus, Polio and Measles. This was introduced to cover the entire population of the country.

- **Eighth Five Year Plan (1992-97):** The eighth five year plan could not be started in 1990 because of political changes at the center and assassination of former Prime Minister of India Rajiv Gandhi. One of the main objectives of this plan was provision of safe drinking water and primary health facilities including immunization so as to be accessible to all villages and entire population and complete elimination of scavenging; The total outlay was fixed at Rs. 4, 34,100 crores. The medical and Public health got the share of Rs. 7, 576 crores and family welfare was invested with Rs.6, 500 crores. As the economy emerges from the crisis and the stabilization measures needed to get us off it, special care must be taken to protect the weakest and poorest segments of the society. There was increase in the outlay allocation for social section particularly to health and education. Many new plans were started to safeguard the health of rural mass. Government made compulsory medical practice in rural areas under new appointment of doctors. Every village with a population of more 500 was given with primary health care

unit with full infrastructure. Under Pulse polio programme, the children 0. 5 years are given two doses of polio vaccine at an interval of six weeks.

- **Ninth Five Year Plan (1997-2002):** The ninth plan was started with "growth with social justice and equity". It aimed at agricultural and rural development, providing safe drinking water, primary health, education, housing facilities, controlling population, ensuring environmental sustainability, and so on The plan outlay was fixed Rs. 21,90,000 crores of which about Rs. 1,82,174 crores was allocated to social services. Community development projects were undertaken to create employment opportunities. Health related projects like Hepatitis project, universal immunization, intensive family welfare programme were launched under Family Planning Scheme to control population.

- **Tenth Five Year Plan (2002-2007):** The tenth plan targeted 8.00 percent of growth in GDP. To increase Per-capita income by 6.4% per annum, to reduce infant mortality rate to 45 per 1000 live birth by 2007, to reduce maternal mortality rate to 2 per 1000 live births, are the objectives relating to health care. The total outlay was fixed at Rs. 26,68,815 crores of which Rs. 3,47,391 crores was to social services including health. Under Hepatitis B project, vaccine for infants was provided by covering 33 districts throughout the country. An intensive program was also launched to combat AIDS. In 2000 there were about 5 lakhs HIV positive patients in India. Government is consistently creating awareness among the public in general and students in particular about the HIV infection preventive measures under National Service Scheme(NSS).

- **Eleventh Five Year Plan (2007-2012):** The eleventh plan was started by Dr Manmohan Singh, the Prime Minister of India with the objective of creating infrastructure for different sectors of the economy. The target of 9% in GDP growth was fixed. Apart from these it also aimed to achieve 4% growth in agriculture, reducing poverty, increasing job opportunities were given importance. In respect of health programs, rural health care infrastructure was given prime emphasis. To provide better health facilities to rural women, health care center, and maternity centers have opened under "Janani Suraksha Scheme" by providing free medical and maternity facilities.

Role of State and Central Governments in Financing Health Care: Health is Wealth. Health is physical, mental and social soundness of human beings. Health plays an important role in economic development of the country. Healthy laborers increase both productivity and production. Healthy soldiers are indispensable for National Defense. For any economic, social or politica activity good health is required. Hence, it is the responsibility of both the Governments to provide good health care amenities to the needy people. As the health comes under State list, the state government with the financial assistance of Central Government is allowed to take required steps to provide disease free environment to its people. Both the Governments are playing an important role by providing necessary health care services. They are:

- Central Government under Directive Principles of State Policy has instructed to start hospitals, dispensaries in all Taluk and Districts to attend the patients.

- Primary Health Care units are encouraged to open under Government programs to meet the needs of rural patients.
- Private Nursing Homes and Laboratories are encouraged under liberalization policy of Government.
- Permission is granted to open Nursing and Medical Colleges throughout the state or country.
- State Governments have made compulsory to all the new doctors who are appointed, to serve at least one year in rural areas.
- Rural health education is provided through awareness programme undertaken through extensions programmes at the school and college levels.
- Safe drinking water and sanitation is being provided to all the people of the state including rural mass.
- Financial assistance is provided through various nationalized banks to private sectors to start pharmaceutical companies, medical shops, ambulance services, etc.
- The Central Government has started universal health programmes under the guidance of WHO (World Health Organization) to completely eradicate Polio disease and other contagious diseases.
- Voluntary counseling centers are opened to counsel HIV positive patients.
- Family Welfare Programme is started to provide child and maternal health services to the entire population of the country.
- Environment protection programs have been launched.

Index

Page numbers followed by *b* refer to box, *f* refer to figure, *fc* refer to flowchart, and *t* refer to table.